Innate Immune Regulation and Cancer Immunotherapy

Rong-Fu Wang
Editor

Innate Immune Regulation and Cancer Immunotherapy

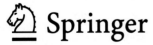

Editor
Rong-Fu Wang
Baylor College of Medicine
Houston, Texas 77030, USA
rongfuw@bcm.edu

ISBN 978-1-4419-9913-9   e-ISBN 978-1-4419-9914-6
DOI 10.1007/978-1-4419-9914-6
Springer New York Dordrecht Heidelberg London

Library of Congress Control Number: 2011939215

© Springer Science+Business Media, LLC 2012
All rights reserved. This work may not be translated or copied in whole or in part without the written permission of the publisher (Springer Science+Business Media, LLC, 233 Spring Street, New York, NY 10013, USA), except for brief excerpts in connection with reviews or scholarly analysis. Use in connection with any form of information storage and retrieval, electronic adaptation, computer software, or by similar or dissimilar methodology now known or hereafter developed is forbidden.
The use in this publication of trade names, trademarks, service marks, and similar terms, even if they are not identified as such, is not to be taken as an expression of opinion as to whether or not they are subject to proprietary rights.

Printed on acid-free paper

Springer is part of Springer Science+Business Media (www.springer.com)

Contents

1. **Introduction** 1
   Rong-Fu Wang

2. **The Role of NKT Cells in the Immune Regulation of Neoplastic Disease** 7
   Jessica J. O'Konek, Masaki Terabe, and Jay A. Berzofsky

3. **γδ T Cells in Cancer** 23
   Lawrence S. Lamb, Jr.

4. **Toll-Like Receptors and Their Regulatory Mechanisms** 39
   Shin-Ichiroh Saitoh

5. **Cytoplasmic Sensing of Viral Double-Stranded RNA and Activation of Innate Immunity by RIG-I-Like Receptors** 51
   Mitsutoshi Yoneyama and Takashi Fujita

6. **Innate Immune Signaling and Negative Regulators in Cancer** 61
   Helen Y. Wang and Rong-Fu Wang

7. **Dendritic Cell Subsets and Immune Regulation** 89
   Meredith O'Keeffe, Mireille H. Lahoud, Irina Caminschi, and Li Wu

8. **Human Dendritic Cells in Cancer** 121
   Gregory Lizée and Michel Gilliet

9. **Regulatory T Cells in Cancer** 147
   Tyler J. Curiel

10. **Relationship Between Th17 and Regulatory T Cells in the Tumor Environment** 175
    Ilona Kryczek, Ke Wu, Ende Zhao, Guobin Wang, and Weiping Zou

11	**Mechanisms and Control of Regulatory T Cells in Cancer**	195
	Bin Li and Rong-Fu Wang	
12	**Myeloid-Derived Suppressor Cells in Cancer**	217
	Wiaam Badn and Vincenzo Bronte	
13	**Myeloid-Derived Suppressive Cells and Their Regulatory Mechanisms in Cancer**	231
	Ge Ma, Ping-Ying Pan, and Shu-Hsia Chen	
14	**Cell Surface Co-signaling Molecules in the Control of Innate and Adaptive Cancer Immunity**..	251
	Stasya Zarling and Lieping Chen	
15	**Negative Regulators of NF-κB Activation and Type I Interferon Pathways**	267
	Caroline Murphy and Luke A.J. O'Neill	
16	**Role of TGF-β in Immune Suppression and Inflammation**	289
	Joanne E. Konkel and WanJun Chen	
17	**Indoleamine 2,3-Dioxygenase and Tumor-Induced Immune Suppression**	303
	David H. Munn	
18	**Myeloid-Derived Suppressor Cells in Cancer: Mechanisms and Therapeutic Perspectives**...	319
	Paulo C. Rodríguez and Augusto C. Ochoa	
19	**Human Tumor Antigens Recognized by T Cells and Their Implications for Cancer Immunotherapy**.........................	335
	Ryo Ueda, Tomonori Yaguchi, and Yutaka Kawakami	
20	**Cancer/Testis Antigens: Potential Targets for Immunotherapy**..	347
	Otavia L. Caballero and Yao-Tseng Chen	
21	**Tumor Antigens and Immune Regulation in Cancer Immunotherapy**...	371
	Rong-Fu Wang and Helen Y. Wang	
22	**Immunotherapy of Cancer**..	391
	Michael Dougan and Glenn Dranoff	
23	**Current Progress in Adoptive T-Cell Therapy of Lymphoma**...........	415
	Kenneth P. Micklethwaite, Helen E. Heslop, and Malcolm K. Brenner	
24	**Adoptive Immunotherapy of Melanoma**...	439
	Seth M. Pollack and Cassian Yee	

Index... 467

Contributors

Jay A. Berzofsky Vaccine Branch, National Cancer Institute, National Institutes of Health, Bethesda, MD 20892, USA

Wiaam Badn Istituto Oncologico Veneto, Via Gattamelata 64, 35128 Padova, Italy

Malcolm K. Brenner Center for Cell and Gene Therapy, Baylor College of Medicine, The Methodist Hospital and Texas Children's Hospital, Houston, TX, USA

Vincenzo Bronte Istituto Oncologico Veneto, Via Gattamelata 64, 35128 Padova, Italy

Otavia L. Caballero Ludwig Institute for Cancer Research, New York Branch at Memorial Sloan-Kettering Cancer Center, New York, NY, USA

Irina Caminschi The Walter and Eliza Hall Institute, 1G Royal Parade, Parkville, VIC 3052, Australia

Lieping Chen Department of Oncology and the Sidney Kimmel Comprehensive Cancer Center, Johns Hopkins University School of Medicine, Baltimore, MD, USA

Shu-Hsia Chen Department of Gene and Cell Medicine, Mount Sinai School of Medicine, 1425 Madison Avenue, Room 13-02, New York, NY 10029-6574, USA

Department of Surgery, Mount Sinai School of Medicine, 1425 Madison Avenue, Room 13-02, New York, NY 10029-6574, USA

WanJun Chen Mucosal Immunology Section, Oral Infection and Immunity Branch, National Institute of Dental and Craniofacial Research, National Institutes of Health, Bethesda, MD 20892, USA

Yao-Tseng Chen Department of Pathology and Laboratory Medicine, Weill Cornell Medical College, New York, NY, USA

Tyler J. Curiel Cancer Therapy and Research Center, University of Texas Health Science Center, San Antonio, TX 78229, USA

Glenn Dranoff Department of Medical Oncology and Cancer Vaccine Center, Dana-Farber Cancer Institute and Department of Medicine, Brigham and Women's Hospital and Harvard Medical School, Boston, MA 02115, USA

Michael Dougan Department of Medical Oncology and Cancer Vaccine Center, Dana-Farber Cancer Institute and Department of Medicine, Brigham and Women's Hospital and Harvard Medical School, Boston, MA 02115, USA

Takashi Fujita Laboratory of Molecular Genetics, Institute for Virus Research, and Laboratory of Molecular Cell Biology, Graduate School of Biostudies, Kyoto University, Kyoto, Japan

Michel Gilliet Department of Dermatology, University Hospital CHUV, CH-1011, Lausanne, Switzerland

Helen E. Heslop Center for Cell and Gene Therapy, Baylor College of Medicine, The Methodist Hospital and Texas Children's Hospital, Houston, TX, USA

Yutaka Kawakami Division of Cellular Signaling, Institute for Advanced Medical Research, Keio University School of Medicine, 35 Shinanomachi Shinjuku-ku, Tokyo 160-8582, Japan

Joanne E. Konkel Mucosal Immunology Section, Oral Infection and Immunity Branch, National Institute of Dental and Craniofacial Research, National Institutes of Health, Bethesda, MD 20892, USA

Ilona Kryczek Department of Surgery, University of Michigan, Ann Arbor, MI 48109, USA

Mireille H. Lahoud The Walter and Eliza Hall Institute, 1G Royal Parade, Parkville, VIC 3052, Australia

Lawrence S. Lamb, Jr. Department of Medicine, Division of Hematology and Oncology, University of Alabama Birmingham, Birmingham, AL, USA

Bin Li Key Laboratory of Molecular Virology and Immunology, Institut Pasteur of Shanghai, Shanghai Institutes for Biological Sciences, Chinese Academy of Sciences, Shanghai 200025, P.R. China

Gregory Lizée Department of Melanoma Medical Oncology, The University of Texas M. D. Anderson Cancer Center, Houston, TX, USA

Department of Immunology, The University of Texas M.D. Anderson Cancer Center, Houston, TX, USA

Ge Ma Department of Gene and Cell Medicine, Mount Sinai School of Medicine, 1425 Madison Avenue, Room 13-02, New York, NY 10029-6574, USA

Kenneth P. Micklethwaite Center for Cell and Gene Therapy, Baylor College of Medicine, The Methodist Hospital and Texas Children's Hospital, Houston, TX, USA

David H. Munn Cancer Immunotherapy Program, Room CN-4141, Augusta, GA 30912, USA

Caroline Murphy School of Biochemistry and Immunology, Trinity College Dublin, Dublin, Ireland

Augusto C. Ochoa Stanley S. Scott Cancer Center, Louisiana State University Health Sciences Center, New Orleans, LA, USA

Department of Pediatrics, Louisiana State University Health Sciences Center, New Orleans, LA, USA

Meredith O'Keeffe Centre for Immunology, Burnet Institute, 85 Commercial Road, Melbourne, VIC 3004, Australia

Jessica J. O'Konek Vaccine Branch, National Cancer Institute, National Institutes of Health, Bethesda, MD 20892, USA

Luke A.J. O'Neill School of Biochemistry and Immunology, Trinity College Dublin, Dublin, Ireland

Ping-Ying Pan Department of Gene and Cell Medicine, Mount Sinai School of Medicine, 1425 Madison Avenue, Room 13-02, New York, NY 10029-6574, USA

Seth M. Pollack Fred Hutchinson Cancer Research Center, University of Washington, 825 Eastlake Avenue East, G3630, Seattle, WA 98109-1023, USA

Paulo C. Rodríguez Department of Microbiology, Immunology and Parasitology, Louisiana State University Health Sciences Center, New Orleans, LA, USA

Stanley S. Scott Cancer Center, Louisiana State University Health Sciences Center, New Orleans, LA, USA

Shin-ichiroh Saitoh Division of Infectious Genetics, The Institute of Medical Science, The University of Tokyo, Shirokanedai, Tokyo 108-8639, Japan

Masaki Terabe Vaccine Branch, National Cancer Institute, National Institutes of Health, Bethesda, MD 20892, USA

Ryo Ueda Division of Cellular Signaling, Institute for Advanced Medical Research, Keio University School of Medicine, 35 Shinanomachi Shinjuku-ku, Tokyo 160-8582, Japan

Guobin Wang Department of Surgery, University of Michigan, Ann Arbor, MI, USA

Helen Y. Wang Department of Pathology and Immunology and Center for Cell and Gene Theraphy, Baylor College of Medicine, Houston, TX 77030, USA

Rong-Fu Wang Department of Pathology and immunology, The Center for Cell and Gene Therapy, Baylor College of Medicine, Houston, TX 77030, USA

Ke Wu Department of Surgery, Union Hospital, Tongji Medical College, Huazhong University of Science and Technology, Wuhan 430022, China

Li Wu The Walter and Eliza Hall Institute, 1G Royal Parade, Parkville, VIC 3052, Australia

Tomonori Yaguchi Division of Cellular Signaling, Institute for Advanced Medical Research, Keio University School of Medicine, 35 Shinanomachi Shinjuku-ku, Tokyo 160-8582, Japan

Cassian Yee Fred Hutchinson Cancer Research Center, University of Washington, 825 Eastlake Avenue East, G3630, Seattle, WA 98109-1023, USA

Mitsutoshi Yoneyama Laboratory of Molecular Genetics, Institute for Virus Research, and Laboratory of Molecular Cell Biology, Graduate School of Biostudies, Kyoto University, Kyoto, Japan

PRESTO, Japan Science and Technology Agency, Saitama, Japan

Stasya Zarling Department of Oncology and the Sidney Kimmel Comprehensive Cancer Center, Johns Hopkins University School of Medicine, Baltimore, MD, USA

Ende Zhao Department of Surgery, University of Michigan, Ann Arbor, MI 48109, USA

Department of Surgery, Union Hospital, Tongji Medical College, Huazhong University of Science and Technology, Wuhan 430022, China

Weiping Zou Department of Surgery, University of Michigan, Ann Arbor, MI 48109, USA

Chapter 1
Introduction

Rong-Fu Wang

1 Brief Historical Background and Recent Progresses

Immune system is composed of innate and adaptive responses and plays critical roles in cancer development and destruction. A century ago, Paul Ehrlich postulated that cancer would be quite common in long-lived organisms if not for the protective effects of immunity. About 50 years later, Burnet and Thomas proposed the concept of cancer immunosurveillance based on the experimental evidence of immune recognition of tumor antigens expressed on tumor cells (Dunn et al. 2004). In 1971, the US Congress created a National Cancer Act – a War on Cancer. Among many tough questions asked were whether the immune system can be manipulated so that it recognizes tumor cells as foreign invaders that must be eliminated from the body and whether viruses play a role in human cancer. In 1980s, Steven Rosenberg and his colleagues developed adoptive cell therapy (ACT) for the treatment of melanoma cancer patients using lymphocyte activated killed (LAK) cells, providing the first direct evidence that the immune system can be manipulated to achieve therapeutic efficacy of cancer treatment (Rosenberg, 2011). In 1990s, many human tumor antigens such as MAGE and NY-ESO-1 have been identified from melanoma and many other types of cancer using tumor-reactive T cells, thus setting the stage for the development of cancer vaccines in the twenty-first century (Wang and Rosenberg, 1999). Indeed, the first dendritic cell (DC)-based vaccine was approved in 2010 by the U.S. Food and Drug Administration (FDA) for the treatment of patients with prostate cancer.

R.-F. Wang (✉)
Center for Cell and Gene Therapy, Baylor College of Medicine, Houston, TX 77030, USA

Department of Pathology and Immunology, Baylor College of Medicine,
Houston, TX 77030, USA
e-mail: rongfuw@bcm.edu

In the last 10 years, a large body of evidence not only supports the concept of cancer immunosurveillance, but also proposes cancer immunoediting – a dynamic interaction between the host immune system and cancer cells. Innate immunity is the first line of host defense against pathogens and transformed tumor cells. Innate immune cells including NK, NKT, and δγT cells have been shown to play a critical role in protecting the host against cancer (Dunn et al. 2004; Smyth et al. 2001). Both macrophages and DCs function as major sensors of invading pathogens and transformed cells via a limited number of germline-encoded pattern recognition receptors (PRRs), and play an important role in modulating inflammation and immune responses (Akira et al. 2006). Adaptive immunity is involved in the elimination of pathogens and transformed tumor cells in the late phase of host defense and generates more specific immunity and immunological memory. This notion is further supported by direct experimental evidence, showing that the immune system can restrain cancer growth in an equilibrium phase (i.e., expansion of transformed cells is held in check by immunity) (Koebel et al. 2007). Thus, both innate and adaptive immune response play a key role in eliminating and controlling tumor growth. However, there is a continuous dynamic battle between immune cells and tumor cells, which, in some circumstances, favors the growth of the latter. The failure of the initial immune responses to control infections/tissue injury leads to chronic inflammation, which in turn modulates tumor growth. The concept that links chronic inflammation and cancer development was proposed long ago. In 1863, Rudolf Virchow first proposed that cancer originates at sites of chronic inflammation. Although the mechanisms by which chronic inflammation directly contributes to cancer are poorly understood, activation of the innate immune response (in particular the NF-κB pathway), through Toll-like receptor (TLR)-mediated recognition of invading pathogens or damaged tissues, serves as a link between chronic inflammation and cancer (Clevers 2004; Condeelis and Pollard 2006; Greten et al. 2004; Karin and Greten 2005). Whether inflammation promotes or suppresses tumor development depends upon many factors, including the cytokine milieu and the presence or absence of other immune cells (Greten et al. 2004; Karin and Greten 2005). For example, IL-1, IL-6, IL-8, and TGF-β released by immune cells and tumor cells promote angiogenesis, tumor growth, and differentiation of Th1, Th17, and Treg cells. Recent studies show that TLR and IRAK sequence polymorphism is an important risk factor for prostate cancer (Sun et al. 2005; Xu et al. 2005). Chronic inflammation induced by *Helicobacter pylori* infection is the leading cause of stomach cancer, while inflammatory bowel diseases including ulcerative colitis and Crohn's disease are closely associated with colon cancer (Coussens and Werb 2002; Karin et al. 2006). Similarly, hepatitis B and C viral infections are the leading factor contributing to liver cancer (Coussens and Werb 2002; Karin et al. 2006). Thus, these studies clearly demonstrate that pathogens including bacteria and viruses can trigger innate immune responses, which in turn affect tumor development, through various innate PRRs. Besides TLRs, NOD-like receptors (NLRs), RIG-I-like receptors (RLRs), AIM2-like receptors, and C-type lectin-like receptors have been identified and characterized as major innate immune receptors or sensors for detecting structure-conserved molecules, so-called pathogen-associated molecular patterns (PAMPs), as well as endogenous ligands released from damaged cells, termed damage-associated molecular patterns (DAMPs). Recognition of PAMPs or DAMPs by PRRs triggers the activation of several key signaling pathways, including NF-κB, type I interferon (IFN), and inflammasome, leading to the production of inflammatory cytokines. Because of the importance of these key signaling pathways, their tight regulation is essential for both innate and adaptive immunities; otherwise, aberrant immune responses may occur, leading to severe or even fatal consequences such as bacterial sepsis, autoimmune, and chronic inflammatory diseases. In the last few years, we have witnessed significant and rapid progress being made in the areas of innate immune signaling and inflammation-associated cancer development. Thus, inflammation mediated by innate immune cells that are designed to fight pathogen infections and tissue damages and heal wounds can result in their inadvertent support of multiple hallmark capabilities associated with cancer, thereby manifesting the now widely appreciated tumor-promoting consequences of inflammatory responses.

Although the first DC-based cancer vaccine (Provenge) has been approved by FDA as a treatment option for prostate cancer patients, it is very expensive and its clinical efficacy remains to be improved (extending only 4 months of patient survival). There are many reasons that could account for relatively ineffectiveness of current cancer vaccines in general. Among them include immunological escape, negative regulations or immune suppression in tumor microenvironment, because all solid tumors are embedded in a stromal environment consisting of immune cells, such as macrophages and lymphocytes, and non-immune cells such as endothelium and fibroblasts. Recent studies suggest that $CD4^+$ regulatory T (Treg) cells and myeloid-derived suppressor cells at tumor sites potently suppress the $CD4^+$ and $CD8^+$ T-cell responses elicited by vaccination, thus promoting tumor growth (Wang and Wang, 2007). In addition, there are many suppressive cytokines and negative signaling molecules in signaling pathways that dampen strong immune responses. Blocking negative signaling molecules on immune cell surface by specific antibody could be one way to enhance antitumor immune response. Recent approval of anti-CTLA-4 antibody by FDA as a treatment for melanoma patient this year is another milestone for T-cell-based immunotherapy of cancer.

2 Parts of the Book

Part I of the book discusses innate immune signaling and inflammatory responses to pathogens and cancer. Chapters 2 and 3 introduce innate lymphocytes, including NKT and gamma–delta T cells and their roles in innate immune response to cancer. Chapters 4 and 5 offer an overview of TLR- and RLR-mediated innate immune signaling and their role in detecting invading pathogens and initiating inflammatory response to pathogen infection. Chapter 6 discusses the innate immune signaling pathways induced by TLRs, RLRs, and NLRs and the control of their immune responses by negative regulators. Activation of these innate immune receptors expressed on many cell types by invading pathogens triggers NF-κB, type I interferon, and inflammasome pathways, leading to production of proinflammatory cytokines. Tight control of these innate immune responses is critical to the maintenance of immune homeostasis. Unchecked immune responses, otherwise, lead to harmful, even fatal consequence to the host.

Part II of the book introduces the concept of immune regulation and cell-mediated immune suppression. Chapters 7 and 8 provide overviews of our current understanding of human and mouse dendritic cell (DC) subsets and their regulatory mechanisms, since DC functions as sensors of invading pathogens and professional antigen-presenting cells to initiate innate and adaptive immune responses. Chapter 9 discusses regulatory T (Treg) cells in cancer and their clinical relevance to cancer therapy. Chapter 10 offers an overview of Treg cells and IL-17-producing T (Th17) cells in cancer, while chapter 11 discusses the regulation and function of Treg and Th17 cells by TLR-mediated signaling. Chapters 12 and 13 introduce and discuss myeloid-derived suppressor cells and their role in cancer.

Part III of the book introduces the concept of negative regulators and immune suppressive molecules that may serve as therapeutic targets of cancer immunotherapy. Chapter 14 provides an overview of co-stimulatory and co-inhibitory molecules in T cell activation. Some of these molecules such as cytotoxic T-lymphocyte antigen 4 (CTLA-4), also known as cluster of differentiation 152 and programmed death receptor 1 (PD-1) have been extensively studied as therapeutic drug targets for cancer treatment. Chapter 15 discusses the negative regulators of NF-κB and type I IFN signaling. Chapter 16 offers an overview of TGF-β signaling pathway and its role in the regulation of Treg and Th17 cells. Chapters 17 and 18 discuss several key immune suppressive molecules such as the catabolic enzymes indoleamine 2,3-dioxygenase (IDO) and arginase in cancer.

Part IV of the book introduces the concept of cancer antigens, cancer vaccines, and adoptive T-cell therapy. Chapters 19–21 provide a broad overview of our understanding of antibody- and T-cell-recognized cancer-associated antigens. Identification of these cancer antigens has set the stage for the development of effective cancer vaccine therapy. Chapter 22 discusses the current strategies of cancer immunotherapy. Chapters 23 and 24 demonstrate the effectiveness of T-cell-based therapy for the treatment of various types of cancer.

In summary, this book highlights emerging concept and research areas about the underlying mechanisms of innate immunity, and signaling regulation and immune suppression and offers novel ideas and strategies to develop therapeutic cancer drugs by blocking these negative signaling pathways, suppressive cells and molecules. Major progresses in the understanding of tumor antigens, immune suppressive molecules, and suppressive cell population have made therapeutic cancer vaccines and drugs a reality. Recent approval of DC-based cancer vaccines and anti-CTLA-4 antibody-based drugs by FDA are two examples in the pipeline of therapeutic anticancer drugs or vaccines that are being developed.

References

Akira S, Uematsu S, Takeuchi O (2006) Pathogen recognition and innate immunity. Cell 124:783–801

Clevers H (2004) At the crossroads of inflammation and cancer. Cell 118:671–674

Condeelis J, Pollard JW (2006) Macrophages: obligate partners for tumor cell migration, invasion, and metastasis. Cell 124:263–266

Coussens LM, Werb Z (2002) Inflammation and cancer. Nature 420:860–867

Dunn GP, Old LJ, Schreiber RD (2004) The immunobiology of cancer immunosurveillance and immunoediting. Immunity 21:137–148

Greten FR, Eckmann L, Greten TF, Park JM, Li ZW, Egan LJ, Kagnoff MF, Karin M (2004) IKKbeta links inflammation and tumorigenesis in a mouse model of colitis-associated cancer. Cell 118:285–296

Karin M, Greten FR (2005) NF-kappaB: linking inflammation and immunity to cancer development and progression. Nat Rev Immunol 5:749–759

Karin M, Lawrence T, Nizet V (2006) Innate immunity gone awry: linking microbial infections to chronic inflammation and cancer. Cell 124:823–835

Koebel CM, Vermi W, Swann JB, Zerafa N, Rodig SJ, Old LJ, Smyth MJ, Schreiber RD (2007) Adaptive immunity maintains occult cancer in an equilibrium state. Nature 450:903–907

Rosenberg SA (2011). Cell transfer immunotherapy for metastatic solid cancer-what clinicians need to know. Nat Rev Clin Oncol

Smyth MJ, Crowe NY, Godfrey DI (2001) NK cells and NKT cells collaborate in host protection from methylcholanthrene-induced fibrosarcoma. Int Immunol 13:459–463

Sun J, Wiklund F, Zheng SL, Chang B, Balter K, Li L, Johansson JE, Li G, Adami HO, Liu W et al (2005) Sequence variants in Toll-like receptor gene cluster (TLR6-TLR1-TLR10) and prostate cancer risk. J Natl Cancer Inst 97:525–532

Wang RF, Rosenberg SA (1999) Human tumor antigens for cancer vaccine development. Immunol Rev 170:85–100

Wang HY, Wang RF (2007) Regulatory T cells and cancer. Curr Opin Immunol 19:217–223

Xu J, Lowey J, Wiklund F, Sun J, Lindmark F, Hsu FC, Dimitrov L, Chang B, Turner AR, Liu W et al (2005) The interaction of four genes in the inflammation pathway significantly predicts prostate cancer risk. Cancer Epidemiol Biomarkers Prev 14:2563–2568

Chapter 2
The Role of NKT Cells in the Immune Regulation of Neoplastic Disease

Jessica J. O'Konek, Masaki Terabe, and Jay A. Berzofsky

1 Definition of NKT Cells

Natural killer T (NKT) cells are a subset of T cells that have phenotypic and functional characteristics of both T cells and NK cells, expressing both a T cell receptor and NK lineage markers (Godfrey et al. 2004). NKT cells are defined by their ability to recognize lipid antigens presented by the non-classical MHC class Ib molecule CD1d (Godfrey et al. 2004; Bendelac et al. 2007; Tupin et al. 2007). Although NKT cells make up only a small percentage of lymphocytes (1–2% of mouse spleen and 0.01–2% of human peripheral blood mononuclear cells), they play very important roles in many aspects of the immune system because they can regulate many other cell types such as macrophages, dendritic cells (DCs), $CD8^+T$, and NK cells and are uniquely equipped to link innate and adaptive immune responses (Taniguchi et al. 2003; Kronenberg 2005; Bendelac et al. 2007).

Upon activation, NKT cells can rapidly release many cytokines, such as IFN-γ, IL-4, IL-13, and IL-17, and also stimulate other cells to produce cytokines, such as IL-12 from CD1d-expressing APCs (Matsuda et al. 2003; Stetson et al. 2003; Michel et al. 2007; Rachitskaya et al. 2008). NKT cells express IFN-γ and IL-4 mRNA, even in the absence of TCR stimulation, suggesting that they are poised to quickly respond once stimulated (Matsuda et al. 2003; Stetson et al. 2003). The balance of cytokines determines which downstream immune cells are activated, and thus NKT cells help to steer the adaptive immune system in the desired direction.

J.J. O'Konek • M. Terabe (✉) • J.A. Berzofsky
Vaccine Branch, National Cancer Institute, National Institutes of Health,
Bethesda, MD 20892, USA
e-mail: okonekj@mail.nih.gov; terabe@mail.nih.gov

1.1 Type I NKT Cells

NKT cells are a heterogeneous population which can be further subdivided into two groups, type I and type II. Type I NKT cells express an invariant TCR receptor α chain (Vα14Jα18 in mice and Vα24Jα18 in humans) which pairs with Vβ2, 7, and 8.2 in mice and Vβ11 in humans (Imai et al. 1986; Koseki et al. 1989; Porcelli et al. 1993; Dellabona et al. 1994; Lantz and Bendelac 1994; Makino et al. 1995; Godfrey et al. 2004). Type I NKT cells often express other markers such as NK1.1, CD44, and CD69; however none of these are expressed on all type I NKT cells and cannot be used to define this population (Chiu et al. 1999; Kronenberg 2005; McNab et al. 2007). Both CD4$^+$ and CD4$^-$CD8$^-$ double negative (DN) populations of type I NKT cells exist in mice, and some express CD8αα or CD8αβ in humans (Bendelac et al. 1994; Gadola et al. 2002). In humans, CD4$^+$ type I NKT cells were found to express both Th1 and Th2 cytokines, while DN type I NKT cells mainly expressed Th1 cytokines (Gumperz et al. 2002; Lee et al. 2002). Tissue distribution has also been implicated in the function of type I NKT cells. NKT cells derived from the liver could stimulate tumor rejection, while those from the thymus or spleen could not (Crowe et al. 2005). The role of type I NKT cells is often investigated in Jα18$^{-/-}$ mice which lack only type I NKT cells. CD1d$^{-/-}$ mice are also useful tools since they lack all NKT cells. There are no known markers specific for type II NKT cells, and a knockout mouse expressing only type I NKT cells and not type II does not exist. NKT cells are often defined by staining with CD1d-tetramers loaded with α-galactosylceramide (α-GalCer) for type I NKT cells or sulfatide for type II cells (Benlagha et al. 2000; Matsuda et al. 2000; Karadimitris et al. 2001; Jahng et al. 2004).

Despite being very limited in their TCRβ repertoire with an invariant TCRα chain, type I NKT cells recognize a range of lipid antigens (Brutkiewicz 2006; Behar and Porcelli 2007; Tupin et al. 2007). Recently discovered NKT cell recognition of a variety of microbial lipids from *Sphingomonas*, *Ehrlichia*, and *Borrelia* organisms suggests that type I NKT cells play a role in host defense (Kinjo et al. 2005; Mattner et al. 2005; Wu et al. 2005; Brutkiewicz 2006; Tupin et al. 2007). Only a few endogenous glycolipid antigens have been discovered to stimulate NKT cells including phosphatidylinositol, isoglobotrihexosylceramide, and disialoganglioside GD3 (Gumperz et al. 2000; De Silva et al. 2002; Wu et al. 2003; Zhou et al. 2004). The most widely investigated antigen for type I NKT cells is α-GalCer, a glycolipid derived from a marine sponge (Kobayashi et al. 1995; Morita et al. 1995; Kawano et al. 1997; Taniguchi et al. 2003). Upon stimulation with α-GalCer, type I NKT cells rapidly release large amounts of both Th1 (IFN-γ) and Th2 (IL-4, IL-13) cytokines and promote anti-tumor immunity. The mechanism of α-GalCer-mediated tumor protection was shown to require IFN-γ and IL-12 (Cui et al. 1997; Fuji et al. 2000; Chiodoni et al. 2001; Hayakawa et al. 2002; Smyth et al. 2002) and involved IFN-γ-activated NK cells (Hayakawa et al. 2001; Smyth et al. 2001; 2002) as well as activated CD4$^+$ and CD8$^+$ T cells (Nakagawa et al. 2004; Osada et al. 2004; Hong et al. 2006).

Distinct from conventional T cells, for which different cytokine profiles can be induced against the same peptide-MHC complex, the structure of antigens seems to play a critical role in determining the cytokine profile induced in type I NKT cells. Modifications of the length and saturation of the lipid chains of α-GalCer can lead to different binding affinities to CD1d as well as altered TCR signaling (McCarthy et al. 2007). Truncation of the lipid chains has been associated with more Th2-skewed immune responses using glycolipids such as OCH (Miyamoto et al. 2001; Oki et al. 2004). More recently, it has been shown that glycolipids modified to include an aromatic ring in their acyl or sphingosine tail were more potent than α-GalCer in activating and expanding human NKT cells (Fujio et al. 2006; Chang et al. 2007).

Although the majority of structure function studies are focusing more on alterations of the lipid portion of α-GalCer, the sugar moiety, as well as its linkage to the ceramide tails, also influences the response of the NKT cells, as this is the portion of the antigen which the TCR interacts with. For example, while α-GalCer is a potent stimulator of cytokine production, α-glucosylceramide can also stimulate type I NKT cells, while β-galactosylceramide has been found to downregulate TCR expression without causing cytokine release or activation of effector cells (Ortaldo et al. 2004). A subsequent study attributed differences in the activity of theses glycolipids to their affinity for theTCR (Sidobre et al. 2002). A C-glycosidic analog of α-GalCer induces more IFN-γ production and is a more potent inhibitor of tumor growth (Schmieg et al. 2003). β-linked glycosylceramides have been shown not to induce significant anti-tumor immune responses, compared with α-linked glycosylceramides (Ortaldo et al. 2004; Parekh et al. 2004). Although IFN-γ has been found to be the key mediator for type I NKT-mediate anti-tumor immunity together with α-GalCer and other type I NKT agonists (Smyth and Godfrey 2000; Berzofsky and Terabe 2008), we have recently discovered that β-mannosylceramide is just as potent in eliciting an anti-tumor immune response similar to α-GalCer, despite failing to induce significant IFN-γ production (O'Konek et al. 2011).

Recently, nonglycosidic lipid antigens, such as threitolceramide, were found to be type I NKT cell agonists (Silk et al. 2008). While these lipid/CD1d complexes were found to have weaker binding affinities for the TCR compare to α-GalCer/CD1d, they could stimulate type I NKT cells to promote DC maturation and activation of antigen-specific T cells. Interestingly, the decreased affinity for TCR resulted in less activation-induced anergy and decreased lysis of DCs presenting the antigen. Thus despite limited TCR usage, NKT cells can discriminate a wide variety of antigen structures to initiate the proper immune response.

As mentioned above, α-GalCer was originally discovered for its anti-tumor properties, as it promotes type I NKT-dependent tumor rejection in a wide variety of mouse models (Kawano et al. 1998; Fuji et al. 2000; Chiodoni et al. 2001; Hayakawa et al. 2001, 2002, 2003; Miyagi et al. 2003; Nakagawa et al. 2004; Osada et al. 2004; Ambrosino et al. 2007). α-GalCer can induce protection against chemical or oncogene-driven tumor formation (Hayakawa et al. 2003). Loading tumor cells with α-GalCer induce antitumor immunity (Chung et al. 2007; Shimizu et al. 2007). Because α-GalCer is such a potent stimulator, it also causes type I NKT cells to become anergic (Wilson et al. 2003; Harada et al. 2004; Parekh et al. 2005). Blockade of the interaction between PD-1 and PD-L during α-GalCer treatment prevented this anergy, and in mice which lacked PD-1, repeated injection of α-GalCer did not induce anergy of type I NKT cells (Parekh et al. 2009). Thus PD-1/PD-L blockade could be a potential therapeutic target to enhance the antitumor effect of α-GalCer, allowing it to be administered repeatedly.

Even in the absence of exogenous stimulation by α-GalCer, type I NKT cells can prevent tumor formation (Cui et al. 1997). Mice lacking type I NKT cells are more susceptible to methylcholanthrene-induced carcinogenesis (Smyth et al. 2000, 2001; Crowe et al. 2002; Nishikawa et al. 2003). Both $J\alpha 18^{-/-}$ and $CD1d^{-/-}$ $p53^{+/-}$ mice exhibit a faster onset of tumorigenesis and decreased survival compared to $p53^{+/-}$ mice, suggesting that type I NKT cells can suppress spontaneous tumorigenesis (Swann et al. 2009).

Although it has been reported that type I NKT cells can kill tumor cells in vitro (Kawano et al. 1998), the immune response initiated by stimulation of type I NKT cells relies on activation of other effector mechanisms to ultimately kill tumor cells (Smyth et al. 2000). Type I NKT cells have been shown to activate NK and $CD8^+$ T cells (Carnaud et al. 1999; Toura et al. 1999; Eberl and MacDonald 2000; Smyth et al. 2002; Fujii et al. 2003b). NKT cells also promote maturation and production of IL-12 by DCs through interaction of CD40L on NKT cells with CD40 on DCs, and α-GalCer can induce DC maturation by mimicking the effect of Toll-like receptor agonists (Fujii et al. 2004). This NKT-mediated anti-tumor response is likely initiated by the production of IFN-γ by activated type I NKT cells, leading to the recruitment of NK and $CD8^+$ T cells which directly lead to tumor cell lysis. The sequential production of IFN-γ by NKT cells followed by NK cells recruitment has been shown to be necessary for tumor protection induced by α-GalCer (Smyth et al. 2002). Additionally, type I NKT cells have been shown to activate B cells, resulting in increased Ig secretion and generation of better antibody responses (Galli et al. 2003). NKT-mediated cytotoxic activity has also been demonstrated to occur through several mechanisms including perforin/granzyme, Fas ligand, and TNF-related apoptosis-inducing ligand (TRAIL) (Kawano et al. 1999; Nieda et al. 2001; Gumperz et al. 2002).

A role for type I NKT cells has also been demonstrated in humans. In vitro it was shown that stimulating human NKT cells with α-GalCer induced NK-mediated lysis of human tumor cells (Ishihara et al. 2000). Studies have reported a decreased type I NKT cell number in the blood of patients with advanced cancer (Tahir et al. 2001; Giaccone et al. 2002; Dhodapkar et al. 2003), and levels of circulating type I NKT cells inversely correlated with survival in patients with head and neck squamous cell carcinoma (Molling et al. 2007). It was also reported that type I NKT cells from cancer patients have decreased capacity to make IFN-γ, proliferate, and respond to α-GalCer when compared to healthy controls (Tahir et al. 2001; Yanagisawa et al. 2002; Dhodapkar et al. 2003; Fujii et al. 2003a; Crough et al. 2004). In colon carcinoma, a correlation was observed between the number of type I NKT cells infiltrating the tumor and survival (Tachibana et al. 2005). It is also important to note that in humans expression of Vα24 alone cannot be used to define type I NKT cells as a population of Vα24-negative cells was found to bind and respond to α-GalCer, possibly suggesting a new subset of NKT cells (Gadola et al. 2002). Both in humans and mice, type I NKT cells are being defined more commonly by staining with CD1d-tetramers loaded with α-GalCer or an analog (Benlagha et al. 2000; Matsuda et al. 2000; Karadimitris et al. 2001).

1.2 Type II NKT Cells

In contrast to type I NKT cells, type II NKT cells express a diverse TCR repertoire (Cardell et al. 1995; Godfrey et al. 2004). Type II NKT cells also are CD1d restricted; however these cells are much less characterized than type I NKT cells, and there are no good markers to define these cells. Type II NKT cells recognize a distinct set of lipid antigens from type I NKT cells. While sulfatide is the prototypical antigen for type II NKT cells (Jahng et al. 2004; Zajonc et al. 2005), some type II NKT cell hybridomas have been reported not to recognize sulfatide (Park et al. 2001; Jahng et al. 2004), suggesting that type II NKT cells may be further subdivided on the basis of antigen recognition. Recently, it was reported that alterations of the fatty acid chain of sulfatide alter the degree to which it can stimulate a type II NKT cell hybridoma (Roy et al. 2008; Blomqvist et al. 2009). This suggests that alternating the structure of sulfatide may influence its action, as has been observed with type I NKT stimulation and modifications of the structure of α-GalCer.

Unlike type I NKT cells, which can be characterized by specific markers (Vα14Jα18 TCR, recognition of α-GalCer), type II NKT cells are far less defined. It has been reported that a subset of type II NKT cells may be stained using CD1d-sulfatide tetramers (Jahng et al. 2004); however, this has not yet seen as widespread use as CD1d-α-GalCer tetramers. Further characterization of type II NKT cells will depend upon future discovery of markers specifically expressed on these cells.

Type II NKT cells have been implicated in suppressing immune responses which result in the development of autoimmune diseases. For example, in the NOD mouse model of type I diabetes, overexpression of type II NKT cells prevented disease onset (Duarte et al. 2004), and similarly type II NKT cells have been found to suppress experimental autoimmune encephalomyelitis, a mouse model of multiple sclerosis (Jahng et al. 2004) and concanavalin A-induced hepatitis (Halder et al. 2007). In contrast to the protective role of type I NKT cells in tumor models, type II NKT cells have been shown to suppress anti-tumor immunity and enhance tumor growth (Moodycliffe et al. 2000; Terabe et al. 2000, 2003a). For example, it has been demonstrated that 15-12RM fibrosarcoma, 4T1 mammary tumors, CT26-L5 subcutaneous tumors, and CT26 lung metastases, which grow well in wild-type and Jα18KO mice, are rejected in CD1d$^{-/-}$ mice (Terabe et al. 2005). Blockade of CD1d with monoclonal antibodies inhibited tumor growth, presumably by inhibiting type II NKT cells (Terabe et al. 2005; Teng et al. 2009a, b). Stimulation of type II NKT cells with the glycolipid sulfatide suppressed immunosurveillance (Ambrosino et al. 2007). In humans, a subset of type II NKT cells which recognize lysophosphatidylcholine has been identified in the blood of patients with multiple myeloma (Chang et al. 2008). In human bone marrow, type II NKT cells have been shown to suppress autoimmune T cell responses by releasing Th2 cytokines (Exley et al. 2001). In a similar manner, type II NKT cells may also suppress anti-tumor immune responses in humans.

1.3 Interaction Between Type I and Type II NKT Cells

A new immunoregulatory axis was discovered in tumor immunity where type I and type II NKT cells not only have opposite roles but also counterregulate each other (Ambrosino et al. 2007; Terabe and Berzofsky 2007, 2008; Ambrosino et al. 2008; Berzofsky and Terabe 2008). When type II NKT cells are activated in vitro with sulfatide, they are able to suppress the proliferation of activated type I NKT cells (Ambrosino et al. 2007). This result was verified in vivo, as sulfatide suppressed α-GalCer induced protection against 15-12RM subcutaneous tumors and CT26 lung metastases (Ambrosino et al. 2007). From these studies, a new immunoregulatory axis was defined in which the interaction between type I and type II NKT cells may be analogous to that of Th1 and Th2 cells. Understanding of the interaction between type I and type II NKT cells is critical, as the success of immunotherapies may depend on which way the balance of this axis is shifted. One goal of future anti-tumor therapies should be to enhance the activity of type I NKT cells while simultaneously blocking type II NKT cells.

1.4 Interaction Between NKT Cells and Other Cell Types

NKT cells have been shown to interact with other immune components (Terabe and Berzofsky 2008). As described above, type I NKT cells can also induce maturation of DCs and activation of NK cells.

$CD4^+CD25^+$ T regulatory (Treg) cells have been well characterized for their ability to suppress other cells of the immune system (Sakaguchi 2004). The interaction between NKT cells and Tregs has not been well-characterized; however, evidence suggests that such crosstalk does exist. In a mouse lung metastasis model, it was reported that Tregs reduced the number of type I NKT cells in tumor-bearing mice, resulting in increased tumor burden (Nishikawa et al. 2003). Human Tregs can suppress proliferation and function of type I NKT cells activated by α-GalCer-loaded DCs (Azuma et al. 2003). Increased number of Tregs and decreased type I NKT cells in cancer correlate with worse prognosis or more advanced cancer (Tahir et al. 2001; Dhodapkar et al. 2003; Curiel et al. 2004; Tachibana et al. 2005; Molling et al. 2007). Interestingly, in the setting of autoimmune disease, type I NKT cells and Tregs cooperate with one another (Roelofs-Haarhuis et al. 2003). Also in autoimmune disease, type I NKT cells appeared to increase Treg cell numbers through IL-2 production (Liu et al. 2005; La Cava et al. 2006). Further characterization of how type I NKT cells as well as type II NKT cells interact with Tregs is needed.

Myeloid-derived suppressor cells (MDSC), which are defined as $CD11b^+Gr-1^+$ cells, are immature myeloid lineage cells capable of producing arginase, nitric oxide, and TGF-β to suppress other immune cells (Gabrilovich 2004; Bronte and Zanovello 2005). Accumulation of MDSCs has been well characterized in many mouse tumor models as well as in human cancer patients (Pak et al. 1995; Almand et al. 2001; Schmielau and Finn 2001; Gabrilovich 2004; Bronte and Zanovello

2005). Type II NKT cells produce IL-13 which, along with TNF-α, stimulates MDSCs to produce TGF-β, resulting in the inhibition of CD8$^+$ T cell-mediated tumor lysis in multiple mouse tumor models (Terabe et al. 2003a, b; Fichtner-Feigl et al. 2005, 2008; Renukaradhya et al. 2008). IL-13, which can be made by type II NKT cells, can also induce arginase expression in MDSCs (Gallina et al. 2006). MDSCs can in turn suppress the function of type I NKT cells. In a B16 melanoma model where MDSCs suppress type I NKT cells, α-GalCer is a poor inducer of anti-tumor immunity; however, if the number of MDSCs was reduced using retinoic acid, α-GalCer was able to protect against tumor formation (Yanagisawa et al. 2006). It has also been reported in a model of influenza that activated type I NKT cells can reduce the suppressive activity of MDSCs in both mice and humans (De Santo et al. 2008). Recently, it was reported that type I NKT cells from human tumors can kill tumor-associated macrophages which are considered to be a subset of MDSCs (Song et al. 2009). Conversely, IL-13 from type II NKT cells can activate tumor-associated macrophages (Sinha et al. 2005). These studies support a role for type I NKT cells in suppressing and type II NKT cells in activating MDSCs.

2 Clinical Trials/Therapeutics

Activation of type I NKT cells using α-GalCer and other glycolipid antigens has generated much preclinical success in mice, leading to several clinical trials in humans (reviewed in (Motohashi and Nakayama 2009)). To date, all of the trials have used α-GalCer to manipulate NKT cells, but preclinical success achieved with other glycolipids suggests that these may progress into the clinic trials. Phase I clinical trials have used soluble α-GalCer (Giaccone et al. 2002), α-GalCer-pulsed autologous DCs (Chang et al. 2005; Ishikawa et al. 2005; Kunii et al. 2009), or adoptive transfer of NKT cells expanded ex vivo with α-GalCer (Motohashi et al. 2006) in patients with melanoma, glioma, lung, breast, colorectal, liver, kidney, prostate, and head and neck cancers. These trials have demonstrated that α-GalCer is well-tolerated with no dose-limiting toxicity (Giaccone et al. 2002; Ishikawa et al. 2005). In some patients, this treatment induced expansion of type I NKT cells as well as an increase in IFN-γ-producing PBMCs and memory CD8$^+$ T cells, suggesting that this may have the potential to induce an anti-tumor immune response.

However, α-GalCer has had limited success so far in patients. A few possible explanations have been suggested. The frequency of type I NKT cells is much lower in humans than in mice (Kronenberg 2005), and as noted above, cancer in advanced stages often correlates with reduced number of type I NKT cells. Patients in these trials also had much more advanced disease than the mice in which α-GalCer showed significant greater therapeutic effect. This therapy may also be hindered by the anergy induced by α-GalCer, since in mice it has been demonstrated that following injection of α-GalCer, type I NKT cells can not be restimulated for at least 1 month (Fujii et al. 2002). The lack of success with α-GalCer in humans compared with mice also may be due in part to the presence of anti-α-linked sugar antibodies in humans which the mouse lacks (Galili et al. 1987, 1988; Yoshimura et al. 2001).

More success has been observed with the adoptive transfer of α-GalCer-pulsed DCs. In contrast to the administration of soluble glycolipid, adoptive transfer of DCs loaded with α-GalCer resulted in prolonged NKT activation in mice without the induction of anergy (Fujii et al. 2002). Several clinical trials have studied the effects of injecting monocyte-derived immature DCs loaded with α-GalCer (Nieda et al. 2004; Chang et al. 2005; Ishikawa et al. 2005). This therapy was also shown to be well-tolerated and gave more promising results compared with soluble α-GalCer. A similar trial using mature DCs showed better NKT expansion in vivo, although these cells displayed diminished ability to secrete IFN-γ (Chang et al. 2005). Because many patients with advanced cancers have defects in NKT cell number or function, an adoptive transfer study was carried out in which in vitro expanded NKT cells were administered to patients with lung cancer (Motohashi et al. 2006). Two out of three patients who received the higher dose of NKT cells showed increased numbers of IFN-γ-producing cells and had stable disease. A recent Phase I/II study of adoptive transfer of whole PBMCs cultured with IL-2 and GM-CSF and subsequently pulsed with α-GalCer for the treatment of non-small cell lung cancer reported that 10 of 17 patients displayed an increased number of IFN-γ producing cells following treatment (Motohashi et al. 2009). The patients who showed increased IFN-γ producing cells had significantly longer median survival. This suggests that IFN-γ production following α-GalCer administration can be a predictive marker of success and may be a useful screening tool for selecting patients who may benefit from this treatment.

Manipulating NKT cells alone may not be sufficient to eradicate tumors in patients, and combinatorial approaches may prove to be more successful. For example, α-GalCer can function as a vaccine adjuvant by promoting the generation of antigen-specific T cells (Gonzalez-Aseguinolaza et al. 2002; Silk et al. 2004) and overcoming oral tolerance by inducing the upregulation of costimulatory molecules on dendritic cells (Chung et al. 2004). Recently, α-GalCer has been shown to be an effective mucosal adjuvant for inducing antigen-specific immune responses following administration of HIV peptides (Courtney et al. 2009) and for inducing protective immunity against sexually transmitted HSV-2 infection in mice (Lindqvist et al. 2009). Because α-GalCer-pulsed DCs can stimulate cytokine production without inducing anergy, they may also be attractive candidates in the adjuvant setting. Combining α-GalCer with monoclonal antibodies against TRAIL and 4-1BB, which induce apoptosis of tumor cells and activation of T cells, respectively, induced regression and complete rejection of established tumors in mice (Teng et al. 2007). Taken together, data from these preclinical mouse models suggest that clinical approaches combining multiple agents which take advantage of the interactions of NKT cells with other immune cells may work better than stimulating NKT cells with α-GalCer alone.

3 Conclusion

NKT cells act as pivotal regulatory as well as effector cells bridging the gap between the innate and adaptive immune systems. The balance along the immunoregulatory axis between type I and type II NKT cells may play a key role in many immune responses, and manipulating this balance may be an important component of immunotherapy for autoimmune, infectious, and neoplastic diseases.

References

Almand B, Clark JI, Nikitina E et al (2001) Increased production of immature myeloid cells in cancer patients: a mechanism of immunosuppression in cancer. J Immunol 166:678–689

Ambrosino E, Terabe M, Halder RC et al (2007) Cross-regulation between type I and type II NKT cells in regulating tumor immunity: a new immunoregulatory axis. J Immunol 179:5126–5136

Ambrosino E, Berzofsky JA, Terabe M (2008) Regulation of tumor immunity: the role of NKT cells. Expert Opin Biol Ther 8:725–734

Azuma T, Takahashi T, Kunisato A et al (2003) Human CD4+ CD25+ regulatory T cells suppress NKT cell functions. Cancer Res 63:4516–4520

Behar SM, Porcelli SA (2007) CD1-restricted T cells in host defense to infectious diseases. Curr Top Microbiol Immunol 314:215–250

Bendelac A, Killeen N, Littman DR et al (1994) A subset of CD4+ thymocytes selected by MHC class I molecules. Science 263:1774–1778

Bendelac A, Savage PB, Teyton L (2007) The biology of NKT cells. Annu Rev Immunol 25:297–336

Benlagha K, Weiss A, Beavis A et al (2000) In vivo identification of glycolipid antigen-specific T cells using fluorescent CD1d tetramers. J Exp Med 191:1895–1903

Berzofsky JA, Terabe M (2008) NKT cells in tumor immunity: opposing subsets define a new immunoregulatory axis. J Immunol 180:3627–3635

Blomqvist M, Rhost S, Teneberg S et al (2009) Multiple tissue-specific isoforms of sulfatide activate CD1d-restricted type II NKT cells. Eur J Immunol 39:1726–1735

Bronte V, Zanovello P (2005) Regulation of immune responses by L-arginine metabolism. Nat Rev Immunol 5:641–654

Brutkiewicz RR (2006) CD1d ligands: the good, the bad, and the ugly. J Immunol 177:769–775

Cardell S, Tangri S, Chan S et al (1995) CD1-restricted CD4+ T cells in major histocompatibility complex class II-deficient mice. J Exp Med 182:993–1004

Carnaud C, Lee D, Donnars O et al (1999) Cutting edge: cross-talk between cells of the innate immune system: NKT cells rapidly activate NK cells. J Immunol 163:4647–4650

Chang DH, Osman K, Connolly J et al (2005) Sustained expansion of NKT cells and antigen-specific T cells after injection of {alpha}-galactosyl-ceramide loaded mature dendritic cells in cancer patients. J Exp Med 201:1503–1517

Chang YJ, Huang JR, Tsai YC et al (2007) Potent immune-modulating and anticancer effects of NKT cell stimulatory glycolipids. Proc Natl Acad Sci USA 104:10299–10304

Chang DH, Deng H, Matthews P et al (2008) Inflammation associated lysophospholipids as ligands for CD1d restricted T cells in human cancer. Blood 112:1308–1316

Chiodoni C, Stoppacciaro A, Sangaletti S et al (2001) Different requirements for alpha-galactosylceramide and recombinant IL-12 antitumor activity in the treatment of C-26 colon carcinoma hepatic metastases. Eur J Immunol 31:3101–3110

Chiu YH, Jayawardena J, Weiss A et al (1999) Distinct subsets of CD1d-restricted T cells recognize self-antigens loaded in different cellular compartments. J Exp Med 189:103–110

Chung Y, Chang WS, Kim S et al (2004) NKT cell ligand alpha-galactosylceramide blocks the induction of oral tolerance by triggering dendritic cell maturation. Eur J Immunol 34:2471–2479

Chung Y, Qin H, Kang CY et al (2007) An NKT-mediated autologous vaccine generates CD4 T-cell dependent potent antilymphoma immunity. Blood 110:2013–2019

Courtney AN, Nehete PN, Nehete BP et al (2009) Alpha-galactosylceramide is an effective mucosal adjuvant for repeated intranasal or oral delivery of HIV peptide antigens. Vaccine 27(25–26):3335–41

Crough T, Purdie DM, Okai M et al (2004) Modulation of human Valpha24(+)Vbeta11(+) NKT cells by age, malignancy and conventional anticancer therapies. Br J Cancer 91:1880–1886

Crowe NY, Smyth MJ, Godfrey DI (2002) A critical role for natural killer T cells in immunosurveillance of methylcholanthrene-induced sarcomas. J Exp Med 196:119–127

Crowe NY, Coquet JM, Berzins SP et al (2005) Differential antitumor immunity mediated by NKT cell subsets in vivo. J Exp Med 202:1279–1288

Cui J, Shin T, Kawano T et al (1997) Requirement for Valpha14 NKT cells in IL-12-mediated rejection of tumors. Science 278:1623–1626

Curiel TJ, Coukos G, Zou L et al (2004) Specific recruitment of regulatory T cells in ovarian carcinoma fosters immune privilege and predicts reduced survival. Nat Med 10:942–949

De Santo C, Salio M, Masri SH et al (2008) Invariant NKT cells reduce the immunosuppressive activity of influenza A virus-induced myeloid-derived suppressor cells in mice and humans. J Clin Invest 118:4036–4048

De Silva AD, Park JJ, Matsuki N et al (2002) Lipid protein interactions: the assembly of CD1d1 with cellular phospholipids occurs in the endoplasmic reticulum. J Immunol 168:723–733

Dellabona P, Padovan E, Casorati G et al (1994) An invariant V alpha 24-J alpha Q/V beta 11 T cell receptor is expressed in all individuals by clonally expanded CD4-8-T cells. J Exp Med 180:1171–1176

Dhodapkar MV, Geller MD, Chang DH et al (2003) A reversible defect in natural killer T cell function characterizes the progression of premalignant to malignant multiple myeloma. J Exp Med 197:1667–1676

Duarte N, Stenstrom M, Campino S et al (2004) Prevention of diabetes in nonobese diabetic mice mediated by CD1d-restricted nonclassical NKT cells. J Immunol 173:3112–3118

Eberl G, MacDonald HR (2000) Selective induction of NK cell proliferation and cytotoxicity by activated NKT cells. Eur J Immunol 30:985–992

Exley MA, Tahir SM, Cheng O et al (2001) A major fraction of human bone marrow lymphocytes are Th2-like CD1d-reactive T cells that can suppress mixed lymphocyte responses. J Immunol 167:5531–5534

Fichtner-Feigl S, Strober W, Kawakami K et al (2005) IL-13 signaling through the IL-13alpha(2) receptor is involved in induction of TGF-beta(1) production and fibrosis. Nat Med 12:99–106

Fichtner-Feigl S, Terabe M, Kitani A et al (2008) Restoration of tumor immunosurveillance via targeting of interleukin-13 receptor-alpha 2. Cancer Res 68:3467–3475

Fuji N, Ueda Y, Fujiwara H et al (2000) Antitumor effect of alpha-galactosylceramide (KRN7000) on spontaneous hepatic metastases requires endogenous interleukin 12 in the liver. Clin Cancer Res 6:3380–3387

Fujii S, Shimizu K, Kronenberg M et al (2002) Prolonged IFN-gamma-producing NKT response induced with alpha-galactosylceramide-loaded DCs. Nat Immunol 3:867–874

Fujii S, Shimizu K, Klimek V et al (2003a) Severe and selective deficiency of interferon-gamma-producing invariant natural killer T cells in patients with myelodysplastic syndromes. Br J Haematol 122:617–622

Fujii S, Shimizu K, Smith C et al (2003b) Activation of natural killer T cells by alpha-galactosyl-ceramide rapidly induces the full maturation of dendritic cells in vivo and thereby acts as an adjuvant for combined CD4 and CD8 T cell immunity to a coadministered protein. J Exp Med 198:267–279

Fujii S, Liu K, Smith C et al (2004) The linkage of innate to adaptive immunity via maturing dendritic cells in vivo requires CD40 ligation in addition to antigen presentation and CD80/86 costimulation. J Exp Med 199:1607–1618

Fujio M, Wu D, Garcia-Navarro R et al (2006) Structure-based discovery of glycolipids for CD1d-mediated NKT cell activation: tuning the adjuvant versus immunosuppression activity. J Am Chem Soc 128:9022–9023

Gabrilovich D (2004) Mechanisms and functional significance of tumour-induced dendritic-cell defects. Nat Rev Immunol 4:941–952

Gadola SD, Dulphy N, Salio M et al (2002) Valpha24-JalphaQ-independent, CD1d-restricted recognition of alpha-galactosylceramide by human CD4(+) and CD8alphabeta(+) T lymphocytes. J Immunol 168:5514–5520

Galili U, Clark MR, Shohet SB et al (1987) Evolutionary relationship between the natural anti-Gal antibody and the Gal alpha 1–3Gal epitope in primates. Proc Natl Acad Sci USA 84:1369–1373

Galili U, Shohet SB, Kobrin E et al (1988) Man, apes, and Old World monkeys differ from other mammals in the expression of alpha-galactosyl epitopes on nucleated cells. J Biol Chem 263: 17755–17762

Galli G, Nuti S, Tavarini S et al (2003) CD1d-restricted help to B cells by human invariant natural killer T lymphocytes. J Exp Med 197:1051–1057

Gallina G, Dolcetti L, Serafini P et al (2006) Tumors induce a subset of inflammatory monocytes with immunosuppressive activity on CD8+ T cells. J Clin Invest 116:2777–2790

Giaccone G, Punt CJ, Ando Y et al (2002) A phase I study of the natural killer T-cell ligand alpha-galactosylceramide (KRN7000) in patients with solid tumors. Clin Cancer Res 8:3702–3709

Godfrey DI, MacDonald HR, Kronenberg M et al (2004) NKT cells: What's in a name? Nat Rev Immunol 4:231–237

Gonzalez-Aseguinolaza G, Van Kaer L, Bergmann CC et al (2002) Natural killer T cell ligand alpha-galactosylceramide enhances protective immunity induced by malaria vaccines. J Exp Med 195:617–624

Gumperz JE, Roy C, Makowska A et al (2000) Murine CD1d-restricted T cell recognition of cellular lipids. Immunity 12:211–221

Gumperz JE, Miyake S, Yamamura T et al (2002) Functionally distinct subsets of CD1d-restricted natural killer T cells revealed by CD1d tetramer staining. J Exp Med 195:625–636

Halder RC, Aguilera C, Maricic I et al (2007) Type II NK T cell-mediated anergy induction in type I NK T cells prevents inflammatory liver disease. J Clin Invest 117:2302–2312

Harada M, Seino K, Wakao H et al (2004) Down-regulation of the invariant Valpha14 antigen receptor in NKT cells upon activation. Int Immunol 16:241–247

Hayakawa Y, Takeda K, Yagita H et al (2001) Differential regulation of Th1 and Th2 functions of NKT cells by CD28 and CD40 costimulatory pathways. J Immunol 166:6012–6018

Hayakawa Y, Takeda K, Yagita H et al (2002) IFN-gamma-mediated inhibition of tumor angiogenesis by natural killer T-cell ligand, alpha-galactosylceramide. Blood 100:1728–1733

Hayakawa Y, Rovero S, Forni G et al (2003) Alpha-galactosylceramide (KRN7000) suppression of chemical- and oncogene-dependent carcinogenesis. Proc Natl Acad Sci USA 100:9464–9469

Hong C, Lee H, Oh M et al (2006) CD4+ T cells in the absence of the CD8+ cytotoxic T cells are critical and sufficient for NKT cell-dependent tumor rejection. J Immunol 177:6747–6757

Imai K, Kanno M, Kimoto H et al (1986) Sequence and expression of transcripts of the T-cell antigen receptor alpha-chain gene in a functional, antigen-specific suppressor-T-cell hybridoma. Proc Natl Acad Sci USA 83.8708–8712

Ishihara S, Nieda M, Kitayama J et al (2000) Alpha-glycosylceramides enhance the antitumor cytotoxicity of hepatic lymphocytes obtained from cancer patients by activating CD3-CD56+ NK cells in vitro. J Immunol 165:1659–1664

Ishikawa A, Motohashi S, Ishikawa E et al (2005) A phase I study of alpha-galactosylceramide (KRN7000)-pulsed dendritic cells in patients with advanced and recurrent non-small cell lung cancer. Clin Cancer Res 11:1910–1917

Jahng A, Maricic I, Aguilera C et al (2004) Prevention of autoimmunity by targeting a distinct, noninvariant CD1d-reactive T cell population reactive to sulfatide. J Exp Med 199:947–957

Karadimitris A, Gadola S, Altamirano M et al (2001) Human CD1d-glycolipid tetramers generated by in vitro oxidative refolding chromatography. Proc Natl Acad Sci USA 98:3294–3298

Kawano T, Cui J, Koezuka Y et al (1997) CD1d-restricted and TCR-mediated activation of valpha14 NKT cells by glycosylceramides. Science 278:1626–1629

Kawano T, Cui J, Koezuka Y et al (1998) Natural killer-like nonspecific tumor cell lysis mediated by specific ligand-activated Valpha14 NKT cells. Proc Natl Acad Sci USA 95:5690–5693

Kawano T, Nakayama T, Kamada N et al (1999) Antitumor cytotoxicity mediated by ligand-activated human V alpha24 NKT cells. Cancer Res 59:5102–5105

Kinjo Y, Wu D, Kim G et al (2005) Recognition of bacterial glycosphingolipids by natural killer T cells. Nature 434:520–525

Kobayashi E, Motoki K, Uchida T et al (1995) KRN7000, a novel immunomodulator, and its antitumor activities. Oncol Res 7:529–534

Koseki H, Imai K, Ichikawa T et al (1989) Predominant use of a particular alpha-chain in suppressor T cell hybridomas specific for keyhole limpet hemocyanin. Int Immunol 1:557–564

Kronenberg M (2005) Toward an understanding of NKT cell biology: progress and paradoxes. Annu Rev Immunol 23:877–900

Kunii N, Horiguchi S, Motohashi S et al (2009) Combination therapy of in vitro-expanded natural killer T cells and alpha-galactosylceramide-pulsed antigen-presenting cells in patients with recurrent head and neck carcinoma. Cancer Sci 100:1092–1098

La Cava A, Van Kaer L, Fu Dong S (2006) CD4+CD25+ Tregs and NKT cells: regulators regulating regulators. Trends Immunol 27:322–327

Lantz O, Bendelac A (1994) An invariant T cell receptor alpha chain is used by a unique subset of major histocompatibility complex class I-specific CD4+ and CD4-8- T cells in mice and humans. J Exp Med 180:1097–1106

Lee PT, Benlagha K, Teyton L et al (2002) Distinct functional lineages of human Va24 natural killer cells. J Exp Med 195:637–641

Lindqvist M, Persson J, Thorn K et al (2009) The mucosal adjuvant effect of alpha-galactosylceramide for induction of protective immunity to sexually transmitted viral infection. J Immunol 182:6435–6443

Liu R, La Cava A, Bai XF et al (2005) Cooperation of invariant NKT cells and CD4+CD25+ T regulatory cells in the prevention of autoimmune myasthenia. J Immunol 175:7898–7904

Makino Y, Kanno R, Ito T et al (1995) Predominant expression of invariant V alpha 14+ TCR alpha chain in NK1.1+ T cell populations. Int Immunol 7:1157–1161

Matsuda JL, Naidenko OV, Gapin L et al (2000) Tracking the response of natural killer T cells to a glycolipid antigen using CD1d tetramers. J Exp Med 192:741–754

Matsuda JL, Gapin L, Baron JL et al (2003) Mouse V alpha 14i natural killer T cells are resistant to cytokine polarization in vivo. Proc Natl Acad Sci USA 100:8395–8400

Mattner J, Debord KL, Ismail N et al (2005) Exogenous and endogenous glycolipid antigens activate NKT cells during microbial infections. Nature 434:525–529

McCarthy C, Shepherd D, Fleire S et al (2007) The length of lipids bound to human CD1d molecules modulates the affinity of NKT cell TCR and the threshold of NKT cell activation. J Exp Med 204:1131–1144

McNab FW, Pellicci DG, Field K et al (2007) Peripheral NK1.1 NKT cells are mature and functionally distinct from their thymic counterparts. J Immunol 179:6630–6637

Michel ML, Keller AC, Paget C et al (2007) Identification of an IL-17-producing NK1.1(neg) iNKT cell population involved in airway neutrophilia. J Exp Med 204:995–1001

Miyagi T, Takehara T, Tatsumi T et al (2003) CD1d-mediated stimulation of natural killer T cells selectively activates hepatic natural killer cells to eliminate experimentally disseminated hepatoma cells in murine liver. Int J Cancer 106:81–89

Miyamoto K, Miyake S, Yamamura T (2001) A synthetic glycolipid prevents autoimmune encephalomyelitis by inducing TH2 bias of natural killer T cells. Nature 413:531–534

Molling JW, Langius JA, Langendijk JA et al (2007) Low levels of circulating invariant natural killer T cells predict poor clinical outcome in patients with head and neck squamous cell carcinoma. J Clin Oncol 25:862–868

Moodycliffe AM, Nghiem D, Clydesdale G et al (2000) Immune suppression and skin cancer development: regulation by NKT cells. Nat Immunol 1:521–525

Morita M, Motoki K, Akimoto K et al (1995) Structure-activity relationship of alpha-galactosylceramides against B16-bearing mice. J Med Chem 38:2176–2187

Motohashi S, Nakayama T (2009) Natural killer T cell-mediated immunotherapy for malignant diseases. Front Biosci (Schol Ed) 1:108–116

Motohashi S, Ishikawa A, Ishikawa E et al (2006) A phase I study of in vitro expanded natural killer T cells in patients with advanced and recurrent non-small cell lung cancer. Clin Cancer Res 12:6079–6086

Motohashi S, Nagato K, Kunii N et al (2009) A phase I-II study of alpha-galactosylceramide-pulsed IL-2/GM-CSF-cultured peripheral blood mononuclear cells in patients with advanced and recurrent non-small cell lung cancer. J Immunol 182:2492–2501

Nakagawa R, Inui T, Nagafune I et al (2004) Essential role of bystander cytotoxic CD122+CD8+ T cells for the antitumor immunity induced in the liver of mice by alpha-galactosylceramide. J Immunol 172:6550–6557

Nieda M, Nicol A, Koezuka Y et al (2001) TRAIL expression by activated human CD4(+)V alpha 24NKT cells induces in vitro and in vivo apoptosis of human acute myeloid leukemia cells. Blood 97:2067–2074

Nieda M, Okai M, Tazbirkova A et al (2004) Therapeutic activation of Valpha24+Vbeta11+ NKT cells in human subjects results in highly coordinated secondary activation of acquired and innate immunity. Blood 103:383–389

Nishikawa H, Kato T, Tanida K et al (2003) CD4+ CD25+ T cells responding to serologically defined autoantigens suppress antitumor immune responses. Proc Natl Acad Sci USA 100:10902–10906

Oki S, Chiba A, Yamamura T et al (2004) The clinical implication and molecular mechanism of preferential IL-4 production by modified glycolipid-stimulated NKT cells. J Clin Invest 113:1631–1640

O'Konek JJ, Illarionov P, Khursigara DS et al (2011) Mouse and human iNKT cell agonist beta-mannosylceramide reveals a distinct mechanism of tumor immunity. J Clin Invest 121:683–694

Ortaldo JR, Young HA, Winkler-Pickett RT et al (2004) Dissociation of NKT stimulation, cytokine induction, and NK activation in vivo by the use of distinct TCR-binding ceramides. J Immunol 172:943–953

Osada T, Nagawa H, Shibata Y (2004) Tumor-infiltrating effector cells of alpha-galactosylceramide-induced antitumor immunity in metastatic liver tumor. J Immune Based Ther Vaccines 2:7

Pak AS, Wright MA, Matthews JP et al (1995) Mechanisms of immune suppression in patients with head and neck cancer: presence of CD34(+) cells which suppress immune functions within cancers that secrete granulocyte-macrophage colony-stimulating factor. Clin Cancer Res 1:95–103

Parekh VV, Singh AK, Wilson MT et al (2004) Quantitative and qualitative differences in the in vivo response of NKT cells to distinct alpha- and beta-anomeric glycolipids. J Immunol 173:3693–3706

Parekh VV, Wilson MT, Olivares-Villagomez D et al (2005) Glycolipid antigen induces long-term natural killer T cell anergy in mice. J Clin Invest 115:2572–2583

Parekh VV, Lalani S, Kim S et al (2009) PD-1/PD-L blockade prevents anergy induction and enhances the anti-tumor activities of glycolipid-activated invariant NKT cells. J Immunol 182:2816–2826

Park SH, Weiss A, Benlagha K et al (2001) The mouse CD1d-restricted repertoire is dominated by a few autoreactive T cell receptor families. J Exp Med 193:893–904

Porcelli S, Yockey CE, Brenner MB et al (1993) Analysis of T cell antigen receptor (TCR) expression by human peripheral blood CD4-8-alpha/beta T cells demonstrates preferential use of several V beta genes and an invariant TCR alpha chain. J Exp Med 178:1–16

Rachitskaya AV, Hansen AM, Horai R et al (2008) Cutting edge: NKT cells constitutively express IL-23 receptor and RORgammat and rapidly produce IL-17 upon receptor ligation in an IL-6-independent fashion. J Immunol 180:5167–5171

Renukaradhya GJ, Khan MA, Vieira M et al (2008) Type I NKT cells protect (and type II NKT cells suppress) the host's innate antitumor immune response to a B-cell lymphoma. Blood 111:5637–5645

Roelofs-Haarhuis K, Wu X, Nowak M et al (2003) Infectious nickel tolerance: a reciprocal interplay of tolerogenic APCs and T suppressor cells that is driven by immunization. J Immunol 171:2863–2872

Roy KC, Maricic I, Khurana A et al (2008) Involvement of secretory and endosomal compartments in presentation of an exogenous self-glycolipid to type II NKT cells. J Immunol 180:2942–2950

Sakaguchi S (2004) Naturally arising CD4+ regulatory t cells for immunologic self-tolerance and negative control of immune responses. Annu Rev Immunol 22:531–562

Schmieg J, Yang G, Franck RW et al (2003) Superior protection against malaria and melanoma metastases by a C-glycoside analogue of the natural killer T cell ligand alpha-Galactosylceramide. J Exp Med 198:1631–1641

Schmielau J, Finn OJ (2001) Activated granulocytes and granulocyte-derived hydrogen peroxide are the underlying mechanism of suppression of T-cell function in advanced cancer patients. Cancer Res 61:4756–4760

Shimizu K, Goto A, Fukui M et al (2007) Tumor cells loaded with alpha-galactosylceramide induce innate NKT and NK cell-dependent resistance to tumor implantation in mice. J Immunol 178:2853–2861

Sidobre S, Naidenko OV, Sim BC et al (2002) The V alpha 14 NKT cell TCR exhibits high-affinity binding to a glycolipid/CD1d complex. J Immunol 169:1340–1348

Silk JD, Hermans IF, Gileadi U et al (2004) Utilizing the adjuvant properties of CD1d-dependent NK T cells in T cell-mediated immunotherapy. J Clin Invest 114:1800–1811

Silk JD, Salio M, Reddy BG et al (2008) Cutting edge: nonglycosidic CD1d lipid ligands activate human and murine invariant NKT cells. J Immunol 180:6452–6456

Sinha P, Clements VK, Ostrand-Rosenberg S (2005) Interleukin-13-regulated M2 macrophages in combination with myeloid suppressor cells block immune surveillance against metastasis. Cancer Res 65:11743–11751

Smyth MJ, Godfrey DI (2000) NKT cells and tumor immunity – a double-edged sword. Nat Immunol 1:459–460

Smyth MJ, Thia KY, Street SE et al (2000) Differential tumor surveillance by natural killer (NK) and NKT cells. J Exp Med 191:661–668

Smyth MJ, Crowe NY, Godfrey DI (2001) NK cells and NKT cells collaborate in host protection from methylcholanthrene-induced fibrosarcoma. Int Immunol 13:459–463

Smyth MJ, Crowe NY, Pellicci DG et al (2002) Sequential production of interferon-gamma by NK1.1(+) T cells and natural killer cells is essential for the antimetastatic effect of alpha-galactosylceramide. Blood 99:1259–1266

Song L, Asgharzadeh S, Salo J et al (2009) Valpha24-invariant NKT cells mediate antitumor activity via killing of tumor-associated macrophages. J Clin Invest 119:1524–1536

Stetson DB, Mohrs M, Reinhardt RL et al (2003) Constitutive cytokine mRNAs mark natural killer (NK) and NK T cells poised for rapid effector function. J Exp Med 198:1069–1076

Swann JB, Uldrich AP, van Dommelen S et al (2009) Type I natural killer T cells suppress tumors caused by p53 loss in mice. Blood 113:6382–6385

Tachibana T, Onodera H, Tsuruyama T et al (2005) Increased intratumor Valpha24-positive natural killer T cells: a prognostic factor for primary colorectal carcinomas. Clin Cancer Res 11:7322–7327

Tahir SM, Cheng O, Shaulov A et al (2001) Loss of IFN-gamma production by invariant NK T cells in advanced cancer. J Immunol 167:4046–4050

Taniguchi M, Harada M, Kojo S et al (2003) The regulatory role of Valpha14 NKT cells in innate and acquired immune response. Annu Rev Immunol 21:483–513

Teng MW, Westwood JA, Darcy PK et al (2007) Combined natural killer T-cell based immunotherapy eradicates established tumors in mice. Cancer Res 67:7495–7504

Teng MW, Sharkey J, McLaughlin NM et al (2009a) CD1d-based combination therapy eradicates established tumors in mice. J Immunol 183:1911–1920

Teng MW, Yue S, Sharkey J et al (2009b) CD1d activation and blockade: a new antitumor strategy. J Immunol 182:3366–3371

Terabe M, Berzofsky JA (2007) NKT cells in immunoregulation of tumor immunity: a new immunoregulatory axis. Trends Immunol 28:491–496

Terabe M, Berzofsky JA (2008) The role of NKT cells in tumor immunity. Adv Cancer Res 101:277–348

Terabe M, Matsui S, Noben-Trauth N et al (2000) NKT cell-mediated repression of tumor immunosurveillance by IL-13 and the IL-4R-STAT6 pathway. Nat Immunol 1:515–520

Terabe M, Matsui S, Park J-M et al (2003a) Transforming growth factor-β production and myeloid cells are an effector mechanism through which CD1d-restricted T cells block cytotoxic T lymphocyte-mediated tumor immunosurveillance: abrogation prevents tumor recurrence. J Exp Med 198:1741–1752

Terabe M, Park JM, Berzofsky JA (2003b) Role of IL-13 in negative regulation of anti-tumor immunity. Cancer Immunol Immunother 53:79–85

Terabe M, Swann J, Ambrosino E et al (2005) A nonclassical non-Va14Ja18 CD1d-restricted (type II) NKT cell is sufficient for down-regulation of tumor immunosurveillance. J Exp Med 202:1627–1633

Toura I, Kawano T, Akutsu Y et al (1999) Cutting edge: inhibition of experimental tumor metastasis by dendritic cells pulsed with alpha-galactosylceramide. J Immunol 163:2387–2391

Tupin E, Kinjo Y, Kronenberg M (2007) The unique role of natural killer T cells in the response to microorganisms. Nat Rev Microbiol 5:405–417

Wilson MT, Johansson C, Olivares-Villagomez D et al (2003) The response of natural killer T cells to glycolipid antigens is characterized by surface receptor down-modulation and expansion. Proc Natl Acad Sci USA 100:10913–10918

Wu DY, Segal NH, Sidobre S et al (2003) Cross-presentation of disialoganglioside GD3 to natural killer T cells. J Exp Med 198:173–181

Wu D, Xing GW, Poles MA et al (2005) Bacterial glycolipids and analogs as antigens for CD1d-restricted NKT cells. Proc Natl Acad Sci USA 102:1351–1356

Yanagisawa K, Seino K, Ishikawa Y et al (2002) Impaired proliferative response of V alpha 24 NKT cells from cancer patients against alpha-galactosylceramide. J Immunol 168:6494–6499

Yanagisawa K, Exley MA, Jiang X et al (2006) Hyporesponsiveness to natural killer T-cell ligand alpha-galactosylceramide in cancer-bearing state mediated by CD11b+ Gr-1+ cells producing nitric oxide. Cancer Res 66:11441–11446

Yoshimura N, Sawada T, Furusawa M et al (2001) Expression of xenoantigen transformed human cancer cells to be susceptible to antibody-mediated cell killing. Cancer Lett 164:155–160

Zajonc DM, Maricic I, Wu D et al (2005) Structural basis for CD1d presentation of a sulfatide derived from myelin and its implications for autoimmunity. J Exp Med 202:1517–1526

Zhou D, Mattner J, Cantu C 3rd et al (2004) Lysosomal glycosphingolipid recognition by NKT cells. Science 306:1786–1789

Chapter 3
γδ T Cells in Cancer

Lawrence S. Lamb, Jr.

The field of cancer immunology and immune therapy has been an important focus of basic and clinical research since early discoveries of tumor antigens and adoptive immunity (Disis et al. 2009; Dougan and Dranoff 2009a, b). As techniques developed that allowed researchers to distinguish various lymphocyte subsets, more specific strategies began to develop, and included such therapies as IL-2 stimulation of autologous lymphokine activated killer (LAK) cells from peripheral blood and ex vivo culture and activation of tumor-infiltrating lymphocytes (TIL). Most of these studies focused on natural killer (NK) cells or cytotoxic T lymphocytes (CTL) as the primary mediators of antitumor immunity (Yannelli et al. 1996; Bloom et al. 1997; Fleischhauer et al. 1997; Kawakami et al. 1998; Kim et al. 1998; Dudley et al. 1999; Mateo et al. 1999; Colella et al. 2000) and although notable successes have been achieved, most CTL- or NK-based immunotherapeutic strategies have delivered mixed results. The contribution of γδ T cells, a minor T cell subset with distinct innate immune recognition properties, has not been explored until recently.

Several lines of evidence support a broad role for γδ T cells in tumor immunosurveillance (Zocchi and Poggi 2004; Kabelitz et al. 2007). Mice lacking γδ T cells are highly susceptible to induction of cutaneous carcinogenesis (Girardi et al. 2001) and to progression of prostate cancer (Liu et al. 2008). In clinical studies, γδ T cells have been shown to infiltrate a variety of tumors including lung cancer (Ferrarini et al. 1994), renal cell carcinoma (Choudhary et al. 1995), seminoma (Zhao et al. 1995), ovarian cancer (Xu et al. 2007), and colon cancer (Corvaisier et al. 2005). In many instances, γδ T cells that are cytotoxic to a specific tumor type will cross-react with other tumors but not with the tumor's nontransformed counterpart (Corvaisier et al. 2005; Xu et al. 2007; Bryant et al. 2009a, b). This chapter will focus on the unique properties of γδ T cells with respect to tumor surveillance and will review

L.S. Lamb Jr. (✉)
Department of Medicine, Division of Hematology and Oncology,
University of Alabama Birmingham, Birmingham, AL, USA
e-mail: Lawrence.Lamb@ccc.uab.edu

the short history and clinical potential for γδ T cell-based adoptive therapies of cancer. Obstacles to the implementation of these therapies will be discussed and future directions explored.

1 Development, Migration, and Recognition Strategies of γδ T Cells

Most mature T cells express the αβ T cell receptor (TCR), reside in the secondary lymphoid organs, and function primarily in adaptive immune responses. A small proportion express the γδ TCR and reside principally in the epithelial tissues such as the skin, intestine, and lung (Haas et al. 1993) where they function as primary responders by recognizing intact structures such as stress-associated proteins, heat shock proteins, and lipids (Haas et al. 1993; Hayday 2000). The developmental pathways of αβ and γδ T cells diverge early during thymic development as the γ and δ proteins are first detected in the DN3 population (Wilson et al. 1999; Prinz et al. 2006; Xiong and Raulet 2007; Taghon and Rothenberg 2008). Their developmental program generally does not include expression of CD4 or CD8β nor do they require the extensive proliferation or multiple TCR recombination events that are characteristic of αβ T cells. There is some evidence for extrathymic development of γδ T cells, particularly intestinal epithelial Vγ5+ T cells (Guy-Grand et al. 1991; Lefrancois and Puddington 1995).

The γδ TCR structure is more similar to immunoglobulins than it is to the αβ TCR and has the potential to recognize a wide variety of antigens. However, many γδ T cell subsets are tissue-specific, having been formed at different stages of ontology in a fixed developmental program that begins in the early fetal thymus. Hence, these cells show little or no TCR diversity (Allison and Havran 1991; Haas et al. 1993). Initial studies in mice indicate that a combination of chemokine receptors, tissue-specific ligands, and other molecules involved in cellular localization combine to pair a particular subset of γδ T cells with the required functional properties into the specific tissues in which they reside.

Activating ligands for γδ T cells as well as the process by which γδ T cells recognize stressed or malignant cells have been recently reviewed (Chien and Konigshofer 2007; O'Brien et al. 2007). These processes are complex and incompletely understood, but are fundamentally different from both αβ T cells and NK cells (Boismenu and Havran 1997; Hayday 2000). Functional characteristics of αβ T cells derive from recognition of peptides that are displayed on MHC Class I or Class II molecules by antigen presenting cells (APCs). Endogenous or exogenous proteins are degraded in the endocytic compartments of APCs, transported to the cell surface, and complexed with the appropriate MHC molecule (Germain and Margulies 1993; Germain 1994; Cresswell 1996). Antigen recognition by γδ T cells, however, is less well defined and is thought to be determined by germline-encoded elements and various combinations of the TCR V, D, and J segments of both γ and δ chains. Antigens that generally fit this pattern include endogenous and synthetic phosphoantigens (Morita et al. 1995; Bukowski et al. 1999; Hayday 2000; Kunzmann et al. 2000; Miyagawa et al. 2001; Gober et al. 2003), heat-shock proteins (Born et al. 1990; Fu et al. 1994; Laad et al. 1999), and stress-associated antigens (Groh et al. 1999; Wu et al. 2002).

NKG2D, a C-type, lectin-like homodimeric activating receptor expressed by NK cells, αβCD8+ T cells, and γδ T cells, is a ligand for MHC class-I like proteins such as MIC-A/B and the UL-16 binding proteins. These NKG2D ligands are upregulated in response to cell stress including infection and malignant transformation (Gleimer and Parham 2003; Raulet 2003). Although there is some controversy regarding the use of NKG2D by γδ T cells, several lines of evidence suggest that the Vδ1 TCR is required for γδ T cells to engage cells that express MIC-A/B. MIC-A tetramers have been shown to bind an NKG2D⁻ cell line transfected with various Vδ1+ TCRs that had previously been shown to react against MIC-A-expressing targets (Wu et al. 2002). Furthermore, Zhao et al. (2006) found that coupled V domains from the MICA-induced T cells expressed as a single polypeptide chain soluble TCR can specifically bind to MIC-A expressed by HeLa cells and to immobilized MICA molecules. NKG2D ligation has been thought to play a costimulatory role in the activation of γδ T cells (Bauer et al. 1999; Das et al. 2001); however, recent findings indicate that NKG2D ligation may be sufficient to independently activate some γδ T cell subsets (Rincon-Orozco et al. 2005; Whang et al. 2009).

2 Vδ1+ T Cells

Vδ1+ T cells are predominant in intestines and skin but comprise only a minor population of circulating γδ T cells (Groh et al. 1998; Ebert et al. 2006). Unlike Vδ2+ cells, they do not preferentially pair with a specific Vγ chain and are not activated by alkylamines, IPP or N-BP (Tanaka et al. 1994, 1995; Bukowski et al. 1995). As discussed above, Vδ1+ T cells are activated by stress-induced self antigens such as MIC-A/B and UL-16 binding proteins, many of which are constitutively expressed by solid tumors as well as some leukemias and lymphomas (Groh et al. 1999; Wu et al. 2002; Poggi et al. 2004a, b). Vδ1+ cells also recognize glycolipids presented by CD1c on the surface of immature dendritic cells and can induce DC to mature and produce IL-12 (Spada et al. 2000; Ismaili et al. 2002; Leslie et al. 2002). Vδ1+ T cells can also exhibit immunosuppressive and regulatory properties, a function which is discussed at greater length below.

Vδ1+ T cells infiltrate and kill a wide variety of lymphoid and myeloid malignancies (Duval et al. 1995; Groh et al. 1999; Dolstra et al. 2001; Lamb et al. 2001; Poggi et al. 2004b; Catellani et al. 2007), neuroblastoma (Schilbach et al. 2008), and cancers of the lung, colon, and pancreas (Maeurer et al. 1995; Ferrarini et al. 1996; Maeurer et al. 1996). Primary myeloid and lymphoid leukemias activate Vδ1+ T cells (Duval et al. 1995; Dolstra et al. 2001; Lamb et al. 2001), which are cytotoxic to both primary leukemia and leukemia cell lines. Vδ1+ T cells show a restricted CDR3 repertoire in patients with leukemia (Meeh et al. 2006). In addition, supra-normal recovery of leukemia-reactive Vδ1+ T cells is associated with long-term leukemia-free survival after allogeneic bone marrow transplantation (Lamb et al. 1996; Godder et al. 2007).

Virus-infected cells are also vulnerable to recognition and lysis by γδ T cells, particularly the Vδ1+ and Vδ3+ subtypes. It has recently been shown that γδ T cells that are reactive against EBV and CMV are cross-reactive to various tumors. Vδ1+ γδ T cells recognize EBV-transformed B cells (Hacker et al. 1992), and expand in vitro and in vivo using clonally restricted δ1 CDR3 repertoire that persists for several years (Fujishima et al. 2007). Vδ1+ γδ T cells are also highly active against CMV-infected cells, and these CMV-reactive cells are cross-reactive against the colon cancer line HT29 (Dechanet et al. 1999; Halary et al. 2005; Pitard et al. 2008). The mechanism of cross-reactivity has not been fully described as yet, but may have therapeutic implications for other malignancies with an EBV or CMV component such as glioblastoma, which has been shown to be vulnerable to γδ T cell response (Fujimiya et al. 1997; Lau et al. 2005; Cobbs et al. 2007; Mitchell et al. 2008; Scheurer et al. 2008; Bryant et al. 2009a, b).

3 Vδ2+ T Cells

Vδ2+ T cells comprise the majority of γδ T cells in the circulation and in secondary lymphoid organs (Parker et al. 1990). The Vδ2+ chain usually pairs with a Vγ9 chain to form the Vγ9/Vδ2 heterodimer. Vγ9/Vδ2+ T cells are thought to be activated via the TCR principally by three groups of non-peptide antigens: alkylphosphates such as isopentenyl pyrophosphate (IPP) generated by eukaryotic isoprenoid biosynthesis using the mevalonate pathway (Morita et al. 1995), alkylamines (Bukowski et al. 1999), and synthetic aminobisphosphonates (N-BP) (Kunzmann et al. 2000; Miyagawa et al. 2001). The first two compounds are naturally occurring in bacteria, plants, and some eukaryotes. Synthetic N-BPs such as Pamidronate and Zoledronate are clinically used to improve bone strength.

Some hematologic malignancies and solid tumors also produce IPP at concentrations that render them vulnerable to recognition and lysis by Vγ9Vδ2+ T cells likely through overexpression of nonpeptidic phosphorylated mevalonate metabolites (Hayday 2000; Gober et al. 2003; Bonneville and Scotet 2006). In addition, N-BP compounds bind and inhibit IPP-consuming enzymes such as farneyl pyrophosphate synthase and geranylgeranyl pyrophosphate synthase (Guo et al. 2007) leading to the accumulation of IPP within the tumor cell, a process that was recently shown to activate Vγ9Vδ2+ T cells (Li et al. 2009). These findings suggest that N-BP compounds have a dual role in the initiation of innate antitumor immune response both by activating and by expanding Vγ9Vδ2+ T cells and by rendering selected tumors more vulnerable to Vγ9Vδ2+ T cell-mediated lysis.

As discussed above, NKG2D activation is also an important factor in tumor recognition and lysis by Vγ9Vδ2+ T cells, potentially playing a costimulatory role in cooperation with TCR-dependent activation (Das et al. 2001; Wrobel et al. 2007), although direct ligation of the Vγ9Vδ2+ receptor by the NKG2D ligand ULBP-4 has been recently reported (Kong et al. 2009). In some situations, NKG2D activation may be the primary stimulus, while TCR stimulation has a secondary role or is not required (Rincon-Orozco et al. 2005; Nitahara et al. 2006).

Vγ9Vδ2+ T cells recognize and kill hematologic malignancies such as Daudi Burkitt's lymphoma (Wright et al. 1989; Freedman et al. 1997) and other non-Hodgkin's lymphomas (Wilhelm et al. 2003), and multiple myeloma (Kunzmann et al. 2000). Vγ9Vδ2+ γδ T cells also recognize and lyse cell lines from glioblastoma (Suzuki et al. 1999), lung cancer (Ferrarini et al. 2002), breast cancer (Gober et al. 2003), bladder cancer (Kato et al. 2001) as well as melanoma and pancreatic cancer (Kabelitz et al. 2004).

4 Regulatory γδ T Cells

Certain subsets or γδ T cells with regulatory/suppressor functions have also been identified (Hayday and Tigelaar 2003; Pennington et al. 2005). A suppressive γδ T cell population of γδ+TIL was recently characterized in breast cancer (Peng et al. 2007) as Vδ1+ T cells that expressed IFN- γ and GM-CSF when stimulated by autologous tumor or anti-CD3. Other cytokines typically expressed by effector γδ T cells such as TGF-β were not expressed by this population. Additionally, suppressor γδ T cells did not express Foxp3. Suppressive activity could be reversed by TLR8 ligands, suggesting a potential immunotherapeutic strategy in breast tumors with a high percentage of suppressive γδ T cells. It has also been recently shown that Foxp3-expressing γδ T cells can be generated from mouse splenocytes following stimulation with anti-TCR-γδ and TGF-β (Kang et al. 2009). These γδ T cells also expressed CD25, TGF-β, and GITR and showed a potent immunosuppressive effect on anti-CD3 stimulated T cell activation and proliferation. A small population of FoxP3-expressing γδ T cells was also identified in human peripheral blood although they could not be expanded with anti-TCR-γδ and TGF-β as in the mouse model.

5 Potential for γδ T Cells as Primary Effectors in Immunotherapy of Cancer

A number of in vitro and in vivo studies suggest that γδ T cells might be ideally suited for immunotherapy via in vivo activation or adoptive cellular therapy within the context of hematopoietic stem cell transplantation (HSCT) and/or as a donor innate lymphocyte infusion (DILI). The potential advantages and disadvantages of autologous vs. allogeneic donors are also a subject of much investigation. Issues with the various strategies are discussed as follows:

5.1 In Vivo Activation and Expansion of γδ T Cells

The most attractive and logistically simple approach would be in vivo expansion and activation of γδ T cells in the cancer patient using pharmacologic agents that are currently available for clinical use. One early trial compared the bisphosphonates Pamidronate, Coldronate, and Ibandronate with respect to their ability to induce proliferation of γδ T cells in patients with multiple myeloma (Kunzmann et al. 2000). Only the N-BP Pamidronate induced γδ T cell expansion. In addition, viable bone marrow plasma cells were significantly reduced following the administration of Pamidronate at 24 h prior to marrow sampling when compared to controls. Wilhelm treated a series of patients with low-grade non-Hodgkin lymphoma using intravenous Pamidronate after determining that their γδ T cells would respond to Pamidronate+IL-2 in vitro. Significant in vivo activation/proliferation of γδ T cells was observed in 5/9 patients, and objective responses were achieved in 3/9 as determined by CT scanning and biopsy (Wilhelm et al. 2003). Dieli compared Zoledronate alone and in combination with IL-2 (ZOL/IL-2) in patients with hormone-refractory prostate cancer. In patients that received the ZOL/IL-2 regimen, the numbers of effector-memory γδ T cells showed a statistically significant correlation with declining prostate-specific antigen levels and objective clinical outcomes that consisted of three instances of partial remission and five of stable disease. By contrast, most patients treated with ZOL alone failed to sustain γδ T cell numbers and did not show a clinical response (Dieli et al. 2007). As of this writing, clinical trials of bromohydrin pyrophosphate, a synthetic phosphoantigen that is a potent activator of Vγ9Vδ2 γδ T cells, are being conducted in patients with follicular lymphoma and chronic myeloid leukemia. Preliminary results have recently been published (Bennouna et al. 2010) showing that the drug is well tolerated and induces a robust expansion of gamma/delta T cells in patients.

5.2 Autologous γδ T Cell Therapy

Although autologous cellular therapy carries with it the advantages of limiting the potential for graft vs. host disease (GvHD) and immunologic rejection of the infused therapeutic cell product, there is evidence that γδ T cells from cancer patients are reduced in number and impaired in their potential for activation and expansion as described in recent findings from patients with melanoma (Argentati et al. 2003), leukemia (Meeh et al. 2006), breast cancer (Gaafar et al. 2009), and glioblastoma (Bryant et al. 2009a, b). Indeed, it has been known as early as 1991 that TCR/CD3 signaling can induce apoptosis (Janssen et al. 1991) in mature γδ T cells. Daudi lymphoma cells, which are killed by Vγ9Vδ+γδ T cells, also induce apoptotic death in the γδ T cell effectors upon TCR triggering (Ferrarini et al. 1995). This is possibly a result of a negative feedback mechanism which may limit the time span of γδ T cell expansions during infectious diseases, even when pathogens are not eliminated and persist in the host.

These findings do not rule out the potential for autologous γδ T cell therapies but may limit their application to patients with sufficient γδ T cell function to warrant the undertaking of a complex cell-manufacturing procedure. Indeed, large numbers of cytotoxic γδ T cell effectors can be obtained from selected cancer patients using either N-BP or phosphoantigen stimulation (Kondo et al. 2008). Two small trials of autologous γδ T cell therapy have been conducted in patients with metastatic renal cell carcinoma, a tumor with documented sensitivity to host immune function. In the first trial (Kobayashi et al. 2007), γδ T cells were expanded and activated using a synthetic phosphoantigen 2-methyl-3-butenyl-1-pyrophosphate (2M3B1-PP). No severe adverse events were seen in this trial, and 3 of 5 patients showed slower tumor progression. Patients in whom a response was documented showed an increase in the peripheral γδ T cell absolute count and a strong in vitro response to phosphoantigen stimulation. In the second trial, ten patients were treated with BrHPP-expanded γδ T cells in a dose-escalation Phase I trial to determine the safety of this therapy and the maximum tolerated dose (Bennouna et al. 2008). Although there was no measurable effect on disease progression in this study, the data indicate that repeated infusions of BrHPP-expanded γδ T cells up to a dose of 8×10^9 total cells, either alone or with IL-2, are well tolerated. These early trials show promise for the development of autologous γδ T cell therapies in eligible patients.

5.3 Allogeneic γδ T Cell Therapy in the Setting of Hematopoietic Stem Cell Transplantation

To date, there have been no studies performed in which γδ T cells have been specifically introduced in HSCT, although some information can be gained from studies in which αβ T cells were specifically depleted from allogeneic grafts, thereby enriching the cell product for γδ T cells and NK cells. One single institution study compared outcomes of patients who received αβ T cell depleted (αβTCD) grafts with patients who received pan T cell-depleted grafts (Lamb et al. 1996, 1999). In this study, a significant number of patients that received αβTCD cells subsequently developed spontaneous increases in the absolute count of circulating γδ T cells during the first year following HSCT. These cells were predominately Vδ1+ and were cytotoxic to primary leukemias and leukemia cell lines in vitro. The patients experienced a significant long-lasting improvement in disease-free survival when compared with similar risk patients (Godder et al. 2007). Conversely, another single-center study of 535 patients who received αβ TCD grafts vs. pan-CD3 TCD (Keever-Taylor et al. 2001) showed no difference in DFS for either TCD method, although patients with increased γδ T cell counts, if present, were not analyzed separately. Renewed interest in preserving innate immunity in HSCT has prompted the development of an immunomagnetic procedure for clinical-scale αβTCD (Chaleff et al. 2007), which is expected to be released for clinical use in Europe in early 2012.

Indeed, both animal and human studies suggest that allogeneic γδ T cells can be safely infused into the setting of HSCT. Although γδ T cells can be activated in the setting of GvHD, there is no evidence to suggest that donor-derived γδ T cells are primary initiators of GvHD (Ellison et al. 1995; Drobyski et al. 2000).

Indeed, large doses of IL-2 expanded γδ T cells can be infused into lethally irradiated MHC-disparate mice (C57BL/6 [H-2^b] → B10.BR [H-2^k] and C57BL/6 [H-2^b] → B6D2F1 [H-2$^{b/d}$]) without causing GvHD (Drobyski et al. 1999). In vitro studies provide evidence that γδ T cells are not substantially activated in the allogeneic mixed lymphocyte culture (Schilbach et al. 2000; Lamb et al. 2001). In addition, animal studies and indirect evidence from human allogeneic transplant studies suggest that γδ T cells can also facilitate alloengraftment (Blazar et al. 1996; Drobyski and Majewski 1997) (Henslee et al. 1987; Kawanishi et al. 1997).

5.4 Donor Innate Lymphocyte Infusion Therapy

Although several examples of the successful application of donor lymphocyte infusions (DLI) for relapsed leukemia have been published (Kolb and Holler 1997; Guglielmi et al. 2002), acute and chronic GvHD remain as major direct complications from DLI (Montero et al. 2006) even with modifications such as T-cell depleted DLI or graded incremental DLI doses (Dazzi et al. 2000). Innate lymphocytes such as γδ T cells may provide an ideal source of allogeneic cellular immunotherapy as they respond to malignancy without the recognition of allo-specific antigens. Given the potentially lower risk for initiation of GvHD by γδ T cells, it may be possible to deliver donor-derived γδ T cells as DLI early after allogeneic HSC transplantation with minimal risk of GvHD. In addition to post-HSCT DLI, allogeneic expanded/activated γδ T cells could be employed directly in combination with lymphodepleting cytoreductive therapy for the treatment of a variety of malignancies in a non-transplant setting as has been recently described for NK cell therapy (Miller et al. 2005).

5.5 Cell Manufacturing Strategies

As discussed above, several investigators have developed procedures for the expansion and activation of γδ T cells for infusion based on their responsiveness to phosphoantigens and N-BPs. As N-BPs are approved in the United States and Europe as bone-strengthening drugs, strategies that employ cGMP-approvable culture methods for γδ T cells with IL-2 and commercially available bisphosphonates such as Zoledronate or Pamidronate could easily be translated for use in both allogeneic and autologous therapies. The synthetic phosphoantigen BrHPP (Phosphostim™; Innate Pharma; Marseille, FR) was developed specifically for innate immune therapy which has recently completed early trials that have shown efficacy in the expansion of γδ T cells with no significant toxicity as discussed previously (Salot et al. 2007; Bennouna et al. 2008). At issue, however, is the finding that both N-BP and phosphoantigen-mediated γδ T cell stimulation expand only the Vγ9Vδ2 γδ T cell subset and do not deliver the potential therapeutic benefit of an expanded Vδ1+ population (Kabelitz et al. 2007; Schilbach et al. 2008).

Lopez and colleagues have developed a procedure for the expansion and activation of γδ T cells based on a CD2-initiated signaling pathway which induces a coordinated downregulation of the IL-2Rα chain and a corresponding upregulation of the IL-15Rα chain on γδ T cells. The γδ T cells stimulated in this manner express tenfold higher levels of mRNA for *bcl*-2 resulting in an inhibition of apoptosis in mitogen-stimulated human γδ T cells and potentially overcoming some of the problems with activation-induced cell death discussed previously. In addition, this procedure activates and expands all δ-chain phenotypes (Lopez et al. 2000; Guo et al. 2002), not only the Vγ9Vδ2 subset. As with N-BP, γδ T cells that are expanded and activated using this method retain potent innate antitumor activity against a wide variety of human hematopoietic and solid primary tumors and cell lines (Lopez et al. 2000; Guo et al. 2001). Potential limitations of this procedure include the requirement for compounds that are not currently approved for clinical use. Since αβ T cells are also expanded in culture, it is also necessary to deplete the αβ T cells or positively select γδ T cells, potentially increasing the cost and complexity of the procedure.

6 Obstacles to Development and Implementation of γδ T Cell Therapies

The potential and actual problems that must be considered when developing γδ T cell-based cellular therapies have recently been reviewed in detail (Martinet et al. 2009b). Two issues that deserve mention have been previously explored in this chapter. The first is the observation that circulating γδ T cells from cancer are reduced in number and show impairment of proliferative function, thus limiting the applicability of autologous infusion therapies or strategies that rely on in vivo stimulation of γδ T cells. A separate though related problem is the sensitivity of normal γδ T cells to activation-induced cell death, which could impact the longevity of ex vivo expanded allogeneic cells once infused.

Other obstacles are those common to most T cell-based therapies. In order to eradicate solid tumors, γδ T cells must be able to traverse the tumor vasculature and migrate into the surrounding parenchyma. To date, clinical trials using ex vivo expanded γδ T cells have not addressed this issue, although γδ T cells express CXCR3 and CCR5 receptors for cytokines such as CXCL9 (MIG), CXCL10 (IP-10), CXCL11 (ITAC), and CCL5 (RANTES) which are generally produced in the tumor inflammatory microenvironment (Glatzel et al. 2002; Dieli et al. 2003; Poggi et al. 2004b, 2007). The tumor vasculature can impair T cell migration via endothelin-B-mediated inhibition of ICAM-1 and abnormal differentiation and morphology of tumor vasculature. Recent studies also suggest that anti-angiogenic agents currently used in cancer therapy can restore normal vascular morphology and thus permit improved T cell migration into the tumor (Martinet et al. 2009b).

A host of tumor-derived inhibitory factors such as TGF-β can effectively paralyze the immune response to tumor via multiple mechanisms such as inhibition of dendritic cell (DC) maturation, antigen presentation, T cell activation, and expansion of CD3+CD4+Foxp3+ regulatory T cells, (Smyth et al. 1991; Inge et al. 1992; Jachimczak et al. 1993), which have recently been implicated in direct suppression of γδ T cell function (Kunzmann et al. 2009). Of particular concern to innate immune responses is the proteolytic shedding of soluble NKG2D ligands from tumors which in turn bind NKG2D (and possibly the γδ TCR) and inhibit both γδ T cell and NK cell functions (Groh et al. 2002). Tumor-derived proinflammatory factors also recruit suppressive cells such as monocyte-derived suppressor cells (MDSC) and mesenchymal stromal cells (MSC) into the tumor microenvironment. Although the impact of MDSC on γδ T cell function remains unclear, it is known that MSC actively suppress Vγ9Vδ2+ T cell responses to phosphoantigen via COX-2 mediated production of PGE-2, which in turn suppresses proliferation, TNF-α and IFN-γ production, and tumor cytolysis (Martinet et al. 2009b).

7 Conclusions and Future Directions

Development of strategies to exploit the innate antitumor properties of human γδ T cells – particularly as an adjuvant to more traditional cancer therapies – may allow treatment of a variety of malignant diseases that are now only partially responsive to HSCT and/or other cell-based immunotherapies. The increasing knowledge of tumor-derived immunosuppression and immune escape will ultimately lead to strategies that will remove some of the barriers to effectiveness of these therapies. Finally, the recent clinical and translational studies highlighted in this chapter illustrate that therapeutic numbers of γδ T cells with significant anti-tumor activity can be expanded with methods that are easily translated to comply with current cell manufacturing regulatory requirements.

For the above reasons, we envision that it will eventually become possible to specifically transfer tumor-reactive donor-derived γδ T cells as part of both allogeneic and autologous transplant strategies for the treatment of a variety of malignancies. Particularly in the setting of lymphodepleting non-myeloablative chemotherapy and/or radiotherapy, evidence strongly suggests that γδ T cell-based innate lymphocyte infusion therapy and/or strategies to augment γδ T cell activation and expansion in vivo can become important tools in the treatment of selected cancers.

References

Allison JP, Havran WL (1991) The immunobiology of T cells with invariant gamma delta antigen receptors. Annu Rev Immunol 9:679–705

Argentati K, Re F et al (2003) Reduced number and impaired function of circulating gamma delta T cells in patients with cutaneous primary melanoma. J Invest Dermatol 120(5):829–834

Bauer S, Groh V et al (1999) Activation of NK cells and T cells by NKG2D, a receptor for stress-inducible MICA [see comments]. Science 285(5428):727–729

Bennouna J, Bompas E et al (2008) Phase-I study of Innacell gammadeltatrade mark, an autologous cell-therapy product highly enriched in gamma9delta2 T lymphocytes, in combination with IL-2, in patients with metastatic renal cell carcinoma. Cancer Immunol Immunother 57(11):1599–1609

Bennouna J, Levy V et al (2010) Phase-I study of bromohydrin pyrophosphate (BrHPP, IPH 1101), a Vgamma9Vdelta2 T lymphocyte agonist in patients with solid tumors. Cancer Immunol Immunother 59(10):1521–1530. Epub 2010 Jun 19

Blazar BR, Taylor PA et al (1996) Murine gamma/delta-expressing T cells affect alloengraftment via the recognition of nonclassical major histocompatibility complex class Ib antigens. Blood 87(10):4463–4472

Bloom MB, Perry-Lalley D et al (1997) Identification of tyrosinase-related protein 2 as a tumor rejection antigen for the B16 melanoma. J Exp Med 185(3):453–459

Boismenu R, Havran WL (1997) An innate view of gamma delta T cells. Curr Opin Immunol 9:57–63

Bonneville M, Scotet E (2006) Human Vgamma9Vdelta2 T cells: promising new leads for immunotherapy of infections and tumors. Curr Opin Immunol 18(5):539–546

Born W, Happ MP et al (1990) Recognition of heat shock proteins and gamma delta cell function. Immunol Today 11(2):40–43

Bryant NL, Suarez-Cuervo C et al (2009a) Characterization and immunotherapeutic potential of γδ T cells in patients with glioblastoma. Neuro-Oncology 11(4):357–67

Bryant NL, Suarez-Cuervo C et al (2009b) Characterization and immunotherapeutic potential of {gamma}{delta} T cells in patients with glioblastoma. Neuro Oncol 11(4):357–67

Bukowski JF, Morita CT et al (1999) Human gamma delta T cells recognize alkylamines derived from microbes, edible plants, and tea: implications for innate immunity. Immunity 11(1):57–65

Bukowski JF, Morita CT et al (1995) V gamma 2V delta 2 TCR-dependent recognition of non-peptide antigens and Daudi cells analyzed by TCR gene transfer. J Immunol 154(3):998–1006

Catellani S, Poggi A et al (2007) Expansion of Vdelta1 T lymphocytes producing IL-4 in low-grade non-Hodgkin lymphomas expressing UL-16-binding proteins. Blood 109(5):2078–2085

Chaleff S, Otto M et al (2007) A large-scale method for the selective depletion of alphabeta T lymphocytes from PBSC for allogeneic transplantation. Cytotherapy 9(8):746–754

Chien YH, Konigshofer Y (2007) Antigen recognition by gammadelta T cells. Immunol Rev 215:46–58

Choudhary A, Davodeau F et al (1995) Selective lysis of autologous tumor cells by recurrent gamma delta tumor-infiltrating lymphocytes from renal carcinoma. J Immunol 154(8):3932–3940

Cobbs CS, Soroceanu L et al (2007) Human cytomegalovirus induces cellular tyrosine kinase signaling and promotes glioma cell invasiveness. J Neurooncol 85(3):271–280

Colella TA, Bullock TN et al (2000) Self-tolerance to the murine homologue of a tyrosinase-derived melanoma antigen: implications for tumor immunotherapy. J Exp Med 191(7):1221–1232

Corvaisier M, Moreau-Aubry A et al (2005) V gamma 9V delta 2 T cell response to colon carcinoma cells. J Immunol 175(8):5481–5488

Cresswell P (1996) Invariant chain structure and MHC class II function. Cell 84(4):505–507

Das H, Groh V et al (2001) MICA engagement by human Vgamma2Vdelta2 T cells enhances their antigen-dependent effector function. Immunity 15(1):83–93

Dazzi F, Szydlo RM et al (2000) Comparison of single-dose and escalating-dose regimens of donor lymphocyte infusion for relapse after allografting for chronic myeloid leukemia [see comment]. Blood 95(1):67–71

Dechanet J, Merville P et al (1999) Implication of gammadelta T cells in the human immune response to cytomegalovirus. J Clin Invest 103(10):1437–1449

Dieli F, Poccia F et al (2003) Differentiation of effector/memory Vdelta2 T cells and migratory routes in lymph nodes or inflammatory sites. J Exp Med 198(3):391–397

Dieli F, Vermijlen D et al (2007) Targeting human {gamma}delta T cells with zoledronate and interleukin-2 for immunotherapy of hormone-refractory prostate cancer. Cancer Res 67(15):7450–7457

Disis ML, Bernhard H et al (2009) Use of tumour-responsive T cells as cancer treatment. Lancet 373(9664):673–683

Dolstra H, Fredrix H et al (2001) TCR gamma delta cytotoxic T lymphocytes expressing the killer cell-inhibitory receptor p58.2 (CD158b) selectively lyse acute myeloid leukemia cells. Bone Marrow Transplant 27(10):1087–1093

Dougan M, Dranoff G (2009) The immune response to tumors. Curr Protoc Immunol. Chap. 20 (Unit 20):11

Dougan M, Dranoff G (2009b) Immune therapy for cancer. Annu Rev Immunol 27:83–117

Drobyski WR, Majewski D (1997) Donor gamma delta T lymphocytes promote allogeneic engraftment across the major histocompatibility barrier in mice. Blood 89(3):1100–1109

Drobyski WR, Majewski D et al (1999) Graft-facilitating doses of ex vivo activated gammadelta T cells do not cause lethal murine graft-vs.-host disease. Biol Blood Marrow Transplant 5(4):222–230

Drobyski WR, Vodanovic-Jankovic S et al (2000) Adoptively transferred gamma delta T cells indirectly regulate murine graft-versus-host reactivity following donor leukocyte infusion therapy in mice. J Immunol 165(3):1634–1640

Dudley ME, Nishimura MI et al (1999) Antitumor immunization with a minimal peptide epitope (G9-209-2M) leads to a functionally heterogeneous CTL response. J Immunother 22(4):288–298

Duval M, Yotnda P et al (1995) Potential antileukemic effect of gamma delta T cells in acute lymphoblastic leukemia. Leukemia 9(5):863–868

Ebert LM, Meuter S et al (2006) Homing and function of human skin gammadelta T cells and NK cells: relevance for tumor surveillance. J Immunol 176(7):4331–4336

Ellison CA, MacDonald GC et al (1995) Gamma delta T cells in the pathobiology of murine acute graft-versus-host disease. Evidence that gamma delta T cells mediate natural killer-like cytotoxicity in the host and that elimination of these cells from donors significantly reduces mortality. J Immunol 155(9):4189–4198

Ferrarini M, Ferrero E et al (2002) Human gammadelta T cells: a nonredundant system in the immune-surveillance against cancer. Trends Immunol 23(1):14–18

Ferrarini M, Heltai S et al (1995) Daudi lymphoma killing triggers the programmed death of cytotoxic V gamma 9/V delta 2 T lymphocytes. J Immunol 154(8):3704–3712

Ferrarini M, Heltai S, Pupa SM, Mernard S, Zocchi R (1996) Killing of laminin receptor-positive human lung cancers by tumor-infiltrating lymphocytes bearing gd+ T-cell receptors. Journal of the National Cancer Institute 88:436–441

Ferrarini M, Pupa SM et al (1994) Distinct pattern of HSP72 and monomeric laminin receptor expression in human lung cancers infiltrated by gamma/delta T lymphocytes. Int J Cancer 57(4):486–490

Fleischhauer K, Tanzarella S et al (1997) Functional heterogeneity of HLA-A*02 subtypes revealed by presentation of a MAGE-3-encoded peptide to cytotoxic T cell clones. J Immunol 159(5): 2513–2521

Freedman MS, D'Souza S et al (1997) gamma delta T-cell-human glial cell interactions. I. In vitro induction of gammadelta T-cell expansion by human glial cells. J Neuroimmunol 74(1–2): 135–142

Fu YX, Vollmer M et al (1994) Structural requirements for peptides that stimulate a subset of gamma delta T cells. J Immunol 152(4):1578–1588

Fujimiya Y, Suzuki Y et al (1997) In vitro interleukin 12 activation of peripheral blood CD3(+) CD56(+) and CD3(+)CD56(−) gammadelta T cells from glioblastoma patients. Clin Cancer Res 3(4):633–643

Fujishima N, Hirokawa M et al (2007) Skewed T cell receptor repertoire of Vdelta1(+) gammadelta T lymphocytes after human allogeneic haematopoietic stem cell transplantation and the potential role for Epstein-Barr virus-infected B cells in clonal restriction. Clin Exp Immunol 149(1): 70–79

Gaafar A, Aljurf MD et al (2009) Defective gammadelta T-cell function and granzyme B gene polymorphism in a cohort of newly diagnosed breast cancer patients. Exp Hematol 37(7):838–848

Germain RN (1994) MHC-dependent antigen processing and peptide presentation: providing ligands for T lymphocyte activation. Cell 76(2):287–299

Germain RN, Margulies DH (1993) The biochemistry and cell biology of antigen processing and presentation. Annu Rev Immunol 11:403–450

Girardi M, Oppenheim DE et al (2001) Regulation of cutaneous malignancy by gammadelta T cells. Science 294(5542):605–609

Glatzel A, Wesch D et al (2002) Patterns of chemokine receptor expression on peripheral blood gamma delta T lymphocytes: strong expression of CCR5 is a selective feature of V delta 2/V gamma 9 gamma delta T cells. J Immunol 168(10):4920–4929

Gleimer M, Parham P (2003) Stress management: MHC class I and class I-like molecules as reporters of cellular stress. Immunity 19(4):469–477

Gober HJ, Kistowska M et al (2003) Human T cell receptor gammadelta cells recognize endogenous mevalonate metabolites in tumor cells. J Exp Med 197(2):163–168

Godder KT, Henslee-Downey PJ et al (2007) Long term disease-free survival in acute leukemia patients recovering with increased gammadelta T cells after partially mismatched related donor bone marrow transplantation. Bone Marrow Transplant 39(12):751–757

Groh V, Rhinehart R et al (1999) Broad tumor-associated expression and recognition by tumor-derived gamma delta T cells of MICA and MICB. Proc Natl Acad Sci USA 96(12):6879–6884

Groh V, Steinle A et al (1998) Recognition of stress-induced MHC molecules by intestinal epithelial gammadelta T cells. Science 279(5357):1737–1740

Groh V, Wu J et al (2002) Tumour-derived soluble MIC ligands impair expression of NKG2D and T-cell activation. Nature 419(6908):734–738

Guglielmi C, Arcese W et al (2002) Donor lymphocyte infusion for relapsed chronic myelogenous leukemia: prognostic relevance of the initial cell dose. Blood 100(2):397–405

Guo B, Hollmig K et al (2001) In vitro activity of apoptosis-resistant human gd-T cells against solid malignances. Journal of Clinical Oncology 20:267 (abstract)

Guo B, Hollmig K et al (2002) Down-regulation of IL-2 receptor a (CD25) characterizes human gd-T cells rendered resistant to apoptosis after CD2 engagement in the presence of IL-12. Cancer Immunol Immunother 50:625–637

Guo RT, Cao R et al (2007) Bisphosphonates target multiple sites in both cis- and trans-prenyltransferases. Proc Natl Acad Sci USA 104(24):10022–10027

Guy-Grand D, Cerf-Bensussan N et al (1991) Two gut intraepithelial CD8+ lymphocyte populations with different T cell receptors: a role for the gut epithelium in T cell differentiation. J Exp Med 173(2):471–481

Haas W, Pereira P et al (1993) Gamma/delta T cells. Annu Rev Immunol 11:637–686

Hacker G, Kromer S et al (1992) V delta 1+ subset of human gamma delta T cells responds to ligands expressed by EBV-infected Burkitt lymphoma cells and transformed B lymphocytes. J Immunol 149(12):3984–3989

Halary F, Pitard V et al (2005) Shared reactivity of V{delta}2(neg) {gamma}{delta} T cells against cytomegalovirus-infected cells and tumor intestinal epithelial cells. J Exp Med 201(10): 1567–1578

Hayday A, Tigelaar R (2003) Immunoregulation in the tissues by gammadelta T cells. Nat Rev Immunol 3(3):233–242

Hayday AC (2000) [gamma][delta] cells: a right time and a right place for a conserved third way of protection. Annu Rev Immunol 18:975–1026

Henslee PJ, Thompson JS et al (1987) T cell depletion of HLA and haploidentical marrow reduces graft-versus-host disease but it may impair a graft-versus-leukemia effect. Transplant Proc 19(1 Pt 3):2701–2706

Inge TH, McCoy KM et al (1992) Immunomodulatory effects of transforming growth factor-beta on T lymphocytes. Induction of CD8 expression in the CTLL-2 cell line and in normal thymocytes. J Immunol 148(12):3847–3856

Ismaili J, Olislagers V et al (2002) Human gamma delta T cells induce dendritic cell maturation. Clin Immunol 103(3 Pt 1):296–302

Jachimczak P, Bogdahn U et al (1993) The effect of transforming growth factor-beta 2-specific phosphorothioate-anti-sense oligodeoxynucleotides in reversing cellular immunosuppression in malignant glioma. J Neurosurg 78(6):944–951

Janssen O, Wesselborg S et al (1991) T cell receptor/CD3-signaling induces death by apoptosis in human T cell receptor gamma delta+T cells. J Immunol 146(1):35–39

Kabelitz D, Wesch D et al (2007) Perspectives of gammadelta T cells in tumor immunology. Cancer Res 67(1):5–8

Kabelitz D, Wesch D et al (2004) Characterization of tumor reactivity of human V gamma 9V delta 2 gamma delta T cells in vitro and in SCID mice in vivo. J Immunol 173(11):6767–6776

Kang N, Tang L et al (2009) Identification and characterization of Foxp3(+) gammadelta T cells in mouse and human. Immunol Lett 125(2):105–113

Kato Y, Tanaka Y et al (2001) Targeting of tumor cells for human gammadelta T cells by nonpeptide antigens. J Immunol 167(9):5092–5098

Kawakami Y, Robbins PF et al (1998) Identification of new melanoma epitopes on melanosomal proteins recognized by tumor infiltrating T lymphocytes restricted by HLA-A1, -A2, and -A3 alleles. J Immunol 161(12):6985–6992

Kawanishi Y, Passweg J et al (1997) Effect of T cell subset dose on outcome of T cell-depleted bone marrow transplantation. Bone Marrow Transplant 19(11):1069–1077

Keever-Taylor CA, Craig A et al (2001) Complement-mediated T-cell depletion of bone marrow: comparison of T10B9.1A-31 and Muromonab-Orthoclone OKT3. Cytotherapy 3(6):467–481

Kim CJ, Parkinson DR et al (1998) Immunodominance across HLA polymorphism: implications for cancer immunotherapy. J Immunother 21(1):1–16

Kobayashi H, Tanaka Y et al (2007) Safety profile and anti-tumor effects of adoptive immunotherapy using gamma-delta T cells against advanced renal cell carcinoma: a pilot study. Cancer Immunol Immunother 56(4):469–476

Kolb HJ, Holler E (1997) Adoptive immunotherapy with donor lymphocyte transfusions. Curr Opin Oncol 9(2):139–145

Kondo M, Sakuta K et al (2008) Zoledronate facilitates large-scale ex vivo expansion of functional gammadelta T cells from cancer patients for use in adoptive immunotherapy. Cytotherapy 10(8):842–856

Kong Y, Cao W et al (2009) The NKG2D ligand ULBP4 binds to TCRgamma9/delta2 and induces cytotoxicity to tumor cells through both TCRgammadelta and NKG2D. Blood 114(2):310–317

Kunzmann V, Bauer E et al (2000) Stimulation of gammadelta T cells by aminobisphosphonates and induction of antiplasma cell activity in multiple myeloma. Blood 96(2):384–392

Kunzmann V, Kimmel B et al (2009) Inhibition of phosphoantigen-mediated gammadelta T-cell proliferation by CD4+ CD25+ FoxP3+ regulatory T cells. Immunology 126(2):256–267

Laad AD, Thomas ML et al (1999) Human gamma delta T cells recognize heat shock protein-60 on oral tumor cells. Int J Cancer 80(5):709–714

Lamb LS Jr, Gee AP, Hazlett LJ, Musk P et al (1999) Influence of T cell depletion method on circulating gd+ T cell reconstitution and potential role in the graft-versus-leukemia effect. Cytotherapy 1:7–19

Lamb LS Jr, Henslee-Downey PJ et al (1996) Increased frequency of TCR gamma delta+ T cells in disease-free survivors following T cell-depleted, partially mismatched, related donor bone marrow transplantation for leukemia. J Hematother 5(5):503–509

Lamb LS Jr, Musk P et al (2001) Human gammadelta(+) T lymphocytes have in vitro graft vs leukemia activity in the absence of an allogeneic response. Bone Marrow Transplant 27(6):601–606

Lau SK, Chen YY et al (2005) Lack of association of cytomegalovirus with human brain tumors. Mod Pathol 18(6):838–843

Lefrancois L, Puddington L (1995) Extrathymic intestinal T-cell development: virtual reality? Immunol Today 16(1):16–21

Leslie DS, Vincent MS et al (2002) CD1-mediated gamma/delta T cell maturation of dendritic cells. J Exp Med 196(12):1575–1584

Li J, Herold MJ et al (2009) Reduced expression of the mevalonate pathway enzyme farnesyl pyrophosphate synthase unveils recognition of tumor cells by Vgamma9Vdelta2 T cells. J Immunol 182(12):8118–8124

Liu Z, Eltoum IE et al (2008) Protective immunosurveillance and therapeutic antitumor activity of gammadelta T cells demonstrated in a mouse model of prostate cancer. J Immunol 180(9):6044–6053

Lopez RD, Xu S et al (2000) CD2-mediated IL-12-dependent signals render human gamma-delta T cells resistant to mitogen-induced apoptosis, permitting the large-scale ex vivo expansion of functionally distinct lymphocytes: implications for the development of adoptive immunotherapy strategies. Blood 96(12):3827–3837

Maeurer M, Zitvogel L et al (1995) Human intestinal V delta 1+ T cells obtained from patients with colon cancer respond exclusively to SEB but not to SEA. Nat Immun 14(4):188–197

Maeurer MJ, Martin D et al (1996) Human intestinal Vdelta1+ lymphocytes recognize tumor cells of epithelial origin. J Exp Med 183(4):1681–1696

Martinet L, Fleury-Cappellesso S et al (2009a) A regulatory cross-talk between Vgamma9Vdelta2 T lymphocytes and mesenchymal stem cells. Eur J Immunol 39(3):752–762

Martinet L, Poupot R et al (2009b) Pitfalls on the roadmap to gammadelta T cell-based cancer immunotherapies. Immunol Lett 124(1):1–8

Mateo L, Gardner J et al (1999) An HLA-A2 polyepitope vaccine for melanoma immunotherapy. J Immunol 163(7):4058–4063

Meeh PF, King M et al (2006) Characterization of the gammadelta T cell response to acute leukemia. Cancer Immunol Immunother 55(9):1072–1080

Miller JS, Soignier Y et al (2005) Successful adoptive transfer and in vivo expansion of human haploidentical NK cells in patients with cancer. Blood 105(8):3051–3057

Mitchell DA, Xie W et al (2008) Sensitive detection of human cytomegalovirus in tumors and peripheral blood of patients diagnosed with glioblastoma. Neuro Oncol 10(1):10–18

Miyagawa F, Tanaka Y et al (2001) Essential contribution of germline-encoded lysine residues in Jgamma1.2 segment to the recognition of nonpeptide antigens by human gammadelta T cells. J Immunol 167(12):6773–6779

Montero A, Savani BN et al (2006) T cell depleted peripheral blood stem cell allotransplantation with T cell add back for patients with hematological malignancies: effect of chronic GVHD on outcome. Biol Blood Marrow Transplant 12(12):1318–1325

Morita CT, Beckman EM et al (1995) Direct presentation of nonpeptide prenyl pyrophosphate antigens to human gamma delta T cells. Immunity 3(4):495–507

Nitahara A, Shimura H et al (2006) NKG2D ligation without T cell receptor engagement triggers both cytotoxicity and cytokine production in dendritic epidermal T cells. J Invest Dermatol 126(5):1052–1058

O'Brien RL, Roark CL et al (2007) gammadelta T-cell receptors: functional correlations. Immunol Rev 215:77–88

Parker CM, Groh V et al (1990) Evidence for extrathymic changes in the T cell receptor gamma/delta repertoire. J Exp Med 171(5):1597–1612

Peng G, Wang HY et al (2007) Tumor-infiltrating gammadelta T cells suppress T and dendritic cell function via mechanisms controlled by a unique toll-like receptor signaling pathway. Immunity 27(2):334–348

Pennington DJ, Vermijlen D et al (2005) The integration of conventional and unconventional T cells that characterizes cell-mediated responses. Adv Immunol 87:27–59

Pitard V, Roumanes D et al (2008) Long-term expansion of effector/memory Vdelta2-gammadelta T cells is a specific blood signature of CMV infection. Blood 112(4):1317–1324

Poggi A, Carosio R et al (2004a) Migration of V delta 1 and V delta 2 T cells in response to CXCR3 and CXCR4 ligands in healthy donors and HIV-1-infected patients: competition by HIV-1 Tat. Blood 103(6):2205–2213

Poggi A, Catellani S et al (2007) Adhesion molecules and kinases involved in gammadelta T cells migratory pathways: Implications for viral and autoimmune diseases. Curr Med Chem 14(30):3166–3170

Poggi A, Venturino C et al (2004b) Vdelta1 T lymphocytes from B-CLL patients recognize ULBP3 expressed on leukemic B cells and up-regulated by trans-retinoic acid. Cancer Res 64(24): 9172–9179

Prinz I, Sansoni A et al (2006) Visualization of the earliest steps of gammadelta T cell development in the adult thymus. Nat Immunol 7(9):995–1003

Raulet DH (2003) Roles of the NKG2D immunoreceptor and its ligands. Nat Rev Immunol 3(10):781–790

Rincon-Orozco B, Kunzmann V et al (2005) Activation of V gamma 9V delta 2 T cells by NKG2D. J Immunol 175(4):2144–2151

Salot S, Laplace C et al (2007) Large scale expansion of gamma 9 delta 2 T lymphocytes: Innacell gamma delta cell therapy product. J Immunol Methods 326(1–2):63–75

Scheurer ME, Bondy ML et al (2008) Detection of human cytomegalovirus in different histological types of gliomas. Acta Neuropathol 116(1):79–86

Schilbach K, Frommer K et al (2008) Immune response of human propagated gammadelta-T-cells to neuroblastoma recommend the Vdelta1+ subset for gammadelta-T-cell-based immunotherapy. J Immunother 31(9):896–905

Schilbach KE, Geiselhart A et al (2000) Human gammadelta T lymphocytes exert natural and IL-2-induced cytotoxicity to neuroblastoma cells. J Immunother 23(5):536–548

Smyth MJ, Strobl SL et al (1991) Regulation of lymphokine-activated killer activity and pore-forming protein gene expression in human peripheral blood CD8+ T lymphocytes. Inhibition by transforming growth factor-beta. J Immunol 146(10):3289–3297

Spada FM, Grant EP et al (2000) Self-recognition of CD1 by gamma/delta T cells: implications for innate immunity. J Exp Med 191(6):937–948

Suzuki Y, Fujimiya Y et al (1999) Enhancing effect of tumor necrosis factor (TNF)-alpha, but not IFN-gamma, on the tumor-specific cytotoxicity of gammadeltaT cells from glioblastoma patients. Cancer Lett 140(1–2):161–167

Taghon T, Rothenberg EV (2008) Molecular mechanisms that control mouse and human TCR-alphabeta and TCR-gammadelta T cell development. Semin Immunopathol 30(4):383–398

Tanaka Y, Morita CT et al (1995) Natural and synthetic non-peptide antigens recognized by human gamma delta T cells. Nature 375(6527):155–158

Tanaka Y, Sano S et al (1994) Nonpeptide ligands for human gamma delta T cells. Proc Natl Acad Sci USA 91(17):8175–8179

Whang MI, Guerra N et al (2009) Costimulation of dendritic epidermal gammadelta T cells by a new NKG2D ligand expressed specifically in the skin. J Immunol 182(8):4557–4564

Wilhelm M, Kunzmann V et al (2003) Gammadelta T cells for immune therapy of patients with lymphoid malignancies. Blood 102(1):200–206

Wilson A, Capone M et al (1999) Unexpectedly late expression of intracellular CD3epsilon and TCR gammadelta proteins during adult thymus development. Int Immunol 11(10):1641–1650

Wright A, Lee JE et al (1989) Cytotoxic T lymphocytes specific for self tumor immunoglobulin express T cell receptor delta chain. J Exp Med 169(5):1557–1564

Wrobel P, Shojaei H et al (2007) Lysis of a broad range of epithelial tumour cells by human gamma delta T cells: involvement of NKG2D ligands and T-cell receptor- versus NKG2D-dependent recognition. Scand J Immunol 66(2–3):320–328

Wu J, Groh V et al (2002) T cell antigen receptor engagement and specificity in the recognition of stress-inducible MHC class I-related chains by human epithelial gamma delta T cells. J Immunol 169(3):1236–1240

Xiong N, Raulet DH (2007) Development and selection of gammadelta T cells. Immunol Rev 215:15–31

Xu C, Zhang H et al (2007) Gammadelta T cells recognize tumor cells via CDR3delta region. Mol Immunol 44(4):302–310

Yannelli JR, Hyatt C et al (1996) Growth of tumor-infiltrating lymphocytes from human solid cancers: summary of a 5-year experience. Int J Cancer 65(4):413–421

Zhao J, Huang J et al (2006) Vdelta1 T cell receptor binds specifically to MHC I chain related A: molecular and biochemical evidences. Biochem Biophys Res Commun 339(1):232–240

Zhao X, Wei YQ et al (1995) Accumulation of gamma/delta T cells in human dysgerminoma and seminoma: roles in autologous tumor killing and granuloma formation. Immunol Invest 24(4):607 618

Zocchi MR, Poggi A (2004) Role of gammadelta T lymphocytes in tumor defense. Front Biosci 9:2588–2604

Chapter 4
Toll-Like Receptors and Their Regulatory Mechanisms

Shin-Ichiroh Saitoh

1 Toll-Like Receptors and Their Signaling Molecules

Infectious diseases are threats to living organisms. Therefore Recognizing invading bacteria and viruses is important to protect us from them. There are sensors in our cells to detect the infection by virus or microbes. Toll-like receptors (TLRs) are one of the sensors to recognize conserved microbial molecules specific for virus and microbes (Janeway and Medzhitov 2002; Takeda et al. 2003). Twelve TLRs have been identified in mammals. TLRs are a conserved membrane-spanning receptor including leucine-rich repeat (LRR) in an extacelluar domain, a transmembrane region, and Toll/IL-1 receptor (TIR) domain in a cytoplasmic domain (Takeda et al. 2003). The LRR binds to pathogen-associated molecular patterns (PAMPs) as foreign ligands. Certain members of the TLR family, including TLR1, TLR2, TLR4, TLR5, and TLR6, sense the protein flagellin (Hayashi et al. 2001) or lipid components (Aliprantis et al. 1999; Medzhitov et al. 1997; Poltorak et al. 1998; Schwandner et al. 1999; Takeuchi et al. 1999) of bacteria and fungi, and are found on the plasma membrane (Fig. 4.1). By contrast, TLR3, TLR7, TLR8, and TLR9, which detect double-stranded RNA (dsRNA) (Alexopoulou et al. 2001), single-stranded RNA (ssRNA) (Heil et al. 2004; Lund et al. 2004a), and un-methylated CpG DNA (Hemmi et al. 2000) respectively, mainly reside in intracellular organelles such as the endoplasmic reticulum (ER), endosomes, and lysosomes (Fig. 4.1).

After their ligands binding, TLRs dimerize and change their conformation (Jin et al. 2007; Kim et al. 2007; Latz et al. 2007; Park et al. 2009). This is followed by recruitment of TIR domain-containing adaptor proteins to TLRs (Fig. 4.1). TIR domain can be found in the cytoplasmic portions of all TLRs. The adaptor proteins with TIR domains have been identified, including myeloid differentiation

---

S.-I. Saitoh (✉)
Division of Infectious Genetics, The Institute of Medical Science, The University of Tokyo, Shirokanedai, Tokyo 108-8639, Japan
e-mail: shinss@ims.u-tokyo.ac.jp

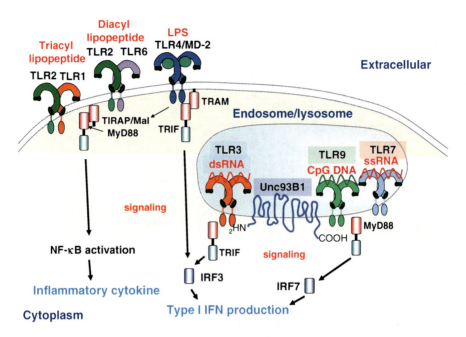

Fig. 4.1 TLR ligands and signaling. Toll-like receptors (TLRs) recognize bacterial and viral components. TLR ligands induce TLRs homodimer or heterodimer to trigger the activation of signaling molecules. Bacterial lipopeptides, Triacyl lipopeptide, and Diacyl lipopeptide are recognized by TLR1 and TLR2 (TLR1/TLR2) and TLR2 and TLR6 (TLR2/TLR6) to induce a heterodimer. TLR4/MD-2 recognizes LPS to form a homodimer. TLR3, TLR7, and TLR9 localize in intracellular compartment and recognize pathogen-derived nucleotides like double-strand RNA, single-strand RNA, and CpG-containing DNA, respectively. TLR1/TLR2, TLR2/TLR6, and TLR4/MD-2 activate MyD88 pathway through TIRAP, which is a membrane-association molecule, to induce inflammatory cytokines. In addition, TLR4/MD-2 activates TRAM and TRIF to induce type I interferon through activating IRF3. TLR3 directly bind TRIF to induce type I interferon and inflammatory cytokines. TLR7 and TLR9 activate MyD88 pathway to induce type I interferon and inflammatory cytokines

factor 88 (MyD88), TIR-domain-containing adaptor protein (TIRAP)/MyD88 adaptor-like (Mal), TIR-domain-containing adaptor inducing interferon-β (TRIF)/TICAM-1, and TRIF-related adaptor molecule (TRAM)/TICAM-2 (Fig. 4.1). These TIR containing adaptor molecules are associated with the TIR domain of TLRs (Akira and Takeda 2004). For example, MyD88 and TRAM are recruited to TLR4 and the TIR domain of the adaptor proteins associates with the TIR domain of TLR4. The activation of TLRs leads to the activation of these adaptor molecules and specificity in TLR signaling. TLR3 activates only TRIF, while other TLRs activate MyD88. TLR4 activates the four TIR-domain-containing adaptors, and TLR2 uses both MyD88 and TIRAP/Mal. TIRAP/Mal contains a phosphatidylinositol 4, 5-bisphosphate (PIP2) binding domain that targets this adaptor to a special region on membrane for signaling where it recruits MyD88 (Kagan and Medzhitov 2006). There are MyD88-dependent and MyD88-independent pathways in TLR signaling (Akira and Takeda 2004). MyD88 is activated on the plasma membrane, where it associates with tumor-necrosis factor (TNF)-receptor-associated factor 6 (TRAF6), interleukin 1 receptor-associated kinase-1 (IRAK-1), and IRAK-4 (Akira and Takeda 2004). MyD88 activation leads to the activation of nuclear factor-κB (NF-κB) to produce inflammatory cytokines. On the other hand, the MyD88-independent pathway leads to the activation of TRAM and TRIF to produce type I interferon (IFN) via the activation of TRAF3 and IFN-regulatory factor-3 (IRF3) (Akira and Takeda 2004; Häcker et al. 2006). Myristoylation of TRAM is important for its function, because a point mutation that leads to loss of myristoylation of TRAM results in failure of TRAM activation by LPS stimulation. (Rowe et al. 2006). These adaptor molecules activate multiple signaling pathways such as NF-κB, mitogen-activated protein kinases (MAPKs), and IRFs to induce the expression of inflammatory cytokines, co-stimulatory molecules, and type I IFN.

2 Activation Mechanism of TLRs

The heterodimer consisting of TLR1 and TLR2 recognizes triacyl lipopeptides, whereas the heterodimer consisting of TLR2 and TLR6 recognizes diacyl lipopeptides. TLR4 recognizes lipopolysaccharide (LPS) on the cell surface (Fig. 4.1). Unlike TLR1, TLR2, and TLR6, the extracellular domain of TLR4 is not satisfactory for LPS recognition because HEK293 cells transfected with TLR4 remain unresponsive. MD-2 is one of the key molecules for the LPS receptor (Shimazu et al. 1999), and MD-2 acts as an extracellular molecule that is associated with the extracellular domain of TLR4. MD-2-deficient mice are similar in phenotype to TLR4-deficient mice, demonstrating that MD-2 is an essential molecule for LPS recognition (Nagai et al. 2002). In particular, MD-2 plays an important role in interaction with LPS and subsequent TLR4 dimerization (Park et al. 2009). MD-2 alone was shown to directly bind to LPS, whereas TLR4 alone did not. MD-2 is the ligand-binding component of the TLR4/MD-2 receptor complex (Kim et al. 2007). LPS binding to TLR4/MD-2 induces TLR4 dimerization, which activates downstream signaling pathway. However, LPS antagonists are able to bind to TLR4/MD-2, but unable to induce TLR4 dimerization (Kim et al. 2007; Saitoh et al. 2004).

3 Immune Function of Nucleotide-Sensing TLRs

TLR3, TLR7, TLR8, and TLR9 are nucleotide-sensing receptors which are located in intracellular compartment. TLR7 and TLR8 recognize ssRNA in human cells. Both TLR7 and TLR9 are mainly expressed in plasmacytoid dendritic cells (pDC) and B cells. TLR7 recognizes guanosine- and uridine-rich single-stranded RNA (ssRNA) in order to detect ssRNA viruses, such as influenza virus and vesicular stomatitis virus (VSV) (Diebold et al. 2004; Heil et al. 2004; Lund et al. 2004b). TLR7 also responds to synthetic imidazoquinoline compounds such as imiquimod and R-848. TLR9 recognizes single-stranded DNA (ssDNA) including unmethylated

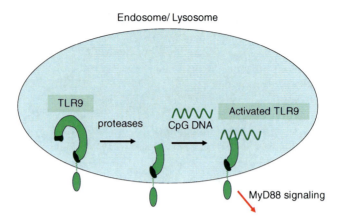

Fig. 4.2 TLR9 cleavage by proteases is required for its ligand recognition. TLR9 is cleaved by cathepsin-like proteases in endosome or lysosome. This cleavage makes TLR9 a functional form to recognize CpG DNA

CpG enabling detection of bacterial and viral DNA (Hemmi et al. 2000). For example, TLR9 senses ssDNA viruses, such as herpes simplex virus1 (HSV1), HSV2, and murine cytomegalovirus (Krug et al. 2004a, b; Lund et al. 2003). TLR3 senses double-stranded RNA (dsRNA) in the intracellular compartment. TLR3 is preferentially expressed in myeloid DCs, intestinal epithelial cells, and fibroblasts. TLR3 seems to play a role in sensing dsRNA virus and dsDNA viruses with dsRNA intermediates. Furthermore, some studies using TLR3-deficient mice have indicated that TLR3 is also capable of sensing ssRNA viruses. It was reported that TLR3 plays an essential role for defense against mouse cytomegalovirus (MCMV, dsDNA virus) (Tabeta et al. 2004). In addition, TLR3 plays a partial role in sensing encephalomyocarditis virus (EMCV), respiratory syncytial virus (RSV), influenza A virus (IAV), and West Nile virus, which are ssRNA viruses. The crystal structure analyses of the human TLR3 ectodomain have revealed that this domain takes the form of a large horseshoe-shaped solenoid, which potentially provides a large surface area for ligand interaction. The ectodomain of TLR3 is also essential for TLR3 homodimerization in order to activate signaling molecules. It was proposed that dsRNA induces a symmetrical dimerization of TLR3.

Synthetic unmethylated CpG directly binds the ectodomain of TLR9 and induces conformational changes to activate signaling. TLR7/TLR8 and TLR9 sense nucleic acids in endolysosomes. In the endolysosomes, the cleavage of TLR9 by proteases such as cathepsins is required for TLR9 activation (Fig. 4.2) (Asagiri et al. 2008; Ewald et al. 2008; Matsumoto et al. 2008; Park et al. 2008; Sepulveda et al. 2009). Signaling via TLR7/8 or TLR9 is dependent on MyD88. TLR7 and TLR9 activation induces the expression of costimulatory molecules, T-helper type 1 (Th1) or Th1-promoting cytokines and chemokine such as type I IFNs, IFN-γ, IFN-inducible protein-10 (IP-10), interleukin-12 (IL-12), and IL-6, but lacks robust induction of Th2 cytokines.

4 Regulatory Mechanism by a Master Chaperone of TLRs, Heat Shock Protein gp96

Gp96, is a 96-kDa glycoprotein, and a ER resident member of HSP90 that is also designated as Grp94 (glucose-regulated protein 94) family. It has 50% homology to its cytosolic counterpart HSP90. Gp96 is the most abundant glycoprotein in the ER. Gp96 is uniformly distributed in the ER lumen and does not associate with the ER membrane. Gp96 is constitutively expressed in virtually all cell types. Its expression is upregulated by interferon and a variety of stress conditions.

In contrast to hundreds of client proteins known for its cytosolic counterpart HSP90, the number of gp96-binding proteins identified so far is very limited. Some of the binding proteins were Ig chains, MHC class II, and integrins, which are critical players in immunity.

The first direct evidence showing gp96 is required for cell surface TLR folding was reported in 2001 (Randow and Seed 2001). A mutant B cell line was generated that is not responsive to LPS stimulation by mutagenesis. This cell line is also not responsive to TLR2 ligands. The mutation corresponding to this phenotype is located in the gp96 locus, resulting in coding of truncated gp96 proteins. In addition, the expression of wild-type gp96 is able to rescue the loss of cell surface TLR1, TLR2, and TLR4 in this mutant cell line (Randow and Seed 2001). In the case of conditional deficiency of gp96 in macrophages, gp96-deficient macrophages developed normally and could be activated through the classic pathway with interferon-γ (IFN-γ) and tumor necrosis factor-α (TNF-α) as well as with interleukin-1β (IL-1β), which is the MyD88-dependent pathway. However, these macrophages failed to produce proinflammatory cytokines in response to agonists of cell surface TLRs, including TLR2–TLR1, TLR4, and TLR5 and intracellular TLRs, TLR7, and TLR9. TLR9 was still expressed in these macrophages (Yang et al. 2007) and biochemical experiment shows that TLR9 associates with gp96 in HEK293 cells. These results indicate that the defects in TLR9 signaling were not due to a lack of TLR9 expression at the transcriptional and translational level, but due to posttranslational folding of TLR9 by gp96 to be functional receptor.

5 Regulatory Mechanism of an ER Resident Molecule, A Protein Associated with Toll-Like Receptor 4, on TLRs Trafficking

The cell surface expression of TLR4 was reported to be regulated by a protein associated with Toll-like receptor 4 (PRAT4A) (Wakabayashi et al. 2006). PRAT4A is about 40 kDa protein and resides in the ER. In PRAT4A-deficient DCs, cell surface TLR4/MD-2 is downregulated and cell surface TLR2 is partially downregulated; however, the expression of cell surface markers such as CD11c, CD14, and MHC class I antigen is normal. PRAT4A specifically regulates the cell surface expression of TLRs (Wakabayashi et al. 2006). When these DCs were stimulated with a variety of TLR ligands, a partial, but substantial, reduction was observed not only in response to a TLR4/MD-2 ligand but also to a TLR1/TLR2 ligand, a TLR2/TLR6 ligand, and a TLR9 ligand. By contrast, responses to TLR3 ligand (poly (I:C)) were not altered in PRAT4A-deficient DCs.

TLR9-dependent responses were completely abolished in bone marrow-derived DCs (BM-DCs) and bone marrow-derived macrophage (BM-macrophages) from mice lacking PRAT4A (Takahashi et al. 2007). Further analyses using PRAT4A knockdown cells showed that TLR9 resides in the ER in resting PRAT4A knockdown cells, but is unable to traffic from the ER to endolysosomes upon ligand stimulation (Takahashi et al. 2007). However, the TLR9 ligand CpG internalizes from the cell surface to endolysosomes normally in PRAT4A knockdown cells. In addition, biochemical experiments showed that PRAT4A is associated with TLR9. These results indicate that PRAT4A regulates the subcellular distribution of TLR9 like a chaperone. As a result, TLR9 responses and signaling are completely abolished in PRAT4A-deficient cells. The mechanisms by which PRAT4A regulates TLR9 trafficking remains to be resolved.

6 UNC93B1 Delivers TLR7 and TLR9 to Endolysosomes

Recently, mutant mice named "triple D" (3d) were generated which are defective in TLR3, TLR7, and TLR9 signaling (Tabeta et al. 2006). The mutation was identified as a single histidine-to-arginine substitution (H412R) in the polytopic membrane protein UNC93B1 (Tabeta et al. 2006). Unc93B1 is a 598 amino acid protein with 12 transmembrane domains that localizes in the ER. UNC93B1 has two putative N-linked glycosylation sites (NXS/T), N251HT and N272KT, and it is glycosylated. The mutation in UNC93B1 clearly caused the defective responses to TLR3, TLR7 and TLR9 ligands. Transfection of wild-type UNC93B1 into BM-DCs from 3d mice corrected the defect.

3d mice are highly susceptible to infection with cytomegalovirus, *Listeria monocytogenes*, and *Staphylococcus aureus* (Tabeta et al. 2006). Notably, the histidine residue affected in the UNC93B1 mutation is invariant for all vertebrate orthologues. In human, homozygous germline mutations in UNC93B1 were reported in 2006, in two unrelated patients (Casrouge et al. 2006). The UNC93B1 deficiency has also been linked to the etiology of herpes simplex virus-1 encephalitis in these human patients (Casrouge et al. 2006). Similar to what was observed in 3d mice, cells from patients with functional null mutations in UNC93B1 show impaired cytokine production upon stimulation of TLR-3, TLR8 and TLR9 without compromising other TLRs.

Recently, biochemical analysis showed that UNC93B1 specifically binds to TLR3, 7, and 9 via the transmembrane domains of the TLRs (Brinkmann et al. 2007). The point mutation of H412R of UNC93B1 in 3d mice abolishes these interactions. The result indicates that the physical interactions between UNC93B1 and TLRs control proper TLR signaling. Finally, it was reported that the function of

UNC93B1 is to deliver the nucleotide sensing receptors TLR7 and TLR9 from the ER to endolysosomes (Kim et al. 2008). In addition, the N-terminal region of Unc93b1 regulates translocation of TLR7 and TLR9 (Fukui et al. 2009). LPS stimulation also causes the translocation of TLR7 and TLR9 from the ER to endolysosomes. Specific signaling pathways might be needed for causing the translocation of TLR7 and TLR9. The detailed mechanism of delivering TLR7 and TLR9 with UNC93B1 remains to be resolved.

7 Negative Regulatory Molecules of TLR Signaling

TLR activation leads to the induction of immune and inflammatory responses. However, excessive activation of the TLR signaling contributes to pathogenesis of autoimmune and chronic inflammatory diseases. TLRs activation is a double-edged sword. TLR signaling therefore must be negatively regulated to maintain immune balance. From the reason, there are a lot of negative regulatory molecules regulating TLR signaling at the multiple steps.

TLR4 exists on the cell surface and recognizes LPS. After LPS recognition, TLR4 internalizes to endosomes and lysosomes (Husebye et al. 2006). Internalization of TLR4 is one of negative regulatory mechanisms to turn off receptor activation. Internalization of TLR4 leads to the activation of TRAM/TRIF signaling pathway in endosomes (Kagan et al. 2008) and also receptor degradation in lysosomes (Husebye et al. 2006). In general, degradation or destabilization of receptor and signaling molecules is one of the principal mechanisms that terminates the activation of signaling pathways. Late endosome/lysosome-associated small Rab GTPase Rab7b, which is expressed selectively in monocytes and dendritic cells, was reported to regulate the translocation of TLR4 into lysosomes for degradation. Silencing of Rab7b expression in macrophages by knockdown potentiates the LPS induced signaling pathway and inflammatory cytokine expression (Wang et al. 2007). TLR is also modified by ubiquitin molecules for degradation by proteosome. A ubiquitin-modifying enzyme triad domain-containing protein 3 (triad3A) interacts with the TIR domain of TLR3, TLR4, TLR5, and TLR9 but not with TLR2. Triad3A acts as an E3 ubiquitin-protein ligase and promotes ubiquitination and proteolitic degradation of these TLRs (Chuang and Ulevitch 2004).

Supressor of cytokine signaling (SOCS)-1 is a negative regulator of the JAK-STAT signaling pathway and TLR2 and TLR4 signaling pathway. TIRAP/Mal is required for MYD88-dependent signaling by TLR2 and TLR4. After TLR2 and TLR4 stimulation, TIRAP leads to activation of MyD88 pathway and TIRAP/Mal is phosphorylated by Bruton's tyrosine kinase (Btk). Phosphorylated TIRAP/Mal is recognized by the SH2 domain of SOCS-1. The association of SOCS-1 with TIRAP/Mal induces the polyubiquitination and proteosomal degradation of TIRAP/Mal (Mansell et al. 2006). Therefore, SOCS-1 is a negative regulator of the TLR2 and TLR4 signaling pathways. Macrophages from SOCS-1-deficient mice developed enhanced production of inflammatory cytokine in response to LPS.

Ubiquitination plays an important role not only in protein degradation of receptors and signaling molecules to attenuate signaling, but also in activation of signaling molecules. K-63-linked ubiquitin chains may induce protein–protein interaction and activation of downstream signaling. Similar to phosphorylation, ubiquitination is a reversible mechanism regulated by ubiquitin enzymes and de-ubiquitination enzymes. Several de-ubiquitination enzymes work as a negative regulators. A20, CYLD, and de-ubiquitinating enzyme A (DUBA) are de-ubiquitination enzymes (Sun 2008), which remove K63-linked polyubiquitin chains from TRAF6 or TRAF3, thereby terminating NF-κB and IRF3 activation.

There are negative regulatory molecules by competitive inhibition in TLR signaling. TLR signaling includes specific TIR domain-containing adaptor proteins such as MyD88, TIRAP, TRIF, and TRAM. Another TIR domain-containing molecule was found, named Armadillo motif-containing protein (SARM). SARM is a negative regulator of TRIF. SARM interacts with TRIF, and interaction is enhanced by LPS stimulation. The complex of SARM and TRIF inhibits TRIF signaling by preventing it from being involved in TIR interactions with TRAM or TLRs. Knockdown of endogenous SARM expression leads to enhanced TRIF-dependent type I interferon expression. IRF5 interacts with MyD88 and induces proinflammatory cytokines. IRF4 is a negative regulator of IRF5, which also interacts with MyD88 and competes with IRF5 for MyD88 interaction (Negishi et al. 2005). The TLR-dependent induction of proinflammatory cytokines is markedly enhanced in peritoneal macrophages from IRF4-deficient mice. A splicing variant of MyD88, MyD88s, has a negative regulatory function as a dominant-negative molecule. MyD88 is composed of three main domains: the N-terminal death domain, the intermediate domain, and the TIR domain. However, MyD88s lacks the intermediate domain. MyD88 strongly interacts with IRAK-4 via the intermediate domain, and this interaction is essential for the phosphorylation of IRAK-1. On that account, MyD88s is not able to interact with IRAK-4, resulting in inhibition of the phosphorylation of IRAK-1 and the subsequent signaling pathway (Burns et al. 2003).

References

Akira S, Takeda K (2004) Toll-like receptor signalling. Nat Rev Immunol 4:499–511
Alexopoulou L, Holt A, Medzhitov R, Flavell R (2001) Recognition of double-stranded RNA and activation of NF-kappaB by Toll-like receptor 3. Nature 413:732–738
Aliprantis A, Yang R, Mark M, Suggett S, Devaux B, Radolf J, Klimpel G, Godowski P, Zychlinsky A (1999) Cell activation and apoptosis by bacterial lipoproteins through toll-like receptor-2. Science 285:736–739
Asagiri M, Hirai T, Kunigami T, Kamano S, Gober H, Okamoto K, Nishikawa K, Latz E, Golenbock D, Aoki K et al (2008) Cathepsin K-dependent toll-like receptor 9 signaling revealed in experimental arthritis. Science 319:624–627
Brinkmann M, Spooner E, Hoebe K, Beutler B, Ploegh H, Kim Y (2007) The interaction between the ER membrane protein UNC93B and TLR3, 7, and 9 is crucial for TLR signaling. J Cell Biol 177:265–275

Burns K, Janssens S, Brissoni B, Olivos N, Beyaert R, Tschopp J (2003) Inhibition of interleukin 1 receptor/Toll-like receptor signaling through the alternatively spliced, short form of MyD88 is due to its failure to recruit IRAK-4. J Exp Med 197:263–268

Casrouge A, Zhang S, Eidenschenk C, Jouanguy E, Puel A, Yang K, Alcais A, Picard C, Mahfoufi N, Nicolas N et al (2006) Herpes simplex virus encephalitis in human UNC-93B deficiency. Science 314:308–312

Chuang T, Ulevitch R (2004) Triad3A, an E3 ubiquitin-protein ligase regulating Toll-like receptors. Nat Immunol 5:495–502

Diebold S, Kaisho T, Hemmi H, Akira S, Reis e Sousa C (2004) Innate antiviral responses by means of TLR7-mediated recognition of single-stranded RNA. Science 303:1529–1531

Ewald S, Lee B, Lau L, Wickliffe K, Shi G, Chapman H, Barton G (2008) The ectodomain of Toll-like receptor 9 is cleaved to generate a functional receptor. Nature 456:658–662

Fukui R, Saitoh S, Matsumoto F, Kozuka-Hata H, Oyama M, Tabeta K, Beutler B, Miyake K (2009) Unc93B1 biases Toll-like receptor responses to nucleic acid in dendritic cells toward DNA – but against RNA-sensing. J Exp Med 206:1339–1350

Häcker H, Redecke V, Blagoev B, Kratchmarova I, Hsu L, Wang G, Kamps M, Raz E, Wagner H, Häcker G et al (2006) Specificity in Toll-like receptor signalling through distinct effector functions of TRAF3 and TRAF6. Nature 439:204–207

Hayashi F, Smith K, Ozinsky A, Hawn T, Yi E, Goodlett D, Eng J, Akira S, Underhill D, Aderem A (2001) The innate immune response to bacterial flagellin is mediated by Toll-like receptor 5. Nature 410:1099–1103

Heil F, Hemmi H, Hochrein H, Ampenberger F, Kirschning C, Akira S, Lipford G, Wagner H, Bauer S (2004) Species-specific recognition of single-stranded RNA via toll-like receptor 7 and 8. Science 303:1526–1529

Hemmi H, Takeuchi O, Kawai T, Kaisho T, Sato S, Sanjo H, Matsumoto M, Hoshino K, Wagner H, Takeda K, Akira S (2000) A Toll-like receptor recognizes bacterial DNA. Nature 408:740–745

Husebye H, Halaas Ø, Stenmark H, Tunheim G, Sandanger Ø, Bogen B, Brech A, Latz E, Espevik T (2006) Endocytic pathways regulate Toll-like receptor 4 signaling and link innate and adaptive immunity. EMBO J 25:683–692

Janeway C, Medzhitov R (2002) Innate immune recognition. Annu Rev Immunol 20:197–216

Jin M, Kim S, Heo J, Lee M, Kim H, Paik S, Lee H, Lee J (2007) Crystal structure of the TLR1-TLR2 heterodimer induced by binding of a tri-acylated lipopeptide. Cell 130:1071–1082

Kagan J, Medzhitov R (2006) Phosphoinositide-mediated adaptor recruitment controls Toll-like receptor signaling. Cell 125:943–955

Kagan J, Su T, Horng T, Chow A, Akira S, Medzhitov R (2008) TRAM couples endocytosis of Toll-like receptor 4 to the induction of interferon-beta. Nat Immunol 9:361–368

Kim H, Park B, Kim J, Kim S, Lee J, Oh S, Enkhbayar P, Matsushima N, Lee H, Yoo O, Lee J (2007) Crystal structure of the TLR4-MD-2 complex with bound endotoxin antagonist Eritoran. Cell 130:906–917

Kim Y, Brinkmann M, Paquet M, Ploegh H (2008) UNC93B1 delivers nucleotide-sensing toll-like receptors to endolysosomes. Nature 452:234–238

Krug A, French A, Barchet W, Fischer J, Dzionek A, Pingel J, Orihuela M, Akira S, Yokoyama W, Colonna M (2004a) TLR9-dependent recognition of MCMV by IPC and DC generates coordinated cytokine responses that activate antiviral NK cell function. Immunity 21:107–119

Krug A, Luker G, Barchet W, Leib D, Akira S, Colonna M (2004b) Herpes simplex virus type 1 activates murine natural interferon-producing cells through toll-like receptor 9. Blood 103:1433–1437

Latz E, Verma A, Visintin A, Gong M, Sirois C, Klein D, Monks B, McKnight C, Lamphier M, Duprex W et al (2007) Ligand-induced conformational changes allosterically activate Toll-like receptor 9. Nat Immunol 8:772–779

Lund J, Sato A, Akira S, Medzhitov R, Iwasaki A (2003) Toll-like receptor 9-mediated recognition of Herpes simplex virus-2 by plasmacytoid dendritic cells. J Exp Med 198:513–520

Lund J, Alexopoulou L, Sato A, Karow M, Adams N, Gale N, Iwasaki A, Flavell R (2004a) Recognition of single-stranded RNA viruses by Toll-like receptor 7. Proc Natl Acad Sci U S A 101:5598–5603

Lund J, Alexopoulou L, Sato A, Karow M, Adams N, Gale N, Iwasaki A, Flavell R (2004b) Recognition of single-stranded RNA viruses by Toll-like receptor 7. Proc Natl Acad Sci USA 101:5598–5603

Mansell A, Smith R, Doyle S, Gray P, Fenner J, Crack P, Nicholson S, Hilton D, O'Neill L, Hertzog P (2006) Suppressor of cytokine signaling 1 negatively regulates Toll-like receptor signaling by mediating Mal degradation. Nat Immunol 7:148–155

Matsumoto F, Saitoh S, Fukui R, Kobayashi T, Tanimura N, Konno K, Kusumoto Y, Akashi-Takamura S, Miyake K (2008) Cathepsins are required for Toll-like receptor 9 responses. Biochem Biophys Res Commun 367:693–699

Medzhitov R, Preston-Hurlburt P, Janeway CJ (1997) A human homologue of the Drosophila Toll protein signals activation of adaptive immunity. Nature 388:394–397

Nagai Y, Akashi S, Nagafuku M, Ogata M, Iwakura Y, Akira S, Kitamura T, Kosugi A, Kimoto M, Miyake K (2002) Essential role of MD-2 in LPS responsiveness and TLR4 distribution. Nat Immunol 3:667–672

Negishi H, Ohba Y, Yanai H, Takaoka A, Honma K, Yui K, Matsuyama T, Taniguchi T, Honda K (2005) Negative regulation of Toll-like-receptor signaling by IRF-4. Proc Natl Acad Sci USA 102:15989–15994

Park B, Brinkmann M, Spooner E, Lee C, Kim Y, Ploegh H (2008) Proteolytic cleavage in an endolysosomal compartment is required for activation of Toll-like receptor 9. Nat Immunol 9:1407–1414

Park B, Song D, Kim H, Choi B, Lee H, Lee J (2009) The structural basis of lipopolysaccharide recognition by the TLR4-MD-2 complex. Nature 458:1191–1195

Poltorak A, He X, Smirnova I, Liu M, Van Huffel C, Du X, Birdwell D, Alejos E, Silva M, Galanos C et al (1998) Defective LPS signaling in C3H/HeJ and C57BL/10ScCr mice: mutations in Tlr4 gene. Science 282:2085–2088

Randow F, Seed B (2001) Endoplasmic reticulum chaperone gp96 is required for innate immunity but not cell viability. Nat Cell Biol 3:891–896

Rowe D, McGettrick A, Latz E, Monks B, Gay N, Yamamoto M, Akira S, O'Neill L, Fitzgerald K, Golenbock D (2006) The myristoylation of TRIF-related adaptor molecule is essential for Toll-like receptor 4 signal transduction. Proc Natl Acad Sci U S A 103:6299–6304

Saitoh S, Akashi S, Yamada T, Tanimura N, Kobayashi M, Konno K, Matsumoto F, Fukase K, Kusumoto S, Nagai Y et al (2004) Lipid A antagonist, lipid IVa, is distinct from lipid A in interaction with Toll-like receptor 4 (TLR4)-MD-2 and ligand-induced TLR4 oligomerization. Int Immunol 16:961–969

Schwandner R, Dziarski R, Wesche H, Rothe M, Kirschning C (1999) Peptidoglycan- and lipoteichoic acid-induced cell activation is mediated by toll-like receptor 2. J Biol Chem 274:17406–17409

Sepulveda F, Maschalidi S, Colisson R, Heslop L, Ghirelli C, Sakka E, Lennon-Duménil A, Amigorena S, Cabanie L, Manoury B (2009) Critical role for asparagine endopeptidase in endocytic Toll-like receptor signaling in dendritic cells. Immunity 31:737–748

Shimazu R, Akashi S, Ogata H, Nagai Y, Fukudome K, Miyake K, Kimoto M (1999) MD-2, a molecule that confers lipopolysaccharide responsiveness on Toll-like receptor 4. J Exp Med 189:1777–1782

Sun S (2008) Deubiquitylation and regulation of the immune response. Nat Rev Immunol 8:501–511

Tabeta K, Georgel P, Janssen E, Du X, Hoebe K, Crozat K, Mudd S, Shamel L, Sovath S, Goode J et al (2004) Toll-like receptors 9 and 3 as essential components of innate immune defense against mouse cytomegalovirus infection. Proc Natl Acad Sci U S A 101:3516–3521

Tabeta K, Hoebe K, Janssen E, Du X, Georgel P, Crozat K, Mudd S, Mann N, Sovath S, Goode J et al (2006) The Unc93b1 mutation 3d disrupts exogenous antigen presentation and signaling via Toll-like receptors 3, 7 and 9. Nat Immunol 7:156–164

Takahashi K, Shibata T, Akashi-Takamura S, Kiyokawa T, Wakabayashi Y, Tanimura N, Kobayashi T, Matsumoto F, Fukui R, Kouro T et al (2007) A protein associated with Toll-like receptor

(TLR) 4 (PRAT4A) is required for TLR-dependent immune responses. J Exp Med 204: 2963–2976

Takeda K, Kaisho T, Akira S (2003) Toll-like receptors. Annu Rev Immunol 21:335–376

Takeuchi O, Hoshino K, Kawai T, Sanjo H, Takada H, Ogawa T, Takeda K, Akira S (1999) Differential roles of TLR2 and TLR4 in recognition of gram-negative and gram-positive bacterial cell wall components. Immunity 443–451:443–451

Wakabayashi Y, Kobayashi M, Akashi-Takamura S, Tanimura N, Konno K, Takahashi K, Ishii T, Mizutani T, Iba H, Kouro T et al (2006) A protein associated with toll-like receptor 4 (PRAT4A) regulates cell surface expression of TLR4. J Immunol 177:1772–1779

Wang Y, Chen T, Han C, He D, Liu H, An H, Cai Z, Cao X (2007) Lysosome-associated small Rab GTPase Rab7b negatively regulates TLR4 signaling in macrophages by promoting lysosomal degradation of TLR4. Blood 110:962–971

Yang Y, Liu B, Dai J, Srivastava P, Zammit D, Lefrançois L, Li Z (2007) Heat shock protein gp96 is a master chaperone for toll-like receptors and is important in the innate function of macrophages. Immunity 26:215–226

Chapter 5
Cytoplasmic Sensing of Viral Double-Stranded RNA and Activation of Innate Immunity by RIG-I-Like Receptors

Mitsutoshi Yoneyama and Takashi Fujita

1 Structure of RLRs

Innate antiviral reactions are induced within hours of a viral infection. These reactions are critical to the activation of adaptive immunity. The major innate antiviral reaction is that mediated by type I and III interferons (IFNs), which activate antiviral genes through cell surface receptors, signal transducers, and transcription factors (Samuel. Clin Microbiol Rev 14:778–809, 2001; Theofilopoulos et al. Annu Rev Immunol 23:307–336, 2005; Uze and Monneron. Biochimie 89:729–734, 2007). Once the antiviral gene products establish an antiviral state, viral replication is selectively repressed. Efficient expression of IFN is observed in cells infected with viruses, suggesting that viral components produced during replication are detected by cellular sensors. A family of RNA helicases termed RIG-I-like receptors (RLRs), including retinoic acid-inducible gene-I (RIG-I), melanoma differentiation associated gene 5 (MDA5), and laboratory of genetics and physiology 2 (LGP2), sense viral double-stranded (ds) RNA and trigger an antiviral program including the production of IFN (Kawai and Akira. Ann N Y Acad Sci 1143:1–20, 2008; Yoneyama and Fujita. Immunol Rev 227:54–65, 2009). We review here the structure and function of RLRs

RIG-I and MDA5 contain tandem repeats of a domain similar to the caspase recruitment and activation domain (CARD) at their N-terminal, however LGP2 lacks these repeats (Fig. 5.1) (Yoneyama et al. 2004; Yoneyama et al. 2005). Forced

M. Yoneyama
Laboratory of Molecular Genetics, Institute for Virus Research, and Laboratory of Molecular Cell Biology, Graduate School of Biostudies, Kyoto University, Kyoto, Japan

PRESTO, Japan Science and Technology Agency, Saitama, Japan

T. Fujita (✉)
Laboratory of Molecular Genetics, Institute for Virus Research, and Laboratory of Molecular Cell Biology, Graduate School of Biostudies, Kyoto University, Kyoto, Japan
e-mail: tfujita@virus.kyoto-u.ac.jp

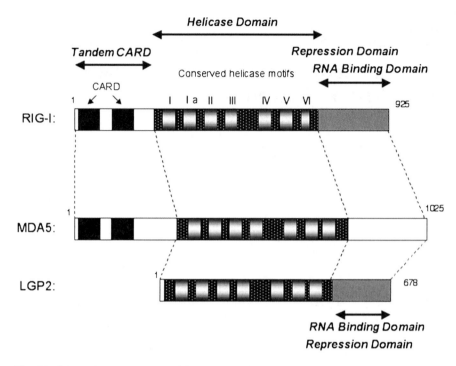

Fig. 5.1 Schematic representation of the domains of RLR. The precise boundary of the repression domain has not been identified

overexpression of the tandem CARD, but not individual CARD, can mimic virus-induced signaling and leads to the production of IFN (Saito et al. 2007). However, full-length RIG-I exhibits much less basal activity (Yoneyama et al. 2004).

The C-terminal region of RIG-I is responsible for this weak basal activity and is termed the repression domain. It has been demonstrated that this domain directly interacts with CARD, which leads to the inactivation of CARD-mediated signaling (Saito et al. 2007). In addition to the intramolecular repression, the isolated repression domain can block activation by wild-type RIG-I. The biological significance of the transrepression is not clear. Full-length and the C-terminal regions of LGP2 also exhibit transrepression; therefore, the function of the repression domain is conserved between RIG-I and LGP2, however the corresponding region of MDA5 does not share this activity. Because LGP2 lacks the signaling domain but retains the repression domain, it can act as a dominant inhibitor when overexpressed in cells (Komuro and Horvath 2006; Rothenfusser et al. 2005; Saito et al. 2007; Yoneyama et al. 2005) (Table 5.1).

The largest domain in the middle part of RLRs is the RNA helicase domain. RNA helicase motifs (I–VI) of DExD/H box RNA helicase are highly conserved. When motif I (Walker's ATP binding site) is mutated, RIG-I and MDA5 are inactivated (Yoneyama et al. 2004, 2005). This mutant acts as a dominant inhibitor for

Table 5.1 Molecules involved in the regulation of RLR-mediated signaling

Name	Positive or Negative	Description of the molecule	References
TRAF2, 3, 6	Positive	Adaptor	Oganesyan et al. (2006); Saha et al. (2006); Xu et al. (2005); Yoshida et al. (2008)
RIP1	Positive	Adaptor	Balachandran et al. (2004); Kawai et al. (2005)
FADD	Positive	Adaptor	Balachandran et al. (2004); Kawai et al. (2005)
TRADD	Positive	Adaptor	Michallet et al. (2008)
TRIM25	Positive	Ub ligase	Gack et al. (2007)
STING/MITA/ MPYS	Positive	4 TM protein	Ishikawa and Barber (2008); Zhong et al. (2008)
RNF135/Riplet/ REUL	Positive	Ub ligase	Gao et al. (2009); Oshiumi et al. (2009)
RNF125	Negative	Ub ligase	Arimoto et al. (2007)
Mfn2	Negative	GTPase	Yasukawa et al. (2009)
NLRX1	Negative	NOD family	Moore et al. (2008)
DAK	Negative	MDA5-specific	Diao et al. (2007)
CYLD	Negative	de-Ub	Friedman et al. (2008); Zhang et al. (2008)
DUBA	Negative	de-Ub	Kayagaki et al. (2007)
A20	Negative	de-Ub/Ub ligase	Lin et al. (2006b)
Atg5, Atg12	Negative	Autophagy regulation	Jounai et al. (2007); Tal et al. (2009)

List of the regulatory molecules in RLR signaling. Positive and negative: Positive and negative regulator of the signaling, respectively. Adaptor: Signaling adaptor; *Ub ligase* Ubiquitin ligase; 4 TM protein: A protein with four transmembrane domains; *de-Ub* deubiquitinase

RIG-I but not for MDA5, consistent with the notion that RIG-I but not MDA5 retains the repression domain (Saito et al. 2007). RIG-I unwinds dsRNA or RNA/DNA duplexes with a >15 nt 3′ RNA overhang in an ATP hydrolysis-dependent manner (Takahasi et al. 2008). However, RNA/DNA duplexes do not activate RIG-I for antiviral signaling, suggesting that helicase activity (unwinding dsRNA) per se is not sufficient for antiviral signaling.

The C-terminal region was also identified as a dsRNA-binding domain (Cui et al. 2008; Takahasi et al. 2008). This domain was discovered because of its strong resistance to digestion by a protease in the presence of dsRNA. The C-terminal region exhibits both a RNA-binding function and a repression function, however RNA-binding-deficient mutants of RIG-I and LGP2 exhibit repression, suggesting that distinct residues are responsible for these activities. The three-dimensional structure of the C-terminal domains of RLRs has been determined (Cui et al. 2008; Li et al. 2009; Pippig et al. 2009; Takahasi et al. 2008). Although the dsRNA-binding of this domain of RIG-I and LGP is strong, the corresponding region of MDA5 exhibits significantly weak binding. These observations are consistent with the structure of the RNA-binding surface of these domains as determined by NMR titration experiments. The RNA-binding surface of RIG-I and LGP2 exhibits a deep basic cleft, however the corresponding cleft of MDA5 is extended.

2 RLR Knockout Mice

Knockout mice without each RLR were established and their antiviral phenotype was analyzed (Kato et al. 2005, 2006; Venkataraman et al. 2007; Wang et al. 2007). RIG-I and MDA5 play a critical role in the production of IFNs and other cytokines in different cell types except plasmocytoid dendritic cells (pDCs), in which the TLR-MyD88-IRF-7 pathway is dominant (Kato et al. 2005, 2006). RIG-I appears to sense Paramyxoviridae (Sendai virus, Newcastle disease virus), Orthomyxoviridae (influenza A virus: IAV), Rhabdoviridae (vesicular stomatitis virus: VSV), Flaviviridae (Japanese encephalitis virus, hepatitis C virus: HCV), and Poxviridae (Myxoma virus) (Kato et al. 2005, 2006; Sumpter et al. 2005; Wang et al. 2008). MDA5 senses encephalomyocarditis virus: EMCV, Theiler's virus, and Mengo virus (Picornaviridae) (Kato et al. 2006). Dengue and West Nile viruses (Flaviviridae) are sensed by both RIG-I and MDA5 (Fredericksen et al. 2008; Loo et al. 2008). There is only one report on the knockout of LGP2. LGP2 knockout mice and cells exhibited enhanced and diminished antiviral responses to VSV and EMCV, respectively (Venkataraman et al. 2007). The mechanism by which CARD-less LGP2 activates EMCV-induced signaling is unknown.

3 Ligands for RLRs

The knockout studies indicated that RIG-I and MDA5 recognize different viruses. The specificity is partly explained by the recognition of different sized dsRNA; long (>1 kbp) dsRNA by MDA5 and short (100–1,000 bp) dsRNA by RIG-I (Kato et al. 2008). However, despite the correlation between the size of the viral dsRNA and the preference of the sensor, this specificity is not simply explained by an affinity for dsRNA of different sizes because MDA5 binds weakly to some long dsRNA (Yoneyama et al. 2005).

Two reports identified 5'-ppp containing RNA as a potent agonist for RIG-I, suggesting a new non-self RNA pattern (Hornung et al. 2006; Pichlmair et al. 2006). This discovery is based on the observation that while RNA transcribed by phage RNA polymerase in vitro is capable of activating antiviral signaling, the corresponding RNA made by chemical synthesis was not active and removal of the 5'-ppp moiety inactivates the transcripts in vitro. This led to the idea that even single-stranded RNA with the 5'-ppp structure is a strong agonist for RIG-I. However, recent reports found that transcription in vitro produces "copy back" (after transcription from the DNA template is completed, transcription resumes using the transcript RNA as template) products with partial double strands and this is critical for

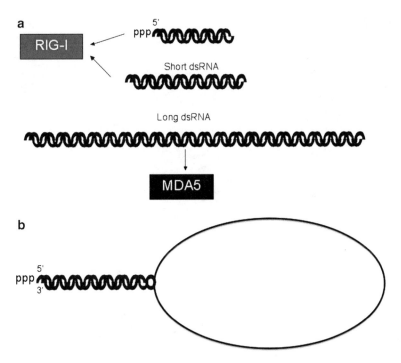

Fig. 5.2 Agonist dsRNA species for RIG-I and MDA5. (**a**) Short dsRNA selectively activates RIG-I. For very short dsRNA (20–50 bp), a 5′-ppp structure is necessary for efficient signaling, however a longer dsRNA (100-1,000 bp), 5′-ppp is not essential. MDA5 detects long dsRNA (>1,000 bp) independent of the 5′ structure. (**b**) Panhandle structure of the IAV genome. Genomic RNA of IAV contains 5′-ppp and complementary sequences at 5′ and 3′ terminus, thus forming a panhandle structure. A similar structure is predicted for other viruses

RIG-I's activation (Schlee et al. 2009; Schmidt et al. 2009). In summary, RIG-I recognizes relatively short dsRNA (<1 kbp) but for very short dsRNA (20–50 bp), an additional structure, 5′-ppp, is necessary for activation (Fig. 5.2a). IAV RNA contains 5′-ppp and forms a double helix with its 5′ and 3′ regions (Fig. 5.2b). This panhandle structure fulfills the requirement of a RIG-I ligand. Other reports have described different features of natural viral ligands. The reason why very long dsRNA does not activate RIG-I is unknown. The requirement of a dual pattern for short RNA suggests dual structural recognition by RIG-I, which presumably facilitates the formation of a dimer (Cui et al. 2008; Schmidt et al. 2009), however further study is required.

More recently it was reported that dsDNA with an alternating AT sequence is transcribed in cells by RNA polymerase III (pol III) and the resultant dsRNA activates RIG-I (Ablasser et al. 2009; Chiu et al. 2009). Some DNA viruses have been shown to activate antiviral responses through the activation of RIG-I, however further study is required to relate this observation to physiological responses against DNA viruses.

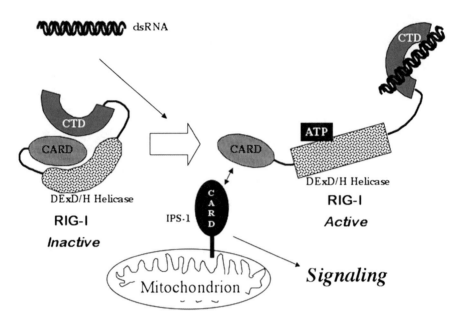

Fig. 5.3 Activation model for RIG-I. In uninfected cells, RIG-I adopts a closed structure in which the CARD is masked. Viral replication produces viral dsRNA to which RIG-I specifically binds and conformational change is induced. The helicase domain is responsible for this conformational change and the ATP-binding site is crucial for this. The exposed CARD relays signals to the mitochondrial adaptor, IPS-1, through physical interaction and the signaling is further transduced

4 Activation of RLRs

RIG-I and MDA5 are similar in structure and both contain a tandem CARD, which is the activation domain, suggesting a similar mechanism of activation. Here, we describe a model for the activation of RIG-I. In unstimulated cells, RIG-I adopts a closed conformation, in which the CARD is masked by the C-terminal repression domain (Fig. 5.3). DsRNA, which accumulates as a consequence of viral replication, binds to RIG-I through the RNA-binding surface of the C-terminal domain. This binding induces a conformational change of RIG-I, thereby exposing the CARD, which in turn transduces signals to downstream molecules through physical interaction (see below). The conformational change requires an intact helicase motif I (ATP-binding motif), suggesting the involvement of either the binding or hydrolysis of ATP. Although RIG-I and MDA5 have major similarities, MDA5 has little affinity for dsRNA and lacks a repression domain. Particularly for the recognition of dsRNA, MDA5 may utilize additional compensatory components, however their identity is unknown.

5 RLR Signaling

The notion that overexpression of the tandem CARD, which is unlikely to retain any enzymatic activity, is sufficient for signaling downstream, suggests that RIG-I and MDA5 transmit signals through physical interaction with downstream molecules. IFN-β promoter stimulator-1, IPS-1; (also known as MAVS, VISA, and Cardif), which contains one copy of CARD at its N-terminus, has been identified as an immediate downstream signaling adaptor (Kawai et al. 2005; Meylan et al. 2005; Seth et al. 2005; Xu et al. 2005). IPS-1 is specifically anchored to the mitochondrial outer membrane by its C-terminal transmembrane domain and exposes the CARD to the cytoplasm. Such a mitochondrial localization is crucial to its function as a signaling adaptor, because the NS3/4 protease of HCV inactivates IPS-1 by releasing it from the mitochondria (Lin et al. 2006a; Loo et al. 2006; Meylan et al. 2005). IPS-1 contains other regulatory regions including those for interaction with tumor necrosis factor receptor-associated factor (TRAF)3 and 6 (Oganesyan et al. 2006; Saha et al. 2006; Xu et al. 2005; Yoshida et al. 2008). TRAF3 activaties the non-canonical IκB kinase (IKK)-related kinases, while TRAF-family member-associated NF-κB activator-binding kinase 1 (TBK1), and IKK-i (IKK-ε), and these kinases activate IFN regulatory factor (IRF)-3 and -7, which are essential for IFN's activation, by specific phosphorylation. TRAF6 activates the canonical IKK complex and then NF-κB, another critical transcriptional activator for IFN genes. Recently, papers describing the regulatory factors for RIG-I-mediated signaling have been published (Table 5.1) (Yoneyama and Fujita 2009). These factors may be involved in the fine-tuning of the mainstream signaling or in providing a supporting role for the signaling. Further study is required to elucidate their physiological significance.

6 Biological Activity Other Than Immune Regulation

The RIG-I knockout mouse line died at the embryonic stage, however those of the other knockout line in which different exons were targeted did not (Kato et al. 2005; Wang et al. 2007). The lethal phenotype is dependent on the genetic background of the mice. A side-by-side comparison of these lines is necessary to elucidate the mechanism underlying the different phenotypes.

RIG-I and MDA5 exhibit structural similarity to *Caenorhabditis elegans*'s Dicer-related helicase (DRH-1), which is crucial for RNA interference (Tabara et al. 2002). Irrespective of this similarity, no report has described the phenotype caused by knocking out RLR with RNA interference in mammals. The IFN system and a true homolog for RLR have not been identified in invertebrates, suggesting that these antiviral systems were acquired during the evolution of vertebrates.

7 Future Perspectives

An outline of RLR function has been described, however several critical problems exist. First, the meaning of the mitochondrial localization of IPS-1 is not entirely clear. Although there have been several reports connecting RLR signaling to apoptosis (Besch et al. 2009), unlike well-defined death-inducing signals, the correlation between RLR's activation and apoptosis is not 100%. The second problem also concerns the intracellular localization of the signaling molecules. Usually viruses hijack cellular components, such as organella, and initiate replication, and therefore viral nucleic acid is localized to certain compartments. This compartmentalization is one of the ways viruses evade immune surveillance. It is not clear how RLR penetrates such places and detects viral dsRNA. Also, the mechanism by which RIG-I and MDA5 sense the length of dsRNA has not been elucidated. Finally, although we proposed a model for auto-repression and de-repression of RIG-I, no clear evidence based on structural biology has been presented.

References

Ablasser A, Bauernfeind F, Hartmann G et al (2009) RIG-I-dependent sensing of poly(dA:dT) through the induction of an RNA polymerase III-transcribed RNA intermediate. Nat Immunol 10(10):1065–1072

Arimoto K, Takahashi H, Hishiki T et al (2007) Negative regulation of the RIG-I signaling by the ubiquitin ligase RNF125. Proc Natl Acad Sci U S A 104:7500–7505

Balachandran S, Thomas E, Barber GN (2004) A FADD-dependent innate immune mechanism in mammalian cells. Nature 432:401–405

Besch R, Poeck H, Hohenauer T et al (2009) Proapoptotic signaling induced by RIG-I and MDA-5 results in type I interferon-independent apoptosis in human melanoma cells. J Clin Invest 119:2399–2411

Chiu YH, Macmillan JB, Chen ZJ (2009) RNA polymerase III detects cytosolic DNA and induces type I interferons through the RIG-I pathway. Cell 138:576–591

Cui S, Eisenacher K, Kirchhofer A et al (2008) The C-terminal regulatory domain is the RNA 5'-triphosphate sensor of RIG-I. Mol Cell 29:169–179

Diao F, Li S, Tian Y et al (2007) Negative regulation of MDA5- but not RIG-I-mediated innate antiviral signaling by the dihydroxyacetone kinase. Proc Natl Acad Sci USA 104:11706–11711

Fredericksen BL, Keller BC, Fornek J et al (2008) Establishment and maintenance of the innate antiviral response to West Nile Virus involves both RIG-I and MDA5 signaling through IPS-1. J Virol 82:609–616

Friedman CS, O'Donnell MA, Legarda-Addison D et al (2008) The tumour suppressor CYLD is a negative regulator of RIG-I-mediated antiviral response. EMBO Rep 9:930–936

Gack MU, Shin YC, Joo CH et al (2007) TRIM25 RING-finger E3 ubiquitin ligase is essential for RIG-I-mediated antiviral activity. Nature 446:916–920

Gao D, Yang YK, Wang RP et al (2009) REUL is a novel E3 ubiquitin ligase and stimulator of retinoic-acid-inducible gene-I. PLoS One 4:e5760

Hornung V, Ellegast J, Kim S et al (2006) 5'-Triphosphate RNA is the ligand for RIG-I. Science 314:994–997

Ishikawa H, Barber GN (2008) STING is an endoplasmic reticulum adaptor that facilitates innate immune signalling. Nature 455:674–678

Jounai N, Takeshita F, Kobiyama K et al (2007) The Atg5 Atg12 conjugate associates with innate antiviral immune responses. Proc Natl Acad Sci USA 104:14050–14055

Kato H, Sato S, Yoneyama M et al (2005) Cell type-specific involvement of RIG-I in antiviral response. Immunity 23:19–28

Kato H, Takeuchi O, Sato S et al (2006) Differential roles of MDA5 and RIG-I helicases in the recognition of RNA viruses. Nature 441:101–105

Kato H, Takeuchi O, Mikamo-Satoh E et al (2008) Length-dependent recognition of double-stranded ribonucleic acids by retinoic acid-inducible gene-I and melanoma differentiation-associated gene 5. J Exp Med 205:1601–1610

Kawai T, Akira S (2008) Toll-like receptor and RIG-I-like receptor signaling. Ann N Y Acad Sci 1143:1–20

Kawai T, Takahashi K, Sato S et al (2005) IPS-1, an adaptor triggering RIG-I- and Mda5-mediated type I interferon induction. Nat Immunol 6:981–988

Kayagaki N, Phung Q, Chan S et al (2007) DUBA: A deubiquitinase that regulates type I interferon production. Science 318:1628–1632

Komuro A, Horvath CM (2006) RNA- and virus-independent inhibition of antiviral signaling by RNA helicase LGP2. J Virol 80:12332–12342

Li X, Lu C, Stewart M et al (2009) Structural basis of double-stranded RNA recognition by the RIG-I like receptor MDA5. Arch Biochem Biophys 488:23–33

Lin R, Lacoste J, Nakhaei P et al (2006a) Dissociation of a MAVS/IPS-1/VISA/Cardif-IKKepsilon molecular complex from the mitochondrial outer membrane by hepatitis C virus NS3-4A proteolytic cleavage. J Virol 80:6072–6083

Lin R, Yang L, Nakhaei P et al (2006b) Negative regulation of the retinoic acid-inducible gene I-induced antiviral state by the ubiquitin-editing protein A20. J Biol Chem 281: 2095–2103

Loo YM, Owen DM, Li K et al (2006) Viral and therapeutic control of IFN-beta promoter stimulator 1 during hepatitis C virus infection. Proc Natl Acad Sci USA 103:6001–6006

Loo YM, Fornek J, Crochet N et al (2008) Distinct RIG-I and MDA5 signaling by RNA viruses in innate immunity. J Virol 82:335–345

Meylan E, Curran J, Hofmann K et al (2005) Cardif is an adaptor protein in the RIG-I antiviral pathway and is targeted by hepatitis C virus. Nature 437:1167–1172

Michallet MC, Meylan E, Ermolaeva MA et al (2008) TRADD protein is an essential component of the RIG-like helicase antiviral pathway. Immunity 28:651–661

Moore CB, Bergstralh DT, Duncan JA et al (2008) NLRX1 is a regulator of mitochondrial antiviral immunity. Nature 451:573–577

Oganesyan G, Saha SK, Guo B et al (2006) Critical role of TRAF3 in the Toll-like receptor-dependent and -independent antiviral response. Nature 439:208–211

Oshiumi H, Matsumoto M, Hatakeyama S et al (2009) Riplet/RNF135, a RING finger protein, ubiquitinates RIG-I to promote interferon-beta induction during the early phase of viral infection. J Biol Chem 284:807–817

Pichlmair A, Schulz O, Tan CP et al (2006) RIG-I-mediated antiviral responses to single-stranded RNA bearing 5'-phosphates. Science 314:997–1001

Pippig DA, Hellmuth JC, Cui S et al (2009) The regulatory domain of the RIG-I family ATPase LGP2 senses double-stranded RNA. Nucleic Acids Res 37:2014–2025

Rothenfusser S, Goutagny N, DiPerna G et al (2005) The RNA helicase Lgp2 inhibits TLR-independent sensing of viral replication by retinoic acid-inducible gene-I. J Immunol 175:5260–5268

Saha SK, Pietras EM, He JQ et al (2006) Regulation of antiviral responses by a direct and specific interaction between TRAF3 and Cardif. EMBO J 25:3257–3263

Saito T, Hirai R, Loo YM et al (2007) Regulation of innate antiviral defenses through a shared repressor domain in RIG-I and LGP2. Proc Natl Acad Sci USA 104:582–587

Samuel CE (2001) Antiviral actions of interferons. Clin Microbiol Rev 14:778–809

Schlee M, Roth A, Hornung V et al (2009) Recognition of 5' triphosphate by RIG-I helicase requires short blunt double-stranded RNA as contained in panhandle of negative-strand virus. Immunity 31:25–34

Schmidt A, Schwerd T, Hamm W et al (2009) 5'-triphosphate RNA requires base-paired structures to activate antiviral signaling via RIG-I. Proc Natl Acad Sci USA 106:12067–12072

Seth RB, Sun L, Ea CK et al (2005) Identification and characterization of MAVS, a mitochondrial antiviral signaling protein that activates NF-kappaB and IRF 3. Cell 122:669–682

Sumpter R Jr, Loo YM, Foy E et al (2005) Regulating intracellular antiviral defense and permissiveness to hepatitis C virus RNA replication through a cellular RNA helicase, RIG-I. J Virol 79:2689–2699

Tabara H, Yigit E, Siomi H et al (2002) The dsRNA binding protein RDE-4 interacts with RDE-1, DCR-1, and a DExH-box helicase to direct RNAi in *C. elegans*. Cell 109:861–871

Takahasi K, Yoneyama M, Nishihori T et al (2008) Nonself RNA-sensing mechanism of RIG-I helicase and activation of antiviral immune responses. Mol Cell 29:428–440

Tal MC, Sasai M, Lee HK et al (2009) Absence of autophagy results in reactive oxygen species-dependent amplification of RLR signaling. Proc Natl Acad Sci U S A 106:2770–2775

Theofilopoulos AN, Baccala R, Beutler B et al (2005) Type I interferons (alpha/beta) in immunity and autoimmunity. Annu Rev Immunol 23:307–336

Uze G, Monneron D (2007) IL-28 and IL-29: Newcomers to the interferon family. Biochimie 89: 729–734

Venkataraman T, Valdes M, Elsby R et al (2007) Loss of DExD/H box RNA helicase LGP2 manifests disparate antiviral responses. J Immunol 178:6444–6455

Wang Y, Zhang HX, Sun YP et al (2007) Rig-I–/– mice develop colitis associated with downregulation of G alpha i2. Cell Res 17:858–868

Wang F, Gao X, Barrett JW et al (2008) RIG-I mediates the co-induction of tumor necrosis factor and type I interferon elicited by myxoma virus in primary human macrophages. PLoS Pathog 4:e1000099

Xu LG, Wang YY, Han KJ et al (2005) VISA is an adapter protein required for virus-triggered IFN-beta signaling. Mol Cell 19:727–740

Yasukawa K, Oshiumi H, Takeda M et al (2009) Mitofusin 2 inhibits mitochondrial antiviral signaling. Sci Signal 2:ra47

Yoneyama M, Fujita T (2009) RNA recognition and signal transduction by RIG-I-like receptors. Immunol Rev 227:54–65

Yoneyama M, Kikuchi M, Natsukawa T et al (2004) The RNA helicase RIG-I has an essential function in double-stranded RNA-induced innate antiviral responses. Nat Immunol 5:730–737

Yoneyama M, Kikuchi M, Matsumoto K et al (2005) Shared and unique functions of the DExD/H-Box helicases RIG-I, MDA5, and LGP2 in antiviral innate immunity. J Immunol 175:2851–2858

Yoshida R, Takaesu G, Yoshida H et al (2008) TRAF6 and MEKK1 play a pivotal role in the RIG-I-like helicase antiviral pathway. J Biol Chem 283:36211–36220

Zhang M, Wu X, Lee AJ et al (2008) Regulation of IkappaB kinase-related kinases and antiviral responses by tumor suppressor CYLD. J Biol Chem 283:18621–18626

Zhong B, Yang Y, Li S et al (2008) The adaptor protein MITA links virus-sensing receptors to IRF3 transcription factor activation. Immunity 29:538–550

Chapter 6
Innate Immune Signaling and Negative Regulators in Cancer

Helen Y. Wang and Rong-Fu Wang

1 Introduction

Toll-like receptors (TLRs), NOD-like receptors (NLRs) and RIG-I-like receptors (RLRs) have emerged as important innate immune receptors or innate Pattern recognition receptors (PRRs) that can detect a variety of invading pathogens and intracellular ligands, thus serving as a first line of defense against infectious pathogens and cancer. These germline-encoded PRRs are expressed in DCs and other immune cells and recognize structure-conserved molecules, so called pathogen-associated molecular patterns (PAMPs) as well as endogenous ligands released from damaged cells, termed damage-associated molecular patterns (DAMPs). Recognition of PAMPs or DAMPs by PRRs triggers the activation of several key signaling pathways, including NF-κB, type I interferon (IFN) and inflammasome, leading to the production of inflammatory cytokines. They secrete proinflammatory cytokines and promote DC maturation programs for the induction of adaptive immune responses (Iwasaki and Medzhitov 2004; Takeda and Akira 2005).

TLRs are type 1 integral membrane glycoproteins characterized by extracellular domains containing variable numbers of leucine-rich-repeat (LRR) motifs and a cytoplasmic Toll/IL-1R homology (TIR) domain. These receptors are expressed on the cell surface (TLR1, TLR2, TLR4, and TLR5) or in the endosome (TLR3, TLR7, TLR8, and TLR9). In addition to these extracellular TLRs, several intracellular pattern recognition receptors have been found to be responsible for the recognition of invading viruses in the cytoplasm. RIG-1 and melanoma differentiation associated gene 5 (MDA5) are IFN-inducible proteins containing caspase recruitment domains (CARDs) and RNA helicase domains that functions as cytoplasmic receptors for

H.Y. Wang • R.-F. Wang (✉)
Departments of Pathology and Immunology, The Center for Cell and Gene Therapy,
Baylor College of Medicine, Houston, TX 77030, USA
e-mail: Rongfuw@bcm.tmc.edu

dsRNA (Akira et al. 2006; Kato et al. 2005; Yoneyama et al. 2004). Ligation of TLRs and RLRs by PAMPs or DAMPs mainly activates NF-κB and type I IFN signaling pathways and produces proinflammatory cytokines such as IL-1, IL-6, TNF-α, IFN-α, and IFN-β, which play critical roles in anti-cancer or antiviral immunity.

Nucleotide-binding oligomerization domain (NOD)-like receptors (NLRs, also called Caterpillars) represent a large family of protein receptors/regulators harboring an initiating signal domain, such as the CARD, pyrin domain (PYRIN), or baculovirus inhibitor-of-apoptosis repeat (BIR) domain, a NOD and an LRR domain. These NLRs have very diverse biological functions. Some of these NLR proteins have been implicated in the recognition of bacterial components (Inohara et al. 2005; Martinon and Tschopp 2005; Ting and Davis 2005), while others function as innate immune regulators of innate immune signaling pathways. Activation of such cytoplasmic receptors by invading pathogens including bacteria and viruses activate inflammasome consisting of caspase-1 and ASC, and leads to the production of proinflammatory cytokines such as IL-1β and IL-18. Thus, TLRs, NLRs, and RLRs are critical in bridging innate and adaptive immune responses by activating several key signaling pathways and producing many important cytokines as mediators. These cytokines have been shown to have a critical role in the differentiation of CD4 T cells (Th1, Th2, and Th17) and controlling the suppressive function of regulatory T (Treg) cells. Thus, they represent a potent means of modulating immune responses in cancer development as well as cancer therapy. In this chapter, we will review recent advances in PRRs research; discuss how distinct PRRs sense invading pathogens; and how these PRRs-induced innate signaling pathways are controlled and linked to inflammation-associated cancer.

2 Toll-like Receptors and Their Specificity of Ligand Recognition

Since the discovery of mammalian TLRs, both natural and synthetic ligands for these receptors have been identified and characterized for their recognition. For example, TLR2 recognizes lipoproteins such as peptidoglycan found in gram-positive bacteria, *Mycoplasma*, fungi, and viruses by forming a heterodimer with either TLR1 or TLR6. The TLR1/TLR2 and TLR2/TLR6 heterodimers respond to triacyl- and diacyl-lipoproteins, respectively. TLR4, along with myeloid differentiation factor 2 (MD2), recognizes lipopolysaccharide (LPS), which is unique to gram-negative bacteria. The crystal structural analysis shows that TLR4-MD2-LPS forms a TLR4 homodimer. Recent studies show that TLR4 can respond to H5N1 avian influenza virus infection by recognizing a DAMP signal, endogenous oxidized phospholipids produced during viral infection. TLR5 expressed in DCs of the lamina propria in the small intestine recognizes flagellin from bacteria. TLR11 has been found to be inactive in humans, but is functional in mice and recognizes a profilin-like molecule from the protozoan parasite *Toxoplasma gondii* (Yarovinsky et al. 2005; Zhang et al. 2004).

In contrast, TLR3, TLR7, TLR8, and TLR9 are DNA/RNA sensors and activate NF-κB and type I IFN signaling pathways. TLR3 recognizes viral double-stranded (ds) RNA in the endolysomes produced during infection as well as synthetic poly(I:C) oligonucleotides. Crystal structural studies demonstrate that TLR3 forms a large horseshoe-shaped solenoid assembled from 23 LRRs. Highly conserved surface residues and a TLR3-specific LRR insertion form a homodimer interface, whereas two patches of positively charged residues and a second insertion would provide an appropriate binding site for double-stranded RNA (Choe et al. 2005). TLR9 recognizes an unmethylated CpG DNA motif of prokaryotic genomes and DNA viruses (Takeda and Akira 2005). TLR7 and TLR8 recognize either single-stranded viral RNAs or guanosine-related analogs (loxoribine and imidazoquinoline) (Diebold et al. 2004; Heil et al. 2004; Lund et al. 2004). Human TLR8 recognizes CpG-A and Poly-G3 oligonucleotides (Peng et al. 2005), but murine TLR8 is not functional (Jurk et al. 2002).

TLR expression has been detected on many types of cells, including different subsets of DCs, macrophages, T cells, neutrophils, eosinophils, mast cells, monocytes, and epithelial cells (Iwasaki and Medzhitov 2004). Some TLRs are expressed by T cells, such as Tregs (Peng et al. 2005; Peng et al. 2007; Sutmuller et al. 2006). Unlike TLR2, 4, 5, and 6, which are expressed on the cell surface, TLR3, 7, 8, and 9 reside in the endosomal compartments (Akira and Takeda 2004; Hemmi et al. 2002; Jurk et al. 2002). Their endosomal localization is thought to be crucial for providing self vs. non-self discrimination, because self-nucleic acids are generally degraded by extracellular or endosomal DNases (Barton et al. 2006). UNC93B1 has been demonstrated to play a role in the translocation of these TLRs from the ER to the endosomal compartment (Kim et al. 2008; Tabeta et al. 2006). Importantly, TLR9 undergoes processing by proteases in the endosomes to generate an active form of TLR9 for CpG-DNA recognition (Asagiri et al. 2008; Ewald et al. 2008; Park et al. 2008). Additionally, TLR3 and TLR7 were recently found to be processed by several proteases (Ewald et al. 2011).

3 Intracellular RLRs and Their Ligands

The RLR family contains RIG-I, MDA5, and LGP2 (Laboratory of Genetics and Physiology-2). Both RIG-I and MDA5 are composed of two CARD domains in the N-terminus a central DEAD box helicase domain and a C-terminal regulatory domain, while LGP2 contains the helicase and regulatory domains, but lacks the CARD domain (Takeuchi and Akira 2008; Yoneyama and Fujita 2009). These receptors are inducible for their expression after viral infection or type I IFN stimulation, localized in the cytoplasm and responsible for recognition of cytoplasmic dsRNA. For RNA-sensing in the cytoplasm, RIG-I was recently shown to recognize relatively short dsRNA and the 5′-end of certain viral RNA genomes, specifically, uncapped 5′-triphosphate RNA (Hornung et al. 2006; Pichlmair et al. 2006). Such 5′-triphosphates are generally removed or modified during post-transcriptional

RNA processing of host RNA species, thereby remaining invisible or silent to innate immunity and providing a structural basis for the distinction of viral RNA from abundant self RNA in the cytoplasm of virally infected cells. It appears that dsRNA with a 5′-triphosphate serves as a better stimulator, compared with synthetic dsRNA lacking 5′-triphosphate, although they are capable of stimulating RIG-I for type I IFN response (Kato et al. 2008; Takahasi et al. 2008). To identify natural RNA stimulus from viruses such as HCV and influenza virus, it has been shown that Poly(U) or poly(A)-rich sequences from the HCV RNA 3′ untranslated region can potently stimulate RIG-I (Saito et al. 2008). Influenza viral genomes bearing 5′-triphosphates, but not short double-stranded RNAs, viral transcripts, or cleaved self-RNA, constitute the physiological source of RIG-I stimulation and IFN induction during infection with negative strand RNA viruses (Rehwinkel et al. 2010).

Unlike RIG-I, MDA-5 recognizes long dsRNA and poly(I:C). Because of these different requirements for RIG-I and MDA5 recognition, it may explain that RIG-I is responsible for the recognition of Newcastle disease virus (NDV) and Sendai virus (SeV), vesticular stomatitis virus (VSV), influenza virus, HCV, and Japanese encephatitis virus (JEV), while MDA5 may be responsible for the recognition of segmented RNA viruses such as reovirus. Both RIG-I and MDA5 can recognize Dengue virus and West Nile virus (Kato et al. 2006; Loo et al. 2008). LGP2 may be a negative regulator of RIG-I and MDA5 due to its lack of CARD domains (Saito et al. 2007). However, a recent study using LGP2−/− mice shows that, LGP2 positively regulates type I IFN response to RNA viruses recognized by RIG-I and MDA5 (Satoh et al. 2010), suggesting that LGP2 may have a role in the modification of RNAs with its helicase and regulatory domains. Interestingly, recent studies show that the C-terminal regulatory domains of RIG-I and LGP2 can bind to the termini of dsRNA through a large basic surface forming an RNA binding loop. By contrast, the C-terminal domain of MDA5 is a large basic, but flat surface conformation. Thus, the binding affinity of RIG-I and LGP2 is higher than that of MDA5. Once RIG-I and MDA5 bind to their ligands, they undergo conformational changes and expose the CARD domains for interaction with downstream molecules such as MAVS and NLRC5 (Cui et al. 2010; Yoneyama and Fujita 2009). A recent study shows that RIG-I activation requires both RNA bearing the 5′-triphosphate and polyubiquitin chains linked through lysine 63 of ubiquitin (Zeng et al. 2010). CARD domains of RIG-I bind to unanchored K63-ubiquitin chain, depends on RNA and ATP (Zeng et al. 2010), suggesting that RNA recognition and the helicase activity of RIG-1 are required for making the CARDs accessible for sensing polyubiquitin chains and downstream signaling activation. These studies indicate that RIG-I functions a sensor for viral RNA bearing 5′-triphosphate and unanchored polyubiquitin chains.

4 Signaling Pathways and Regulation of TLRs and RLRs

The current model of TLR signaling pathways predicts that TLR1, 2, 5, 7, 8, and 9 use MyD88 as their sole receptor-proximal adaptor to transduce signals (Fig. 6.1). Thus, MyD88 is essential for the signaling of most TLRs to MyD88-IRAK4 and

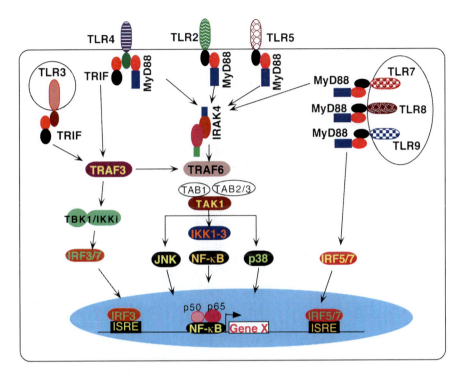

Fig. 6.1 A schematic presentation of TLR signaling pathway. TLR2, TLR4 and TLR5 are cell surface molecules, while TLR3, TLR7, TLR8 and TLR9 are localized in endosomes. Most TLRs use MyD88 as a central adaptor molecule, and TLR3 uses TRIF as an adaptor for downstream signaling. TLR4 use both MyD88 and TRIF adaptor molecules to activate NF-κB and type I interferon pathways

other downstream molecules. After the MyD88-IRAK4-IRAK1 complex activates TNFR-associated factor 6 (TRAF6), a ubiquination protein ligase (E3), together with a ubiquitination E2 enzyme complex consisting of UBC13 and UEV1A, the TRAF6 complex catalyzes the formation of a K63-linked polyubiquitin chain on TRAF6 itself and on NEMO, a subunit of IKK complex. Meanwhile, the recruitment of TGF-β-activated kinase 1 (TAK1) and its binding proteins (TAB1, TAB2, and TAB3) leads to the phosphorylation of IKK-β and MAP kinase 6 (MKK6) and then activation of NF-κB and MAP kinase pathways for the production of inflammatory cytokines. Recent studies also suggest that MyD88 may also interact with IRF-5 and IRF-7 for the induction of proinflammatory cytokines or type-I interferon (IFN-α and IFN-β) response (Honda et al. 2005a; Honda et al. 2005b; Takaoka et al. 2005). TLR3 relies on a MyD88-independent, but TRIF-mediated pathway for the production of IFN-β in response to pathogen recognition, while TLR4 is linked to both MyD88-dependent and TRIF-dependent pathways (Akira and Takeda 2004; Takeda and Akira 2005). Activation of TLR3 leads to recruitment of receptor-interacting protein 1 (RIP1), TRAF3 and TRAF6, which activates TRAF family-member-associated NF–κB activator (TANK) binding kinase 1 (TBK1) and/or inducible IkB kinase (IKK-i), which directly phosphorylate IRF3 and IRF7 for the production of type-I interferon cytokines (Akira et al. 2006).

The adaptor molecule IPS-1/MAVS/VISA/CARDIF that interacts with the RIG-1/MDA5 receptor for recognition of cytoplasmic dsRNA has been independently identified by several groups (Kawai et al. 2005; Meylan et al. 2005; Seth et al. 2005; Xu et al. 2005). MAVS is present in the outer mitochondrial membrane, and the cleavage of this protein at the C-terminus by the NS3/4A protease of hepatitis C virus inactivates its ability to transduce signals to TBK1 and IKKi (Meylan et al. 2005; Seth et al. 2005). Recently, STING (stimulator of interferon genes, also known as MITA) appears essential for effective innate immune signaling after intracellular B-form DNA stimulation and non-CpG intracellular DNA species produced by various DNA viral pathogens (Ishikawa and Barber 2008; Ishikawa et al. 2009; Zhong et al. 2008). In the presence of intracellular DNA, STING interacts with TBK1 from the endoplasmic reticulum to perinuclear vesicles and mediates its phosphorylation, thus activating IRF3 (Ishikawa et al. 2009; Zhong et al. 2008). Interestingly, STING is regulated by two ubiquitin E3 ligases RNF5 and TRIM56, resulting in two complete opposite effects on STING stability and function (Tsuchida et al. 2010; Zhong et al. 2009). More recently, IFI16, a PYHIN protein, has been identified as an intracellular DNA sensor that mediates the induction of IFN-β and interacts with STING in response to DNA stimulation (Fig. 6.2). Knockdown of IFI16 or its mouse ortholog p204 by RNA-mediated interference inhibited gene induction and activation of the transcription factors IRF3 and NF-κB induced by DNA and herpes simplex virus type 1 (HSV-1) (Unterholzner et al. 2010). Recently, it was found that during Kaposi sarcoma-associated herpes virus (KSHV) infection, IFI16 interacts with ASC and procaspase-1 to form a functional inflammasome (Kerur et al. 2011). AIM-2 has been identified as a cytoplasmic double-stranded DNA sensor that activate the inflammasome pathway (Burckstummer et al. 2009; Fernandes-Alnemri et al. 2009; Hornung et al. 2009; Roberts et al. 2009). Thus, the PYHIN proteins IFI16 and AIM2 form a new family of innate DNA sensors to activate IFN and inflammasome pathways.

5 NOD-like Receptors and Their Ligand Recognition

NLRs comprise a large number of intracellular receptor family, consisting of 22 NLR proteins in humans and 34 genes in mice. This protein family is characterized by the following features (1) an N-terminal CARD, PYD, acidic transactivating domain, or baculovirus inhibitor repeat (BIR) domain; (2) a central NOD domain; and (3) a C-terminal LRR domain (Fig. 6.3). The N-terminal domain of NLRs is critical for transducing signals to downstream adaptor molecules. For example, the CARD domain of NLRs is involved in the interaction with CARD-containing proteins such as caspase-1 and ASC (adaptor protein apoptosis speck protein with caspase recruitment) in inflammasome activation. The PYD domain of NLRs is homologous to CARD and interacts with other PYD-containing proteins during

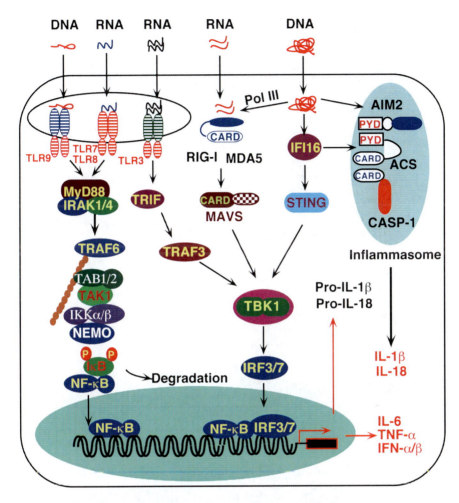

Fig. 6.2 DNA and RNA sensors of innate immune signaling. TLR3 recognizes double-stranded RNA, while TLR7 and TLR8 respond to single-stranded RNA in endosomes for initiating downstream signaling pathway. However, RIG-I and MDA-5 recognize cytosolic RNAs derived from viruses. TLR9 recognizes methylated DNA from pathogens in endosomes, while IFI16 (interferon induced gene 16) and AIM-2 (antigen in melanoma 2) recognize viral DNA and cytosolic DNA for initiating type I IFN and inflammasome pathways. MAVS and STING are key adaptor molecules for RNA and DNA sensor-induced signaling pathways. Inflammasome-activated caspase-1 is responsible for the cleavage of pro-IL-1beta and pro-IL-18 to generate mature IL-1beta and IL-18

signaling transduction. The BIR domain of NLRs contains two major groups: inhibitor of apoptosis proteins (IAPs) and neuronal apoptosis inhibitor proteins (NAIPs). Thus, the CARD, PYD, or BIR domain of NLRs is involved in apoptosis and inflammation. NOD is important for self-oligomerization during inflammasome activation, while LRR functions as ligand sensors to detect PAMPs or plays a

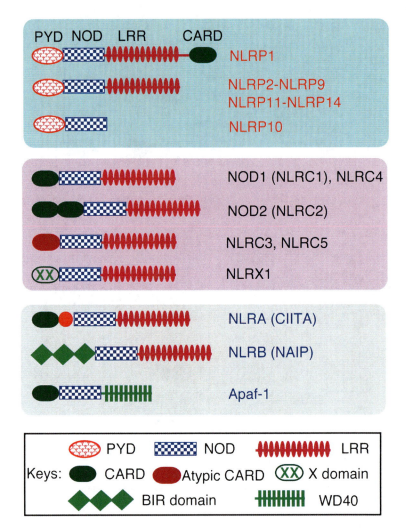

Fig. 6.3 Domain organization of the human NLR protein family. The members of the human NLRA, NLRB, NLRC, NLRP and NLRX are shown

regulatory role in innate immune signaling through protein-protein interactions. Because all NLR family members contain the evolutionarily conserved NOD and LRR domains, but differ in the N-terminal domains, these NLRs are divided into several subfamilies: a NLRA protein (CIITA), a NLRB protein (NAIP), 5 CARD-containing NLRC proteins (NLRC1, NLRC2, NLRC3, NLRC4 and NLRC5), 14 PYD-containing NLRP proteins (NLRP1-14), and an X domain containing NLRX1 (Fig. 6.3).

Although NLRs are expressed in various cell types and tissues, their expression patterns are different. For example, NLRX1 and NLRP1 are widely expressed in many tissues or cell types, while NOD1, NOD2, NLRP3, and NAIP are highly expressed in immune cells and epithelial cells. NLRP4, NLRP5, NLRP7, NLRP8, NLRP10, and NLRP11 are strongly expressed in germ cells (testis) or specific tissues. For example, we recently found that NLRP4 is highly expressed in testis and pancreatic tissue (unpublished data). Expression of some NLRs such as NOD1, NOD2, NLRP3, and NLRC5 is inducible by cytokine or NF-κB signaling (Becker and O'Neill 2007; Benko et al. 2010; Cui et al. 2010; Kuenzel et al. 2010; Meissner et al. 2010; Neerincx et al. 2010).

Among the large number of NLR family members, NOD1 and NOD2 recognize bacteria-derived g-D-glutamyl-meso-diaminopimelic acid (iE-DAP) and muramyl dipeptide (MDP), respectively. However, NALP3 can recognize many ligands, including bacterial RNA, ATP and uric-acid crystals, silica and asbestos (Dostert et al. 2008; Duncan et al. 2007; Eisenbarth et al. 2008; Kanneganti et al. 2006; Mariathasan et al. 2006; Martinon et al. 2006; Sutterwala et al. 2006). Despite of these extensive studies, a direct interaction between specific ligands and their corresponding NLRs has not been demonstrated. Thus, it is likely that NLR activation by their ligands or pathogens is indirect, or may involve another host molecule for their recognition. Specific ligands for other NOD-LRR family members remain to be identified.

6 Diverse Biological Functions and Signaling Pathways of NLRs

NLR family proteins are involved in many biological processes and have very diverse biological functions, including their roles in expression of major histocompatibility complex (MHC) class I and II molecules, apoptosis, NF-κB and MAPK signaling and inflammasome activation.

6.1 NF-κB and MAPK Signaling Activation and Autophagy Induction by NOD1 and NOD2

Ligand binding to NOD1 and NOD2 induces their oligomerization and recruits RIP2/RICK to the complex, leading to activation of the NF-κB and MAPK pathways and the production of inflammatory cytokines (Akira et al. 2006; Inohara et al. 2005; Martinon and Tschopp 2005; Ting and Davis 2005). NOD2 is required for T cell differentiation in response to *Toxoplasma gondii* infection (Shaw et al. 2009). A recent study shows that NOD1 and NOD2 are critical for the autophagic response to invasive bacteria. By a mechanism independent of the adaptor RIP2 and transcription factor NF-κB, NOD1 and NOD2 recruit the autophagy protein ATG16L1 to the plasma membrane at the bacterial entry sites for the induction of autophagy (Travassos et al. 2010), thus providing a functional role for NOD1/2 in autophagy-mediated immunity against invading bacteria. Furthermore, NOD2 interacts with ATG5, ATG7, and ATG16L for autophagy induction and is required for anti-bacterial immunity and generation of MHC class II antigen-specific CD4 T cell responses (Cooney et al. 2010). In addition to its role in defense against bacteria, a recent study indicates that NOD2 can function as a cytoplasmic viral PRR and trigger activation of IRF3 and production of IFN-β by interacting with MAVS (Sabbah et al. 2009), suggesting that NOD2 functions as a viral PRR in host antiviral defense mechanisms. However, it is not known whether NOD2 directly binds to viral ssRNA.

6.2 Inflammasome Activation by NLRs

Activation of NLRs such as NALP3 recruits apoptosis-associated speck-like protein containing a CARD (ASC) through a homotypic interaction between the PYRIN domains. ASC then recruits procaspase-1 via its CARD, leading to the activation of caspase-1 (Chen et al. 2009; Schroder and Tschopp 2010). Active caspase-1 then cleaves pro-IL-1β for release from cells. It appears that TLR signaling is required for the production of pro-IL-1β. Hence, signaling via both TLRs and NLRs pathways is needed to achieve the maximal production of IL-1β (Mariathasan and Monack 2007; Schroder and Tschopp 2010). Although the detailed biochemical mechanisms and specificity of inflammasome activation are not completely understood, there are four types of inflammasomes: NLRP1 inflammasome, NLRP3 inflammasome, NLRC4 inflammasome, and AIM-2 inflammasome (Fig. 6.4).

(1) NLRP1 inflammasome is the first to be demonstrated in the activation of caspase-1. Human NLRP1 contains a C-terminal CARD domain that can directly interact with procaspase-1, without the participation of ASC, thus activating caspase-1 to process pro-IL-1β to release IL-1β. NLRP1 can be activated by microbes and specific ligands (Fig. 6.4).
(2) NLRP3 inflammasome is most extensively studied and consists of ASC and procaspase-1. Upon exposure to invading pathogens or diverse PAMPs, DAMPs and environmental irritates through the LRR domain of NLRP3, NLRP3 activation leads to oligomerization and recruits ASC through the PYD domain. The CARD domain of ASC in turn interacts with the CARD domain of procaspase-1. Clustering of procaspase-1 leads to autocleavage to generate an active caspase-1 (p10/p20 tetramer), which processes pro-IL-1β to generate the active and mature form of IL-β. Mature IL-1β is then released from cells by an unknown protein secretion pathway (Fig. 6.4). Since many structurally diverse molecules can activate NLRP3, at least three models have been put forward to explain the NLRP3 inflammasome activation. The first model is that pore formation induced by triggering K+efflux and pannexin-1 membrane pore formation allows extracellular NLRP3 agonists to access the cytosol and directly activate NLRP3. The second model is that all NLRP3 agonists such as MSU,

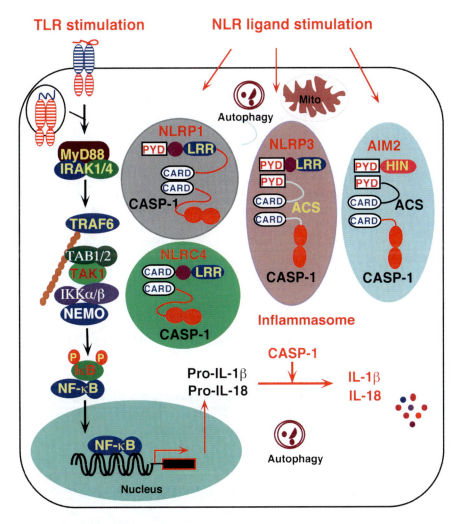

Fig. 6.4 A schematic presentation of inflammasomes mediated by NLRP1, NLRC4, NLRP3 and AIM-2. Inflammasome also contains ASC and procaspase-1 (also known as interleukin-converting enzyme)

silica, asbestos, alum, and β-amyloid polypeptide directly activate NLRP3 (Dostert et al. 2008; Eisenbarth et al. 2008; Kanneganti et al. 2006; Mariathasan et al. 2006; Martinon et al. 2006; Masters et al. 2010; Sutterwala et al. 2006), but these interactions have not been demonstrated. The third possibility is that all NLRP3 agonists either directly or indirectly trigger the generation of reactive oxygen species (ROS), which in turn activates NLRP3 inflammasome activation. Recent studies show that the accumulation of damaged, ROS-generating mitochondria by blocking autophagy processing activates the NLRP3 inflammasome (Nakahira et al. 2011; Zhou et al. 2011).

(3) NLRC4 inflammasome consists of NLRC4 and procaspase-1, since NLRC4 contains a CARD domain, which interacts with the CARD domain of procaspase-1. Activation of NLRC4 requires ligands that are different from NLRP3 (Fig. 6.4).
(4) AIM2 inflammasome is the most recently identified member of the HIN-200 family member. AIM2 functions as a cytosolic DNA sensor. Once activation of AIM2 by cytosolic DNA happens, it interacts with ASC through the PYD domain, while the CARD domain of ASC recruits and interacts with the CARD domain of procaspase-1. Active caspase-1 processes pro-IL-1β to produce mature IL-β for secretion (Burckstummer et al. 2009; Fernandes-Alnemri et al. 2009; Hornung et al. 2009; Roberts et al. 2009). AIM2-deficient mice are extremely susceptible to *Francisella tularensis* infection, with greater mortality and bacterial burden than that of wild-type mice. Caspase-1-dependent maturation of IL-1beta and IL-18 are absent in AIM2-deficient macrophages in response to *F. tularensis* infection or to synthetic double-stranded DNA (Fernandes-Alnemri et al. 2010; Rathinam et al. 2010). Thus, AIM2 is a DNA sensor that activates the inflammasome for IL-1beta and IL-18 production (Fig. 6.4).

7 Tight Control of Innate Immune Signaling by Positive and Negative Regulators

Innate immune responses are the first defense system against invading pathogens (bacteria, viruses, and fungi) through NF-κB, type I IFN and inflammasome activation. Tight regulation of these key signaling pathways is essential for both innate and adaptive immunity; otherwise, aberrant immune responses may occur, leading to severe or even fatal consequences such as bacterial sepsis, autoimmune, and chronic inflammatory diseases. In the last few years, many positive and negative regulators have been identified to control these signaling pathways through different mechanisms or at multiple levels (Fig. 6.5).

7.1 Negative Regulators of TLR-mediated NF-κB Signaling

SIGIRR: SIGIRR is a membrane protein containing a single extracellular immunoglobulin domain and a cytoplasmic TIR domain (Thomassen et al. 1999). SIGIRR is highly expressed in epithelial cells and immature DCs, but not in macrophages, and it interacts with IRAK and TRAF6 molecules. SIGIRR-deficient mice are more susceptibile to LPS-induced septic shock (Wald et al. 2003). Specific deletion of SIGIRR in T cells resulted in increased Th17 cell polarization in vivo upon myelin oligodendrocyte glycoprotein (MOG35-55) peptide immunization. IL-1-induced proliferation was abolished in mTOR-deficient Th17 cells, suggesting that

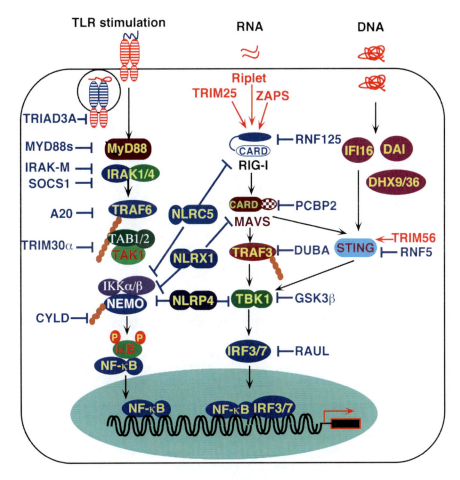

Fig. 6.5 Positive and negative regulators of NF-κB and type I IFN pathways. Each layer of key signaling pathways is tightly regulated by positive and/or negative regulators to maintain the balance of immune homeostasis in response to invading pathogens and endogenous ligand stimulators

IL-1 signaling and mTOR activation play a critical role in Th17 differentiation and expansion (Gulen et al. 2010). Furthermore, SIGIRR-deficient colonic epithelial cells displayed commensal bacteria-dependent homeostatic defects and increased inflammatory responses to dextran sulfate sodium (DSS) challenge, and increased Azoxymethane (AOM)+DSS-induced colitis-associated tumorigenesis (Xiao et al. 2007).

TRIAD3A: TRIAD3A is a member of the TRIAD3 family of RING-finger E3 ligase and binds to TLR4 and TLR9, but not TLR2, which leads to ubiquitination-mediated degradation of TLR4 and TLR9 (Chuang and Ulevitch 2004). However, the physiological relevance of TRIAD3A has not been determined.

IRAKM: The IRAK family of kinases is comprised of four members (IRAK1, IRAK2, IRAK4, and IRAKM). While IRAK1 and IRAK4 are important signaling molecules activating TRAF6 in the TLR pathway (Suzuki et al. 2002), IRAKM is predominantly expressed in peripheral blood cells (Janssens and Beyaert 2003; Wesche et al. 1999). IRAKM deficient mice produce more inflammatory cytokines in response to LPS treatment (Kobayashi et al. 2002). IRAKM mediates critical aspects of innate immunity that result in an immunocompromised state during sepsis (Deng et al. 2006). These studies indicate that IRAKM plays a critical role in the control of TLR-induced NF-κB signaling.

SOCS1: SOCS1 is a member of the SOCS (suppressing cytokine signaling) family that consists of SOCS1, SOCS2, SOCS3, SOCS4, SOCS5, SOCS6, SOCS7, and SOCS8 proteins (Alexander and Hilton 2004; Starr et al. 1997). SOCS1 inhibits TLR-induced NF-κB signaling by targeting IRAK1. SOCS1 knockout mice die within 3 weeks due to extensive inflammation, in particular IFN-γ production (Alexander et al. 1999; Marine et al. 1999). SOCS1 deficient mice increase the susceptibility to LPS-induced septic shock (Kinjyo et al. 2002; Nakagawa et al. 2002).

A20: A20 is a deubiquitynating enzyme that removes ubiquitin from the polyubiquitin chains of TRAF6, thus blocking NF-κB signaling. A20 was initially identified as a TNF-induced zinc-finger protein that inhibits TNF-mediated NF-κB activation (Opipari et al. 1990). A20-deficient mice develop severe inflammation, and are hypersensitive to both lipopolysaccharide and TNF, and die prematurely (Lee et al. 2000). A20 contains a N-terminal OTU (ovarian tumor) for deubiquitinating (DUB) enzyme activity to remove K63-linked ubiquitin chains from RIP1 (an essential mediator of the proximal TNF receptor 1 (TNFR1) signaling complex), and a C-terminal seven C2/C2 zinc finger domain as a ubiquitin ligase by polyubiquitinating RIP with K48-linked ubiquitin chains (Wertz et al. 2004). Thus, A20 removes activating chains of ubiquitin molecules linked together by a K63 linkage, and facilitates the addition of similar chains with a K48 linkage, thus targeting RIP1 for proteasomal degradation (Sun 2008). A20 zinc finger 4 (ZnF4) can bind mono-Ub and K63-linked poly-Ub (Bosanac et al. 2010). Recently, several A20-interacting proteins, including Itch, RNF11, and TAX1BP1 have been identified that regulate A20 function for control ubiquitination and proteasome-dependent degradation (Shembade et al. 2008; Shembade et al. 2010; Shembade et al. 2009). It was recently reported that A20 binds to TRAF6, thus disrupting its interactions with a key E2 enzyme Ubc13 or Ubc5 that controls activation of the IKK complex in different cell types (Shembade et al. 2010).

CYLD: The familial cylindromatosis tumor suppressor gene (*CYLD*) was originally identified as a tumor suppressor by detecting germline mutations in 21 cylindromatosis families and somatic mutations in 1 sporadic and 5 familial cylindroma cases (Bignell et al. 2000). CYLD contains a DUB domain with a deubiquitinase activity critically important for its inhibitory function in NF-κB signaling that removes lysine 63-linked ubiquitin chains from TRAF2 and inhibits NF-κB activation, thus negatively regulating NF-κB signaling (Brummelkamp et al. 2003; Kovalenko et al. 2003; Trompouki et al. 2003). CYLD-deficient mice are highly susceptible to chemically induced skin tumors. The elevated cyclin D1 in CYLD-deficient cells is caused by increased nuclear activity of Bcl-3-associated NF-κB p50 and p52 (Massoumi et al. 2006). It has been demonstrated that CYLD negatively regulates TLR- or TNF-α-induced NF-κB activation and type I IFN signaling by targeting TRAF2, TRAF6, RIP1, TAK1, NEMO, RIG-I, and TBK1 in T cells and other immune cells (Friedman et al. 2008; Lee et al. 2010; Reiley et al. 2007; Reiley et al. 2006; Sun 2008). The specificity of CYLD for targeting these important signaling proteins relies on its ubiquitin-specific protease (USP) domain that recognizes K63-linked polyubiquitin chains (Komander et al. 2008). Thus, it is likely that CYLD requires both USPs for recognizing ubiquitin chains on target proteins and DUB to remove the ubiquitin chains, thus blocking NF-κB and type I IFN signaling.

NLRX1: Although most NLRs are thought to function as intracellular receptors for detecting various microbial products/ligands, several NLRs have been identified as negative regulators of NF-κB activation. NLRX1 is a member of NLR protein family and contains an uncharacterized N-terminal X domain with mitochondria targeting signal, followed by NOD and LRR domains. NLRX1 was originally identified as a negative regulator of type I IFN signaling by targeting MAVS (Moore et al. 2008), and is involved in reactive oxygen species production in the mitochondria (Arnoult et al. 2009; Tattoli et al. 2008). NLRX1 enhances ROS production following infection with *chlamydial trachomatis* through NADPH oxidase (Abdul-Sater et al. 2010). Recently, we found that NLRX1 negatively regulates NF-κB signaling by interacting with TRAF6 and IKK complex in a signaling-dependent manner (Xia et al. 2011). NLRX1 interacts with TRAF6 in unstimulated cells. Upon LPS stimulation, NLRX1 is rapidly ubiquitinated, disassociates from TRAF6 and then binds to the IKK complex, resulting in inhibition of IKKα/IKKβ phosphorylation and NF-κB activation. Knockdown of NLRX1 in cells and in mice enhances IKK phosphorylation and NF-κB signaling, and produces more inflammatory cytokines such as IL-6, compared with wild type mice. NLRX1 knockdown in mice markedly enhances susceptibility to LPS-induced septic shock and plasma IL-6 levels (Xia et al. 2011), suggesting that NLRX1 is a negative regulator of NF-κB activation.

NLRC5: NLRC5 is another member of the NLR protein family, and contains a CARD domain at the N-terminus, a NOD domain at the center and a long LRR domain at the C-terminus. Unlike NLRX1, NLRC5 expression is up-regulated by many cytokines such as IFN-γ and TLR ligands such as LPS (Benko et al. 2010; Cui et al. 2010; Kuenzel et al. 2010). NLRC5 inhibits both NF-κB and type I IFN signaling (Cui et al. 2010) (Benko et al. 2010). Importantly, NLRC5 inhibits NF-κB activation by interacting with IKKα and IKKβ, but not NEMO, while it blocks type I IFN signaling by targeting RIG-I/MDA5, but not MAVS (Cui et al. 2010). Consistent with these results, knockdown of NLRC5 enhances IKK phosphorylation and secretion of inflammatory cytokines such as IL-6, TNF-α IL-1β, IL-10 and IFN-β (Benko et al. 2010; Cui et al. 2010). In addition, NLRC5 modulates inflammasome activation and functions as a transcriptional regulator of MHC class I genes (Davis et al.

2011; Meissner et al. 2010). NLRC5 is predominantly localized in the cytosol, but can shuttle between the cytosol and nucleus of a cell in a CrmA-dependent manner (Benko et al. 2010; Meissner et al. 2010). These studies indicate that NLRC5 may have multiple regulatory functions in innate and adaptive immune responses.

7.2 Regulators of the Type I IFN Signaling Pathway

Upon binding to viral RNA, RIG-I and MDA5 undergo conformational changes such that the CARD domain is exposed to recruit the mitochondrial adaptor protein MAVS, which in turn interacts with TRAF3 or STING (also known as MITA) (Ishikawa and Barber 2008; Saha et al. 2006; Zhong et al. 2008). A recent study shows that a cytosol DNA sensor IFI16 recruits STING, but not MAVS, for downstream signal activation of type I IFN pathway (Unterholzner et al. 2010). Thus, MAVS or STING acts as a scaffolding protein to recruit the kinase TBK1 to promote TBK1-IRF3 association, leading to phosphorylation and activation of IRF3 (Ishikawa and Barber 2008; Zhong et al. 2008). Because of its importance in antiviral immunity, many signaling molecules in the type I IFN pathway are tightly controlled by positive and negative regulators. Thus, we discuss these regulators at each molecular level (Fig. 6.5).

Regulators of RIG-I and MDA5: RIG-I and MDA5 are key receptors for detecting viral RNAs and induce potent type I IFN antiviral immunity. RIG-I is tightly regulated by multiple regulators, including TRIM25, Riplet and ZAPS (PARP-13 shorter isoform). TRIM25, Riplet, and ZAPS function as positive regulators for the type I IFN signaling pathway. TRIM25 mediates K63-linked polyubiquitination at Lys172 of RIG-I CARDs (Gack et al. 2007). K63-linked polyubiquitination induces interaction between RIG-I and MAVS CARD domains, leading to the activation of signaling (Gack et al. 2007), but its role in vivo remains to be determined. By contrast, Riplet deficiency abolishes RIG-I activation during RNA virus infection, and increases susceptibility to vesicular stomatitis virus infection (Oshiumi et al. 2010), suggesting that Riplet is essential for RIG-I-mediated antiviral immunity. ZAPS is found to be associated with RIG-I to promote the oligomerization and ATPase activity of RIG-I, leading to robust activation of IRF3. Disruption of ZAPS results in impaired induction of interferon and other cytokines after viral infection (Hayakawa et al. 2010), indicating that ZAPS is a key regulator of RIG-I signaling during the innate antiviral immune response. Interestingly, RIG-I CARDs are required for binding to the unanchored K63-linked polyubiquitin chains for RIG-I activation (Zeng et al. 2010). On the other hand, RNF125 and NLRC5 serve as negative regulators of RIG-I-mediated signaling. Specifically, RNF125 mediates K48-linked polyubiquitination of RIG-I, leading to protein degradation by the proteasome (Arimoto et al. 2007). We recently showed that NLRC5 inhibits type I IFN signaling by interacting with RIG-I and MDA5, thus blocking their interactions with MAVS (Cui et al. 2010).

Regulators of MAVS: MAVS is critical in innate antiviral immunity as the key adaptor for RIG-I and MDA5. NLRX1 negatively regulates type I IFN signaling by interacting with MAVS (Moore et al. 2008). A recent study identifies PCBP2 as another negative regulator in MAVS-mediated type I IFN signaling. PCBP2 interacts with MAVS and recruits a HECT domain-containing E3 ligase AIP4 to ubiquitinate MAVS for proteasomal degradation (You et al. 2009), suggesting that PCBP2-AIP4 negatively controls MAVS for the "fine tuning" of antiviral innate immunity.

Regulators of STING: STING was recently identified as a critical adaptor molecule for NF-κB and type I IFN signaling (Ishikawa and Barber 2008; Zhong et al. 2008). STING ablation abrogates the ability of intracellular DNA, as well as members of the herpes virus family to induce IFN-β, but did not significantly affect the TLR pathway (Ishikawa et al. 2009). STING is required for transduction of a signal from DNA sensor IFI16 to TBK1 (Unterholzner et al. 2010). STING protein is controlled by RNF5 and interferon-inducible tripartite-motif (TRIM) 56 through ubiquitination of the same amino acid. RNF5 ubiqitinates STING with a K48-linked ubiquitin chain for protein degradation. Virus-induced ubiquitination and degradation of STING by RNF5 occurred in the mitochondria (Zhong et al. 2009). These findings suggest that RNF5 negatively regulates virus-triggered signaling by targeting STING for ubiquitination and degradation at the mitochondria. By contrast, TRIM56 interacts with STING and targets it for K63 linked ubiquitination (Tsuchida et al. 2010). Overexpression of TRIM56 enhances IFN-beta promoter activation after double-stranded DNA stimulation, whereas TRIM56 knockdown reduces its activity (Tsuchida et al. 2010), thus serving as a positive regulator of DNA-mediated innate type I IFN immune responses.

Regulators of TRAF3: Deubiquitynating enzyme A (DUBA, also known as OTUD5) was found to remove K63-linked polyubiquitin chains of TRAF3, but not TRAF6, thus functioning as a negative regulator of type I IFN signaling pathway (Kayagaki et al. 2007). However, its physiological relevance to negative regulation of type I IFN signaling has not been determined. A recent study shows that IL-1R regulates DUBA expression and is essential for TLR9-dependent activation of TRAF3 and for production of the anti-inflammatory cytokines IL-10 and type I IFN. DUBA is up-regulated in the absence of IL-1R1 signaling (Gonzalez-Navajas et al. 2010).

Regulators of TBK1/IKKi: It is known that TBK1 can interact with several proteins, including TANK (TRAF family member-associated NF-κB activator), NAP1 (NAK-associated protein) and SINTBAD (similar to NAP1 TBK1 adaptor) for its activation (Chau et al. 2008). Although NAP1 and SINTBAD are important for TBK1 activation (Ryzhakov and Randow 2007), a recent study with TANK-deficient mice suggests that TANK is not involved in interferon responses and is a negative regulator of proinflammatory cytokine production induced by TLR signaling by possibly interacting with TRAF6 (Kawagoe et al. 2009). Both MAVS and STING can interact with TBK1, which further phosphorylates and activates IRF3 for type I IFN-responsive gene expression. It has been demonstrated that TBK1 and NF-κB signaling play critical roles in *Kras*-mediated tumor development (Barbie et al. 2009; Meylan et al. 2009). Thus, tight control of TBK1 protein is important for inflammation and cancer development. Recently, GSK3β was shown to interact with TBK1 in a viral infection-dependent manner. GSK3β enhances TBK1 self-association and autophosphorylation at Ser172, which is critical for virus-induced IRF3 activation and IFN-β induction. By contrast, we recently found that NLRP4 inhibits type 1 IFN signaling by targeting TBK1 for degradation (unpublished data). These studies suggest that both positive and negative regulators control TBK1 activation and protein level.

Regulators of IRF3/IRF7: IRF3 and IRF7 are master transcriptional factors that control type I IFN genes (IFN-α and IFN-β) expression and antiviral immunity (Honda and Taniguchi 2006). While IRF3 is activated by TLR3 and TLR4 ligand stimulation, IRF7 is induced by TLR7 and TLR9 and essential for type I IFN-responsive gene expression in conventional DCs. IRF7 is constitutively expressed in pDCs (Honda and Taniguchi 2006). Thus, the balance between activated IRF3/7 and degradation is important to type I IFN signaling. It has been reported that the KSHV immediate-early lytic cycle triggers protein RTA (RNA transcriptional activator) that can target IRF7 for degradation (Yu et al. 2005). A recent study shows that RAUL, (an RTA-associated E3 ubiquitin ligase, also known as KIAA10 or UBE3C) regulates type I IFN by targeting both IRF7 and IRF3 for lysine 48-linked ubiquitination and degradation (Yu and Hayward 2010). Furthermore, RAUL is positively regulated by a deubiquitinating enzyme ubiquitin-specific processing protease 7 (Usp7, also known as HAUSP) (Yu and Hayward 2010). Thus, both viral protein RTA and cellular RAUL E3 ligases play a critical role in the negative regulation of host antiviral immunity.

8 Innate Immunity Links Inflammation and Cancer

Activation of the innate immune response (in particular the NF-κB pathway and inflammasome), through TLR-mediated recognition of invading pathogens or damaged tissues, serves as a link between chronic inflammation and cancer (Clevers 2004; Condeelis and Pollard 2006; Greten et al. 2004; Karin and Greten 2005). There is increasing evidence showing chronic inflammation as a major driving force in cancer development (De Marzo et al. 2007; El-Omar et al. 2008; Haverkamp et al. 2008). It has been estimated that chronic infection or chronic inflammation has caused about 20% of human cancers (Coussens and Werb 2002; De Marzo et al. 2007). For example, chronic inflammation induced by *Helicobacter pylori* infection is the leading cause of stomach cancer, while inflammatory bowel diseases including ulcerative colitis and Crohn's disease are closely associated with colon cancer (Coussens and Werb 2002; Karin et al. 2006). Similarly, hepatitis B virus (HBV) and HCV infection of liver cells is a primary factor in the development of liver cancer (Coussens and Werb 2002; Karin et al. 2006; Peto

2001). Recent studies have found a significant association between prostate cancer and TLR4 sequence variants, suggesting that TLR sequence polymorphism is an important risk factor for prostate cancer (El-Omar et al. 2008; Sun et al. 2005; Zheng et al. 2004). One possible interpretation of these results is that innate immune receptors are sensors of immune cells including macrophages, DCs and T cells, and the activation of these receptors by bacteria, viruses, or damaged tissues can stimulate the NF-κB pathway, type I IFN and/or inflammasome pathways to secrete proinflammatory cytokines. Thus, chronic inflammation is linked to cancer through innate receptors-mediated cytokines and inflammatory cells (Greten et al. 2004; Lin and Karin 2007; Luo et al. 2004; Maeda et al. 2005b; Pikarsky et al. 2004).

Recent studies show that TLR-mediated signaling is required for damage or tissue repair. MyD88-deficient mice are susceptible to cytotoxic agent dextran sulfate sodium (DSS) (Rakoff-Nahoum et al. 2004). Pretreatment of MyD88-deficient mice with commensal bacteria enhances their ability to repair tissue and survive after DSS treatment. Similarly, ASC1 KO, caspase-1 KO, and NLRP3 KO mice are susceptible to DSS-induce tissue injury (Allen et al. 2010; Dupaul-Chicoine et al. 2010; Zaki et al. 2010). Recent studies demonstrate the important role of MyD88 in tumor development and promotion. For example, MyD88 deficiency reduces the incidence of cancer in mice with heterozygous mutation in the adenomatous polyposis coli ($APC^{min/+}$) background and in an AOM-DSS-induced colon cancer model (Rakoff-Nahoum and Medzhitov 2007). MyD88 deficiency also reduces chemically induced skin cancer or liver cancer development (Naugler et al. 2007; Swann et al. 2008). These studies suggest that MyD88-mediated signaling plays a critical role in promoting tumor development and progression. However, a recent study shows that MyD88 deficiency increases tumor incidence in AOM-DSS-induced model, due to the reduced ability to heal ulcers and repair DNA damage (Salcedo et al. 2010). Similarly, NLRP3 deficiency also increases tumor incidence and development (Allen et al. 2010; Dupaul-Chicoine et al. 2010). These studies indicate that innate immune signaling-mediated inflammation may have more complicated roles in tissue injury/damage repair and tumor development.

9 Mutations in Signaling Adaptors and Regulators in Cancer

NOD2 mutation has been found to be associated with inflammation-linked colitis and cancer (Hugot et al. 2001; Ogura et al. 2001). NOD2 mutations increase NF-κB activation and IL-1beta secretion (Maeda et al. 2005a). More recently, mutations in A20 have been identified in lymphoma (Kato et al. 2009; Schmitz et al. 2009), while CYLD mutations have been identified (Kovalenko et al. 2003). Thus, both A20 and CYLD function as tumor suppressors and inhibit tumor development. TBK1 is a key molecule for both the type IFN and NF-κB pathways and has been shown to play a critical role in cancer development (Barbie et al. 2009; Meylan et al. 2009).

10 Conclusions

Since their discovery a decade ago, TLRs have been shown to be critical for efficient innate and adaptive immunity and the framework of TLR-mediated signaling pathways has been elucidated. In contrast, many NLRs, their recognized ligands and their signaling pathways remain to be determined. These innate immune receptors are clearly important in host response against infectious diseases and autoimmune diseases. Thus the role of NLRs and RLRs in cancer immunosurveillance remains to be determined. Increasing evidence indicates that immune suppression and inflammation in the tumor microenvironment is a major obstacle to the development of effective therapeutic cancer vaccines. Understanding of innate immune receptor-mediated signaling, cytokine production and their regulatory mechanisms of adaptive immune responses in cancer will be critically important for development of effective therapeutic drugs for cancer treatment and prevention.

Acknowledgements This work is in part supported by grants from National Institutes of Health and Cancer Research Institute.

References

Abdul-Sater AA, Said-Sadier N, Lam VM, Singh B, Pettengill MA, Soares F, Tattoli I, Lipinski S, Girardin SE, Rosenstiel P et al (2010) Enhancement of reactive oxygen species production and chlamydial infection by the mitochondrial Nod-like family member NLRX1. J Biol Chem 285:41637–41645

Akira S, Takeda K (2004) Toll-like receptor signalling. Nat Rev Immunol 4:499–511

Akira S, Uematsu S, Takeuchi O (2006) Pathogen recognition and innate immunity. Cell 124:783–801

Alexander WS, Hilton DJ (2004) The role of suppressors of cytokine signaling (SOCS) proteins in regulation of the immune response. Annu Rev Immunol 22:503–529

Alexander WS, Starr R, Fenner JE, Scott CL, Handman E, Sprigg NS, Corbin JE, Cornish AL, Darwiche R, Owczarek CM et al (1999) SOCS1 is a critical inhibitor of interferon gamma signaling and prevents the potentially fatal neonatal actions of this cytokine. Cell 98:597–608

Allen IC, TeKippe EM, Woodford RM, Uronis JM, Holl EK, Rogers AB, Herfarth HH, Jobin C, Ting JP (2010) The NLRP3 inflammasome functions as a negative regulator of tumorigenesis during colitis-associated cancer. J Exp Med 207:1045–1056

Arimoto K, Takahashi H, Hishiki T, Konishi H, Fujita T, Shimotohno K (2007) Negative regulation of the RIG-I signaling by the ubiquitin ligase RNF125. Proc Natl Acad Sci USA 104: 7500–7505

Arnoult D, Soares F, Tattoli I, Castanier C, Philpott DJ, Girardin SE (2009) An N-terminal addressing sequence targets NLRX1 to the mitochondrial matrix. J Cell Sci 122:3161–3168

Asagiri M, Hirai T, Kunigami T, Kamano S, Gober HJ, Okamoto K, Nishikawa K, Latz E, Golenbock DT, Aoki K et al (2008) Cathepsin K-dependent toll-like receptor 9 signaling revealed in experimental arthritis. Science 319:624–627

Barbie DA, Tamayo P, Boehm JS, Kim SY, Moody SE, Dunn IF, Schinzel AC, Sandy P, Meylan E, Scholl C et al (2009) Systematic RNA interference reveals that oncogenic KRAS-driven cancers require TBK1. Nature 462:108–112

Barton GM, Kagan JC, Medzhitov R (2006) Intracellular localization of Toll-like receptor 9 prevents recognition of self DNA but facilitates access to viral DNA. Nat Immunol 7:49–56

Becker CE, O'Neill LA (2007) Inflammasomes in inflammatory disorders: the role of TLRs and their interactions with NLRs. Semin Immunopathol 29:239–248

Benko S, Magalhaes JG, Philpott DJ, Girardin SE (2010) NLRC5 Limits the Activation of Inflammatory Pathways. J Immunol 185:1681–1691

Bignell GR, Warren W, Seal S, Takahashi M, Rapley E, Barfoot R, Green H, Brown C, Biggs PJ, Lakhani SR et al (2000) Identification of the familial cylindromatosis tumour-suppressor gene. Nat Genet 25:160–165

Bosanac I, Wertz IE, Pan B, Yu C, Kusam S, Lam C, Phu L, Phung Q, Maurer B, Arnott D et al (2010) Ubiquitin binding to A20 ZnF4 is required for modulation of NF-kappaB signaling. Mol Cell 40:548–557

Brummelkamp TR, Nijman SM, Dirac AM, Bernards R (2003) Loss of the cylindromatosis tumour suppressor inhibits apoptosis by activating NF-kappaB. Nature 424:797–801

Burckstummer T, Baumann C, Bluml S, Dixit E, Durnberger G, Jahn H, Planyavsky M, Bilban M, Colinge J, Bennett KL (2009) An orthogonal proteomic-genomic screen identifies AIM2 as a cytoplasmic DNA sensor for the inflammasome. Nat Immunol

Chau TL, Gioia R, Gatot JS, Patrascu F, Carpentier I, Chapelle JP, O'Neill L, Beyaert R, Piette J, Chariot A (2008) Are the IKKs and IKK-related kinases TBK1 and IKK-epsilon similarly activated? Trends Biochem Sci 33:171–180

Chen G, Shaw MH, Kim YG, Nunez G (2009) NOD-like receptors: role in innate immunity and inflammatory disease. Annu Rev Pathol 4:365–398

Choe J, Kelker MS, Wilson IA (2005) Crystal structure of human toll-like receptor 3 (TLR3) ectodomain. Science 309:581–585

Chuang TH, Ulevitch RJ (2004) Triad3A, an E3 ubiquitin-protein ligase regulating Toll-like receptors. Nat Immunol 5:495–502

Clevers H (2004) At the crossroads of inflammation and cancer. Cell 118:671–674

Condeelis J, Pollard JW (2006) Macrophages: obligate partners for tumor cell migration, invasion, and metastasis. Cell 124:263–266

Cooney R, Baker J, Brain O, Danis B, Pichulik T, Allan P, Ferguson DJ, Campbell BJ, Jewell D, Simmons A (2010) NOD2 stimulation induces autophagy in dendritic cells influencing bacterial handling and antigen presentation. Nat Med 16:90–97

Coussens LM, Werb Z (2002) Inflammation and cancer. Nature 420:860–867

Cui J, Zhu L, Xia X, Wang HY, Legras X, Hong J, Ji J, Shen P, Zheng S, Chen ZJ et al (2010) NLRC5 negatively regulates the NF-kappaB and type I interferon signaling pathways. Cell 141:483–496

Davis BK, Roberts RA, Huang MT, Willingham SB, Conti BJ, Brickey WJ, Barker BR, Kwan M, Taxman DJ, Accavitti-Loper MA et al (2011) Cutting Edge: NLRC5-Dependent Activation of the Inflammasome. J Immunol 186:1333–1337

De Marzo AM, Platz EA, Sutcliffe S, Xu J, Gronberg H, Drake CG, Nakai Y, Isaacs WB, Nelson WG (2007) Inflammation in prostate carcinogenesis. Nat Rev Cancer 7:256–269

Deng JC, Cheng G, Newstead MW, Zeng X, Kobayashi K, Flavell RA, Standiford TJ (2006) Sepsis-induced suppression of lung innate immunity is mediated by IRAK-M. J Clin Invest 116:2532–2542

Diebold SS, Kaisho T, Hemmi H, Akira S, Reis e Sousa C (2004) Innate antiviral responses by means of TLR7-mediated recognition of single-stranded RNA. Science 303:1529–1531

Dostert C, Petrilli V, Van Bruggen R, Steele C, Mossman BT, Tschopp J (2008) Innate immune activation through Nalp3 inflammasome sensing of asbestos and silica. Science 320:674–677

Duncan JA, Bergstralh DT, Wang Y, Willingham SB, Ye Z, Zimmermann AG, Ting JP (2007) Cryopyrin/NALP3 binds ATP/dATP, is an ATPase, and requires ATP binding to mediate inflammatory signaling. Proc Natl Acad Sci USA 104:8041–8046

Dupaul-Chicoine J, Yeretssian G, Doiron K, Bergstrom KS, McIntire CR, LeBlanc PM, Meunier C, Turbide C, Gros P, Beauchemin N et al (2010) Control of intestinal homeostasis, colitis, and colitis-associated colorectal cancer by the inflammatory caspases. Immunity 32:367–378

Eisenbarth SC, Colegio OR, O'Connor W, Sutterwala FS, Flavell RA (2008) Crucial role for the Nalp3 inflammasome in the immunostimulatory properties of aluminium adjuvants. Nature 453:1122–1126

El-Omar EM, Ng MT, Hold GL (2008) Polymorphisms in Toll-like receptor genes and risk of cancer. Oncogene 27:244–252

Ewald SE, Lee BL, Lau L, Wickliffe KE, Shi GP, Chapman HA, Barton GM (2008) The ectodomain of Toll-like receptor 9 is cleaved to generate a functional receptor. Nature 456:658–662

Ewald SE, Engel A, Lee J, Wang M, Bogyo M, Barton GM (2011) Nucleic acid recognition by Toll-like receptors is coupled to stepwise processing by cathepsins and asparagine endopeptidase. J Exp Med

Fernandes-Alnemri T, Yu JW, Datta P, Wu J, Alnemri ES (2009) AIM2 activates the inflammasome and cell death in response to cytoplasmic DNA. Nature

Fernandes-Alnemri T, Yu JW, Juliana C, Solorzano L, Kang S, Wu J, Datta P, McCormick M, Huang L, McDermott E et al (2010) The AIM2 inflammasome is critical for innate immunity to Francisella tularensis. Nat Immunol 11:385–393

Friedman CS, O'Donnell MA, Legarda-Addison D, Ng A, Cardenas WB, Yount JS, Moran TM, Basler CF, Komuro A, Horvath CM et al (2008) The tumour suppressor CYLD is a negative regulator of RIG-I-mediated antiviral response. EMBO Rep 9:930–936

Gack MU, Shin YC, Joo CH, Urano T, Liang C, Sun L, Takeuchi O, Akira S, Chen Z, Inoue S et al (2007) TRIM25 RING-finger E3 ubiquitin ligase is essential for RIG-I-mediated antiviral activity. Nature 446:916–920

Gonzalez-Navajas JM, Law J, Nguyen KP, Bhargava M, Corr MP, Varki N, Eckmann L, Hoffman HM, Lee J, Raz E (2010) Interleukin 1 receptor signaling regulates DUBA expression and facilitates Toll-like receptor 9-driven antiinflammatory cytokine production. J Exp Med 207:2799–2807

Greten FR, Eckmann L, Greten TF, Park JM, Li ZW, Egan LJ, Kagnoff MF, Karin M (2004) IKKbeta links inflammation and tumorigenesis in a mouse model of colitis-associated cancer. Cell 118:285–296

Gulen MF, Kang Z, Bulek K, Youzhong W, Kim TW, Chen Y, Altuntas CZ, Sass Bak-Jensen K, McGeachy MJ, Do JS et al (2010) The receptor SIGIRR suppresses Th17 cell proliferation via inhibition of the interleukin-1 receptor pathway and mTOR kinase activation. Immunity 32:54–66

Haverkamp J, Charbonneau B, Ratliff TL (2008) Prostate inflammation and its potential impact on prostate cancer: a current review. J Cell Biochem 103:1344–1353

Hayakawa S, Shiratori S, Yamato H, Kameyama T, Kitatsuji C, Kashigi F, Goto S, Kameoka S, Fujikura D, Yamada T et al (2010) ZAPS is a potent stimulator of signaling mediated by the RNA helicase RIG-I during antiviral responses. Nat Immunol 12:37–44

Heil F, Hemmi H, Hochrein H, Ampenberger F, Kirschning C, Akira S, Lipford G, Wagner H, Bauer S (2004) Species-specific recognition of single-stranded RNA via toll-like receptor 7 and 8. Science 303:1526–1529

Hemmi H, Kaisho T, Takeuchi O, Sato S, Sanjo H, Hoshino K, Horiuchi T, Tomizawa H, Takeda K, Akira S (2002) Small anti-viral compounds activate immune cells via the TLR7 MyD88-dependent signaling pathway. Nat Immunol 3:196–200

Honda K, Taniguchi T (2006) IRFs: master regulators of signalling by Toll-like receptors and cytosolic pattern-recognition receptors. Nat Rev Immunol 6:644–658

Honda K, Ohba Y, Yanai H, Negishi H, Mizutani T, Takaoka A, Taya C, Taniguchi T (2005a) Spatiotemporal regulation of MyD88-IRF-7 signalling for robust type-I interferon induction. Nature 434:1035–1040

Honda K, Yanai H, Negishi H, Asagiri M, Sato M, Mizutani T, Shimada N, Ohba Y, Takaoka A, Yoshida N et al (2005b) IRF-7 is the master regulator of type-I interferon-dependent immune responses. Nature 434:772–777

Hornung V, Ellegast J, Kim S, Brzozka K, Jung A, Kato H, Poeck H, Akira S, Conzelmann KK, Schlee M et al (2006) 5'-Triphosphate RNA is the ligand for RIG-I. Science 314:994–997

Hornung V, Ablasser A, Charrel-Dennis M, Bauernfeind F, Horvath G, Caffrey DR, Latz E, Fitzgerald KA (2009) AIM2 recognizes cytosolic dsDNA and forms a caspase-1-activating inflammasome with ASC. Nature

Hugot JP, Chamaillard M, Zouali H, Lesage S, Cezard JP, Belaiche J, Almer S, Tysk C, O'Morain CA, Gassull M et al (2001) Association of NOD2 leucine-rich repeat variants with susceptibility to Crohn's disease. Nature 411:599–603

Inohara C, McDonald C, Nunez G (2005) NOD-LRR proteins: role in host-microbial interactions and inflammatory disease. Annu Rev Biochem 74:355–383

Ishikawa H, Barber GN (2008) STING is an endoplasmic reticulum adaptor that facilitates innate immune signalling. Nature 455:674–678

Ishikawa H, Ma Z, Barber GN (2009) STING regulates intracellular DNA-mediated, type I interferon-dependent innate immunity. Nature 461:788–792

Iwasaki A, Medzhitov R (2004) Toll-like receptor control of the adaptive immune responses. Nat Immunol 5:987–995

Janssens S, Beyaert R (2003) Functional diversity and regulation of different interleukin-1 receptor-associated kinase (IRAK) family members. Mol Cell 11:293–302

Jurk M, Heil F, Vollmer J, Schetter C, Krieg AM, Wagner H, Lipford G, Bauer S (2002) Human TLR7 or TLR8 independently confer responsiveness to the antiviral compound R-848. Nat Immunol 3:499

Kanneganti TD, Ozoren N, Body-Malapel M, Amer A, Park JH, Franchi L, Whitfield J, Barchet W, Colonna M, Vandenabeele P et al (2006) Bacterial RNA and small antiviral compounds activate caspase-1 through cryopyrin/Nalp3. Nature 440:233–236

Karin M, Greten FR (2005) NF-kappaB: linking inflammation and immunity to cancer development and progression. Nat Rev Immunol 5:749–759

Karin M, Lawrence T, Nizet V (2006) Innate immunity gone awry: linking microbial infections to chronic inflammation and cancer. Cell 124:823–835

Kato H, Sato S, Yoneyama M, Yamamoto M, Uematsu S, Matsui K, Tsujimura T, Takeda K, Fujita T, Takeuchi O et al (2005) Cell type-specific involvement of RIG-I in antiviral response. Immunity 23:19–28

Kato H, Takeuchi O, Sato S, Yoneyama M, Yamamoto M, Matsui K, Uematsu S, Jung A, Kawai T, Ishii KJ et al (2006) Differential roles of MDA5 and RIG-I helicases in the recognition of RNA viruses. Nature 441:101–105

Kato H, Takeuchi O, Mikamo-Satoh E, Hirai R, Kawai T, Matsushita K, Hiiragi A, Dermody TS, Fujita T, Akira S (2008) Length-dependent recognition of double-stranded ribonucleic acids by retinoic acid-inducible gene-I and melanoma differentiation-associated gene 5. J Exp Med 205:1601–1610

Kato M, Sanada M, Kato I, Sato Y, Takita J, Takeuchi K, Niwa A, Chen Y, Nakazaki K, Nomoto J et al (2009) Frequent inactivation of A20 in B-cell lymphomas. Nature 459:712–716

Kawagoe T, Takeuchi O, Takabatake Y, Kato H, Isaka Y, Tsujimura T, Akira S (2009) TANK is a negative regulator of Toll-like receptor signaling and is critical for the prevention of autoimmune nephritis. Nat Immunol 10:965–972

Kawai T, Takahashi K, Sato S, Coban C, Kumar H, Kato H, Ishii KJ, Takeuchi O, Akira S (2005) IPS-1, an adaptor triggering RIG-I- and Mda5-mediated type I interferon induction. Nat Immunol 6:981–988

Kayagaki N, Phung Q, Chan S, Chaudhari R, Quan C, O'Rourke KM, Eby M, Pietras E, Cheng G, Bazan JF et al (2007) DUBA: a deubiquitinase that regulates type I interferon production. Science 318:1628–1632

Kerur N, Veettil MV, Sharma-Walia N, Bottero V, Sadagopan S, Otageri P, Chandran B (2011) IFI16 Acts as a Nuclear Pathogen Sensor to Induce the Inflammasome in Response to Kaposi Sarcoma-Associated Herpesvirus Infection. Cell Host Microbe 9:363–375

Kim YM, Brinkmann MM, Paquet ME, Ploegh HL (2008) UNC93B1 delivers nucleotide-sensing toll-like receptors to endolysosomes. Nature 452:234–238

Kinjyo I, Hanada T, Inagaki-Ohara K, Mori H, Aki D, Ohishi M, Yoshida H, Kubo M, Yoshimura A (2002) SOCS1/JAB is a negative regulator of LPS-induced macrophage activation. Immunity 17:583–591

Kobayashi K, Hernandez LD, Galan JE, Janeway CA Jr, Medzhitov R, Flavell RA (2002) IRAK-M is a negative regulator of Toll-like receptor signaling. Cell 110:191–202

Komander D, Lord CJ, Scheel H, Swift S, Hofmann K, Ashworth A, Barford D (2008) The structure of the CYLD USP domain explains its specificity for Lys63-linked polyubiquitin and reveals a B box module. Mol Cell 29:451–464

Kovalenko A, Chable-Bessia C, Cantarella G, Israel A, Wallach D, Courtois G (2003) The tumour suppressor CYLD negatively regulates NF-kappaB signalling by deubiquitination. Nature 424:801–805

Kuenzel S, Till A, Winkler M, Hasler R, Lipinski S, Jung S, Grotzinger J, Fickenscher H, Schreiber S, Rosenstiel P (2010) The nucleotide-binding oligomerization domain-like receptor NLRC5 is involved in IFN-dependent antiviral immune responses. J Immunol 184:1990–2000

Lee EG, Boone DL, Chai S, Libby SL, Chien M, Lodolce JP, Ma A (2000) Failure to regulate TNF-induced NF-kappaB and cell death responses in A20-deficient mice. Science 289:2350–2354

Lee AJ, Zhou X, Chang M, Hunzeker J, Bonneau RH, Zhou D, Sun SC (2010) Regulation of natural killer T-cell development by deubiquitinase CYLD. EMBO J 29:1600–1612

Lin WW, Karin M (2007) A cytokine-mediated link between innate immunity, inflammation, and cancer. J Clin Invest 117:1175–1183

Loo YM, Fornek J, Crochet N, Bajwa G, Perwitasari O, Martinez-Sobrido L, Akira S, Gill MA, Garcia-Sastre A, Katze MG et al (2008) Distinct RIG-I and MDA5 signaling by RNA viruses in innate immunity. J Virol 82:335–345

Lund JM, Alexopoulou L, Sato A, Karow M, Adams NC, Gale NW, Iwasaki A, Flavell RA (2004) Recognition of single-stranded RNA viruses by Toll-like receptor 7. Proc Natl Acad Sci USA 101:5598–5603

Luo JL, Maeda S, Hsu LC, Yagita H, Karin M (2004) Inhibition of NF-kappaB in cancer cells converts inflammation- induced tumor growth mediated by TNFalpha to TRAIL-mediated tumor regression. Cancer Cell 6:297–305

Maeda S, Hsu LC, Liu H, Bankston LA, Iimura M, Kagnoff MF, Eckmann L, Karin M (2005a) Nod2 mutation in Crohn's disease potentiates NF-kappaB activity and IL-1beta processing. Science 307:734–738

Maeda S, Kamata H, Luo JL, Leffert H, Karin M (2005b) IKKbeta couples hepatocyte death to cytokine-driven compensatory proliferation that promotes chemical hepatocarcinogenesis. Cell 121:977–990

Mariathasan S, Monack DM (2007) Inflammasome adaptors and sensors: intracellular regulators of infection and inflammation. Nat Rev Immunol 7:31–40

Mariathasan S, Weiss DS, Newton K, McBride J, O'Rourke K, Roose-Girma M, Lee WP, Weinrauch Y, Monack DM, Dixit VM (2006) Cryopyrin activates the inflammasome in response to toxins and ATP. Nature 440:228–232

Marine JC, Topham DJ, McKay C, Wang D, Parganas E, Stravopodis D, Yoshimura A, Ihle JN (1999) SOCS1 deficiency causes a lymphocyte-dependent perinatal lethality. Cell 98:609–616

Martinon F, Tschopp J (2005) NLRs join TLRs as innate sensors of pathogens. Trends Immunol 26:447–454

Martinon F, Petrilli V, Mayor A, Tardivel A, Tschopp J (2006) Gout-associated uric acid crystals activate the NALP3 inflammasome. Nature 440:237–241

Massoumi R, Chmielarska K, Hennecke K, Pfeifer A, Fassler R (2006) Cyld inhibits tumor cell proliferation by blocking Bcl-3-dependent NF-kappaB signaling. Cell 125:665–677

Masters SL, Dunne A, Subramanian SL, Hull RL, Tannahill GM, Sharp FA, Becker C, Franchi L, Yoshihara E, Chen Z et al (2010) Activation of the NLRP3 inflammasome by islet amyloid polypeptide provides a mechanism for enhanced IL-1beta in type 2 diabetes. Nat Immunol 11:897–904

Meissner TB, Li A, Biswas A, Lee KH, Liu YJ, Bayir E, Iliopoulos D, van den Elsen PJ, Kobayashi KS (2010) NLR family member NLRC5 is a transcriptional regulator of MHC class I genes. Proc Natl Acad Sci USA

Meylan E, Curran J, Hofmann K, Moradpour D, Binder M, Bartenschlager R, Tschopp J (2005) Cardif is an adaptor protein in the RIG-I antiviral pathway and is targeted by hepatitis C virus. Nature 437:1167–1172

Meylan E, Dooley AL, Feldser DM, Shen L, Turk E, Ouyang C, Jacks T (2009) Requirement for NF-kappaB signalling in a mouse model of lung adenocarcinoma. Nature 462:104–107

Moore CB, Bergstralh DT, Duncan JA, Lei Y, Morrison TE, Zimmermann AG, Accavitti-Loper MA, Madden VJ, Sun L, Ye Z et al (2008) NLRX1 is a regulator of mitochondrial antiviral immunity. Nature 451:573–577

Nakagawa R, Naka T, Tsutsui H, Fujimoto M, Kimura A, Abe T, Seki E, Sato S, Takeuchi O, Takeda K et al (2002) SOCS-1 participates in negative regulation of LPS responses. Immunity 17:677–687

Nakahira K, Haspel JA, Rathinam VA, Lee SJ, Dolinay T, Lam HC, Englert JA, Rabinovitch M, Cernadas M, Kim HP et al (2011) Autophagy proteins regulate innate immune responses by inhibiting the release of mitochondrial DNA mediated by the NALP3 inflammasome. Nat Immunol 12:222–230

Naugler WE, Sakurai T, Kim S, Maeda S, Kim K, Elsharkawy AM, Karin M (2007) Gender disparity in liver cancer due to sex differences in MyD88-dependent IL-6 production. Science 317:121–124

Neerincx A, Lautz K, Menning M, Kremmer E, Zigrino P, Hosel M, Buning H, Schwarzenbacher R, Kufer TA (2010) A role for the human nucleotide-binding domain, leucine-rich repeat-containing family member NLRC5 in antiviral responses. J Biol Chem 285:26223–26232

Ogura Y, Bonen DK, Inohara N, Nicolae DL, Chen FF, Ramos R, Britton H, Moran T, Karaliuskas R, Duerr RH et al (2001) A frameshift mutation in NOD2 associated with susceptibility to Crohn's disease. Nature 411:603–606

Opipari AW Jr, Boguski MS, Dixit VM (1990) The A20 cDNA induced by tumor necrosis factor alpha encodes a novel type of zinc finger protein. J Biol Chem 265:14705–14708

Oshiumi H, Miyashita M, Inoue N, Okabe M, Matsumoto M, Seya T (2010) The Ubiquitin Ligase Riplet Is Essential for RIG-I-Dependent Innate Immune Responses to RNA Virus Infection. Cell Host Microbe 8:496–509

Park B, Brinkmann MM, Spooner E, Lee CC, Kim YM, Ploegh HL (2008) Proteolytic cleavage in an endolysosomal compartment is required for activation of Toll-like receptor 9. Nat Immunol 9:1407–1414

Peng G, Guo Z, Kiniwa Y, Voo KS, Peng W, Fu T, Wang DY, Li Y, Wang HY, Wang R-F (2005) Toll-like receptor 8 mediated-reversal of CD4+ regulatory T cell function. Science 309:1380–1384

Peng G, Wang HY, Peng W, Kiniwa Y, Seo K, Wang R-F (2007) Tumor-infiltrating gamma-delta T cells suppress T and dendritic cell function via mechanisms controlled by a unique Toll-like receptor signaling pathway. Immunity 27:334–348

Peto J (2001) Cancer epidemiology in the last century and the next decade. Nature 411:390–395

Pichlmair A, Schulz O, Tan CP, Naslund TI, Liljestrom P, Weber F, Reis e Sousa C (2006) RIG-I-mediated antiviral responses to single-stranded RNA bearing 5'-phosphates. Science 314:997–1001

Pikarsky E, Porat RM, Stein I, Abramovitch R, Amit S, Kasem S, Gutkovich-Pyest E, Urieli-Shoval S, Galun E, Ben-Neriah Y (2004) NF-kappaB functions as a tumour promoter in inflammation-associated cancer. Nature 431:461–466

Rakoff-Nahoum S, Medzhitov R (2007) Regulation of spontaneous intestinal tumorigenesis through the adaptor protein MyD88. Science 317:124–127

Rakoff-Nahoum S, Paglino J, Eslami-Varzaneh F, Edberg S, Medzhitov R (2004) Recognition of commensal microflora by toll-like receptors is required for intestinal homeostasis. Cell 118:229–241

Rathinam VA, Jiang Z, Waggoner SN, Sharma S, Cole LE, Waggoner L, Vanaja SK, Monks BG, Ganesan S, Latz E et al (2010) The AIM2 inflammasome is essential for host defense against cytosolic bacteria and DNA viruses. Nat Immunol 11:395–402

Rehwinkel J, Tan CP, Goubau D, Schulz O, Pichlmair A, Bier K, Robb N, Vreede F, Barclay W, Fodor E et al (2010) RIG-I detects viral genomic RNA during negative-strand RNA virus infection. Cell 140:397–408

Reiley WW, Zhang M, Jin W, Losiewicz M, Donohue KB, Norbury CC, Sun SC (2006) Regulation of T cell development by the deubiquitinating enzyme CYLD. Nat Immunol 7:411–417

Reiley WW, Jin W, Lee AJ, Wright A, Wu X, Tewalt EF, Leonard TO, Norbury CC, Fitzpatrick L, Zhang M et al (2007) Deubiquitinating enzyme CYLD negatively regulates the ubiquitin-dependent kinase Tak1 and prevents abnormal T cell responses. J Exp Med 204:1475–1485

Roberts TL, Idris A, Dunn JA, Kelly GM, Burnton CM, Hodgson S, Hardy LL, Garceau V, Sweet MJ, Ross IL (2009) HIN-200 Proteins Regulate Caspase Activation in Response to Foreign Cytoplasmic DNA. Science

Ryzhakov G, Randow F (2007) SINTBAD, a novel component of innate antiviral immunity, shares a TBK1-binding domain with NAP1 and TANK. EMBO J 26:3180–3190

Sabbah A, Chang TH, Harnack R, Frohlich V, Tominaga K, Dube PH, Xiang Y, Bose S (2009) Activation of innate immune antiviral responses by Nod2. Nat Immunol 10:1073–1080

Saha SK, Pietras EM, He JQ, Kang JR, Liu SY, Oganesyan G, Shahangian A, Zarnegar B, Shiba TL, Wang Y et al (2006) Regulation of antiviral responses by a direct and specific interaction between TRAF3 and Cardif. EMBO J 25:3257–3263

Saito T, Hirai R, Loo YM, Owen D, Johnson CL, Sinha SC, Akira S, Fujita T, Gale M Jr (2007) Regulation of innate antiviral defenses through a shared repressor domain in RIG-I and LGP2. Proc Natl Acad Sci USA 104:582–587

Saito T, Owen DM, Jiang F, Marcotrigiano J, Gale M Jr (2008) Innate immunity induced by composition-dependent RIG-I recognition of hepatitis C virus RNA. Nature 454:523–527

Salcedo R, Worschech A, Cardone M, Jones Y, Gyulai Z, Dai RM, Wang E, Ma W, Haines D, O'HUigin C et al (2010) MyD88-mediated signaling prevents development of adenocarcinomas of the colon: role of interleukin 18. J Exp Med 207:1625–1636

Satoh T, Kato H, Kumagai Y, Yoneyama M, Sato S, Matsushita K, Tsujimura T, Fujita T, Akira S, Takeuchi O (2010) LGP2 is a positive regulator of RIG-I- and MDA5-mediated antiviral responses. Proc Natl Acad Sci USA 107:1512–1517

Schmitz R, Hansmann ML, Bohle V, Martin-Subero JI, Hartmann S, Mechtersheimer G, Klapper W, Vater I, Giefing M, Gesk S et al (2009) TNFAIP3 (A20) is a tumor suppressor gene in Hodgkin lymphoma and primary mediastinal B cell lymphoma. J Exp Med 206:981–989

Schroder K, Tschopp J (2010) The inflammasomes. Cell 140:821–832

Seth RB, Sun L, Ea CK, Chen ZJ (2005) Identification and Characterization of MAVS, a Mitochondrial Antiviral Signaling Protein that Activates NF-kappaB and IRF3. Cell 122:669–682

Shaw MH, Reimer T, Sanchez-Valdepenas C, Warner N, Kim YG, Fresno M, Nunez G (2009) T cell-intrinsic role of Nod2 in promoting type 1 immunity to Toxoplasma gondii. Nat Immunol 10:1267–1274

Shembade N, Harhaj NS, Parvatiyar K, Copeland NG, Jenkins NA, Matesic LE, Harhaj EW (2008) The E3 ligase Itch negatively regulates inflammatory signaling pathways by controlling the function of the ubiquitin-editing enzyme A20. Nat Immunol 9:254–262

Shembade N, Parvatiyar K, Harhaj NS, Harhaj EW (2009) The ubiquitin-editing enzyme A20 requires RNF11 to downregulate NF-kappaB signalling. EMBO J 28:513–522

Shembade N, Ma A, Harhaj EW (2010) Inhibition of NF-kappaB signaling by A20 through disruption of ubiquitin enzyme complexes. Science 327:1135–1139

Starr R, Willson TA, Viney EM, Murray LJ, Rayner JR, Jenkins BJ, Gonda TJ, Alexander WS, Metcalf D, Nicola NA et al (1997) A family of cytokine-inducible inhibitors of signalling. Nature 387:917–921

Sun SC (2008) Deubiquitylation and regulation of the immune response. Nat Rev Immunol 8:501–511

Sun J, Wiklund F, Zheng SL, Chang B, Balter K, Li L, Johansson JE, Li G, Adami HO, Liu W et al (2005) Sequence variants in Toll-like receptor gene cluster (TLR6-TLR1-TLR10) and prostate cancer risk. J Natl Cancer Inst 97:525–532

Sutmuller RP, Morgan ME, Netea MG, Grauer O, Adema GJ (2006) Toll-like receptors on regulatory T cells: expanding immune regulation. Trends Immunol 27:387–393

Sutterwala FS, Ogura Y, Szczepanik M, Lara-Tejero M, Lichtenberger GS, Grant EP, Bertin J, Coyle AJ, Galan JE, Askenase PW et al (2006) Critical role for NALP3/CIAS1/Cryopyrin

in innate and adaptive immunity through its regulation of caspase-1. Immunity 24: 317–327
Suzuki N, Suzuki S, Duncan GS, Millar DG, Wada T, Mirtsos C, Takada H, Wakeham A, Itie A, Li S et al (2002) Severe impairment of interleukin-1 and Toll-like receptor signalling in mice lacking IRAK-4. Nature 416:750–756
Swann JB, Vesely MD, Silva A, Sharkey J, Akira S, Schreiber RD, Smyth MJ (2008) Demonstration of inflammation-induced cancer and cancer immunoediting during primary tumorigenesis. Proc Natl Acad Sci USA 105:652–656
Tabeta K, Hoebe K, Janssen EM, Du X, Georgel P, Crozat K, Mudd S, Mann N, Sovath S, Goode J et al (2006) The Unc93b1 mutation 3d disrupts exogenous antigen presentation and signaling via Toll-like receptors 3, 7 and 9. Nat Immunol 7:156–164
Takahasi K, Yoneyama M, Nishihori T, Hirai R, Kumeta H, Narita R, Gale M Jr, Inagaki F, Fujita T (2008) Nonself RNA-sensing mechanism of RIG-I helicase and activation of antiviral immune responses. Mol Cell 29:428–440
Takaoka A, Yanai H, Kondo S, Duncan G, Negishi H, Mizutani T, Kano S, Honda K, Ohba Y, Mak TW et al (2005) Integral role of IRF-5 in the gene induction programme activated by Toll-like receptors. Nature 434:243–249
Takeda K, Akira S (2005) Toll-like receptors in innate immunity. Int Immunol 17:1–14
Takeuchi O, Akira S (2008) MDA5/RIG-I and virus recognition. Curr Opin Immunol 20:17–22
Tattoli I, Carneiro LA, Jehanno M, Magalhaes JG, Shu Y, Philpott DJ, Arnoult D, Girardin SE (2008) NLRX1 is a mitochondrial NOD-like receptor that amplifies NF-kappaB and JNK pathways by inducing reactive oxygen species production. EMBO Rep 9:293–300
Thomassen E, Renshaw BR, Sims JE (1999) Identification and characterization of SIGIRR, a molecule representing a novel subtype of the IL-1R superfamily. Cytokine 11:389–399
Ting JP, Davis BK (2005) CATERPILLER: a novel gene family important in immunity, cell death, and diseases. Annu Rev Immunol 23:387–414
Travassos LH, Carneiro LA, Ramjeet M, Hussey S, Kim YG, Magalhaes JG, Yuan L, Soares F, Chea E, Le Bourhis L et al (2010) Nod1 and Nod2 direct autophagy by recruiting ATG16L1 to the plasma membrane at the site of bacterial entry. Nat Immunol 11:55–62
Trompouki E, Hatzivassiliou E, Tsichritzis T, Farmer H, Ashworth A, Mosialos G (2003) CYLD is a deubiquitinating enzyme that negatively regulates NF-kappaB activation by TNFR family members. Nature 424:793–796
Tsuchida T, Zou J, Saitoh T, Kumar H, Abe T, Matsuura Y, Kawai T, Akira S (2010) The ubiquitin ligase TRIM56 regulates innate immune responses to intracellular double-stranded DNA. Immunity 33:765–776
Unterholzner L, Keating SE, Baran M, Horan KA, Jensen SB, Sharma S, Sirois CM, Jin T, Latz E, Xiao TS et al (2010) IFI16 is an innate immune sensor for intracellular DNA. Nat Immunol 11:997–1004
Wald D, Qin J, Zhao Z, Qian Y, Naramura M, Tian L, Towne J, Sims JE, Stark GR, Li X (2003) SIGIRR, a negative regulator of Toll-like receptor-interleukin 1 receptor signaling. Nat Immunol 4:920–927
Wertz IE, O'Rourke KM, Zhou H, Eby M, Aravind L, Seshagiri S, Wu P, Wiesmann C, Baker R, Boone DL et al (2004) De-ubiquitination and ubiquitin ligase domains of A20 downregulate NF-kappaB signalling. Nature 430:694–699
Wesche H, Gao X, Li X, Kirschning CJ, Stark GR, Cao Z (1999) IRAK-M is a novel member of the Pelle/interleukin-1 receptor-associated kinase (IRAK) family. J Biol Chem 274:19403–19410
Xia X, Cui J, Wang HY, Zhu L, Matsueda S, Wang Q, Yang X, Hong J, Songyang Z, Chen Z et al (2011) NLRX1 negatively regulates TLR-induced NF-κB signaling by targeting TRAF6 and IKK. Immunity 34(6):843–853
Xiao H, Gulen MF, Qin J, Yao J, Bulek K, Kish D, Altuntas CZ, Wald D, Ma C, Zhou H et al (2007) The Toll-interleukin-1 receptor member SIGIRR regulates colonic epithelial homeostasis, inflammation, and tumorigenesis. Immunity 26:461–475
Xu LG, Wang YY, Han KJ, Li LY, Zhai Z, Shu HB (2005) VISA is an adapter protein required for virus-triggered IFN-beta signaling. Mol Cell 19:727–740

Yarovinsky F, Zhang D, Andersen JF, Bannenberg GL, Serhan CN, Hayden MS, Hieny S, Sutterwala FS, Flavell RA, Ghosh S et al (2005) TLR11 activation of dendritic cells by a protozoan profilin-like protein. Science 308:1626–1629

Yoneyama M, Fujita T (2009) RNA recognition and signal transduction by RIG-I-like receptors. Immunol Rev 227:54–65

Yoneyama M, Kikuchi M, Natsukawa T, Shinobu N, Imaizumi T, Miyagishi M, Taira K, Akira S, Fujita T (2004) The RNA helicase RIG-I has an essential function in double-stranded RNA-induced innate antiviral responses. Nat Immunol 5:730–737

You F, Sun H, Zhou X, Sun W, Liang S, Zhai Z, Jiang Z (2009) PCBP2 mediates degradation of the adaptor MAVS via the HECT ubiquitin ligase AIP4. Nat Immunol 10:1300–1308

Yu Y, Hayward GS (2010) The ubiquitin E3 ligase RAUL negatively regulates type i interferon through ubiquitination of the transcription factors IRF7 and IRF3. Immunity 33:863–877

Yu Y, Wang SE, Hayward GS (2005) The KSHV immediate-early transcription factor RTA encodes ubiquitin E3 ligase activity that targets IRF7 for proteosome-mediated degradation. Immunity 22:59–70

Zaki MH, Boyd KL, Vogel P, Kastan MB, Lamkanfi M, Kanneganti TD (2010) The NLRP3 inflammasome protects against loss of epithelial integrity and mortality during experimental colitis. Immunity 32:379–391

Zeng W, Sun L, Jiang X, Chen X, Hou F, Adhikari A, Xu M, Chen ZJ (2010) Reconstitution of the RIG-I pathway reveals a signaling role of unanchored polyubiquitin chains in innate immunity. Cell 141:315–330

Zhang D, Zhang G, Hayden MS, Greenblatt MB, Bussey C, Flavell RA, Ghosh S (2004) A toll-like receptor that prevents infection by uropathogenic bacteria. Science 303:1522–1526

Zheng SL, Augustsson-Balter K, Chang B, Hedelin M, Li L, Adami HO, Bensen J, Li G, Johnasson JE, Turner AR et al (2004) Sequence variants of toll-like receptor 4 are associated with prostate cancer risk: results from the CAncer Prostate in Sweden Study. Cancer Res 64:2918–2922

Zhong B, Yang Y, Li S, Wang YY, Li Y, Diao F, Lei C, He X, Zhang L, Tien P et al (2008) The adaptor protein MITA links virus-sensing receptors to IRF3 transcription factor activation. Immunity 29:538–550

Zhong B, Zhang L, Lei C, Li Y, Mao AP, Yang Y, Wang YY, Zhang XL, Shu HB (2009) The ubiquitin ligase RNF5 regulates antiviral responses by mediating degradation of the adaptor protein MITA. Immunity 30:397–407

Zhou R, Yazdi AS, Menu P, Tschopp J (2011) A role for mitochondria in NLRP3 inflammasome activation. Nature 469:221–225

Chapter 7
Dendritic Cell Subsets and Immune Regulation

Meredith O'Keeffe, Mireille H. Lahoud, Irina Caminschi, and Li Wu

1 Introduction

Dendritic cells (DC) are bone marrow (BM)-derived cells. They represent a sparsely distributed population of immune cells. DCs are antigen-presenting cells crucial for the innate and adaptive immune responses to foreign antigens and for maintaining immune tolerance to self-tissues (Banchereau and Steinman 1998). Although sharing many common features, multiple subtypes of DC with distinct phenotypes and immune functions have been identified (Shortman and Liu 2002; Shortman and Naik 2007). In steady state, the DC subtypes found in mouse and in human include type-1 interferon (IFN-I) producing plasmacytoid DC (pDC), the lymphoid tissue resident conventional DC (cDC) and the migratory cDC that develop in peripheral tissues and can migrate to draining lymph nodes (LN) via lymphatics. The lymphoid tissues, including thymus, spleen and LN, contain phenotypically and functionally different cDC subsets. In non-lymphoid tissues, cDC can also be divided into subsets according to their phenotype and tissue localisations. These include Langerhans cells (LC) in epidermis and dermal DC in dermal areas of skin, mucosal tissue associated DC and interstitial tissue DC such as DC in liver and lung. Tissue microenvironments appear to have major impact on the function of these DC. Moreover, DC that are not found in the steady state, but develop following infection or inflammation include the monocyte derived DC (moDC) and the TNF and iNOS producing DC (TipDC), representing the "inflammatory DC" (Geissmann et al. 1998; Randolph et al. 1999; Serbina et al. 2003; Naik et al. 2006) and pDC-derived mature DC (Grouard et al. 1997; O'Keeffe et al. 2002; Zuniga et al. 2004).

M. O'Keeffe
Centre for Immunology, Burnet Institute, 85 Commercial Road, Melbourne, VIC 3004, Australia

M.H. Lahoud • I. Caminschi • L. Wu (✉)
The Walter and Eliza Hall Institute, 1G Royal Parade, Parkville, VIC 3052, Australia
e-mail: wu@wehi.edu.au

In this chapter, we review the recent progress on the roles of different DC subsets in immune regulation and their potential application in developing effective immunotherapies.

2 Development of DC

2.1 DC Precursors

2.1.1 Early Precursors for Steady-State DC

The ultimate origin of all DC is BM haematopoietic stem cells (HSC). Differing from other haematopoietic cell lineages, DC can develop through both myeloid and lymphoid pathways (Fig. 7.1). In a steady-state mouse, the early DC precursors include both BM derived myeloid (Lin$^-$CD34$^+$c-kit^{hi}CD16/32^{int}) and lymphoid (Lin$^-$c-kit^{int}Sca-1^{lo}IL-7Rα^+) restricted progenitors that have high proliferative capacity and can efficiently differentiate into both cDC (CD11c$^+$CD45RA$^-$) and pDC (CD11c^{int}CD45RA$^+$) in lymphoid tissues along with all myeloid and lymphoid cells respectively (Traver et al. 2000; Manz et al. 2001; Wu et al. 2001). The surface expression of fms-like tyrosine kinase receptor 3(Flt3) by these early progenitors is a crucial requirement for DC precursor activity (D'Amico and Wu 2003; Karsunky et al. 2003). These Flt3 expressing precursors develop into pDC and cDC via more restricted macrophage/DC precursor (MDP, Lin$^-$c-Kit^{hi}CD115$^+$CX3CR1$^+$Flt3$^+$) (Fogg et al. 2006; Liu et al. 2007; Waskow et al. 2008) and the common DC precursor (CDP, Lin$^-$c-Kit^{int}CD115$^+$Flt3$^+$) stages (Naik et al. 2007; Onai et al. 2007; Liu et al. 2009). They can also differentiate in vitro into pDC and cDC subsets equivalent to those found in the spleen of a steady-state mouse in the presence of Flt3 ligand (FL) (Brasel et al. 2000; Naik et al. 2005). Moreover, the Flt3$^+$ myeloid progenitors also serve as the main source of LC (Mende et al. 2006; Merad et al. 2008).

Similar to mouse, myeloid and lymphoid committed progenitors have also been identified in human BM and cord blood (Hao et al. 2001; Manz et al. 2002). The CD34$^+$ human myeloid and lymphoid progenitors can give rise to both cDC and pDC in vitro in the presence of FL (Galy et al. 1995; Blom et al. 2000; Chen et al. 2004; Chicha et al. 2004) and in humanised mouse models (Traggiai et al. 2004; Chicha et al. 2005; Lepus et al. 2009). However, it is not clear whether they generate these DC via a DC restricted precursor stage. Human CD34$^+$ progenitors can also give rise to both LC and dermal DC in culture in the presence of granulocyte-macrophage colony-stimulating factor (GM-CSF), TNF-α and TGF-β (Caux et al. 1992; Strobl et al. 1996, 1997; Strunk et al. 1997).

2.1.2 Late DC Precursors

A precursor that is at a developmental stage just before the formation of a phenotypically identifiable DC, is defined as an immediate or late DC precursor.

7 Dendritic Cell Subsets and Immune Regulation

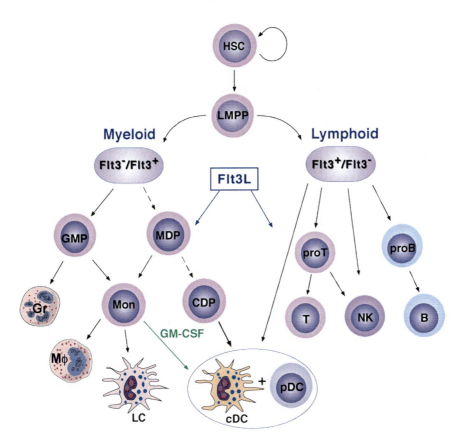

Fig. 7.1 A developmental scheme of mouse DC development from BM haemopoietic stem cells and lineage committed progenitors. Both cDC and pDC can be generated from the Flt3 expressing early myeloid or lymphoid progenitors. FLt3L is essential for the development of steady-state DC populations. Under inflammatory conditions, i.e. in the presence of GM-CSF, monocytes can differentiate into cDC. *HSC* haemopoietic stem cell; *LMPP* lymphoid-primed multipotent progenitors; *GMP* granulocyte and macrophage precursors; *MDP* macrophage and DC precursors; *CDP* common DC precursors. *Dash lines* represent pathways yet to be confirmed by direct evidence

These precursors can be found in mouse blood, BM and spleen and have a capacity to differentiate into mature subsets of DC with limited proliferation capacity (O'Keeffe et al. 2003; Diao et al. 2006; Naik et al. 2006; Liu et al. 2007, 2009). In mouse blood, the CD45RA⁻CD11c^{int}CD11b⁺ population represents immature cDC that acquire the morphology of mature cDC in the presence of TNF-α and the ability to stimulate T cells and to produce IL-12 in response to microbial stimuli. The CD45RA⁺CD11c^{int}CD11b⁻ population represents pDC. These cells mature into cDC-like cells only in the presence of stimuli such as CpG and GM-CSF and produce large quantities of IFN-I (Asselin-Paturel et al. 2001; Nakano et al. 2001; Martin et al. 2002; O'Keeffe et al. 2002). Although they can differentiate into cDC-like cells, their poor antigen presenting capabilities make them distinct from mature cDC (Krug et al. 2003).

The DC in peripheral lymphoid organs are continually replaced by blood-borne precursors. A precursor population with the phenotype MHC Class II$^{-/\text{lo}}$CD11c^{int}CD45RA^{lo}CD43^{int}Sirpα^{int}Flt3$^+$ has been identified in mouse BM, blood, spleen and LN as pre-cDC. These pre-cDC can differentiate into cDC in situ with a limited number of cell divisions and represent the most immediate precursors for steady-state cDC (Diao et al. 2006; Naik et al. 2006; Liu et al. 2007, 2009). These pre-cDC are distinct from monocytes as monocytes do not generate significant number of steady-state cDC in lymphoid tissues (Naik et al. 2006). Monocytes have been suggested to be the immediate precursors for inflammatory cDC as they can differentiate into cDC under GM-CSF-mediated inflammatory conditions (Naik et al. 2006).

2.2 Cytokine Requirement for DC Development

Several cytokines have been shown to be the major factors required for DC development in vivo and in vitro. FL is a growth factor for haematopoietic progenitors and is essential for the development of steady-state DC populations in lymphoid tissues. FL supports the in vitro differentiation of both cDC and pDC populations equivalent to that found in lymphoid tissues (Blom et al. 2000; Brasel et al. 2000; Gilliet et al. 2002; Naik et al. 2005). Administration of FL in vivo leads to dramatic increases in the numbers of both cDC and pDC in both mouse and human (Maraskovsky et al. 1996; Pulendran et al. 2000; Bjorck 2001).

GM-CSF is a crucial cytokine for the development of myeloid cells in both mouse and human. GM-CSF is an important factor for in vitro DC differentiation from monocytes and from haematopoietic progenitors (Inaba et al. 1992), but it blocks the development of pDC (Esashi et al. 2008). GM-CSF also plays an important role in DC differentiation during inflammation (Shortman and Naik 2007; Hamilton 2008) and therefore GM-CSF induced DC potentially represent the inflammatory DC.

Transforming growth factor β1 (TGF-β1) is a cytokine specifically required for epidermal LC development. Mice deficient in TGF-β1 fail to generate skin LC (Borkowski et al. 1996; Kaplan et al. 2007). TGF-β1 can also support LC development in vitro from human haematopoietic progenitors (Strobl et al. 1996).

Macrophage colony stimulating factor (M-CSF) can induce cDC and pDC differentiation from haematopoietic progenitors independently of FL and was required for LC differentiation from monocytes (Ginhoux et al. 2006; Fancke et al. 2008). The expression of M-CSF receptor has been used recently to identify DC restricted precursors in mouse BM (Naik et al. 2007; Onai et al. 2007), suggesting a role in the early stage of DC development.

3 DC Types

The DC network is heterogeneous and is composed of several distinct subtypes (Shortman and Naik 2007). While all DC are characterised by the ability to take up antigen, process it and present it to activate naive T cells, the DC subtypes exhibit very distinct differences in phenotype and ultimately in subset-specific functions (Villadangos and Schnorrer 2007). Broadly, DC can be initially segregated into pDC and cDC. pDC are a circulatory DC subset that only develop into DC-like cells upon activation. They are characterised by poor antigen presentation, but high IFN-I (IFN-α and IFN-β) production after stimulation as further discussed in Sect. 3.4 (Hochrein et al. 2002; O'Keeffe et al. 2002). In contrast, cDC have the morphology of classical DC with efficient antigen presentation ability.

As sentinels of the immune system, DC play an essential role in immune surveillance by surveying their environment from multiple locations in an attempt to maximise their chance at antigen capture from both self tissues and invading pathogens. The following section attempts to summarise some of the DC subtypes found in the mouse and human.

3.1 DC Subsets in Non-Lymphoid Tissues

DC are found in multiple non-lymphoid tissues such as the skin, reproductive tract, gut, lung, kidney and liver where they interface with the environment and serve as antigen-sampling sentinels. In the skin epidermal layer, LC are characterised as MHC Class II$^+$Langerin (CD207)^{hi}. The LC are long-lived, radioresistant cells which are the major carriers of peripheral antigens to the draining LN, although it has been suggested that LC themselves may not present the antigens directly to T cells in the LN (Allan et al. 2003). In the dermal layer of the skin, and in organs including the lung, kidney and gut, there are at least two further populations of interstitial DC which include a CD103$^+$ subset (MHC Class II$^+$CD207$^+$CD11b$^+$CD103$^+$) and a CD103$^-$ subset (MHC Class II$^+$CD207$^-$CD11b^{hi}CD103$^-$ DC) as reviewed in (Merad et al. 2008; Merad and Manz 2009).

The role of these subsets in the non-lymphoid tissue is currently the focus of many studies, they have been suggested to play a critical role in the balance between the maintenance of tolerance to innocuous environmental agents, and the induction of immunity to pathogens. During inflammation or in response to pathogens, these tissue interstitial DC migrate through the lymph to the LN in order to present the antigens they captured in the periphery to T cells in the LN (Bell et al. 1999; Huang and MacPherson 2001). As such, these DC are often referred to as migratory DC. The epidermal LC and dermal DC are good examples of the migratory DC (Schuler and Steinman 1985; Romani et al. 2003). Typically, these migratory DC have a less mature phenotype in the peripheral tissues where they actively sample antigens, and they mature and shut down antigen uptake en route to the LN. In the steady state, migration of DC to the LN also occurs, but at a lower rate (Huang and MacPherson 2001).

3.2 DC Subsets in Lymphoid Tissues

Lymphoid tissues contain both tissue resident and migratory DC. Lymphoid tissue resident DC are found in spleen, LN and thymus. The splenic and LN tissue resident

DC do not migrate, but rather survey their environment from their position in the lymphoid tissue by monitoring antigen that comes in via the blood or the lymph. In addition, LN also contain migratory DC, these are the DC that are initially found in the peripheral tissues, such as the skin, gut and lungs, that can capture antigen from the periphery and traffic it to the LN. The thymus similarly contains tissue resident and migratory DC populations, although the function of the thymic DC is mainly for the induction of tolerance rather than immunity.

The mouse thymus contains both pDC (CD11c^{int}CD45RA$^+$) and cDC (CD11c$^+$CD45RA$^-$) (Fig. 7.2a). The cDC can be segregated into a major subset of tissue resident DC that is generated within the thymus from intrathymic precursors and characterised as CD8^{hi} Sirpα (CD172a)^{lo} (Fig. 7.2a). A minor DC subset, that is CD8^{lo}Sirpα^{hi} (Fig. 7.2a), represents the DC migrated from the periphery into the thymus (Lahoud et al. 2006; Proietto et al. 2008a, b; Li et al. 2009). The CD8^{lo}Sirpα^{hi} cDC have been suggested to carry peripheral tissue antigens into the thymus and to play an important role in the deletion of thymocytes reactive to these self-antigens (Bonasio et al. 2006; Proietto et al. 2008b). This is also the thymic cDC subset capable of efficiently inducing the natural occurring T-regulatory cells (Proietto et al. 2008b). The CD8^{hi}Sirpα^{lo} thymic resident cDC subset has been implicated in presenting self-antigens taken up from thymic medullary epithelial cells to developing thymocytes and to facilitate the deletion of self-reactive thymocytes (Gallegos and Bevan 2004; Koble and Kyewski 2009).

In the mouse spleen and LN, we similarly find both pDC (CD11c^{int}CD45RA$^+$) and cDC (CD11c$^+$CD45RA$^-$) (Fig. 7.2b). Mouse splenic cDC can be further segregated based on their expression of the surface markers CD4 and CD8, into the CD4$^+$8$^-$ (CD4$^+$) cDC which constitute 50–60% of the splenic cDC, the CD4$^-$8$^-$ (DN) cDC which constitute 20–25% of splenic cDC and the CD4$^-$8$^+$ (CD8$^+$) which constitute 20–25% of the splenic cDC (Vremec et al. 2000). The CD4$^+$ and the DN cDC appear to be more closely related in phenotype based on gene expression profiles, cell surface markers, antigen presentation capacity and production of cytokines and chemokines; hence they are often referred to as a pooled splenic CD8$^-$ cDC subset (Vremec et al. 2000; Edwards et al. 2003a, b; Proietto et al. 2004; Lahoud et al. 2006; Schnorrer et al. 2006). In contrast, the CD8$^+$ splenic cDC subset are distinct based on the above parameters.

In the LN, in addition to the tissue resident DC subsets similar to those found in the spleen, there are also the migratory DC populations described above that have trafficked to the LN. In the mesenteric LN, the migratory population of DC is often referred to as interstitial DC and has been characterised as CD8$^-$CD205^{lo}. In subcutaneous LN, there are at least three populations of migratory DC, the LC that have migrated from the epidermal layer of the skin (CD8$^-$CD103$^-$CD326$^+$CD205^{hi}; Fig. 7.2c), the dermal DC (CD8$^-$CD103$^-$CD326$^-$CD205^{int}; Fig. 7.2c) and the recently characterised CD103$^+$ migratory DC (CD8$^-$CD205^{hi}CD103$^+$; Fig. 7.2c) (Henri et al. 2001; Belz et al. 2004; Merad et al. 2008; Bedoui et al. 2009b; Merad and Manz 2009).

The functional properties of different DC subsets in mouse lymphoid tissues have been studied thoroughly. It has been shown that CD8$^+$ cDC can prime Th1

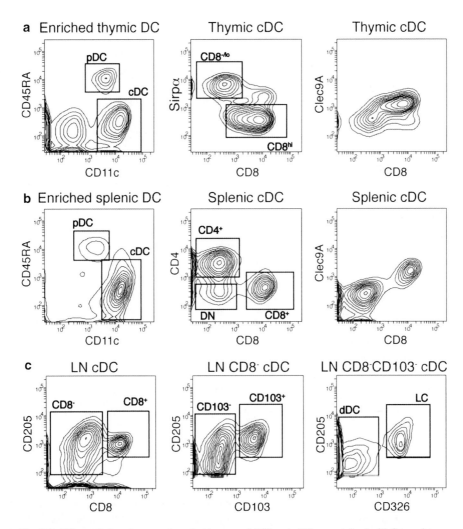

Fig. 7.2 DC populations in mouse lymphoid organs. (**a**) Thymic DC were stained with fluorochrome conjugated antibodies to CD11c, CD45RA, Sirpα, CD8α and Clec9A. Thymic pDC are gated as CD11c^{int} CD45RA^{hi}. Thymic cDC are gated as CD11c^{hi} CD45RA$^-$. Thymic cDC can be further segregated based on their expression of Sirpα and CD8 into Sirpα^{lo} CD8^{hi} and Sirpα^{hi} CD8$^{-/lo}$. Thymic Sirpα^{lo} CD8^{hi} cDC co-express Clec9A. (**b**) Splenic DC were stained with fluorochrome conjugated antibodies to CD11c, CD45RA, CD4, CD8α and Clec9A. Splenic pDC are gated as CD11c^{int} CD45RA^{hi}. Splenic cDC are gated as CD11c^{hi} CD45RA$^-$. Splenic cDC can be further segregated based on their expression of CD4 and CD8α into CD4$^-$ CD8$^-$ (often referred to as double negative or DN), CD4$^+$ CD8$^-$ and CD4$^-$ CD8$^+$. Splenic CD8$^+$ cDC co-express Clec9A. (**c**) Subcutaneous LN DC were stained with fluorochrome conjugated antibodies to CD11c, CD205, CD8, CD103 and CD326. LN cDC are gated as CD11c^{hi}, and can be further segregated into a CD8$^+$ CD205$^+$ (CD8$^+$) lymphoid tissue resident cDC population and a CD8$^-$ cDC population. The CD8$^-$ cDC can be further segregated based on their expression of CD103 and CD326 into a CD8$^-$CD103$^+$CD205$^+$ migratory DC population (CD103$^+$), a CD8$^-$CD103$^-$CD205^{int}CD326$^-$ dermal derived DC (dDC) population and a CD8$^-$CD103$^-$CD205^{hi}CD326$^+$ Langerhans cell derived (LC) population

responses through production of large amounts of IL-12, whereas CD8⁻ cDC prime Th2 responses (Pulendran et al. 1999; Moser and Murphy 2000; Maldonado-López 2001; Hochrein et al. 2001). The CD8⁺ cDC can present self-antigen by endocytosing apoptotic cells in vivo in the steady state and tolerise self-reactive T cells in the periphery (Iyoda et al. 2002). They also have a unique ability to cross-present exogenous antigen for CD8⁺ T cell responses in vivo (den Haan et al. 2000). This function has been suggested to be responsible for the ability of CD8⁺ cDC to induce peripheral tolerance to tissue-associated antigens (Belz et al. 2002) and is also important in viral immunity (Heath and Carbone 2001).

Cytokine production by DC subsets is dependent upon the activation of the DC by ligands to appropriately expressed pattern recognition receptors (PRR) and the genetic makeup of each individual DC subset. pDC are professional high producers of IFN-I in a TLR7, 8 or 9 dependent manner but in general, most pro-inflammatory cytokines can be produced to some extent by each of the known DC subsets. Thus although CD8⁺ cDC are the major producers of IL-12 isoforms in most circumstances, in response to ligands of TLR-7, the CD8⁺ cDC do not respond and make no IL-12 and the lower levels of IL-12 made by CD8⁻ cDC, suddenly become significant. As the knowledge of all PRRs expressed by DC is still incomplete, the documented ability of DC subsets to produce cytokines is restricted by the stimuli that have been used to activate them. Table 7.1 summarises the current literature and our own findings on differential cytokine production by DC subsets.

To further complicate matters, certain cytokines are expressed constitutively by distinct DC subsets, in the absence of known activation. Constitutively expressed cytokines include TGF-β by CD8⁺ mouse cDC and are also listed in Table 7.1.

3.3 Inflammatory DC

DC generated from GM-CSF and IL-4 (Inaba et al. 1992, Scheicher et al. 1992) are thought to represent DC derived from monocytes in blood and spleen under inflammatory conditions (Randolph et al. 1999; Auffray et al. 2009b; Swirski et al. 2009).

The TNF-α and iNOS producing DC (TipDC) correspond to activated monocytes recruited into the spleen and LN in a CCR2 (Serbina et al. 2003) and CX3CR1-dependent fashion. In mice they have been demonstrated to express iNOS, TNFα and reactive oxygen intermediates during *Listeria monocytogenes* and other bacterial infections (Serbina et al. 2003; Engel et al. 2006; Auffray et al. 2009a), *Leishmania major* infection (De Trez et al. 2009) and influenza infections (Aldridge et al. 2009). A similar pro-inflammatory cell type has been implicated in autoimmune pathology in the brain of mice with experimental autoimmune encephalitis (Dogan et al. 2008) and in skin of patients with psoriasis (Lowes et al. 2005).

Whilst it is clear that TipDC develop in a GM-CSF-rich inflammatory milieu (Naik et al. 2006) it is not yet clarified whether TipDC are GM-CSF dependent and whether in fact they are the in vivo corollary of GM-CSF/IL-4 in vitro generated DC. Elucidation of the nature of the growth factor(s) required for TipDC generation

Table 7.1 Differential cytokine production by DC subsets

DC type	IFN-α	IFN-β	IL-2	IL-6	IL-10	IL-12p70	IL-12p40/ IL-23p40	IL-15	TGF-β	TNF-α
pDC mouse and human (Shortman and Liu 2002)	++++	+++								
pDC-Peyers patch (Contractor et al. 2007)	+				++					
Mouse CD8+ cDC (Shortman and Liu 2002; Yamazaki and Steinman 2009)		+		++		++++	++++		+	
Mouse CD8− cDC (Rothfuchs et al. 2009)				++		+	++++			
Peyer's patch CD11b+ DC (Iwasaki and Kelsall 2001)				++++						
Langerhans-human (Mathers et al. 2009)								+		
Human thymic CD11b^{lo} DC (Vandenabeele et al. 2001; Shortman and Liu 2002)						+++				
TipDC (Serbina et al. 2003)										+++
Human CD1a+ mo-derived (Cernadas et al. 2009)						++++				

may be particularly of relevance for tumour therapies. It has been recently demonstrated that infiltrating TipDC can kill tumour cells in an iNOS-dependent manner in a mouse breast cancer model (Parajuli et al. 2010).

It is also not clear what other growth factors may influence the DC present in inflammatory situations. FL and M-CSF, growth factors known to be involved in the development of DC from non-monocytes (Xu et al. 2007; Fancke et al. 2008) in the steady state, are both increased during inflammation. Whether they in turn have an influence on the DC populations present in an inflammatory environment is not yet clear.

3.4 Plasmacytoid DC (pDC)

The classification of pDC as DC is somewhat contradictory as they generally exhibit poor T cell stimulating capacity in the steady state. However, at the global transcriptome level it is clear that pDC belong to the DC "family" in both mouse and human systems (Robbins et al. 2008).

The pDC are present at low levels in all lymphoid organs and have also been reported in non-lymphoid organs including the gut. The innate functions of pDC are well conserved between mouse and human including their unique ability to produce enormous amounts of IFN-I in response to pathogens and analogues that mimic viral nucleic acids. The response of pDC relies largely on stimulation via endosomal-located Toll-like receptors (TLR) that recognise either ssRNA (TLR7, 8) or ssDNA (TLR9). pDC are the only known cell type that possesses the necessary signalling machinery for IFN-I production as a consequence of TLR7 or 9 ligation (Akira and Hemmi 2003). The IFN-I induces a plethora of host-mediated anti-viral mechanisms that include the activation of innate cells and of B and T lymphocytes. Indeed IFN-I are potent at expanding and activating CTL (Cousens et al. 1999; Kolumam et al. 2005). Thus pDC are extremely important during responses to viral infections and also potentially in inducing anti-tumour CTL.

On the other hand, it has recently come to light that the high IFN-I producing capacity of pDC can be detrimental in autoimmune diseases. In lupus, pDC produce high levels of IFN-I in response to FcR-mediated uptake of immune complexes containing self nucleic acids. The IFN-I leads to exacerbation of disease via the continual activation of self-reactive B and T cells (reviewed in (Ronnblom and Pascual 2008)). Similarly in psoriasis, pDC are activated via self DNA that is bound by a self anti-microbial peptide (Lande et al. 2007). In both of these cases normally non-stimulatory self nucleic acids are delivered to the pDC in a complexed form that allows their transport to endosomes and recognition via TLR7, 8 or 9 and subsequent disease exacerbation. The clinical use of activated pDC in tumour eradication would need to proceed with caution, particularly in immunosuppressed patients, to avoid potential deleterious anaemia-inducing effects of IFN-I and other inflammatory cytokines produced by activated pDC.

pDC have been implicated as important cells in maintaining oral (Goubier et al. 2008) and transplant tolerance (Abe et al. 2005; Ochando et al. 2006) and in suppressing airway inflammation (Kool et al. 2009) and dampening allergic responses (Lambrecht and Hammad 2008). They also potentially play a deleterious tolerogenic role in various cancers (Zou et al. 2001; Gerlini et al. 2007). In the BM pDC are the predominant DC population in both mouse and man and they have been implicated as important facilitating cells that support engraftment of donor BM (Fugier-Vivier et al. 2005). Mechanisms of tolerance induction and/or immunosuppression by non-activated pDC probably include, but are not limited to, their ability to produce IDO (Fallarino et al. 2007) and to induce regulatory T cells (Ochando et al. 2006; Hadeiba et al. 2008).

3.5 Blood DC

Mouse blood DC are predominantly pDC (about 0.03% of PBMC) and very few cells display the expression level of CD11c and MHC II of tissue cDC. These cDC found in the blood are $CD4^-CD8^-$ and mainly $CD11b^+$ (O'Keeffe et al. 2003) and about 20% of these cells are $Clec9A^+CD24^+$, similar to $CD8\alpha^+$ mouse spleen DC (Caminschi et al. 2008).

Immature $CD11c^{int}MHC\ II^{lo/-}\ CD11b^+CD4^-CD8^-$ DC are also present in mouse blood and these cells upregulate MHC II and co-stimulation markers after overnight culture and maturation is further enhanced with GM-CSF and/or TNFα (O'Keeffe et al. 2003).

3.6 Human DC Subsets

Due to the difficulties faced in obtaining tissues and ethical considerations, the majority of studies on human DC are derived from in vitro generated DC. As in the murine system, human monocyte-derived cDC can be generated from PBMC or BM cells in the presence of GM-CSF and IL-4 (Sallusto and Lanzavecchia 1994). These in vitro cultures generate high numbers of cDC and have been the method of choice for most human DC researchers. A different cytokine cocktail is used to drive $CD1a^+$ LC and dermal or interstitial cDC from $CD34^+$ haematopoietic progenitors. This cocktail contains GM-CSF, TNF-α, SCF and FL, with the addition of TNF-α for LC generation, or IL-4 for interstitial DC generation (Caux et al. 1996). Human pDC and cDC can also be driven from $CD34^+$ precursors with FL (Blom et al. 2000).

The group of Derek Hart has pioneered the characterisation of human DC subsets in blood (MacDonald et al. 2002) and tonsils (Summers et al. 2001). They identified four cDC subsets that differ in surface phenotype ($CD11c^+CD16^-$ DC, $CD11c^+CD16^+$ DC, CD1c (BDCA-1) $^+$ DC and CD141 (BDCA-3)$^+$ DC), and the $CD11c^-CD123^+$ pDC. $BDCA-1^+$ and $CD141^+$ expression markers are now commonly used to separate human cDC. Several lines of evidence from transcriptome analyses (Lindstedt et al. 2005) and surface phenotype (Demedts et al. 2005; Masten et al. 2006) suggest that in organs including tonsils and lung, BDCA1+ and CD141+ DC may differ from blood DC subsets and possibly be composed of heterogeneous DC populations.

Studies in the human thymus indicate that the expression of CD11b is able to delineate (at least) two different subsets of cDC (Bendriss-Vermare et al. 2001; Vandenabeele et al. 2001). Those cDC that do not express CD11b are major producers of bioactive IL-12p70, reminiscent of the CD8+CD11b− cDC in the mouse. Freshly isolated CD11b+ cDC express high levels of MIP-1α mRNA, as do the CD8− cDC of mouse. Further evidence linking mouse and human cDC subsets comes from the recent finding that an antibody to Nectin-like protein 2 (Necl2), a molecule specific for CD141+ human cDC in blood and T cell areas in spleen, also specifically recognises the CD8+ cDC in mouse spleen (Galibert et al. 2005). The expression of Clec9A, a C-type lectin-like molecule recognising dead cells, is also specifically shared by both CD141+ and mouse CD8+ cDC (Caminschi et al. 2008; Huysamen et al. 2008; Sancho et al. 2008, 2009). Moreover, at the global transcriptome level the CD141+ and CD8+ mouse DC subsets appear closely related (Robbins et al. 2008). Recently it has also been shown that CD141+ human cDC are the functional correlates of mouse CD8+ cDC with a potent ability to cross-present antigen (Jongbloed et al. 2010; Bachem et al. 2010; Crozat et al. 2010; Poulin et al. 2010; Mittag et al. 2011).

4 Pattern Recognition Receptor Types and Their Different Expression in DC Subsets

DC link the ancient innate and "modern" adaptive immune systems and a major basis for this is their expression of multiple members of the ancient TLR family and other evolutionarily conserved PRR. Pathogen recognition and immune responses resulting in autoimmune pathologies in diseases such as lupus and psoriasis involve direct stimulation via TLR and other PRR.

Functionally distinct DC subsets express distinct members of the TLR family. A recent review detailed TLR expression by the known subsets of mouse, human, and rat ex vivo isolated and in vitro generated DC (Hochrein and O'Keeffe 2008). The major difference between mouse and human DC subsets is the expression of TLR9 in all mouse DC but its restricted expression to only the pDC subset in humans. This is of important functional relevance in designing human TLR9-based tumour therapies since whilst CpG-ODN TLR-9 ligands demonstrate encouraging anti-tumour activity in mouse models, their activity in humans, where only the pDC will be activated, remains to be elucidated (reviewed in (Vollmer and Krieg 2009))

Recent data also shows a potential functional alignment of mouse CD8+ cDC and human CD141+ cDC in that both express high levels of TLR3 and no TLR7 (Robbins et al. 2008).

5 Immune Regulation by DC

5.1 DC in T-Cell Activation

The Steinman definition of a DC is a cell that can induce naïve T cells into cycle (Steinman 1991), thus by definition DC present antigen to T cells. As discussed above, even with stimulation the pDC are poor antigen presenters when compared side by side with cDC.

DC have the ability to cross-present antigen, that is to present exogenous antigen via the MHC Class I pathway. Numerous studies have variously shown that pDC and different cDC subsets of mouse and human origin can cross-present to some extent. In mouse the $CD8^+$ cDC subset, and its immediate $CD8^-$ precursor (Bedoui et al. 2009a) is the most efficient and indeed appears specialised to cross-present antigen (Villadangos and Schnorrer 2007). The $CD103^+$ DC within the dermis and lung also show efficient cross-presenting activity. Cross-presented antigen leads to cross priming or cross tolerance of $CD8^+$ T cells. The cross priming pathway is thought to be particularly important for the presentation of viral peptides by non-infected cells and the induction of CTL. Cross-presentation of tumour antigens likely leads to cross tolerance in the absence of a danger signal. The cytoplasmic machinery that endows the $CD8^+$ DC with superior cross-presenting ability is currently unknown. As discussed above, the human equivalent of the mouse $CD8^+$ DC is likely the $CD141^+$ DC.

T regulatory cells (Treg) are a major drawback to overcome in therapeutic tumour interventions as they inhibit efficient effector responses in the tumour environment. At least two different sets of Treg exist in vivo, Treg that are selected in the thymus as a distinct cell lineage (often called natural T reg) and those T cells that are converted to Treg in the periphery (reviewed in Curotto de Lafaille and Lafaille 2009). In the context of tumour environments many studies report the accumulation of Treg at the tumour site. Whether these are always migrated thymic Treg or cells that have been converted to Treg in the periphery or a combination is not clear.

Different DC subsets have been implicated in Treg selection in the thymus and their conversion in the periphery. The $Sirp\alpha^{hi}CD8^{lo}$ migrating DC found in the thymus are efficient at selecting Treg (Proietto et al. 2008b).

In mouse gut and lung, certain subsets of $CD103^+$ DC that express TGF-β have been shown to convert naïve T cells into Treg. Within the spleen the $CD8^+$ DC subset has been shown to convert antigen-specific naïve T cells to Treg, depending upon endogenous TGF-β production, whereas the splenic $CD8^-$ DC more potently stimulated thymic-selected Treg (Yamazaki et al. 2008). Several reports have also suggested pDC can be potent Treg converters (reviewed in Yamazaki and Steinman 2009).

Overall the data indicates that most DC subsets have the ability to stimulate and/or convert Treg. The clarification of the specific involvement of particular DC subsets in different tumour or autoimmune settings will determine the therapeutic measures, such as targeted activation or targeted antigen delivery to skew the ability of these DC subsets to induce or suppress Treg stimulation as required.

5.2 DC Interaction with Other Immune Cells

The ability of DC to produce cytokines in direct response to danger signals allows their indirect interaction with other cells of the immune system. IL-12 produced by cDC and IFN-I produced by pDC are both potent activators of NK cells (Reschner et al. 2008; Ferlazzo and Munz 2009).

B cells can also be activated by DC-derived cytokines such as IL-12 or IFN-I. The response of human B cells to TLR7, 8 and 9 ligands is increased by IFN-I produced by pDC, enhancing their differentiation into antibody secreting cells (Douagi et al. 2009). IL-6 is an important factor in B cell survival and differentiation. During an antibody response within the mouse LN $CD8^-$ DC are thought to substantially contribute to IL-6 and APRIL production (Mohr et al. 2009). IL-6 and retinoic acid are also important mediators produced by gut DC that induce gut homing receptors and T cell-independent IgA production from B cells (Mora et al. 2006). The B cell antibody response to Influenza virus in human blood was shown to be dependent upon IL-6 and IFN-I production by pDC (Jego et al. 2003). It has also been shown that DC have an important role in the initiation of Ab synthesis by direct interaction with B cells (Wykes et al. 1998; Qi et al. 2006). Moreover, DC can play a role in homeostasis of B cell populations. DC within the BM promote the survival of recirculating B cells in the steady state by the production of macrophage migration inhibitory factor (Sapoznikov et al. 2008).

5.3 Immune Modulation by Targeting DC

5.3.1 DC Functional Related Molecules

DC use numerous cell surface molecules to survey and interact with their environment and to carry out specific functions such as pathogen recognition, antigen capture, migration and interaction with T cells. Thus, cell surface molecules which are selectively expressed on the surface of particular DC subsets are particularly important as these molecules form the basis of the functional characteristics of these DC subsets. C-type lectin-like molecules (Geijtenbeek and Gringhuis 2009; Huysamen and Brown 2009), such as CD205, DCIR-2, Clec9A and Clec12A, and the Signal Regulatory Protein (Sirp) molecules (Barclay and Brown 2006; Matozaki et al. 2009) including Sirpα and Sirpβ1 have been particularly important for the segregation of DC subtypes, alignment of DC between mice and human and for the targeted delivery of antigens to DC in vivo. Table 7.2 summarises some of the key features and references pertaining to some of these molecules and their expression by mouse DC subsets.

C-Type Lectin-Like Molecules

C-type lectin or C-type lectin-like molecules are molecules containing extracellular C-type lectin or C-type lectin-like domains (CTLD). Classical C-type lectins, such as

Table 7.2 Selected C-type lectin-like and Sirp molecules that are differentially expressed in mouse splenic DC subsets

	Type of membrane protein; extracellular recognition domains	Signalling motifs (location)	Expression on mouse cells	Expression on mouse splenic DC subsets	Expression on migratory or non-lymphoid tissue DC	Expression on human cells	References
Clec9A	Type II; 1 CTLD	YxxL; ITAM-like (Cyt)	DC	CD8⁺ DC: + CD8⁻DC: − pDC: +	–	CD141+ blood DC, Low levels on B cells, few monocytes	Caminschi et al. (2008), Huysamen et al. (2008), Sancho et al. (2008)
CD205 (Dec-205, Ly75)	Type I; 10 CTLD	FxxxxY	DC, thymic and intestinal epithelial cells, some B cells	CD8⁺ DC: ++ CD8⁻ DC: +/− (low to absent) pDC: −	Dermal derived DC, Langerhans cells	DC, monocytes, B cells, NK cells, pDC and T cells	Inaba et al. (1995), Witmer-Pack et al. (1995), Vremec et al. (2000), O'Keeffe et al. (2002), Bonifaz et al. (2004), Kato et al. (2006), Robinson et al. (2006)
Clec12A (Micl, CLL-1, DCAL-2, KLRL1)	Type II; 1 CTLD	ITIM (Cyt)	DC, macrophages, monocytes	CD8⁺ DC: ++ CD8⁻ DC: +/− pDC: +	Not reported	DC, monocytes, macrophages, granulocytes	Marshall et al. (2004), Chen et al. (2006), Pyz et al. (2008), Lahoud et al. (2009), Huysamen and Brown (2009)
Cire (CD209a)	Type II; 1 CTLD	Not reported	DC, monocytes, macrophages, some B cells	CD8⁺ DC: − CD8⁻ DC: + (small proportion) pDC: +	Not reported	The closely related molecule DC-SIGN is expressed on DC and macrophages	Caminschi et al. (2001, 2006), Robinson et al. (2006), den Dunnen et al. (2009)

(continued)

Table 7.2 (continued)

	Type of membrane protein; extracellular recognition domains	Signalling motifs (location)	Expression on mouse cells	Expression on mouse splenic DC subsets	Expression on migratory or non-lymphoid tissue DC	Expression on human cells	References
Clec4a4 DCIR-2, 33D1	Type II; 1 CTLD	ITIM (Cyt)	DC, Small proportion of splenocytes	CD8+: – CD8−: + pDC: –	Not reported	Not clear orthologue	Flornes et al. (2004), Dudziak et al. (2007)
Clec7a (Dectin1)	Type II; 1 CTLD	YxxL; ITAM-like (Cyt)	DC, macrophages, monocytes, neutrophils, some T cells	CD8+: – CD8−: + pDC: +/–	Langerhans cells	DC, monocytes, macrophages, neutrophils, microglia, low levels on T cells, B cells, mast cells, eosinophils	Ariizumi et al. (2000), Taylor et al. (2002), Reid et al. (2004), Carter et al. (2006b), Robinson et al. (2006), Huysamen and Brown (2009)
Sirpα (CD172a)	Type I: 1 IgV + 2 IgC domains	ITIM (Cyt)	DC, macrophages, Monocytes, neurons	CD8+: + CD8−: +++ pDC: ++	Dermal derived DC, Langerhans cells	DC, macrophages, granulocytes, mast cells, Haemopoietic stem cells	Chuang and Lagenaur (1990), Sano et al. (1999), Fukunaga et al. (2004), Lahoud et al. (2006), van Beek et al. (2005), Barclay and Brown (2006), Matozaki et al. (2009)

| Sirpβ1 | Type I; 1 IgV + 2 IgC domains | K (TM) | mediates interaction with ITAM bearing molecules | DC, macrophages | CD8+: – CD8−: + pDC: – | – | DC, monocytes, granulocytes | Hayashi et al. (2004), van Beek et al. (2005), Lahoud et al. (2006) |

Alternative names are provided in brackets. "X" denotes any amino acid
Clec C-type lectin domain family member; *CTLD* C-type lectin-like domain; *Cyt* cytoplasmic; *TM* transmembrane; *ITAM* immunoreceptor tyrosine based activation motif; *ITIM* immunoreceptor tyrosine based irhibition motif

the mannose receptor, recognise carbohydrate residues in a calcium-dependent manner. However, more recently, many C-type lectin-like molecules have been identified that have domains that are highly similar to the C-type lectin domain but lack the residues thought to be required for carbohydrate recognition, hence these domains have been termed CTLD. Of these, the best known is the endocytic receptor CD205 (Dec205) which has been commonly used as a marker for segregating mouse DC subsets, and as an antigen delivery target (see Sect. 5.3.2) (Mahnke et al. 2000; Bonifaz et al. 2002, 2004). In the mouse, CD205 is predominantly expressed on $CD8^+$ lymphoid tissue resident DC, on migratory DC subsets including dermal DC and LC in the LN and on epithelial cells and some B cells (Table 7.2). In the human, while CD205 is similarly expressed at high levels on blood DC, it has a much broader expression pattern, including monocytes, B cells, NK cells, pDC and T cells (Kato et al. 2006). As a result, CD205 appears to be of limited use for the alignment of mouse and human DC subsets. CD205 is an endocytic recycling receptor but little else is known about its function (Mahnke et al. 2000). Its ligand has not been identified to date, although it has been proposed to play a role in the recognition of dead cells (Shrimpton et al. 2009) and pathogens such as the Gram-negative bacterium *Yersinia pestis* (Zhang et al. 2008).

The recently identified Clec9A (Dngr1) is selectively expressed on the surface of mouse $CD8^+$ DC and pDC, on a subset of primate DC and on $CD141^+$ human blood DC (Caminschi et al. 2008; Huysamen et al. 2008; Sancho et al. 2008). This molecule holds promise for use in segregating DC subsets across different animal species as the *Clec9A* gene appears to be conserved across several species including rodents, large animals and primates; and the expression profile to date appears to be almost exclusive to DC. It is also highly efficient as an antigen delivery target (Caminschi et al. 2008; Sancho et al. 2008) (see Sect. 5.3.2). Although the ligand has not been identified to date, Clec9A binds to a protein or protein-bound intracellular component of cells that is only revealed upon cell death. Furthermore, DC from $Clec9A^{-/-}$ mice show reduced cross presentation of antigens derived from dead cells (Sancho et al. 2009). As such, it is believed to play a key role in the recognition, processing and presentation of antigens derived from dead cells.

DC-SIGN and Dectin-1 are particularly interesting, as they act as pathogen recognition receptors, and again show great promise as antigen delivery targets (see Sect. 5.3.2). Cire was originally identified as a possible mouse homologue to human DC-SIGN(Caminschi et al. 2001) based on its genomic localisation, amino acid similarity, predicted protein structure and DC expression (Table 7.2) (Caminschi et al. 2001, 2006). However, while both Cire and DC-SIGN bound mannosylated residues, Cire was unable to bind to most pathogens previously found to bind to human DC-SIGN (Caminschi et al. 2006; Yang et al. 2008), suggesting that while it is closely related to human DC-SIGN, it may not be the functional homologue.

On the other hand, Dectin1 (Clec7A), which is expressed in mouse and human, has been found to recognise β-glucans, polysaccharides found primarily in fungal pathogens (Brown and Gordon 2001; Robinson et al. 2006), and indeed mice that lack expression of Dectin1 show impaired responses to fungal infections (Taylor et al. 2007). Interestingly, within the mouse splenic cDC compartment, both Cire and Dectin1 are preferentially expressed by the $CD8^-$ cDC (Table 7.2), indicating a role for the $CD8^-$ DC subset in the recognition of certain pathogens.

Clec12A (DCAL2/MICL/CLL1) is also expressed by mouse and human DC. In the mouse, it is preferentially expressed on mouse $CD8^+$ DC and pDC and on a smaller proportion of $CD8^-$ DC (Lahoud et al. 2009). In contrast, human CLEC12A appears to be expressed on monocytes and all blood DC subsets examined (Table 7.2). The ligand for Clec12A has not been identified, but it has been proposed to bind to an endogenous ligand (Pyz et al. 2008). In human DC, mAb cross-linking of CLEC12A was found to induce receptor internalisation and modulate the DC responses to other maturation signals; although the effects were dependent on the maturation signals analysed (Chen et al. 2006). In mouse, although Clec12A ligation using mAb also resulted in receptor internalisation, no effects on DC maturation were observed (Lahoud et al. 2009). The differences in the behaviour of mouse and human DC in response to cross-linking using anti-Clec12A mAb may reflect species differences between mouse and human Clec12A, the DC subsets used in the investigations or the epitopes ligated by the Ab. Nevertheless, Clec12A promises to be an effective target for antigen delivery as described below.

Sirp Molecules

The Sirp molecules are cell surface molecules that contain extracellular immunoglobulin (Ig)-like domains. The Sirpα molecules are characterised by long cytoplasmic domains (110-113aa) containing two potential immunoreceptor inhibitory motifs (ITIM)-signalling motifs whereas Sirpβ molecules are characterised by short cytoplasmic domains (~5aa) that lack signalling motifs, but have a transmembrane domain with a charged motif that mediate an interaction with ITAM containing adaptor proteins such as Dap12 (Dietrich et al. 2000; Tomasello et al. 2000; Anfossi et al. 2003; Hayashi et al. 2004; Lahoud et al. 2006). In the mouse, both Sirpα and the three mouse Sirpβ molecules (Sirpβ1, Sirpβ2 and Sirpβ4) are preferentially expressed by the $CD8^-$ splenic DC and macrophages (Hayashi et al. 2004; Lahoud et al. 2006).

In macrophages and DC, Sirpα has been implicated in playing an important role in cell migration, phagocytosis and cytokine production. One example is the binding of Sirpα (on macrophages and DC) to CD47 (on the surface of interacting cells) which mediates self recognition and delivers a "dont eat me" signal to the macrophage or DC (reviewed in van Beek et al. 2005; Barclay and Brown 2006; Matozaki et al. 2009). To date, no direct ligand has been identified for Sirpβ molecules. However, Ab-mediated ligation of Sirpβ1 has been revealed to play an important role in the uptake of opsonised red blood cells and pathogens such as Leishmania (Hayashi et al. 2004; Lahoud et al. 2006), thus it has been postulated to play a role in the recognition of modified self or pathogens, and to deliver an "eat me" signal to macrophages and DC.

5.3.2 DC Targeting

The fact that DC initiate and control immune responses, naturally leads to the concept of utilising these cells to enhance vaccination procedure. Furthermore, since the DC network consists of multiple subtypes that have specialised function and are able to bias the type of immune response generated, it becomes theoretically possible to immunise via distinct DC subtypes and elicit the type of immune response predicted to be most efficient against the pathogen of interest.

In vivo antigen has been delivered to DC using mAb that specifically recognise certain cell surface proteins present on DC or DC-subsets. This experimental approach has yielded much data and revealed some of the rules that govern immunological outcomes.

Antigen Delivery for the Induction of Immunity

The paradigm in DC biology proposes that immature (quiescent) DC present antigen in a tolerogenic manner, whilst mature (activated) DC present antigen in an immunogenic manner. This model is supported by a large body of evidence, though exceptions appear to exist. Using mAb specific for cell surface molecules found on DC subsets, antigen could be delivered to DC under steady-state or inflammatory conditions. The outcomes of these experiments can be summarised in terms of the parameters examined: humoral or cellular immunity.

Multiple studies have shown that targeting antigen to cell surface molecules expressed on DC (and other APC) resulted in potent antibody responses. Thus, targeting antigen to MHC class II, MHC class I, FcγRII, CD45RA, CD45, CD4, CD11c and the mannose receptor induced potent antibody responses in the absence of added adjuvants (Carayanniotis and Barber 1987; Snider et al. 1990; Skea and Barber 1993; Wang et al. 2000; He et al. 2007). One caveat to these studies is the possibility that trace amounts of endotoxins within the antibody preparations acted as adjuvants. We have found as little as 10 ng of LPS synergised with targeting Ag to Clec12A to increase the Ab response by 50-fold (Lahoud et al. 2009). In that vein, when targeting antigen to FIRE, CIRE (Corbett et al. 2005) and Clec9A (data not shown), molecules expressed on different DC subsets, strong Ab responses were elicited in the absence of detectable endotoxins. Furthermore, TLR4 deficient mice and MyD88–/–TRIF–/– deficient mice, which cannot respond to LPS, had strong Ab responses when targeted with anti-FIRE mAb (data not shown) and anti-Clec9A mAb (Caminschi et al. 2008; and data not shown). Thus, there are instances where potent Ab responses can be induced in the absence of adjuvants. However, not all molecules expressed on DC can be targeted to induce strong antibody responses: CD205, Clec12A, DCIR-2 and Dectin-1 require adjuvants (Finkelman et al. 1996; Boscardin et al. 2006; Carter et al. 2006b; Lahoud et al. 2009), Fig. 7.3.

In contrast to generating Ab responses, priming a cellular immune response, particularly cytotoxic T lymphocytes (CTL), is largely dependent on the presence of adjuvants. Thus, targeting antigen to CD205, DCIR-2, Dectin-1, Clec12A, mannose receptor, CD11c and MHC class II requires adjuvant to induce functional CD8 T cell responses (Bonifaz et al. 2002, 2004; Carter et al. 2006b; Dudziak et al. 2007; He et al. 2007; Castro et al. 2008; Lahoud et al. 2009). Even targeting Clec9A requires adjuvants for the induction of in vivo CTL, despite the fact that Ab production was independent of co-activators (Caminschi et al. 2008).

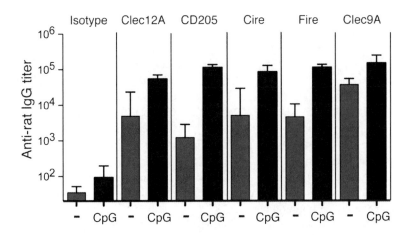

Fig. 7.3 Induction of humoral immunity by delivering Ag to different DC surface molecules utilising specific mAbs. C57BL/6 mice were injected i.v. with 10 μg of the mAb against Clec12A (5D3), CD205 (NLDC-145), Cire (5H10), Fire (6F12), Clec9A (10B4) and isotype control (GL117) respectively in the presence or absence (−) of 5 nm CpG (1668). The anti-rat IgG humoral response was measured 4 weeks later by ELISA. Each group contains five mice and data is depicted as the geometric mean with 95% CI

Antigen Delivery for the Induction of Tolerance

The importance of maturation factors when targeting antigens to DC was first shown by Finkelman et al. using DCIR-2 (Finkelman et al. 1996). In the absence of inflammatory signals, antigen targeted to DCIR-2 induced T and B cell tolerance, but in the presence of inflammatory signals such as IL-1, targeting to DCIR-2 induced immunity (Finkelman et al. 1996). The best example of inducing antigen-specific tolerance by targeting immature or steady-state DC has been documented using mAb against CD205. In the absence of maturation signals, targeting Ag to CD205 results in antigen presentation that activates Ag-specific transgenic T cells into transient proliferation, but ultimately leads to the deletion of both CD8 and CD4 antigen-specific T cells, and the few remaining transgenic CD4 T cells were unresponsive to rechallenge (Hawiger et al. 2001; Bonifaz et al. 2002). There is also evidence of the induction of Treg cells (Mahnke et al. 2003; Kretschmer et al. 2005; Yamazaki et al. 2008). Thus, targeting CD205 has emerged as a potential strategy to induce antigen-specific tolerance, a concept that has been successfully used to delay the onset and progression of autoimmune diabetes (Bruder et al. 2005; Mukhopadhaya et al. 2008).

Targeting DC-Subsets Biases Immune Outcomes

Using mAb to target DC subsets has confirmed the original observations that CD8⁺ DCs, are intrinsically superior at MHC class II presentation. Thus, when mAb were used to shuttle model antigen ovalbumin to CD8⁻ DC via the receptors DCIR-2 and Dectin-1, stronger MHC class II restricted responses were induced compared to when targeting CD8⁺ DC via CD205 (Carter et al. 2006a; Dudziak et al. 2007). Conversely, targeting CD205 induced more potent MHC class I restricted responses than targeting with Dectin-1 or DCIR-2 as evidenced by a stronger proliferative response of OVA-specific transgenic CD8 T cells (Carter et al. 2006a; Dudziak et al. 2007). The mechanism whereby CD8⁺ DC and CD8⁻ DC activate CD4⁺ T cells may differ, for example, when LACK antigen from *Leishmania major* was targeted to CD8⁻ DC using DCIR-2, CD4⁺ T cells were induced to produce IFN-γ in an IL-12 dependent manner (Soares et al. 2007). However, when LACK was targeted to CD8⁺ DC using CD205, CD4⁺ T cells were primed to produce IFN-γ in an IL-12 independent manner, instead, this pathway was entirely reliant on membrane-associated tumour necrosis family member CD70 (Soares et al. 2007). Similarly, DC subsets employ different strategies for the induction of Treg cells, a property that may become important when tolerance induction is sought (Yamazaki et al. 2008).

6 Potential of DC in Cancer Immunotherapy

As professional antigen presenting cells with innate cytokine producing capability, the potential role for DC in cancer immunotherapy is enormous. Tumour cells typically avoid immune attack by attracting Treg, secreting suppressive agents or inducing angiogenesis by VEGF secretion. VEGF also inhibits the generation of inflammatory DC (Johnson et al. 2009). The high expression of pro-survival molecules by tumour cells can also limit their subsequent eradication. The challenge is to overcome the inhibitory environment caused by the tumour.

It follows then that to be successful, therapeutic DC-based therapies will likely need to be carried out in conjunction with studies aimed at reducing the suppressive tumour environment in each specific patient. Inducing anti-angiogenic and pro-death molecules and an inflammatory environment hindering Treg development will be factors to consider alongside the exact type of DC and activation mode of that DC subset to target to optimally induce CTL and NK cell activity.

7 Concluding Remarks

To date, DC have been tested as anti-tumour immunotherapies in pilot and clinical studies without overwhelming success. Understanding the complexities of the DC network, the exquisite functional specificity of certain subsets and how to best target and/or activate these cells in different tumour environments will improve the future of DC-based immunotherapies.

References

Abe M, Colvin BL, Thomson AW (2005) Plasmacytoid dendritic cells: in vivo regulators of alloimmune reactivity? Transplant Proc 37:4119–4121

Akira S, Hemmi H (2003) Recognition of pathogen-associated molecular patterns by TLR family. Immunol Lett 85:85–95

Aldridge JR Jr, Moseley CE, Boltz DA et al (2009) TNF/iNOS-producing dendritic cells are the necessary evil of lethal influenza virus infection. Proc Natl Acad Sci USA 106:5306–5311

Allan RS, Smith CM, Belz GT et al (2003) Epidermal viral immunity induced by CD8alpha$^+$ dendritic cells but not by Langerhans cells. Science 301:1925–1928

Anfossi N, Lucas M, Diefenbach A et al (2003) Contrasting roles of DAP10 and KARAP/DAP12 signaling adaptors in activation of the RBL-2H3 leukemic mast cell line. Eur J Immunol 33:3514–3522

Ariizumi K, Shen GL, Shikano S et al (2000) Identification of a novel, dendritic cell-associated molecule, dectin-1, by subtractive cDNA cloning. J Biol Chem 275:20157–20167

Asselin-Paturel C, Boonstra A, Dalod M et al (2001) Mouse type I IFN-producing cells are immature APCs with plasmacytoid morphology. Nat Immunol 2:1144–1150

Auffray C, Fogg DK, Narni-Mancinelli E et al (2009a) CX3CR1+ CD115+ CD135+ common macrophage/DC precursors and the role of CX3CR1 in their response to inflammation. J Exp Med 206:595–606

Auffray C, Sieweke MH, Geissmann F (2009b) Blood monocytes: development, heterogeneity, and relationship with dendritic cells. Annu Rev Immunol 27:669–692

Bachem A, Güttler S, Hartung E et al (2010) Superior antigen cross-presentation and XCR1 expression define human CD11c$^+$CD141$^+$ cells as homologues of mouse CD8+ dendritic cells. J Exp Med 7;207(6):1273–1281.

Banchereau J, Steinman RM (1998) Dendritic cells and the control of immunity. Nature 392:245–252

Barclay AN, Brown MH (2006) The SIRP family of receptors and immune regulation. Nat Rev Immunol 6:457–464

Bedoui S, Prato S, Mintern J et al (2009a) Characterization of an immediate splenic precursor of CD8$^+$ dendritic cells capable of inducing antiviral T cell responses. J Immunol 182:4200–4207

Bedoui S, Whitney PG, Waithman J et al (2009b) Cross-presentation of viral and self antigens by skin-derived CD103+ dendritic cells. Nat Immunol 10:488–495

Bell D, Young JW, Banchereau J (1999) Dendritic cells. Adv Immunol 72:255–324

Belz GT, Behrens GM, Smith CM et al (2002) The CD8α^+ dendritic cell is responsible for inducing peripheral self-tolerance to tissue-associated antigens. J Exp Med 196:1099–1104

Belz GT, Smith CM, Kleinert L et al (2004) Distinct migrating and nonmigrating dendritic cell populations are involved in MHC class I-restricted antigen presentation after lung infection with virus. Proc Natl Acad Sci USA 101:8670–8675

Bendriss-Vermare N, Barthelemy C, Durand I et al (2001) Human thymus contains IFN-α-producing CD11c$^-$, myeloid CD11c$^+$, and mature interdigitating dendritic cells. J Clin Invest 108:1237

Bjorck P (2001) Isolation and characterization of plasmacytoid dendritic cells from Flt3 ligand and granulocyte-macrophage colony-stimulating factor- treated mice. Blood 98:3520–3526

Blom B, Ho S, Antonenko S et al (2000) Generation of interferon alpha-producing predendritic cell (Pre-DC)2 from human CD34(+) hematopoietic stem cells. J Exp Med 192:1785–1796

Bonasio R, Scimone ML, Schaerli P et al (2006) Clonal deletion of thymocytes by circulating dendritic cells homing to the thymus. Nat Immunol 7:1092–1100

Bonifaz L, Bonnyay D, Mahnke K et al (2002) Efficient targeting of protein antigen to the dendritic cell receptor DEC-205 in the steady state leads to antigen presentation on major histocompatibility complex class I products and peripheral CD8$^+$ T cell tolerance. J Exp Med 196:1627–1638

Bonifaz LC, Bonnyay DP, Charalambous A et al (2004) In vivo targeting of antigens to maturing dendritic cells via the DEC-205 receptor improves T cell vaccination. J Exp Med 199:815–824

Borkowski TA, Letterio JJ, Farr AG et al (1996) A role for endogenous transforming growth factor β1 in Langerhans cell biology: the skin of transforming growth factor β1 null mice is devoid of epidermal Langerhans cells. J Exp Med 184:2417–2422

Boscardin SB, Hafalla JC, Masilamani RF et al (2006) Antigen targeting to dendritic cells elicits long-lived T cell help for antibody responses. J Exp Med 203:599–606

Brasel K, De Smedt T, Smith JL et al (2000) Generation of murine dendritic cells from flt-3-ligand-supplemented bone marrow cultures. Blood 96:3029–3039

Brown GD, Gordon S (2001) Immune recognition. A new receptor for beta-glucans. Nature 413:36–37

Bruder D, Westendorf AM, Hansen W et al (2005) On the edge of autoimmunity: T-cell stimulation by steady-state dendritic cells prevents autoimmune diabetes. Diabetes 54:3395–3401

Caminschi I, Lucas KM, O'Keeffe MA et al (2001) Molecular cloning of a C-type lectin superfamily protein differentially expressed by CD8α⁻ splenic dendritic cells. Mol Immunol 38:365–373

Caminschi I, Corbett AJ, Zahra C et al (2006) Functional comparison of mouse CIRE/mouse DC-SIGN and human DC-SIGN. Int Immunol 18:741–753

Caminschi I, Proietto AI, Ahmet F et al (2008) The dendritic cell subtype-restricted C-type lectin Clec9A is a target for vaccine enhancement. Blood 112:3264–3273

Carayanniotis G, Barber BH (1987) Adjuvant-free IgG responses induced with antigen coupled to antibodies against class II MHC. Nature 327:59–61

Carter RW, Thompson C, Reid DM et al (2006a) Induction of CD8⁺ T cell responses through targeting of antigen to Dectin-2. Cell Immunol 239:87–91

Carter RW, Thompson C, Reid DM et al (2006b) Preferential induction of CD4+ T cell responses through in vivo targeting of antigen to dendritic cell-associated C-type lectin-1. J Immunol 177:2276–2284

Castro FV, Tutt AL, White AL et al (2008) CD11c provides an effective immunotarget for the generation of both CD4 and CD8 T cell responses. Eur J Immunol 38:2263–2273

Caux C, Dezutter-Dambuyant C, Schmitt D et al (1992) GM-CSF and TNF-α cooperate in the generation of dendritic Langerhans cells. Nature 360:258–261

Caux C, Vanbervliet B, Massacrier C et al (1996) Interleukin-3 cooperates with tumor necrosis factor α for the development of human dendritic/Langerhans cells from cord blood CD34+ hematopoietic progenitor cells. Blood 87:2376–2385

Cernadas M, Lu J, Watts G et al (2009) CD1a expression defines an interleukin-12 producing population of human dendritic cells. Clin Exp Immunol 155:523–533

Chen W, Antonenko S, Sederstrom JM et al (2004) Thrombopoietin cooperates with FLT3-ligand in the generation of plasmacytoid dendritic cell precursors from human hematopoietic progenitors. Blood 103:2547–2553

Chen CH, Floyd H, Olson NE et al (2006) Dendritic-cell-associated C-type lectin 2 (DCAL-2) alters dendritic-cell maturation and cytokine production. Blood 107:1459–1467

Chicha L, Jarrossay D, Manz MG (2004) Clonal type I interferon-producing and dendritic cell precursors are contained in both human lymphoid and myeloid progenitor populations. J Exp Med 200:1519–1524

Chicha L, Tussiwand R, Traggiai E et al (2005) Human adaptive immune system Rag2-/-gamma(c)-/- mice. Ann N Y Acad Sci 1044:236–243

Chuang W, Lagenaur CF (1990) Central nervous system antigen P84 can serve as a substrate for neurite outgrowth. Dev Biol 137:219–232

Contractor N, Louten J, Kim L et al (2007) Cutting edge: Peyer's patch plasmacytoid dendritic cells (pDCs) produce low levels of type I interferons: possible role for IL-10, TGF-β, and prostaglandin E2 in conditioning a unique mucosal pDC phenotype. J Immunol 179:2690–2694

Corbett AJ, Caminschi I, McKenzie BS et al (2005) Antigen delivery via two molecules on the CD8⁻ dendritic cell subset induces humoral immunity in the absence of conventional "danger". Eur J Immunol 35:2815–2825

Cousens LP, Peterson R, Hsu S et al (1999) Two roads diverged: interferon alpha/beta- and interleukin 12-mediated pathways in promoting T cell interferon gamma responses during viral infection. J Exp Med 189:1315–1328

Crozat K, Guiton R, Contreras V et al (2010) The XC chemokine receptor 1 is a conserved selective marker of mammalian cells homologous to mouse CD8α⁺ dendritic cells. J Exp Med 7;207(6):1283–1292.

Curotto de Lafaille MA, Lafaille JJ (2009) Natural and adaptive foxp3+ regulatory T cells: more of the same or a division of labor? Immunity 30:626–635

D'Amico A, Wu L (2003) The early progenitors of mouse dendritic cells and plasmacytoid predendritic cells are within the bone marrow hemopoietic precursors expressing Flt3. J Exp Med 198:293–303

De Trez C, Magez S, Akira S et al (2009) iNOS-producing inflammatory dendritic cells constitute the major infected cell type during the chronic Leishmania major infection phase of C57BL/6 resistant mice. PLoS Pathog 5:e1000494

Demedts IK, Brusselle GG, Vermaelen KY et al (2005) Identification and characterization of human pulmonary dendritic cells. Am J Respir Cell Mol Biol 32:177–184

den Dunnen J, Gringhuis SI, Geijtenbeek TB (2009) Innate signaling by the C-type lectin DC-SIGN dictates immune responses. Cancer Immunol Immunother 58:1149–1157

den Haan JM, Lehar SM, Bevan MJ (2000) CD8⁺ but not CD8⁻ dendritic cells cross-prime cytotoxic T cells in vivo. J Exp Med 192:1685–1696

Diao J, Winter E, Cantin C et al (2006) In situ replication of immediate dendritic cell (DC) precursors contributes to conventional DC homeostasis in lymphoid tissue. J Immunol 176: 7196–7206

Dietrich J, Cella M, Seiffert M et al (2000) Cutting edge: signal-regulatory protein beta 1 is a DAP12-associated activating receptor expressed in myeloid cells. J Immunol 164:9–12

Dogan RN, Elhofy A, Karpus WJ (2008) Production of CCL2 by central nervous system cells regulates development of murine experimental autoimmune encephalomyelitis through the recruitment of TNF- and iNOS-expressing macrophages and myeloid dendritic cells. J Immunol 180:7376–7384

Douagi I, Gujer C, Sundling C et al (2009) Human B cell responses to TLR ligands are differentially modulated by myeloid and plasmacytoid dendritic cells. J Immunol 182:1991–2001

Dudziak D, Kamphorst AO, Heidkamp GF et al (2007) Differential antigen processing by dendritic cell subsets in vivo. Science 315:107–111

Edwards AD, Chaussabel D, Tomlinson S et al (2003a) Relationships among murine CD11c(high) dendritic cell subsets as revealed by baseline gene expression patterns. J Immunol 171:47–60

Edwards AD, Diebold SS, Slack EM et al (2003b) Toll-like receptor expression in murine DC subsets: lack of TLR7 expression by CD8α⁺ DC correlates with unresponsiveness to imidazoquinolines. Eur J Immunol 33:827–833

Engel D, Dobrindt U, Tittel A et al (2006) Tumor necrosis factor alpha- and inducible nitric oxide synthase-producing dendritic cells are rapidly recruited to the bladder in urinary tract infection but are dispensable for bacterial clearance. Infect Immun 74:6100–6107

Esashi E, Wang YH, Perng O et al (2008) The signal transducer STAT5 inhibits plasmacytoid dendritic cell development by suppressing transcription factor IRF8. Immunity 28:509–520

Fallarino F, Gizzi S, Mosci P et al (2007) Tryptophan catabolism in IDO+ plasmacytoid dendritic cells. Curr Drug Metab 8:209–216

Fancke B, Suter M, Hochrein H et al (2008) M-CSF: a novel plasmacytoid and conventional dendritic cell poietin. Blood 111:150–159

Ferlazzo G, Munz C (2009) Dendritic cell interactions with NK cells from different tissues. J Clin Immunol 29:265–273

Finkelman FD, Lees A, Birnbaum R et al (1996) Dendritic cells can present antigen in vivo in a tolerogenic or immunogenic fashion. J Immunol 157:1406–1414

Flornes LM, Bryceson YT, Spurkland A et al (2004) Identification of lectin-like receptors expressed by antigen presenting cells and neutrophils and their mapping to a novel gene complex. Immunogenetics 56:506–517

Fogg DK, Sibon C, Miled C et al (2006) A clonogenic bone marrow progenitor specific for macrophages and dendritic cells. Science 311:83–87

Fugier-Vivier IJ, Rezzoug F, Huang Y et al (2005) Plasmacytoid precursor dendritic cells facilitate allogeneic hematopoietic stem cell engraftment. J Exp Med 201:373–383

Fukunaga A, Nagai H, Noguchi T et al (2004) Src homology 2 domain-containing protein tyrosine phosphatase substrate 1 regulates the migration of Langerhans cells from the epidermis to draining lymph nodes. J Immunol 172:4091–4099

Galibert L, Diemer GS, Liu Z et al (2005) Nectin-like protein 2 defines a subset of T-cell zone dendritic cells and is a ligand for class-I-restricted T-cell-associated molecule. J Biol Chem 280:21955–21964

Gallegos AM, Bevan MJ (2004) Central tolerance to tissue-specific antigens mediated by direct and indirect antigen presentation. J Exp Med 200:1039–1049

Galy A, Travis M, Cen D et al (1995) Human T, B, natural killer and dendritic cells arise from a common bone marrow progenitor cell subset. Immunity 3:459–473

Geijtenbeek TB, Gringhuis SI (2009) Signalling through C-type lectin receptors: shaping immune responses. Nat Rev Immunol 9:465–479

Geissmann F, Prost C, Monnet JP et al (1998) Transforming growth factor $\beta 1$, in the presence of granulocyte/macrophage colony-stimulating factor and interleukin 4, induces differentiation of human peripheral blood monocytes into dendritic Langerhans cells. J Exp Med 187:961–966

Gerlini G, Urso C, Mariotti G et al (2007) Plasmacytoid dendritic cells represent a major dendritic cell subset in sentinel lymph nodes of melanoma patients and accumulate in metastatic nodes. Clin Immunol 125:184–193

Gilliet M, Boonstra A, Paturel C et al (2002) The development of murine plasmacytoid dendritic cell precursors is differentially regulated by FLT3-ligand and granulocyte/macrophage colony-stimulating factor. J Exp Med 195:953–958

Ginhoux F, Tacke F, Angeli V et al (2006) Langerhans cells arise from monocytes in vivo. Nat Immunol 7:265–273

Goubier A, Dubois B, Gheit H et al (2008) Plasmacytoid dendritic cells mediate oral tolerance. Immunity 29:464–475

Grouard G, Rissoan MC, Filgueira L et al (1997) The enigmatic plasmacytoid T cells develop into dendritic cells with interleukin (IL)-3 and CD40-ligand. J Exp Med 185:1101–1111

Hadeiba H, Sato T, Habtezion A et al (2008) CCR9 expression defines tolerogenic plasmacytoid dendritic cells able to suppress acute graft-versus-host disease. Nat Immunol 9:1253–1260

Hamilton JA (2008) Colony-stimulating factors in inflammation and autoimmunity. Nat Rev Immunol 8:533–544

Hao QL, Zhu J, Price MA et al (2001) Identification of a novel, human multilymphoid progenitor in cord blood. Blood 97:3683–3690

Hawiger D, Inaba K, Dorsett Y et al (2001) Dendritic cells induce peripheral T cell unresponsiveness under steady state conditions in vivo. J Exp Med 194:769–779

Hayashi A, Ohnishi H, Okazawa H et al (2004) Positive regulation of phagocytosis by SIRPbeta and its signaling mechanism in macrophages. J Biol Chem 279:29450–29460

He LZ, Crocker A, Lee J et al (2007) Antigenic targeting of the human mannose receptor induces tumor immunity. J Immunol 178:6259–6267

Heath WR, Carbone FR (2001) Cross-presentation in viral immunity and self tolerance-dual roles for dendritic cells. Nat Rev Immunol 1:126–134

Henri S, Vremec D, Kamath A et al (2001) The dendritic populations of mouse lymph nodes. J Immunol 167:741–748

Hochrein H, O'Keeffe M (2008) Dendritic cell subsets and toll-like receptors. Handb Exp Pharmacol 183:153–179

Hochrein H, Shortman K, Vremec D et al (2001) Differential production of IL-12, IFN-α, and IFN-γ by mouse dendritic cell subsets. J Immunol 166:5448–5455

Hochrein H, O'Keeffe M, Wagner H (2002) Human and mouse plasmacytoid dendritic cells. Hum Immunol 63:1103–1110

Huang FP, MacPherson GG (2001) Continuing education of the immune system – dendritic cells, immune regulation and tolerance. Curr Mol Med 1:457–468

Huysamen C, Brown GD (2009) The fungal pattern recognition receptor, Dectin-1, and the associated cluster of C-type lectin-like receptors. FEMS Microbiol Lett 290:121–128

Huysamen C, Willment JA, Dennehy KM et al (2008) CLEC9A is a novel activation C-type lectin-like receptor expressed on BDCA3+ dendritic cells and a subset of monocytes. J Biol Chem 283:16693–16701

Inaba K, Inaba M, Romani N et al (1992) Generation of large numbers of dendritic cells from mouse bone marrow cultures supplemented with granulocyte/macrophage colony-stimulating factor. J Exp Med 176:1693–1702

Inaba K, Swiggard WJ, Inaba M et al (1995) Tissue distribution of the DEC-205 protein that is detected by the monoclonal antibody NLDC-145.I. Expression on dendritic cells and other subsets of mouse leukocytes. Cell Immunol 163:148–156

Iwasaki A, Kelsall BL (2001) Unique functions of CD11β^+, CD8α^+, and double-negative Peyer's patch dendritic cells. J Immunol 166:4884–4890

Iyoda T, Shimoyama S, Liu K et al (2002) The CD8$^+$ dendritic cell subset selectively endocytoses dying cells in culture and in vivo. J Exp Med 195:1289–1302

Jego G, Palucka AK, Blanck JP et al (2003) Plasmacytoid dendritic cells induce plasma cell differentiation through type I interferon and interleukin 6. Immunity 19:225–234

Johnson B, Osada T, Clay T et al (2009) Physiology and therapeutics of vascular endothelial growth factor in tumor immunosuppression. Curr Mol Med 9:702–707

Jongbloed SL, Kassianos AJ, McDonald KJ et al (2010) Human CD141$^+$ (BDCA-3)$^+$ dendritic cells (DCs) represent a unique myeloid DC subset that cross-presents necrotic cell antigens. J Exp Med 7;207(6):1247–1260.

Kaplan DH, Li MO, Jenison MC et al (2007) Autocrine/paracrine TGF-β1 is required for the development of epidermal Langerhans cells. J Exp Med 204:2545–2552

Karsunky H, Merad M, Cozzio A et al (2003) Flt3 ligand regulates dendritic cell development from Flt3$^+$ lymphoid and myeloid-committed progenitors to Flt3$^+$ dendritic cells in vivo. J Exp Med 198:305–313

Kato M, McDonald KJ, Khan S et al (2006) Expression of human DEC-205 (CD205) multilectin receptor on leukocytes. Int Immunol 18:857–869

Koble C, Kyewski B (2009) The thymic medulla: a unique microenvironment for intercellular self-antigen transfer. J Exp Med 206:1505–1513

Kolumam GA, Thomas S, Thompson LJ et al (2005) Type I interferons act directly on CD8 T cells to allow clonal expansion and memory formation in response to viral infection. J Exp Med 202:637–650

Kool M, van Nimwegen M, Willart MA et al (2009) An anti-inflammatory role for plasmacytoid dendritic cells in allergic airway inflammation. J Immunol 183:1074–1082

Kretschmer K, Apostolou I, Hawiger D et al (2005) Inducing and expanding regulatory T cell populations by foreign antigen. Nat Immunol 6:1219–1227

Krug A, Veeraswamy R, Pekosz A et al (2003) Interferon-producing cells fail to induce proliferation of naive T cells but can promote expansion and T helper 1 differentiation of antigen-experienced unpolarized T cells. J Exp Med 197:899–906

Lahoud MH, Proietto AI, Gartlan KH et al (2006) Signal regulatory protein molecules are differentially expressed by CD8$^-$ dendritic cells. J Immunol 177:372–382

Lahoud MH, Proietto AI, Ahmet F et al (2009) The C-type lectin Clec12A present on mouse and human dendritic cells can serve as a target for antigen delivery and enhancement of antibody responses. J Immunol 182:7587–7594

Lambrecht BN, Hammad H (2008) Lung dendritic cells: targets for therapy in allergic disease. Chem Immunol Allergy 94:189–200

Lande R, Gregorio J, Facchinetti V et al (2007) Plasmacytoid dendritic cells sense self-DNA coupled with antimicrobial peptide. Nature 449:564–569

Lepus CM, Gibson TF, Gerber SA et al (2009) Comparison of human fetal liver, umbilical cord blood, and adult blood: hematopoietic stem cell engraftment in NOD-scid/gammac(−/−), Balb/c-Rag2(−/−)gammac(−/−), and C.B-17-scid/bg immunodeficient mice. Hum Immunol 70(10):790–802

Li J, Park J, Foss D et al (2009) Thymus-homing peripheral dendritic cells constitute two of the three major subsets of dendritic cells in the steady-state thymus. J Exp Med 206:607–622

Lindstedt M, Lundberg K, Borrebaeck CA (2005) Gene family clustering identifies functionally associated subsets of human in vivo blood and tonsillar dendritic cells. J Immunol 175:4839–4846

Liu K, Waskow C, Liu X et al (2007) Origin of dendritic cells in peripheral lymphoid organs of mice. Nat Immunol 8:578–583

Liu K, Victora GD, Schwickert TA et al (2009) In vivo analysis of dendritic cell development and homeostasis. Science 324:392–397

Lowes MA, Chamian F, Abello MV et al (2005) Increase in TNF-alpha and inducible nitric oxide synthase-expressing dendritic cells in psoriasis and reduction with efalizumab (anti-CD11a). Proc Natl Acad Sci USA 102:19057–19062

MacDonald KP, Munster DJ, Clark GJ et al (2002) Characterization of human blood dendritic cell subsets. Blood 100:4512–4520

Maldonado-López R, Maliszewski C, Urbain J, Moser M (2001) Cytokines regulate the capacity of $CD8\alpha^+$ and $CD8\alpha^-$ dendritic cells to prime Th1/Th2 cells in vivo. J Immunol 15;167(8): 4345–4350

Mahnke K, Guo M, Lee S et al (2000) The dendritic cell receptor for endocytosis, DEC-205, can recycle and enhance antigen presentation via major histocompatibility complex class II-positive lysosomal compartments. J Cell Biol 151:673–684

Mahnke K, Qian Y, Knop J et al (2003) Induction of CD4+/CD25+ regulatory T cells by targeting of antigens to immature dendritic cells. Blood 101:4862–4869

Manz MG, Traver D, Miyamoto T et al (2001) Dendritic cell potentials of early lymphoid and myeloid progenitors. Blood 97:3333–3341

Manz MG, Miyamoto T, Akashi K et al (2002) Prospective isolation of human clonogenic common myeloid progenitors. Proc Natl Acad Sci USA 99:11872–11877

Maraskovsky E, Brasel K, Teepe M et al (1996) Dramatic increase in the numbers of functionally mature dendritic cells in Flt3 ligand-treated mice: multiple dendritic cell subpopulations identified. J Exp Med 184:1953–1962

Marshall AS, Willment JA, Lin HH et al (2004) Identification and characterization of a novel human myeloid inhibitory C-type lectin-like receptor (MICL) that is predominantly expressed on granulocytes and monocytes. J Biol Chem 279:14792–14802

Martin P, Del Hoyo GM, Anjuere F et al (2002) Characterization of a new subpopulation of mouse $CD8\alpha^+$ $B220^+$ dendritic cells endowed with type 1 interferon production capacity and tolerogenic potential. Blood 100:383–390

Masten BJ, Olson GK, Tarleton CA et al (2006) Characterization of myeloid and plasmacytoid dendritic cells in human lung. J Immunol 177:7784–7793

Mathers AR, Janelsins BM, Rubin JP et al (2009) Differential capability of human cutaneous dendritic cell subsets to initiate Th17 responses. J Immunol 182:921–933

Matozaki T, Murata Y, Okazawa H et al (2009) Functions and molecular mechanisms of the CD47-SIRPalpha signalling pathway. Trends Cell Biol 19:72–80

Mende I, Karsunky H, Weissman IL et al (2006) Flk2+ myeloid progenitors are the main source of Langerhans cells. Blood 107:1383–1390

Merad M, Manz MG (2009) Dendritic cell homeostasis. Blood 113:3418–3427

Merad M, Ginhoux F, Collin M (2008) Origin, homeostasis and function of Langerhans cells and other langerin-expressing dendritic cells. Nat Rev Immunol 8:935–947

Mittag D, Proietto AI, Loudovaris T et al (2011) Human DC subsets from spleen and blood are similar in phenotype and function, but modified by donor health status. J Immunol 186:6207–6217

Mohr E, Serre K, Manz RA et al (2009) Dendritic cells and monocyte/macrophages that create the IL-6/APRIL-rich lymph node microenvironments where plasmablasts mature. J Immunol 182:2113–2123

Mora JR, Iwata M, Eksteen B et al (2006) Generation of gut-homing IgA-secreting B cells by intestinal dendritic cells. Science 314:1157–1160

Moser M, Murphy KM (2000) Dendritic cell regulation of TH1-TH2 development. Nature Immunol 1:199–205

Mukhopadhaya A, Hanafusa T, Jarchum I et al (2008) Selective delivery of beta cell antigen to dendritic cells in vivo leads to deletion and tolerance of autoreactive CD8+ T cells in NOD mice. Proc Natl Acad Sci USA 105:6374–6379

Naik SH, Proietto AI, Wilson NS et al (2005) Cutting edge: generation of splenic CD8+ and CD8− dendritic cell equivalents in Fms-like tyrosine kinase 3 ligand bone marrow cultures. J Immunol 174:6592–6597

Naik SH, Metcalf D, van Nieuwenhuijze A et al (2006) Intrasplenic steady-state dendritic cell precursors that are distinct from monocytes. Nat Immunol 7:663–671

Naik SH, Sathe P, Park HY et al (2007) Development of plasmacytoid and conventional dendritic cell subtypes from single precursor cells derived in vitro and in vivo. Nat Immunol 8:1217–1226

Nakano H, Yanagita M, Gunn MD (2001) CD11c+B220+Gr-1+ cells in mouse lymph nodes and spleen display characteristics of plasmacytoid dendritic cells. J Exp Med 194:1171–1178

O'Keeffe M, Hochrein H, Vremec D et al (2002) Mouse plasmacytoid cells: long-lived cells, heterogeneous in surface phenotype and function, that differentiate into CD8+ dendritic cells only after microbial stimulus. J Exp Med 196:1307–1319

O'Keeffe M, Hochrein H, Vremec D et al (2003) Dendritic cell precursor populations of mouse blood: identification of the murine homologues of human blood plasmacytoid pre-DC2 and CD11c+ DC1 precursors. Blood 101:1453–1459

Ochando JC, Homma C, Yang Y et al (2006) Alloantigen-presenting plasmacytoid dendritic cells mediate tolerance to vascularized grafts. Nat Immunol 7:652–662

Onai N, Obata-Onai A, Schmid MA et al (2007) Identification of clonogenic common Flt3+ M-CSFR+ plasmacytoid and conventional dendritic cell progenitors in mouse bone marrow. Nat Immunol 8:1207–1216

Parajuli N, Muller-Holzner E, Bock G et al (2010) Infiltrating CD11b+ CD11c+ cells have the potential to mediate inducible nitric oxide synthase dependent cell death in mammary carcinomas of HER-2/neu transgenic mice. Int J Cancer 126(4):896–908

Poulin LF, Salio M, Griessinger E et al (2010) Characterization of human DNGR-1+ BDCA3+ leukocytes as putative equivalents of mouse CD8α+ dendritic cells. J Exp Med 7;207(6):1261–1271

Proietto AI, O'Keeffe M, Gartlan K et al (2004) Differential production of inflammatory chemokines by murine dendritic cell subsets. Immunobiology 209:163–172

Proietto AI, Lahoud MH, Wu L (2008a) Distinct functional capacities of mouse thymic and splenic dendritic cell populations. Immunol Cell Biol 86:700–708

Proietto AI, van Dommelen S, Zhou P et al (2008b) Dendritic cells in the thymus contribute to T-regulatory cell induction. Proc Natl Acad Sci USA 105:19869–19874

Pulendran B, Smith JL, Caspary G et al (1999) Distinct dendritic cell subsets differentially regulate the class of immune response in vivo. Proc Natl Acad Sci USA 96:1036–1041

Pulendran B, Banchereau J, Burkeholder S et al (2000) Flt3-ligand and granulocyte colony-stimulating factor mobilize distinct human dendritic cell subsets in vivo. J Immunol 165:566–572

Pyz E, Huysamen C, Marshall AS et al (2008) Characterisation of murine MICL (CLEC12A) and evidence for an endogenous ligand. Eur J Immunol 38:1157–1163

Qi H, Egen JG, Huang AY et al (2006) Extrafollicular activation of lymph node B cells by antigen-bearing dendritic cells. Science 312:1672–1676

Randolph GJ, Inaba K, Robbiani DF et al (1999) Differentiation of phagocytic monocytes into lymph node dendritic cells in vivo. Immunity 11:753–761

Reid DM, Montoya M, Taylor PR et al (2004) Expression of the beta-glucan receptor, Dectin-1, on murine leukocytes in situ correlates with its function in pathogen recognition and reveals potential roles in leukocyte interactions. J Leukoc Biol 76:86–94

Reschner A, Hubert P, Delvenne P et al (2008) Innate lymphocyte and dendritic cell cross-talk: a key factor in the regulation of the immune response. Clin Exp Immunol 152:219–226

Robbins SH, Walzer T, Dembele D et al (2008) Novel insights into the relationships between dendritic cell subsets in human and mouse revealed by genome-wide expression profiling. Genome Biol 9:R17

Robinson MJ, Sancho D, Slack EC et al (2006) Myeloid C-type lectins in innate immunity. Nat Immunol 7:1258–1265

Romani N, Holzmann S, Tripp CH et al (2003) Langerhans cells – dendritic cells of the epidermis. APMIS 111:725–740

Ronnblom L, Pascual V (2008) The innate immune system in SLE: type I interferons and dendritic cells. Lupus 17:394–399

Rothfuchs AG, Egen JG, Feng CG et al (2009) In situ IL-12/23p40 production during mycobacterial infection is sustained by CD11bhigh dendritic cells localized in tissue sites distinct from those harboring bacilli. J Immunol 182:6915–6925

Sallusto F, Lanzavecchia A (1994) Efficient presentation of soluble antigen by cultured human dendritic cells is maintained by granulocyte/macrophage colony-stimulating factor plus interleukin 4 and downregulated by tumor necrosis factor α. J Exp Med 179:1109–1118

Sancho D, Mourao-Sa D, Joffre OP et al (2008) Tumor therapy in mice via antigen targeting to a novel, DC-restricted C-type lectin. J Clin Invest 118:2098–2110

Sancho D, Joffre OP, Keller AM et al (2009) Identification of a dendritic cell receptor that couples sensing of necrosis to immunity. Nature 458:899–903

Sano S, Ohnishi H, Kubota M (1999) Gene structure of mouse BIT/SHPS-1. Biochem J 344(Pt 3):667–675

Sapoznikov A, Pewzner-Jung Y, Kalchenko V et al (2008) Perivascular clusters of dendritic cells provide critical survival signals to B cells in bone marrow niches. Nat Immunol 9:388–395

Scheicher C, Mehlig M, Zecher R, Reske K (1992) Dendritic cells from mouse bone marrow: in vitro differentiation using low doses of recombinant granulocyte-macrophage colony-stimulating factor. J Immunol Methods 2;154(2):253–264

Schnorrer P, Behrens GM, Wilson NS et al (2006) The dominant role of CD8$^+$ dendritic cells in cross-presentation is not dictated by antigen capture. Proc Natl Acad Sci USA 103:10729–10734

Schuler G, Steinman RM (1985) Murine epidermal Langerhans cells mature into potent immunostimulatory dendritic cells in vitro. J Exp Med 161:526–546

Serbina NV, Salazar-Mather TP, Biron CA et al (2003) TNF/iNOS-producing dendritic cells mediate innate immune defense against bacterial infection. Immunity 19:59–70

Shortman K, Liu Y-J (2002) Mouse and human dendritic cell subtypes. Nat Rev Immunol 2:153–163

Shortman K, Naik SH (2007) Steady-state and inflammatory dendritic-cell development. Nat Rev Immunol 7:19–30

Shrimpton RE, Butler M, Morel AS et al (2009) CD205 (DEC-205): a recognition receptor for apoptotic and necrotic self. Mol Immunol 46:1229–1239

Skea DL, Barber BH (1993) Studies of the adjuvant-independent antibody response to immunotargeting. Target structure dependence, isotype distribution, and induction of long term memory. J Immunol 151:3557–3568

Snider DP, Kaubisch A, Segal DM (1990) Enhanced antigen immunogenicity induced by bispecific antibodies. J Exp Med 171:1957–1963

Soares H, Waechter H, Glaichenhaus N et al (2007) A subset of dendritic cells induces CD4+ T cells to produce IFN-gamma by an IL-12-independent but CD70-dependent mechanism in vivo. J Exp Med 204:1095–1106

Steinman RM (1991) The dendritic cell system and its role in immunogenicity. Annu Rev Immunol 9:271–296

Strobl H, Riedl E, Scheinecker C et al (1996) TGF-β1 promotes in vitro development of dendritic cells from CD34$^+$ hemopoietic progenitors. J Immunol 157:1499–1507

Strobl H, Riedl E, Scheinecker C et al (1997) TGF-β1 dependent generation of LAG+ dendritic cells from CD34$^+$ progenitors in serum-free medium. Adv Exp Med Biol 417:161–165

Strunk D, Egger C, Leitner G et al (1997) A skin homing molecule defines the Langerhans cell progenitor in human peripheral blood. J Exp Med 185:1131–1136

Summers KL, Hock BD, McKenzie JL et al (2001) Phenotypic characterization of five dendritic cell subsets in human tonsils. Am J Pathol 159:285–295

Swirski FK, Nahrendorf M, Etzrodt M et al (2009) Identification of splenic reservoir monocytes and their deployment to inflammatory sites. Science 325:612–616

Taylor PR, Brown GD, Reid DM et al (2002) The beta-glucan receptor, dectin-1, is predominantly expressed on the surface of cells of the monocyte/macrophage and neutrophil lineages. J Immunol 169:3876–3882

Taylor PR, Tsoni SV, Willment JA et al (2007) Dectin-1 is required for beta-glucan recognition and control of fungal infection. Nat Immunol 8:31–38

Tomasello E, Cant C, Buhring HJ et al (2000) Association of signal-regulatory proteins beta with KARAP/DAP-12. Eur J Immunol 30:2147–2156

Traggiai E, Chicha L, Mazzucchelli L et al (2004) Development of a human adaptive immune system in cord blood cell-transplanted mice. Science 304:104–107

Traver D, Akashi K, Manz M et al (2000) Development of $CD8\alpha^+$ dendritic cells from a common myeloid progenitor. Science 290:2152–2154

van Beek EM, Cochrane F, Barclay AN et al (2005) Signal regulatory proteins in the immune system. J Immunol 175:7781–7787

Vandenabeele S, Hochrein H, Mavaddat N et al (2001) Human thymus contains 2 distinct dendritic cell populations. Blood 97:1733–1741

Villadangos JA, Schnorrer P (2007) Intrinsic and cooperative antigen-presenting functions of dendritic-cell subsets in vivo. Nat Rev Immunol 7:543–555

Vollmer J, Krieg AM (2009) Immunotherapeutic applications of CpG oligodeoxynucleotide TLR9 agonists. Adv Drug Deliv Rev 61:195–204

Vremec D, Pooley J, Hochrein H et al (2000) CD4 and CD8 expression by dendritic cell subtypes in mouse thymus and spleen. J Immunol 164:2978–2986

Wang H, Griffiths MN, Burton DR et al (2000) Rapid antibody responses by low-dose, single-step, dendritic cell-targeted immunization. Proc Natl Acad Sci USA 97:847–852

Waskow C, Liu K, Darrasse-Jeze G et al (2008) The receptor tyrosine kinase Flt3 is required for dendritic cell development in peripheral lymphoid tissues. Nat Immunol 9:676–683

Witmer-Pack MD, Swiggard WJ, Mirza A et al (1995) Tissue distribution of the DEC-205 protein that is detected by the monoclonal antibody NLDC-145. II. Expression in situ in lymphoid and nonlymphoid tissues. Cell Immunol 163:157–162

Wu L, D'Amico A, Hochrein H et al (2001) Development of thymic and splenic dendritic cell populations from different hemopoietic precursors. Blood 98:3376–3382

Wykes M, Pombo A, Jenkins C et al (1998) Dendritic cells interact directly with naive B lymphocytes to transfer antigen and initiate class switching in a primary T-dependent response. J Immunol 161:1313–1319

Xu Y, Zhan Y, Lew AM et al (2007) Differential development of murine dendritic cells by GM-CSF versus Flt3 ligand has implications for inflammation and trafficking. J Immunol 179:7577–7584

Yamazaki S, Steinman RM (2009) Dendritic cells as controllers of antigen-specific Foxp3+ regulatory T cells. J Dermatol Sci 54:69–75

Yamazaki S, Dudziak D, Heidkamp GF et al (2008) $CD8^+$ $CD205^+$ splenic dendritic cells are specialized to induce Foxp3+ regulatory T cells. J Immunol 181:6923–6933

Yang L, Yang H, Rideout K et al (2008) Engineered lentivector targeting of dendritic cells for in vivo immunization. Nat Biotechnol 26:326–334

Zhang SS, Park CG, Zhang P et al (2008) Plasminogen activator Pla of Yersinia pestis utilizes murine DEC-205 (CD205) as a receptor to promote dissemination. J Biol Chem 283:31511–31521

Zou W, Machelon V, Coulomb-L'Hermin A et al (2001) Stromal-derived factor-1 in human tumors recruits and alters the function of plasmacytoid precursor dendritic cells. Nat Med 7:1339–1346

Zuniga EI, McGavern DB, Pruneda-Paz JL et al (2004) Bone marrow plasmacytoid dendritic cells can differentiate into myeloid dendritic cells upon virus infection. Nat Immunol 5:1227–1234

Chapter 8
Human Dendritic Cells in Cancer

Gregory Lizée and Michel Gilliet

1 Introduction

1.1 DCs Control the Balance Between Immune Tolerance and Activation

Dendritic cells (DCs) are currently considered to be of utmost importance for orchestrating appropriate immune responses in vivo, and play critical roles in maintaining the distinction between self and non-self. They are distributed throughout most tissues of the body, where they are well positioned to act as innate sentinel cells that can detect and rapidly respond to pathogenic challenges. DCs are known as professional antigen-presenting cells (APCs) because they sample antigens present within the surrounding tissue microenvironment and process these antigens for presentation to cells of the adaptive immune system, such as T and B lymphocytes. By virtue of their activation status, DCs provide either stimulatory or inhibitory signals to lymphocytes, and thus provide a crucial nexus point by which innate and adaptive immune responses are linked.

In the steady state (i.e., absence of infection), DCs continuously process and present cellular ("self") antigens to adaptive immune cells, which results in the maintenance of

G. Lizée
Department of Melanoma Medical Oncology, The University of Texas M.D. Anderson Cancer Center, Houston, TX, USA

Department of Immunology, The University of Texas M.D. Anderson Cancer Center, Houston, TX, USA
e-mail: glizee@mdanderson.org

M. Gilliet (✉)
Department of Dermatology, University Hospital CHUV, CH-1011, Lausanne, Switzerland
e-mail: michel.gilliet@chuv.ch

immune tolerance, through either inhibiting the activation of self-reactive effector cells or promoting the activation of immunosuppressive regulatory cells. By contrast, during pathogen infections DCs rapidly differentiate into a mature state in which their ability to stimulate productive, pathogen-specific adaptive immunity increases dramatically, due in large part to increased inflammatory cytokine production and upregulated antigen presentation function. Thus, DCs act as a crucial switch that determines whether adaptive immune responses are initiated, and how they are ultimately manifested in vivo.

1.2 Two Distinct Human DC Subsets: Conventional and Plasmacytoid DCs

In humans, two principal DC subsets have been described: conventional dendritic cells (cDCs) and plasmacytoid dendritic cells (pDCs). These two subsets can be readily distinguished by their surface phenotype, tissue localization, cytokine secretion, antigen presentation function, and developmental origin. However, they share the ability to sense microbial infection and undergo maturation into cells with dendritic cell morphology that stimulates adaptive immunity. Importantly, since cDCs and pDCs can also induce immune suppression, both cell types have been implicated in the development and progression of human cancer.

Conventional DCs are broadly defined as CD11c$^+$ myeloid-derived hematopoietic cells that typically seed in peripheral tissues under steady-state conditions. They can also be generated in vitro from peripheral blood monocytes with the use of granulocyte-monocyte colony-stimulating factor (GM-CSF) and interleukin (IL)-4 (Inaba et al. 2001). Conventional DCs were initially noted for their ability to induce potent mixed lymphocyte responses, and are now recognized to be the most potent immune cell type for initiating the priming of antigen-specific T lymphocyte responses (Steinman et al. 1974; Banchereau and Steinman 1998; Banchereau et al. 2000). This is due in large part to their unparalleled ability to internalize and process large amounts of antigens from the extracellular milieu. In addition, cDCs express high levels of major histocompatibility complex (MHC)-I and MHC-II molecules and CD1 upon activation, facilitating the efficient presentation of both peptide and glycolipid antigens (Harding 1996; Vyas et al. 2008; Yewdell et al. 1999). Upon full maturation, cDCs express elevated levels of the costimulatory molecules CD80 and CD86 and produce IL-12, which together provide signals that are critical for the priming and activation of naïve T cells (Heath and Carbone 2009).

pDCs, by contrast, are defined as CD11c-negative, lymphoid-related cells that express CD4 and CD123 (IL-3 receptor-α chain), and lack lineage markers for B-cells, T-cells, myeloid cells, and NK-cells. pDCs are round-shaped cells and usually make up only 0.2–0.8% of peripheral blood leukocytes that colonize secondary lymphoid organs, but are normally absent from most peripheral tissues. pDCs are specialized in sensing nucleic acids through the intracellular expression of TLR7 and 9. Upon viral infection, pDCs can rapidly migrate to infected tissues where they produce large amounts of type I interferons (IFNs). Through the production of type I IFNs, pDCs are capable of activating a myriad of immune cell types that express the IFN-α receptor, including T and B lymphocytes, natural killer (NK) cells, and cDCs (Liu 2005; Lande and Gilliet 2010), thus serving to amplify the speed and magnitude of the immune responses against the viruses. Upon activation, pDCs also upregulate costimulatory molecules and differentiate into mature DCs. In contrast to cDCs, as APC, maturing pDC appear to be involved in immune tolerance and may therefore contribute to the contraction of the effector phase of T-cell responses against viruses.

2 Conventional DCs in Immune Tolerance

Conventional DCs play a critically important role in inducing immunological tolerance to self-antigens in the steady state. This key attribute makes them an important player in the induction of T-cell tolerance against tumor-associated antigens, which shall be discussed in more detail later. Conventional DCs are found in almost all normal tissues of the body, often forming intricate networks of interdigitating "sentinel" cells in and around common sites of pathogen entry (i.e., skin, lungs, gut). Subtypes of cDCs are often distinguished by anatomic location within the skin, cDCs are referred to as Langerhans cells, whereas in the brain, they are thought to constitute a subset of glial cells. In the immature state, tissue cDCs are capable of sampling large quantities of antigens from the surrounding extracellular milieu. This is facilitated in part by dendritic processes extending outward in all directions that allow antigens to be sampled from a sizable volume of tissue. More importantly, cDCs are endowed with several mechanisms to internalize antigens, including pinocytosis, phagocytosis, and receptor-mediated endocytosis by a variety of surface receptors. Relevant surface receptors that facilitate antigen presentation in cDCs include a myriad of scavenger receptors, as well as Fc receptors that specifically bind to multimeric antibody–antigen immune complexes.

It is believed that cDCs normally sample tissue antigens for 1–2 days before dissociating from the tissues and migrating through the draining lymphatics to the regional lymph nodes (LN, Fig. 8.1). Following proteolytic processing, internalized tissue antigens are presented at the cDC surface in the context of MHC-I, MHC-II, and CD1 molecules for presentation to $CD8^+$ T cells, $CD4^+$ T cells, and natural killer (NK) T cells, respectively. In this steady-state context, self-antigen presentation by cDCs typically results in the tolerization or anergization of antigen-specific lymphocytes (Lutz and Kurts 2009; Mueller 2010). As discussed in the next section, effective priming and activation of naïve T and NKT cells requires other costimulatory signals that are only induced in cDCs following their activation by pathogen-derived components.

Although they generally have a suppressive effect on effector $CD4^+$ and $CD8^+$ T cells, nonactivated cDCs migrating to LN have, by contrast, been shown to activate $CD4^+Foxp3^+$ regulatory T cells (Treg, Fig. 8.1). Through a mechanism involving

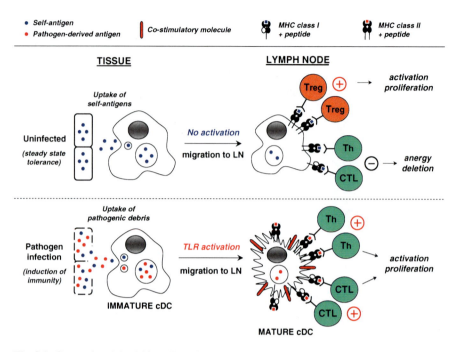

Fig. 8.1 Conventional dendritic cell (cDC) in immunity and tolerance

MHC-II-mediated antigen presentation and IL-10 secretion, steady-state migratory cDCs can stimulate the priming and proliferation of self antigen-specific Treg cells within LN (Yamazaki and Steinman 2009). These Treg cells in turn control the proliferation and function of self antigen-specific effector CD4$^+$ and CD8$^+$ T cells, facilitating immune suppression and providing protection from autoimmunity (Sakaguchi et al. 2009). However, since the prevalence of Treg cells in tumors has been shown to be an adverse prognostic factor in ovarian and pancreatic cancers, steady-state antigen presentation by nonactivated DCs derived from tumor tissues is likely to be an important mechanism contributing to tumor progression, as will be discussed later (Beyer and Schultze 2008; Gallimore and Godkin 2008).

3 Conventional DCs in Protective Immunity to Pathogens

During the course of an infection, viral or bacterial components invariably make contact with tissue-resident cDCs. A wide variety of pathogens are capable of potently triggering cDC activation, which is mediated largely through the expression of Toll-like receptors (TLRs) by cDCs (Iwasaki and Medzhitov 2004). Ligands for different cDC TLRs include viral RNA (TLR3), viral DNA (TLR9), bacterial lipopolysaccharide (LPS, TLR4), and flagellin (TLR5). Tissue debris is internalized by cDCs for antigen processing and presentation, but the simultaneous triggering of TLRs by pathogen-derived TLR ligands provides a strong additional maturation signal for cDCs (Fig. 8.1). TLR signals lead to increases in the expression of antigen processing components and surface MHC-I and MHC-II by cDCs, in addition to inducing expression of the costimulatory molecules CD80 and CD86. Maturation of cDCs also results in upregulated secretion of inflammatory cytokines, such as IFN-α and IL-12 (Medzhitov 2008).

TLR-activated cDCs next migrate to the draining LN, where they present pathogen-derived antigens to naive $CD4^+$ and $CD8^+$ T cells (Banchereau et al. 2000). Due to the maturation-induced expression of costimulatory molecules and IL-12 by cDCs, antigen presentation in this context leads to potent priming and activation of pathogen-specific helper and cytotoxic effector T cells (Fig. 8.1). These effector T cells can then migrate to other sites of tissue infection, where they can specifically target infected cells for destruction. Unlike nonactivated DCs, mature cDCs are not effective at inducing the activation or proliferation of suppressive Treg cells (Yamazaki and Steinman 2009). As will be discussed later, the ability of cDCs to generate potent and specific antitumor T-cell responses is a highly desirable attribute for therapeutic cancer vaccines.

4 Conventional DCs in Cancer

As described above, cDCs play a dual role in immunity: not only are they capable of suppressing immune responses in the steady state, but they are also potent activators of anti-pathogen immune responses during infections. Because tumors often develop in the absence of acute, pathogen-induced inflammation, cDCs presenting antigens derived from the tumor microenvironment tend to naturally promote immune tolerance against tumor antigens rather than inducing active immunity (Seya et al. 2010). However, due to their inherent genetic instability, tumor cells often accumulate mutations that create "neo-epitopes," or tumor-specific altered peptides that can be recognized as foreign by the immune system. Thus, in order to escape immune recognition, tumors often produce additional factors that can further suppress antitumor immunity, above and beyond the mechanisms that normally control self-tolerance. As discussed in the following sections, these tumor-derived factors promote the development of tolerogenic cDCs while simultaneously preventing their activation. In turn, tumor-conditioned, tolerogenic DCs can actively suppress antitumor immunity both within the tumor microenvironment and within the tumor-draining LN.

4.1 Tumor-Derived Factors Promote the Development of Tolerogenic Conventional DCs and Myeloid-Derived Suppressor Cells

Much evidence has accumulated in recent years to support the notion that, in many cancers, tumors actively suppress the antitumor immune responses through multiple mechanisms (Lizee et al. 2006). Some of these mechanisms act directly on immature

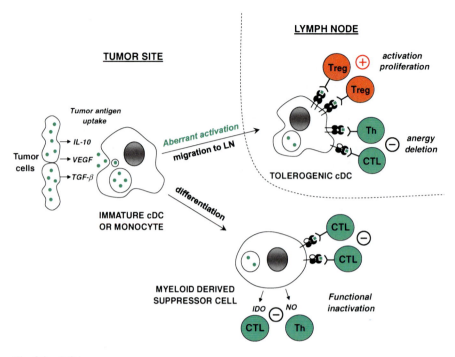

Fig. 8.2 cDC in cancer

cDCs within tumor stroma to prevent their activation and enhance their tolerogenic potential. Secretion of the anti-inflammatory cytokines interleukin (IL)-10, transforming growth factor (TGF)-β, and vascular endothelial growth factor (VEGF) by tumor cells is frequently observed in many cancers (Fig. 8.2). These factors inhibit the differentiation of myeloid cells in vivo, leading to decreased levels of functionally competent, mature APCs and accumulation of iDCs that are unable to upregulate MHC class II and costimulatory molecules or produce appropriate cytokines. IL-10 can suppress T-cell responses indirectly through the inhibition of MHC and costimulatory molecule expression and cytokine production by APCs, including DCs, Langerhans cells, and macrophages (Moore et al. 2001; Mosser and Zhang 2008). TGF-β can also inhibit APC function by suppressing maturation and IFN-γ production and inducing MHC class II downregulation (Gorelik and Flavell 2002; Letterio and Roberts 1998; Bierie and Moses 2006). VEGF appears to be a major mediator of disrupted DC differentiation, and tumors often secrete large amounts of VEGF that is detectable in the serum of cancer patients (Claffey and Robinson 1996; Gabrilovich et al. 1996). Studies have shown that such levels of VEGF can block DC maturation in vitro, whereas VEGF blockade can restore normal DC differentiation and function (Gabrilovich et al. 1999).

Many tumors also produce factors that result in the differentiation and accumulation of myeloid-derived suppressor cells (MDSCs), which are a heterogeneous population that includes immature cells of the granulocyte and monocyte/macrophage lineage that act to suppress antitumor immune responses (Gabrilovich and Nagaraj 2009). Although not well characterized, these cells are thought to represent aberrantly differentiated myeloid cells derived from monocyte precursors that migrate into the tumor microenvironment in response to chemokines such as IL-8 and monocyte chemotactic protein (MCP-1). Once in tumors, they can be induced to differentiate into MDSCs by VEGF and GM-CSF produced by tumor cells (Almand et al. 2001; Kusmartsev and Gabrilovich 2002). In many cancers, these cells are found directly interacting with tumor cells and form an integral part of the tumor stroma. In Hodgkin's lymphoma, MDSCs are associated with poorer prognosis; similarly, levels of MDSCs within melanoma tumor-draining lymph nodes are adversely associated with overall survival (Steidl et al. 2010; Lizee et al. 2010). These cells have also been shown to accumulate in the peripheral blood of patients with melanoma, Hodgkin's lymphoma, breast, lung, or head and neck cancer, and this accumulation is often associated with a decrease in DC numbers (Almand et al. 2000). Similar to the case with immature DCs, circulating levels of MDSCs have been well correlated with stage of disease and poorer prognosis, and surgical resection of tumors has been shown to decrease the number of peripheral blood MDSCs in both humans and animal models (Salvadori et al. 2000; Danna et al. 2004).

4.2 Mechanisms Used by cDCs and MDSCs to Suppress Antitumor Immune Responses

Through suppressing cDC activation and maturation, tumors can take advantage of the natural propensity of immature cDCs to promote tolerance, as discussed above. Therefore, cDCs that acquire self- or tumor-specific antigens in the tumor microenvironment will process these antigens and present them on MHC-I and MHC-II molecules to CD4$^+$ and CD8$^+$ T lymphocytes within tumor-draining lymph nodes. The absence of costimulation and activation-induced inflammatory cytokine secretion by cDCs leads to the induction of tumor antigen-specific T-cell anergy and tolerance (Fig. 8.2).

Furthermore, following their migration to the tumor-draining LN, tumor-conditioned cDCs have been shown to favor the priming of CD4$^+$Foxp3$^+$ Treg cells over priming of CD4$^+$ T-helper cells. This skewing toward Treg-mediated immune suppression requires the expression of TGF-β and retinoic acid by a subset of cDCs, which can also be derived from tumor cells (Yamazaki et al. 2008). In addition, Treg priming is thought to result from presentation of MHC-II-restricted self/tumor antigens by tolerogenic cDCs, implying that suppression is tumor antigen-specific (Wang et al. 2004; Wang and Wang 2007). Primed Treg cells can in turn suppress the proliferation and function of both CD4$^+$ and CD8$^+$ effector cells in both the tumor-draining LN and at the tumor site (Baecher-Allan et al. 2004; Sakaguchi 2005). Elevated levels of Treg cells have been found in several cancer types, including ovarian, pancreatic, and head and neck cancer, and are almost invariably associated with poor prognosis (Curiel et al. 2004a; Liyanage et al. 2002; Wolf et al. 2003).

MDSCs mediate their immunosuppressive activity through the inhibition of IFN-γ production by CD8⁺ T cells in response to MHC class I-associated peptide epitopes presented on the MDSC surface (Gabrilovich et al. 2001). This effect requires direct cell-to-cell contact and is mediated by reactive oxygen and nitrogen species, such as hydrogen peroxide (H_2O_2) and nitric oxide (NO), secreted by the MDSCs in close proximity to the T cell (Kusmartsev et al. 2004; Schmielau and Finn 2001). Although the precise mechanism of action on T cells has yet to be fully elucidated, there is some indication that immature MDSCs (iMCs) act in part through downregulation of the CD3ζ chain on responding CD8⁺ T cells (Otsuji et al. 1996). Recently, a population of iMCs has been described in the peripheral blood of cancer patients having high arginase-1 activity capable of depleting local arginine levels and down-modulating CD3ζ levels on T cells. Depletion of this iMC subset in vitro restored CD3ζ expression and normal T-cell responses (Rodriguez et al. 2004; Zea et al. 2005). Although freshly isolated iMCs do not appear capable of suppressing CD4⁺ T cells, cultured iMCs have been shown to induce CD4⁺ T-cell apoptosis through the production of arginase and NO (Bronte et al. 2003).

5 Plasmacytoid DCs in Protective Immunity to Pathogens

pDCs represent a unique hematopoietic cell type produced within the bone marrow and released into the blood stream. Under steady-state conditions, pDCs spontaneously enter the lymph nodes and colonize the T cell-rich areas, but are normally absent from most peripheral tissues. Upon viral infection, pDCs can however migrate from the blood into infected peripheral tissues and accumulate in draining lymph nodes where they sense viral nucleic acids through TLR7 and 9 and rapidly produce large amounts of type I IFNs. Although constituting only 0.2–0.8% of human blood cells, pDCs were found to produce over 95% of type I IFNs by peripheral blood mononuclear cells in response to many viruses. Within 6 h of activation, human pDCs dedicate 60% of the induced transcriptome to type I IFN genes producing 200–1,000 times more type I IFNs than any other blood cell type.

Type I IFNs induce a cellular anti-viral response that limits the spread of viral infection, but also initiates a network of cellular and molecular events that are crucial to the generation of protective immune responses against viruses (Theofilopoulos et al. 2005) (Fig. 8.3). Type I IFNs strongly activate immature cDCs to produce IL-12, IL-15, IL-18, and IL-23 cytokines that are not produced by human pDCs themselves (Santini et al. 2000; Paquette et al. 1998; Luft et al. 1998). Moreover, type I IFNs differentiate monocytes into cDCs, which subsequently induce strong Th1-mediated immune responses (Santini et al. 2000; Paquette et al. 1998; Santodonato et al. 2003; Blanco et al. 2001). Type I IFNs also increase the ability of mDC to cross-present antigens to CD8 T cells (Le Bon et al. 2003), promote CD8 T cell survival and clonal expansion (Tough et al. 1996; Marrack et al. 1999), and polarize CD4 T cells into Th1 cells (Hibbert et al. 2003). pDC-derived type I IFNs also stimulate activation of natural killer cells (Gerosa et al. 2005) and differentiation

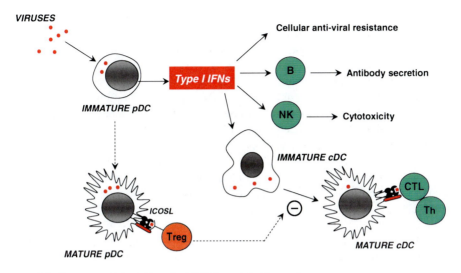

Fig. 8.3 Plasmacytoid dendritic cells (pDC) in antiviral immunity

of B cells into antibody-secreting plasma cells (Jego et al. 2003). The extraordinary ability of pDCs to mount a robust type I IFN response is linked to three unique features of pDCs (Gilliet et al. 2008). First, pDCs selectively express TLR7 and TLR9, but not other TLRs. This is in contrast to cDCs, which express TLR1, TLR2, TLR3, TLR4, TLR5, and TLR8 (Jarrossay et al. 2001; Kadowaki et al. 2001). TLR7 and TLR9 belong to a subset of TLRs expressed exclusively in intracellular compartments. TLR7 recognizes guanosine- and uridine-rich single-stranded RNA, as well as synthetic imidazoquinolines and guanosine analogues (Hemmi et al. 2002; Lund et al. 2004; Heil et al. 2004; Diebold et al. 2004). Through endosomal TLR7, pDCs detect viruses containing ssRNA genomes, such as influenza virus and vesicular stomatitis virus (VSV) (Lund et al. 2004; Heil et al. 2004; Diebold et al. 2004). On the other hand, endosomal TLR9 detects the phosphodiester backbone in natural DNA or unmethylated CpG-oligonucleotides (CpG-ODN) in synthetic phosphothioate DNA (Haas et al. 2008; Hemmi et al. 2000). Through endosomal TLR9, pDCs detect viruses containing dsDNA genomes, such as HSV and murine cytomegalovirus (Lund et al. 2003; Krug et al. 2004). The second important feature that makes pDCs professional type I IFN producing cells is their constitutive high expression levels of the interferon-regulatory factor (IRF)7, the master transcription factor for the induction of type I IFNs in pDCs (Honda et al. 2005; Kawai et al. 2004). This allows the rapid assembly of the MyD88 signal transduction complex and its translocation into the nucleus to rapidly initiate the transcription of type I IFN genes (Honda et al. 2004; Hoshino et al. 2006; Uematsu et al. 2005; Shinohara et al. 2006; Guiducci et al. 2008; Cao et al. 2008). By contrast, other cell types including cDC do not express IRF7 constitutively but require its upregulation in response to IFN-β feedback signaling following virus-induced activation of IRF3 (Taniguchi and Takaoka 2002).

The third reason for the extraordinary ability of pDC to produce high levels of type I IFNs is related to their unique ability to retain DNA in early endosomes for extended periods of time, which allows a sustained activation of IRF7 by the MyD88 signal transduction complex with induction of type I IFNs.

Given the importance of type I IFNs in activating a wide range of immune cells, it becomes clear that IFN production by pDCs has to be under tight control to prevent aberrant immune responses that could harm the host. Indeed, a number of surface receptors that modulate the type I IFN response by pDCs have been identified. BDCA2 and ILT-7 both associate with the γ-chain of the high-affinity Fc receptor for IgE (FcεRI), activate pDCs through an immunoreceptor-based tyrosine activation motif (ITAM)-mediated signaling pathway (Cao et al. 2006, 2007), and suppress the ability of pDCs to produce type I IFNs in response to TLR ligands (Cao et al. 2006; Dzionek et al. 2001). Other receptors that inhibit type I IFN production by human pDCs include the high affinity IgE receptor FcεRIα, which couples with FcεRIγ (Novak et al. 2004), and NKp44, a receptor that signals through the ITAM-bearing adaptor DAP12 (Fuchs et al. 2005). There is recent evidence that both viruses and tumors express ligands for such regulatory receptors on pDCs, suggesting that inhibition of pDC activation with downmodulation of type I IFN production may represent an active immune escape mechanism.

6 Plasmacytoid DCs in Immune Tolerance

Nonactivated (or immature) pDCs are incapable of inducing significant activation of naive T cells as they express low to undetectable levels of CD80 and CD86 (Grouard et al. 1997; Krug et al. 2003; Boonstra et al. 2003). Immature pDCs however express high levels of inducible costimulator ligand (ICOS-L) (Ito et al. 2007), which promotes survival, expansion, and IL-10 production of a subset of Foxp3+ T regulatory cells expressing ICOS (Ito et al. 2008). These findings suggest a specialized role of immature pDCs in peripheral tolerance. Accordingly, pDCs with an immature phenotype can suppress inflammatory responses to inhaled allergens (de Heer et al. 2004), promote allogeneic stem-cell engraftment (Fugier-Vivier et al. 2005), inhibit acute graft vs. host disease (Hadeiba et al. 2008), and mediate tolerance to solid grafts by inducing T regulatory cells (Ochando et al. 2006). pDCs also mediate oral tolerance to antigen feeding by inducing anergy and deletion of antigen-specific T cells in the liver (Goubier et al. 2008).

Upon activation, pDCs not only produce type I IFNs, but also acquire dendritic morphology and upregulate expression of MHC and T-cell costimulatory molecules, which enables them to directly engage and activate naive T cells (Grouard et al. 1997). In response to TLR7 or TLR9 activation, human pDCs produce IFN-α and TNF-α, and differentiate into mature DCs that prime naive CD4 T cells to produce IFN-γ and IL-10 (Kadowaki et al. 2000). The IFN-γ response appears to be partially dependent on IFN-α produced by pDC (Kadowaki et al. 2000). Human pDCs also mature into DC in culture with IL-3 or IL-3 plus CD40L (Grouard et al. 1997).

pDCs activated by IL-3 and CD40L do not produce significant amounts of IFN-α but upregulate the costimulatory molecule OX40L, which leads to an IL-4-independent priming of T-cells secreting Th2 cytokines IL-4, IL-5, and IL-10 (Rissoan et al. 1999; Ito et al. 2004). Thus, like classical cDCs, pDCs display functional plasticity with the ability to prime different effector T-cell responses, depending on the type of maturation signal. However, in contrast to cDCs, human pDCs activated through both TLR and IL-3-dependent pathway, have an intrinsic capacity to prime a population of IL-10-producing T cells with regulatory function (Ito et al. 2007; Gilliet and Liu 2002; Moseman et al. 2004; Kawamura et al. 2006). The molecular basis for this phenomenon was recently identified: upon maturation, pDCs but not cDCs upregulate the expression of ICOS-L, which drives the generation of IL-10-producing regulatory cells in the context of both Th1 and Th2 responses (Ito et al. 2007). These studies suggest that human pDCs have a specialized property to inhibit immune responses by inducing IL-10 producing T regulatory cells even at a mature differentiation stage. These IL-10 producing T regulatory cells induced by maturing pDCs may prevent excessive inflammation, which could damage the host (Fig. 8.3). In support of this hypothesis, pDC depletion during viral infection has been found to exacerbate immunopathology of the host (Smit et al. 2006).

7 Plasmacytoid DCs in Cancer

pDCs have been found in many solid human tumors including head and neck cancer, breast cancer, ovarian cancer, lung cancer, and skin tumors. In these tumors, pDCs are present as immature cells or cells which have been activated but do not secrete type I IFNs and have been implicated in the development of an immunosuppressive tumor microenvironment.

In ovarian cancer, high numbers of pDCs but not cDCs are detected in the malignant ascites (Zou et al. 2001). The recruitment of pDCs into the tumor environment resulted from the high expression of stromal-derived factor (SDF)-1 by the tumor (Zou et al. 2001). These tumor-associated pDCs were immature, expressing low levels of costimulatory molecules and incapable of activating T cells but able to induce IL-10 production by T cells, which promoted the immunosuppressive tumor microenvironment. In follow-up studies, it was found that these tumor pDCs induced IL-10-producing $CD8^+$ T regulatory cells that inhibited the induction of antitumor immunity (Wei et al. 2005). Tumor pDCs did not produce type I IFNs, but instead were found to produce tumor necrosis factor-α and interleukin 8 (IL-8), which directly stimulated neovascularization and tumor progression (Curiel et al. 2004b).

In breast cancer, immature pDCs were found in a subset of primary tumors and strongly correlated with an increased risk of tumor dissemination and relapse (Treilleux et al. 2004). Interestingly, breast cancer cells were found to express bone marrow stromal cell antigen 2 (BST2; CD317) protein, the ligand for ILT-7, the pDC-specific regulatory receptor that inhibits type I IFN in pDCs (Cao et al. 2009).

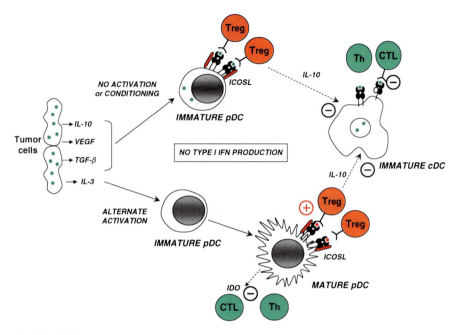

Fig. 8.4 pDC in cancer

In squamous head and neck cancer, Hartmann et al. (2003) demonstrated that pDCs infiltrate the tumor environment. These tumor pDCs had diminished ability to produce type I IFNs upon TLR stimulation ex-vivo (Hartmann et al. 2003). One mechanism likely contributing to the impaired tumor pDC function was found to be tumor-derived prostaglandin E2 (PGE-2) and transforming growth factor-β (TGF-β), which can induce IL-8 but synergistically inhibit IFN-α production of TLR-stimulated pDC (Bekeredjian-Ding et al. 2009).

pDCs were also found in the peritumoral areas of primary skin melanoma and were associated with the lack of type I IFN production (Vermi et al. 2003). Furthermore, pDCs were shown to accumulate in tumor-involved draining lymph nodes of melanoma patients in the vicinity of tumor nests (Gerlini et al. 2010). These pDCs expressed indoleamine 2,3-dioxygenase (IDO), which may contribute to a suppressive microenvironment that inhibits the generation of antitumor T-cell responses (Sharma et al. 2007).

In addition, increased numbers of pDCs were found in the bone marrow of patients with multiple myeloma. pDCs were found to promote tumor growth and the tumor was found to enhance pDC survival in the tumor microenvironment (Chauhan et al. 2009). The pDC–tumor interactions were contact-dependent, which enhanced the secretion of soluble factors including IL-3 (Chauhan et al. 2009). There is increasing evidence for the presence of pDCs in many other cancers including lung cancer (Perrot et al. 2007), T-cell lymphomas, basal cell carcinomas, and squamous cell carcinomas of the skin (Urosevic et al. 2005). In all of these tumors, pDCs exhibited an immature phenotype and were associated with a lack of type I IFN production, suggesting that they may contribute to the establishment of an immunosuppressive microenvironment. Thus, pDCs accumulate in a variety of human tumors and their presence is associated with a lack or inhibition of activation to produce type I IFNs and the induction of a T regulatory cell-mediated immunosuppressive microenvironment that inhibits the induction of antitumor immune responses and promotes tumor growth (Fig. 8.4).

8 Use of DCs for Therapeutic Induction of Antitumor Immunity

As described above, depending on their prior conditioning and activation status, cDCs and pDCs can either promote or suppress T-cell-mediated immune responses. Having now gained a basic understanding of the factors that influence these outcomes, it is becoming possible to develop rational therapeutic strategies that will skew the immune response toward favoring antitumor immunity (Steinman and Banchereau 2007). As discussed below, most current strategies fall into three broad categories: (1) vaccination using in vitro-activated and antigen-loaded DCs, (2) in vivo targeting of DCs to enhance their activation and stimulatory potential, and (3) interfering with mechanisms of DC-mediated immune suppression.

8.1 DC-Based Cancer Vaccines

Over the past decade, several human clinical trials have been performed to test the antitumor efficacy of a number of different DC formulations (Kalinski et al. 2009; Banchereau et al. 2009). In general, DC cancer vaccines have been very successful at generating antigen-specific T cells in the peripheral blood of patients; however, they have been equally unsuccessful at inducing complete regression of established solid tumors, except in a small minority of patients treated (Rosenberg et al. 2004; Palucka et al. 2009). Despite the lack of clinical success up to this point, there are many positive indications that current DC-based cancer vaccines can be improved upon further, and can also be combined with other interventions to improve objective response rates in cancer patients

Most trials have utilized DCs derived from blood monocyte precursors (differentiated using GM-CSF and IL-4), but some have used DCs differentiated from G-CSF-mobilized CD34$^+$ stem cells (Banchereau et al. 2001). Once autologous patient DCs are generated, two key components are required for optimal antitumor efficacy: (1) Loading of DCs with appropriate tumor antigens; (2) Adjuvant-induced maturation of DCs to increase MHC and costimulatory molecules, and in turn T-cell stimulatory capacity (discussed below).

DCs can be loaded with tumor antigens by a number of methods that fall into three broad categories: peptide-pulsing, whole protein-pulsing, or genetic modification. Peptide-pulsing involves using short, defined peptide antigens known to bind to specific HLA molecules. For example, melanoma-specific peptide antigens MART-1(27-35) and gp100(208-217) have been frequently used to stimulate tumor-reactive T cells in melanoma patients, but these peptides are restricted to those people who express HLA-A*0201, which is found in a minority of the general population (Valmori et al. 2002; Rosenberg et al. 1998). DCs pulsed with MHC-II-restricted peptides have also been utilized to generate helper T-cell immunity, but in some settings these have been shown to generate CD4$^+$Foxp3$^+$ Treg cells (Wong et al. 2004; Banerjee et al. 2006; Nakai et al. 2009). Current peptide-pulsed DC vaccines are restricted to a limited number of HLA molecules and relatively few tumor antigens compared to the overall MHC/tumor antigen repertoire.

DCs can also be loaded with whole proteins or tumor cells in order to generate antitumor immune responses. Since this approach relies on DCs to process the tumor antigens prior to their "cross-presentation" to T cells, this approach has the advantage of not being limited by HLA restriction and can theoretically be used to treat all patients (Yewdell et al. 1999; Lizee et al. 2005). In addition, this approach also allows for the potential induction of multiple T-cell specificities, known or unknown, shared among patients or unique to some patients. Examples of trials that have utilized whole protein DC loading approaches include the use of NY-ESO protein-pulsed DCs to vaccinate patients with bladder cancer, and the use of autologous or allogeneic tumor cell lysates to load DCs for stimulating antitumor immunity in melanoma and patients with other types of advanced cancer (Nestle et al. 1998; Chang et al. 2002; Ovali et al. 2007).

A third approach to DC tumor antigen loading utilizes viral vector transductions or nucleic acid (DNA or RNA) transfections to express specific proteins in DCs, where they are efficiently processed and presented on MHC-I and MHC-II molecules. This method has the advantages of including patients of any HLA haplotype and can generate T-cell specificities restricted to multiple HLA molecules, but is limited to known, commonly shared tumor antigens. DCs genetically modified to express tumor antigens have been used to treat bladder cancer, breast cancer, pancreatic cancer, and melanoma patients (Nair et al. 2002; Ponsaerts et al. 2003; Tyagi et al. 2009).

Cancer vaccines that directly inject purified antigenic peptides or killed tumor cells in order to elicit antitumor immunity likely work through endogenous DCs that process and/or present the tumor antigens to prime specific T cells. However, antigenic peptides bound and presented by non-DC types can often induce anergy in responding T cells. In order to address this problem of inappropriate antigen presentation, DC vaccines that utilize whole protein tumor antigens fused to ligands of DC-specific receptors or to antibodies that bind to such receptors have been developed. Some tumor antigen fusion proteins have targeted DEC-205 and other DC chemokine or scavenger receptors in order to specifically deliver tumor antigens to DCs in vivo (Bonifaz et al. 2004; Wang et al. 2009). Similarly, Fc receptors on DCs can be targeted using simple immune complexes of tumor antigens with specific antibody (Rafiq et al. 2002).

These receptor-targeted DC vaccines have shown significantly improved efficacy, requiring ~100-fold less antigen to stimulate similar T-cell responses as for unconjugated antigen (Kalergis and Ravetch 2002; Steinman and Hemmi 2006).

8.2 Intratumoral Activation of cDCs by TLR Ligands

Since mature, activated DCs stimulate the best T-cell responses, there has been much recent interest in the development of TLR ligands for use in cancer therapy. TLR4 (LPS) has been frequently used to activate and mature DCs in vitro prior to injection, but its high toxicity negates its use as a systemic adjuvant. TLR9 (CpG) has been tested as a systemic adjuvant in cancer patients, but response rates were disappointing (Pashenkov et al. 2006; Manegold et al. 2008). More recent evidence has shown that TLR ligands may have a much more potent effect when used to activate DCs locally within the tumor microenvironment (Hofmann et al. 2008). TLR3 (poly I:C) has been shown to promote cross-priming, suggesting that its application directly at the tumor site may act to enhance tumor antigen cross-presentation and priming of antitumor $CD8^+$ T-cell responses (Levine et al. 1979; Schulz et al. 2005; Butowski et al. 2009).

Tumor antigens have also been directly conjugated with TLR ligands in order to stimulate tumor antigen-specific T-cell priming and DC maturation simultaneously (Wagner 2009; Khan et al. 2007). These strategies have been particularly effective for TLR3 and TLR9, which both activate endosomal TLR receptors (Kuznik et al. 2010). There is accumulating evidence that endosomal TLR triggering leads to enhanced antigen cross-presentation, and facilitates the cross-priming of antigen-specific T cells (Basha et al. 2008; Burgdorf et al. 2008). Finally, tumor antigen/TLR ligand conjugates have been coupled with monoclonal antibodies specific for DC receptors in order to enhance specific uptake of these conjugates by DCs (Ramakrishna et al. 2007; Grossmann et al. 2009). Although still in the early stages, several new methods that target DCs in vivo are currently under development, and the next decade is likely to bring a major increase in the number of new DC vaccines being used clinically, and in their antitumor efficacy.

8.3 Intratumoral Activation of pDCs by TLR Ligands

Tumor pDCs fail to produce type I IFNs, which would contribute to a protective antitumor immune response. This is because the tumor lacks the appropriate stimuli to trigger TLR7 and TLR9 or even actively inhibits TLR7 and TLR9 activation. However, tumor pDCs have been found to respond to synthetic TLR7 or TLR9 agonists and produce high levels of type I IFNs, which promote antitumor immunity. Imiquimod is a synthetic nucleoside analogue that triggers endosomal TLR7 in pDCs (Ito et al. 2002). Topical application of imiquimod has been shown to be efficacious in the treatment of superficial basal cell carcinoma and CTCL. In these skin tumors, topical imiquimod treatment induced an accumulation of pDCs, and their activation to produce type I IFNs, which correlated with the induction of an inflammatory response that cleared the tumors (Urosevic et al. 2005; Palamara et al. 2004). Therapeutic pDC activation in tumors can also be achieved by synthetic ODN containing CpG motifs, which trigger TLR9 in pDCs. Intratumoral injection of CpG-ODNs showed tumor regression in patients with basal cell carcinoma and melanoma skin metastases (Hofmann et al. 2008). In a mouse tumor model, Vicari et al. (2002) showed that CpG-ODNs plus anti-IL-10 neutralizing antibodies could activate the tumor infiltrating DCs to induce robust antitumor cytotoxic T-cell responses and tumor rejection in vivo. TLR-activated pDCs in the tumor stimulate NK cell activity and elicit potent CD8 T-cell-mediated antitumor immunity by driving maturation of cDC that cross-present tumor antigens (Liu et al. 2008). TLR-activated pDCs also upregulate the expression of tumor necrosis factor-related apoptosis inducing ligand (TRAIL) and acquire the ability to kill tumor cells via TRAIL in vitro, suggesting an additional mechanism by which activated pDCs may induce antitumor activity (Stary et al. 2007). CpG-activation can reverse the pDC-induced tumor growth of multiple myeloma tumor cells.

8.4 Interfering with DC-Associated Immune Suppression

Since immune suppression is frequently manifested through the secretion of cytokines and the expression of co-inhibitory molecules, there has been much interest in developing clinical agents that are capable of blocking or neutralizing these molecules. These include monoclonal antibodies against VEGF, IL-10, and TGF-β (Mosser and Zhang 2008; Lu et al. 2010; Tuma 2005; Akhurst 2006; Dumont and Arteaga 2003; Midgley and Kerr 2005). These antibodies act by neutralizing the cytokines before they can contact both cDCs and pDCs and induce their suppression. In addition, antibodies against PD-1 and PD-L1 are currently being tested clinically (Blank et al. 2005; Iwai et al. 2005; Okudaira et al. 2009; Pilon-Thomas et al. 2010). By blocking the interaction between PD-1 and its ligands, it is expected that inhibitory signaling through PD-1 can be reduced and antitumor T-cell activity augmented accordingly.

9 Conclusions and Future Directions

As described above, cDCs and pDCs act as powerful modulators of immunity, and can specifically orchestrate appropriate cell-mediated immune responses. Depending on their activation status and prior conditioning, both DC types can alternatively drive tolerance or activation of a productive effector immune response. By understanding the immune modulators that affect DC activation status, it has become possible to design rational therapeutic strategies that will skew immune responses away from tumor antigen-specific tolerance toward antitumor immunity. Several strategies that augment DC-mediated T-cell priming are currently being tested in clinical trials, while other approaches act to reduce the potential tolerogenic effects of DCs in vivo. Future therapies will likely employ combination strategies to obtain optimal antitumor responses; for example, pDCs and cDCs have demonstrated synergistic antitumor effects when combined together in a murine DC vaccine model. It is also likely that future vaccine regimens will combine DC augmentation strategies with interventions that block the induction of DC-mediated tolerance. Although clinical response rates to the first generation of DC-based cancer vaccines were generally disappointing, they still demonstrated a potent ability to prime antitumor T-cell responses. This attribute makes it likely that DC-based vaccines will have an important place in future cancer therapies, as the next generation of DC-based vaccines promises to demonstrate greater antitumor efficacy and improved objective response rates for cancer patients.

References

Akhurst RJ (2006) Large- and small-molecule inhibitors of transforming growth factor-beta signaling. Curr Opin Investig Drugs 7:513–521
Almand B, Resser JR, Lindman B, Nadaf S, Clark JI, Kwon ED, Carbone DP, Gabrilovich DI (2000) Clinical significance of defective dendritic cell differentiation in cancer. Clin Cancer Res 6:1755–1766
Almand B, Clark JI, Nikitina E, van Beynen J, English NR, Knight SC, Carbone DP, Gabrilovich DI (2001) Increased production of immature myeloid cells in cancer patients: a mechanism of immunosuppression in cancer. J Immunol 166:678–689
Baecher-Allan C, Viglietta V, Hafler DA (2004) Human CD4+CD25+ regulatory T cells. Semin Immunol 16:89–98
Banchereau J, Steinman RM (1998) Dendritic cells and the control of immunity. Nature 392: 245–252
Banchereau J, Briere F, Caux C, Davoust J, Lebecque S, Liu YJ, Pulendran B, Palucka K (2000) Immunobiology of dendritic cells. Annu Rev Immunol 18:767–811
Banchereau J, Palucka AK, Dhodapkar M, Burkeholder S, Taquet N, Rolland A, Taquet S, Coquery S, Wittkowski KM, Bhardwaj N, Pineiro L, Steinman R, Fay J (2001) Immune and clinical responses in patients with metastatic melanoma to CD34(+) progenitor-derived dendritic cell vaccine. Cancer Res 61:6451–6458
Banchereau J, Klechevsky E, Schmitt N, Morita R, Palucka K, Ueno H (2009) Harnessing human dendritic cell subsets to design novel vaccines. Ann N Y Acad Sci 1174:24–32
Banerjee DK, Dhodapkar MV, Matayeva E, Steinman RM, Dhodapkar KM (2006) Expansion of FOXP3high regulatory T cells by human dendritic cells (DCs) in vitro and after injection of cytokine-matured DCs in myeloma patients. Blood 108:2655–2661
Basha G, Lizee G, Reinicke AT, Seipp RP, Omilusik KD, Jefferies WA (2008) MHC class I endosomal and lysosomal trafficking coincides with exogenous antigen loading in dendritic cells. PLoS One 3:e3247
Bekeredjian-Ding I, Schafer M, Hartmann E, Pries R, Parcina M, Schneider P, Giese T, Endres S, Wollenberg B, Hartmann G (2009) Tumour-derived prostaglandin E and transforming growth factor-beta synergize to inhibit plasmacytoid dendritic cell-derived interferon-alpha. Immunology 128:439–450

Beyer M, Schultze JL (2008) Immunoregulatory T cells: role and potential as a target in malignancy. Curr Oncol Rep 10:130–136

Bierie B, Moses HL (2006) Tumour microenvironment: TGFbeta: the molecular Jekyll and Hyde of cancer. Nat Rev Cancer 6:506–520

Blanco P, Palucka AK, Gill M, Pascual V, Banchereau J (2001) Induction of dendritic cell differentiation by IFN-alpha in systemic lupus erythematosus. Science 294:1540–1543

Blank C, Gajewski TF, Mackensen A (2005) Interaction of PD-L1 on tumor cells with PD-1 on tumor-specific T cells as a mechanism of immune evasion: implications for tumor immunotherapy. Cancer Immunol Immunother 54:307–314

Bonifaz LC, Bonnyay DP, Charalambous A, Darguste DI, Fujii S, Soares H, Brimnes MK, Moltedo B, Moran TM, Steinman RM (2004) In vivo targeting of antigens to maturing dendritic cells via the DEC-205 receptor improves T cell vaccination. J Exp Med 199:815–824

Boonstra A, Asselin-Paturel C, Gilliet M, Crain C, Trinchieri G, Liu YJ, O'Garra A (2003) Flexibility of mouse classical and plasmacytoid-derived dendritic cells in directing T helper type 1 and 2 cell development: dependency on antigen dose and differential toll-like receptor ligation. J Exp Med 197:101–109

Bronte V, Serafini P, De Santo C, Marigo I, Tosello V, Mazzoni A, Segal DM, Staib C, Lowel M, Sutter G, Colombo MP, Zanovello P (2003) IL-4-induced arginase 1 suppresses alloreactive T cells in tumor-bearing mice. J Immunol 170:270–278

Burgdorf S, Scholz C, Kautz A, Tampe R, Kurts C (2008) Spatial and mechanistic separation of cross-presentation and endogenous antigen presentation. Nat Immunol 9:558–566

Butowski N, Lamborn KR, Lee BL, Prados MD, Cloughesy T, DeAngelis LM, Abrey L, Fink K, Lieberman F, Mehta M, Ian Robins H, Junck L, Salazar AM, Chang SM (2009) A North American brain tumor consortium phase II study of poly-ICLC for adult patients with recurrent anaplastic gliomas. J Neurooncol 91:183–189

Cao W, Rosen DB, Ito T, Bover L, Bao M, Watanabe G, Yao Z, Zhang L, Lanier LL, Liu YJ (2006) Plasmacytoid dendritic cell-specific receptor ILT7-Fc epsilonRI gamma inhibits toll-like receptor-induced interferon production. J Exp Med 203:1399–1405

Cao W, Zhang L, Rosen DB, Bover L, Watanabe G, Bao M, Lanier LL, Liu YJ (2007) BDCA2/Fc epsilon RI gamma complex signals through a novel BCR-like pathway in human plasmacytoid dendritic cells. PLoS Biol 5:e248

Cao W, Manicassamy S, Tang H, Kasturi SP, Pirani A, Murthy N, Pulendran B (2008) Toll-like receptor-mediated induction of type I interferon in plasmacytoid dendritic cells requires the rapamycin-sensitive PI(3)K-mTOR-p70S6K pathway. Nat Immunol 9:1157–1164

Cao W, Bover L, Cho M, Wen X, Hanabuchi S, Bao M, Rosen DB, Wang YH, Shaw JL, Du Q, Li C, Arai N, Yao Z, Lanier LL, Liu YJ (2009) Regulation of TLR7/9 responses in plasmacytoid dendritic cells by BST2 and ILT7 receptor interaction. J Exp Med 206:1603–1614

Chang AE, Redman BG, Whitfield JR, Nickoloff BJ, Braun TM, Lee PP, Geiger JD, Mule JJ (2002) A phase I trial of tumor lysate-pulsed dendritic cells in the treatment of advanced cancer. Clin Cancer Res 8:1021–1032

Chauhan D, Singh AV, Brahmandam M, Carrasco R, Bandi M, Hideshima T, Bianchi G, Podar K, Tai YT, Mitsiades C, Raje N, Jaye DL, Kumar SK, Richardson P, Munshi N, Anderson KC (2009) Functional interaction of plasmacytoid dendritic cells with multiple myeloma cells: a therapeutic target. Cancer Cell 16:309–323

Claffey KP, Robinson GS (1996) Regulation of VEGF/VPF expression in tumor cells: consequences for tumor growth and metastasis. Cancer Metastasis Rev 15:165–176

Curiel TJ, Coukos G, Zou L, Alvarez X, Cheng P, Mottram P, Evdemon-Hogan M, Conejo-Garcia JR, Zhang L, Burow M, Zhu Y, Wei S, Kryczek I, Daniel B, Gordon A, Myers L, Lackner A, Disis ML, Knutson KL, Chen L, Zou W (2004a) Specific recruitment of regulatory T cells in ovarian carcinoma fosters immune privilege and predicts reduced survival. Nat Med 10:942–949

Curiel TJ, Cheng P, Mottram P, Alvarez X, Moons L, Evdemon-Hogan M, Wei S, Zou L, Kryczek I, Hoyle G, Lackner A, Carmeliet P, Zou W (2004b) Dendritic cell subsets differentially regulate angiogenesis in human ovarian cancer. Cancer Res 64:5535–5538

Danna EA, Sinha P, Gilbert M, Clements VK, Pulaski BA, Ostrand-Rosenberg S (2004) Surgical removal of primary tumor reverses tumor-induced immunosuppression despite the presence of metastatic disease. Cancer Res 64:2205–2211

de Heer HJ, Hammad H, Soullie T, Hijdra D, Vos N, Willart MA, Hoogsteden HC, Lambrecht BN (2004) Essential role of lung plasmacytoid dendritic cells in preventing asthmatic reactions to harmless inhaled antigen. J Exp Med 200:89–98

Diebold SS, Kaisho T, Hemmi H, Akira S, Reis e Sousa C (2004) Innate antiviral responses by means of TLR7-mediated recognition of single-stranded RNA. Science 303:1529–1531

Dumont N, Arteaga CL (2003) Targeting the TGF beta signaling network in human neoplasia. Cancer Cell 3:531–536

Dzionek A, Sohma Y, Nagafune J, Cella M, Colonna M, Facchetti F, Gunther G, Johnston I, Lanzavecchia A, Nagasaka T, Okada T, Vermi W, Winkels G, Yamamoto T, Zysk M, Yamaguchi Y, Schmitz J (2001) BDCA-2, a novel plasmacytoid dendritic cell-specific type II C-type lectin, mediates antigen capture and is a potent inhibitor of interferon alpha/beta induction [see comment]. J Exp Med 194:1823–1834

Fuchs A, Cella M, Kondo T, Colonna M (2005) Paradoxic inhibition of human natural interferon-producing cells by the activating receptor NKp44. Blood 106:2076–2082

Fugier-Vivier IJ, Rezzoug F, Huang Y, Graul-Layman AJ, Schanie CL, Xu H, Chilton PM, Ildstad ST (2005) Plasmacytoid precursor dendritic cells facilitate allogeneic hematopoietic stem cell engraftment. J Exp Med 201:373–383

Gabrilovich DI, Nagaraj S (2009) Myeloid-derived suppressor cells as regulators of the immune system. Nat Rev Immunol 9:162–174

Gabrilovich DI, Chen HL, Girgis KR, Cunningham HT, Meny GM, Nadaf S, Kavanaugh D, Carbone DP (1996) Production of vascular endothelial growth factor by human tumors inhibits the functional maturation of dendritic cells. Nat Med 2:1096–1103

Gabrilovich DI, Ishida T, Nadaf S, Ohm JE, Carbone DP (1999) Antibodies to vascular endothelial growth factor enhance the efficacy of cancer immunotherapy by improving endogenous dendritic cell function. Clin Cancer Res 5:2963–2970

Gabrilovich DI, Velders MP, Sotomayor EM, Kast WM (2001) Mechanism of immune dysfunction in cancer mediated by immature Gr-1+ myeloid cells. J Immunol 166:5398–5406

Gallimore A, Godkin A (2008) Regulatory T cells and tumour immunity – observations in mice and men. Immunology 123:157–163

Gerlini G, Di Gennaro P, Mariotti G, Urso C, Chiarugi A, Pimpinelli N, Borgognoni L (2010) Indoleamine 2,3-dioxygenase+ cells correspond to the BDCA2+ plasmacytoid dendritic cells in human melanoma sentinel nodes. J Invest Dermatol 130:898–901

Gerosa F, Gobbi A, Zorzi P, Burg S, Briere F, Carra G, Trinchieri G (2005) The reciprocal interaction of NK cells with plasmacytoid or myeloid dendritic cells profoundly affects innate resistance functions. J Immunol 174:727–734

Gilliet M, Liu YJ (2002) Generation of human CD8 T regulatory cells by CD40 ligand-activated plasmacytoid dendritic cells. J Exp Med 195:695–704

Gilliet M, Cao W, Liu YJ (2008) Plasmacytoid dendritic cells: sensing nucleic acids in viral infection and autoimmune diseases. Nat Rev Immunol 8:594–606

Gorelik L, Flavell RA (2002) Transforming growth factor-beta in T-cell biology. Nat Rev Immunol 2:46–53

Goubier A, Dubois B, Gheit H, Joubert G, Villard-Truc F, Asselin-Paturel C, Trinchieri G, Kaiserlian D (2008) Plasmacytoid dendritic cells mediate oral tolerance. Immunity 29:464–475

Grossmann C, Tenbusch M, Nchinda G, Temchura V, Nabi G, Stone GW, Kornbluth RS, Uberla K (2009) Enhancement of the priming efficacy of DNA vaccines encoding dendritic cell-targeted antigens by synergistic toll-like receptor ligands. BMC Immunol 10:43

Grouard G, Rissoan MC, Filgueira L, Durand I, Banchereau J, Liu YJ (1997) The enigmatic plasmacytoid T cells develop into dendritic cells with interleukin (IL)-3 and CD40-ligand. J Exp Med 185:1101–1111

Guiducci C, Ghirelli C, Marloie-Provost MA, Matray T, Coffman RL, Liu YJ, Barrat FJ, Soumelis V (2008) PI3K is critical for the nuclear translocation of IRF-7 and type I IFN production by human plasmacytoid predendritic cells in response to TLR activation. J Exp Med 205:315–322

Haas T, Metzger J, Schmitz F, Heit A, Muller T, Latz E, Wagner H (2008) The DNA sugar backbone 2' deoxyribose determines toll-like receptor 9 activation [see comment]. Immunity 28:315–323

Hadeiba H, Sato T, Habtezion A, Oderup C, Pan J, Butcher EC (2008) CCR9 expression defines tolerogenic plasmacytoid dendritic cells able to suppress acute graft-versus-host disease. Nat Immunol 9:1253–1260

Harding CV (1996) Class II antigen processing: analysis of compartments and functions. Crit Rev Immunol 16:13–29

Hartmann E, Wollenberg B, Rothenfusser S, Wagner M, Wellisch D, Mack B, Giese T, Gires O, Endres S, Hartmann G (2003) Identification and functional analysis of tumor-infiltrating plasmacytoid dendritic cells in head and neck cancer. Cancer Res 63:6478–6487

Heath WR, Carbone FR (2009) Dendritic cell subsets in primary and secondary T cell responses at body surfaces. Nat Immunol 10:1237–1244

Heil F, Hemmi H, Hochrein H, Ampenberger F, Kirschning C, Akira S, Lipford G, Wagner H, Bauer S (2004) Species-specific recognition of single-stranded RNA via toll-like receptor 7 and 8 [see comment]. Science 303:1526–1529

Hemmi H, Takeuchi O, Kawai T, Kaisho T, Sato S, Sanjo H, Matsumoto M, Hoshino K, Wagner H, Takeda K, Akira S (2000) A toll-like receptor recognizes bacterial DNA. Nature 408:740–745

Hemmi H, Kaisho T, Takeuchi O, Sato S, Sanjo H, Hoshino K, Horiuchi T, Tomizawa H, Takeda K, Akira S (2002) Small anti-viral compounds activate immune cells via the TLR7 MyD88-dependent signaling pathway [see comment]. Nat Immunol 3:196–200

Hibbert L, Pflanz S, De Waal Malefyt R, Kastelein RA (2003) IL-27 and IFN-alpha signal via Stat1 and Stat3 and induce T-Bet and IL-12Rbeta2 in naive T cells. J Interferon Cytokine Res 23:513–522

Hofmann MA, Kors C, Audring H, Walden P, Sterry W, Trefzer U (2008) Phase 1 evaluation of intralesionally injected TLR9-agonist PF-3512676 in patients with basal cell carcinoma or metastatic melanoma. J Immunother 31:520–527

Honda K, Yanai H, Mizutani T, Negishi H, Shimada N, Suzuki N, Ohba Y, Takaoka A, Yeh WC, Taniguchi T (2004) Role of a transductional-transcriptional processor complex involving MyD88 and IRF-7 in toll-like receptor signaling. Proc Natl Acad Sci U S A 101:15416–15421

Honda K, Yanai H, Negishi H, Asagiri M, Sato M, Mizutani T, Shimada N, Ohba Y, Takaoka A, Yoshida N, Taniguchi T (2005) IRF-7 is the master regulator of type-I interferon-dependent immune responses. Nature 434:772–777

Hoshino K, Sugiyama T, Matsumoto M, Tanaka T, Saito M, Hemmi H, Ohara O, Akira S, Kaisho T (2006) IkappaB kinase-alpha is critical for interferon-alpha production induced by toll-like receptors 7 and 9. Nature 440:949–953

Inaba K, Swiggard WJ, Steinman RM, Romani N, Schuler G (2001) Isolation of dendritic cells. Curr Protoc Immunol Chapter 3:Unit 3.7

Ito T, Amakawa R, Kaisho T, Hemmi H, Tajima K, Uehira K, Ozaki Y, Tomizawa H, Akira S, Fukuhara S (2002) Interferon-alpha and interleukin-12 are induced differentially by toll-like receptor 7 ligands in human blood dendritic cell subsets. J Exp Med 195:1507–1512

Ito T, Amakawa R, Inaba M, Hori T, Ota M, Nakamura K, Takebayashi M, Miyaji M, Yoshimura T, Inaba K, Fukuhara S (2004) Plasmacytoid dendritic cells regulate Th cell responses through OX40 ligand and type I IFNs. J Immunol 172:4253–4259

Ito T, Yang M, Wang YH, Lande R, Gregorio J, Perng OA, Qin XF, Liu YJ, Gilliet M (2007) Plasmacytoid dendritic cells prime IL-10-producing T regulatory cells by inducible costimulator ligand. J Exp Med 204:105–115

Ito T, Hanabuchi S, Wang YH, Park WR, Arima K, Bover L, Qin FX, Gilliet M, Liu YJ (2008) Two functional subsets of FOXP3+ regulatory T cells in human thymus and periphery. Immunity 28:870–880

Iwai Y, Terawaki S, Honjo T (2005) PD-1 blockade inhibits hematogenous spread of poorly immunogenic tumor cells by enhanced recruitment of effector T cells. Int Immunol 17:133–144

Iwasaki A, Medzhitov R (2004) Toll-like receptor control of the adaptive immune responses. Nat Immunol 5:987–995

Jarrossay D, Napolitani G, Colonna M, Sallusto F, Lanzavecchia A (2001) Specialization and complementarity in microbial molecule recognition by human myeloid and plasmacytoid dendritic cells. Eur J Immunol 31:3388–3393

Jego G, Palucka AK, Blanck JP, Chalouni C, Pascual V, Banchereau J (2003) Plasmacytoid dendritic cells induce plasma cell differentiation through type I interferon and interleukin 6. Immunity 19:225–234

Kadowaki N, Antonenko S, Lau JY, Liu YJ (2000) Natural interferon alpha/beta-producing cells link innate and adaptive immunity. J Exp Med 192:219–226

Kadowaki N, Ho S, Antonenko S, Malefyt RW, Kastelein RA, Bazan F, Liu YJ (2001) Subsets of human dendritic cell precursors express different toll-like receptors and respond to different microbial antigens. J Exp Med 194:863–869

Kalergis AM, Ravetch JV (2002) Inducing tumor immunity through the selective engagement of activating Fcgamma receptors on dendritic cells. J Exp Med 195:1653–1659

Kalinski P, Urban J, Narang R, Berk E, Wieckowski E, Muthuswamy R (2009) Dendritic cell-based therapeutic cancer vaccines: what we have and what we need. Future Oncol 5:379–390

Kawai T, Sato S, Ishii KJ, Coban C, Hemmi H, Yamamoto M, Terai K, Matsuda M, Inoue J, Uematsu S, Takeuchi O, Akira S (2004) Interferon-alpha induction through toll-like receptors involves a direct interaction of IRF7 with MyD88 and TRAF6. Nat Immunol 5: 1061–1068

Kawamura K, Kadowaki N, Kitawaki T, Uchiyama T (2006) Virus-stimulated plasmacytoid dendritic cells induce CD4+ cytotoxic regulatory T cells. Blood 107:1031–1038

Khan S, Bijker MS, Weterings JJ, Tanke HJ, Adema GJ, van Hall T, Drijfhout JW, Melief CJ, Overkleeft HS, van der Marel GA, Filippov DV, van der Burg SH, Ossendorp F (2007) Distinct uptake mechanisms but similar intracellular processing of two different toll-like receptor ligand-peptide conjugates in dendritic cells. J Biol Chem 282:21145–21159

Krug A, Veeraswamy R, Pekosz A, Kanagawa O, Unanue ER, Colonna M, Cella M (2003) Interferon-producing cells fail to induce proliferation of naive T cells but can promote expansion and T helper 1 differentiation of antigen-experienced unpolarized T cells. J Exp Med 197:899–906

Krug A, Luker GD, Barchet W, Leib DA, Akira S, Colonna M (2004) Herpes simplex virus type 1 activates murine natural interferon-producing cells through toll-like receptor 9. Blood 103:1433–1437

Kusmartsev S, Gabrilovich DI (2002) Immature myeloid cells and cancer-associated immune suppression. Cancer Immunol Immunother 51:293–298

Kusmartsev S, Nefedova Y, Yoder D, Gabrilovich DI (2004) Antigen-specific inhibition of CD8+ T cell response by immature myeloid cells in cancer is mediated by reactive oxygen species. J Immunol 172:989–999

Kuznik A, Panter G, Jerala R (2010) Recognition of nucleic acids by toll-like receptors and development of immunomodulatory drugs. Curr Med Chem 17(18):1899–1914

Lande R, Gilliet M (2010) Plasmacytoid dendritic cells: key players in the initiation and regulation of immune responses. Ann N Y Acad Sci 1183:89–103

Le Bon A, Etchart N, Rossmann C, Ashton M, Hou S, Gewert D, Borrow P, Tough DF (2003) Cross-priming of CD8+ T cells stimulated by virus-induced type I interferon [see comment]. Nat Immunol 4:1009–1015

Letterio JJ, Roberts AB (1998) Regulation of immune responses by TGF-beta. Annu Rev Immunol 16:137–161

Levine AS, Sivulich M, Wiernik PH, Levy HB (1979) Initial clinical trials in cancer patients of polyriboinosinic-polyribocytidylic acid stabilized with poly-L-lysine, in carboxymethylcellulose [poly(ICLC)], a highly effective interferon inducer. Cancer Res 39:1645–1650

Liu YJ (2005) IPC: professional type 1 interferon-producing cells and plasmacytoid dendritic cell precursors. Annu Rev Immunol 23:275–306

Liu C, Lou Y, Lizee G, Qin H, Liu S, Rabinovich B, Kim GJ, Wang YH, Ye Y, Sikora AG, Overwijk WW, Liu YJ, Wang G, Hwu P (2008) Plasmacytoid dendritic cells induce NK cell-dependent, tumor antigen-specific T cell cross-priming and tumor regression in mice. J Clin Investig 118:1165–1175

Liyanage UK, Moore TT, Joo HG, Tanaka Y, Herrmann V, Doherty G, Drebin JA, Strasberg SM, Eberlein TJ, Goedegebuure PS, Linehan DC (2002) Prevalence of regulatory T cells is increased in peripheral blood and tumor microenvironment of patients with pancreas or breast adenocarcinoma. J Immunol 169:2756–2761

Lizee G, Basha G, Jefferies WA (2005) Tails of wonder: endocytic-sorting motifs key for exogenous antigen presentation. Trends Immunol 26:141–149

Lizee G, Radvanyi LG, Overwijk WW, Hwu P (2006) Improving antitumor immune responses by circumventing immunoregulatory cells and mechanisms. Clin Cancer Res 12:4794–4803

Lizee G, Whittington MA, Chen JF, Greene VR, Bassett RL, Prieto VG, Radvanyi LG, Grimm EA, Hwu P, Gershenwald JE (2010) Prevalence of CD68+ macrophages within tumor-draining lymph node basins correlates with poorer overall survival in Stage II melanoma patients. American Society of Clinical Oncologists Meeting Abstracts 2010. J Clin Oncol 28 (suppl; e21034)

Lu H, Wagner WM, Gad E, Yang Y, Duan H, Amon LM, Van Denend N, Larson ER, Chang A, Tufvesson H, Disis ML (2010) Treatment failure of a TLR-7 agonist occurs due to self-regulation of acute inflammation and can be overcome by IL-10 blockade. J Immunol 184(9): 5360–5367

Luft T, Pang KC, Thomas E, Hertzog P, Hart DN, Trapani J, Cebon J (1998) Type I IFNs enhance the terminal differentiation of dendritic cells. J Immunol 161:1947–1953

Lund J, Sato A, Akira S, Medzhitov R, Iwasaki A (2003) Toll-like receptor 9-mediated recognition of Herpes simplex virus-2 by plasmacytoid dendritic cells. J Exp Med 198:513–520

Lund JM, Alexopoulou L, Sato A, Karow M, Adams NC, Gale NW, Iwasaki A, Flavell RA (2004) Recognition of single-stranded RNA viruses by toll-like receptor 7 [see comment]. Proc Natl Acad Sci U S A 101:5598–5603

Lutz MB, Kurts C (2009) Induction of peripheral CD4+ T-cell tolerance and CD8+ T-cell cross-tolerance by dendritic cells. Eur J Immunol 39:2325–2330

Manegold C, Gravenor D, Woytowitz D, Mezger J, Hirsh V, Albert G, Al-Adhami M, Readett D, Krieg AM, Leichman CG (2008) Randomized phase II trial of a toll-like receptor 9 agonist oligodeoxynucleotide, PF-3512676, in combination with first-line taxane plus platinum chemotherapy for advanced-stage non-small-cell lung cancer. J Clin Oncol 26:3979–3986

Marrack P, Kappler J, Mitchell T (1999) Type I interferons keep activated T cells alive. J Exp Med 189:521–530

Medzhitov R (2008) Origin and physiological roles of inflammation. Nature 454:428–435

Midgley R, Kerr D (2005) Bevacizumab – current status and future directions. Ann Oncol 16:999–1004

Moore KW, de Waal Malefyt R, Coffman RL, O'Garra A (2001) Interleukin-10 and the interleukin-10 receptor. Annu Rev Immunol 19:683–765

Moseman EA, Liang X, Dawson AJ, Panoskaltsis-Mortari A, Krieg AM, Liu YJ, Blazar BR, Chen W (2004) Human plasmacytoid dendritic cells activated by CpG oligodeoxynucleotides induce the generation of CD4+CD25+ regulatory T cells. J Immunol 173:4433–4442

Mosser DM, Zhang X (2008) Interleukin-10: new perspectives on an old cytokine. Immunol Rev 226:205–218

Mueller DL (2010) Mechanisms maintaining peripheral tolerance. Nat Immunol 11:21–27

Nair SK, Morse M, Boczkowski D, Cumming RI, Vasovic L, Gilboa E, Lyerly HK (2002) Induction of tumor-specific cytotoxic T lymphocytes in cancer patients by autologous tumor RNA-transfected dendritic cells. Ann Surg 235:540–549

Nakai N, Katoh N, Kitagawa T, Ueda E, Takenaka H, Kishimoto S (2009) Immunoregulatory T cells in the peripheral blood of melanoma patients treated with melanoma antigen-pulsed mature monocyte-derived dendritic cell vaccination. J Dermatol Sci 54:31–37

Nestle FO, Alijagic S, Gilliet M, Sun Y, Grabbe S, Dummer R, Burg G, Schadendorf D (1998) Vaccination of melanoma patients with peptide- or tumor lysate-pulsed dendritic cells. Nat Med 4:328–332

Novak N, Allam JP, Hagemann T, Jenneck C, Laffer S, Valenta R, Kochan J, Bieber T (2004) Characterization of FcepsilonRI-bearing CD123 blood dendritic cell antigen-2 plasmacytoid dendritic cells in atopic dermatitis. J Allergy Clin Immunol 114:364–370

Ochando JC, Homma C, Yang Y, Hidalgo A, Garin A, Tacke F, Angeli V, Li Y, Boros P, Ding Y, Jessberger R, Trinchieri G, Lira SA, Randolph GJ, Bromberg JS (2006) Alloantigen-presenting plasmacytoid dendritic cells mediate tolerance to vascularized grafts [see comment]. Nat Immunol 7:652–662

Okudaira K, Hokari R, Tsuzuki Y, Okada Y, Komoto S, Watanabe C, Kurihara C, Kawaguchi A, Nagao S, Azuma M, Yagita H, Miura S (2009) Blockade of B7-H1 or B7-DC induces an antitumor effect in a mouse pancreatic cancer model. Int J Oncol 35:741–749

Otsuji M, Kimura Y, Aoe T, Okamoto Y, Saito T (1996) Oxidative stress by tumor-derived macrophages suppresses the expression of CD3 zeta chain of T-cell receptor complex and antigen-specific T-cell responses. Proc Natl Acad Sci U S A 93:13119–13124

Ovali E, Dikmen T, Sonmez M, Yilmaz M, Unal A, Dalbasti T, Kuzeyli K, Erturk M, Omay SB (2007) Active immunotherapy for cancer patients using tumor lysate pulsed dendritic cell vaccine: a safety study. J Exp Clin Cancer Res 26:209–214

Palamara F, Meindl S, Holcmann M, Luhrs P, Stingl G, Sibilia M (2004) Identification and characterization of pDC-like cells in normal mouse skin and melanomas treated with imiquimod. J Immunol 173:3051–3061

Palucka K, Ueno H, Fay J, Banchereau J (2009) Harnessing dendritic cells to generate cancer vaccines. Ann N Y Acad Sci 1174:88–98

Paquette RL, Hsu NC, Kiertscher SM, Park AN, Tran L, Roth MD, Glaspy JA (1998) Interferon-alpha and granulocyte-macrophage colony-stimulating factor differentiate peripheral blood monocytes into potent antigen-presenting cells. J Leukoc Biol 64:358–367

Pashenkov M, Goess G, Wagner C, Hormann M, Jandl T, Moser A, Britten CM, Smolle J, Koller S, Mauch C, Tantcheva-Poor I, Grabbe S, Loquai C, Esser S, Franckson T, Schneeberger A, Haarmann C, Krieg AM, Stingl G, Wagner SN (2006) Phase II trial of a toll-like receptor 9-activating oligonucleotide in patients with metastatic melanoma. J Clin Oncol 24:5716–5724

Perrot I, Blanchard D, Freymond N, Isaac S, Guibert B, Pacheco Y, Lebecque S (2007) Dendritic cells infiltrating human non-small cell lung cancer are blocked at immature stage. J Immunol 178:2763–2769

Pilon-Thomas S, Mackay A, Vohra N, Mule JJ (2010) Blockade of programmed death ligand 1 enhances the therapeutic efficacy of combination immunotherapy against melanoma. J Immunol 184:3442–3449

Ponsaerts P, Van Tendeloo VF, Berneman ZN (2003) Cancer immunotherapy using RNA loaded dendritic cells. Clin Exp Immunol 134:378–384

Rafiq K, Bergtold A, Clynes R (2002) Immune complex-mediated antigen presentation induces tumor immunity. J Clin Invest 110:71–79

Ramakrishna V, Vasilakos JP, Tario JD Jr, Berger MA, Wallace PK, Keler T (2007) Toll-like receptor activation enhances cell-mediated immunity induced by an antibody vaccine targeting human dendritic cells. J Transl Med 5:5

Rissoan MC, Soumelis V, Kadowaki N, Grouard G, Briere F, de Waal Malefyt R, Liu YJ (1999) Reciprocal control of T helper cell and dendritic cell differentiation [see comment]. Science 283:1183–1186

Rodriguez PC, Quiceno DG, Zabaleta J, Ortiz B, Zea AH, Piazuelo MB, Delgado A, Correa P, Brayer J, Sotomayor EM, Antonia S, Ochoa JB, Ochoa AC (2004) Arginase I production in the tumor microenvironment by mature myeloid cells inhibits T-cell receptor expression and antigen-specific T-cell responses. Cancer Res 64:5839–5849

Rosenberg SA, Yang JC, Schwartzentruber DJ, Hwu P, Marincola FM, Topalian SL, Restifo NP, Dudley ME, Schwarz SL, Spiess PJ, Wunderlich JR, Parkhurst MR, Kawakami Y, Seipp CA, Einhorn JH, White DE (1998) Immunologic and therapeutic evaluation of a synthetic peptide vaccine for the treatment of patients with metastatic melanoma. Nat Med 4:321–327

Rosenberg SA, Yang JC, Restifo NP (2004) Cancer immunotherapy: moving beyond current vaccines. Nat Med 10:909–915

Sakaguchi S (2005) Naturally arising Foxp3-expressing CD25+CD4+ regulatory T cells in immunological tolerance to self and non-self. Nat Immunol 6:345–352

Sakaguchi S, Wing K, Onishi Y, Prieto-Martin P, Yamaguchi T (2009) Regulatory T cells: how do they suppress immune responses? Int Immunol 21:1105–1111

Salvadori S, Martinelli G, Zier K (2000) Resection of solid tumors reverses T cell defects and restores protective immunity. J Immunol 164:2214–2220

Santini SM, Lapenta C, Logozzi M, Parlato S, Spada M, Di Pucchio T, Belardelli F (2000) Type I interferon as a powerful adjuvant for monocyte-derived dendritic cell development and activity in vitro and in Hu-PBL-SCID mice. J Exp Med 191:1777–1788

Santodonato L, D'Agostino G, Nisini R, Mariotti S, Monque DM, Spada M, Lattanzi L, Perrone MP, Andreotti M, Belardelli F, Ferrantini M (2003) Monocyte-derived dendritic cells generated after a short-term culture with IFN-alpha and granulocyte-macrophage colony-stimulating factor stimulate a potent Epstein-Barr virus-specific CD8+ T cell response. J Immunol 170:5195–5202

Schmielau J, Finn OJ (2001) Activated granulocytes and granulocyte-derived hydrogen peroxide are the underlying mechanism of suppression of T-cell function in advanced cancer patients. Cancer Res 61:4756–4760

Schulz O, Diebold SS, Chen M, Naslund TI, Nolte MA, Alexopoulou L, Azuma YT, Flavell RA, Liljestrom P, Reis e Sousa C (2005) Toll-like receptor 3 promotes cross-priming to virus-infected cells. Nature 433:887–892

Seya T, Shime H, Ebihara T, Oshiumi H, Matsumoto M (2010) Pattern recognition receptors of innate immunity and their application to tumor immunotherapy. Cancer Sci 101:313–320

Sharma MD, Baban B, Chandler P, Hou DY, Singh N, Yagita H, Azuma M, Blazar BR, Mellor AL, Munn DH (2007) Plasmacytoid dendritic cells from mouse tumor-draining lymph nodes directly activate mature Tregs via indoleamine 2,3-dioxygenase. J Clin Investig 117:2570–2582

Shinohara ML, Lu L, Bu J, Werneck MB, Kobayashi KS, Glimcher LH, Cantor H (2006) Osteopontin expression is essential for interferon-alpha production by plasmacytoid dendritic cells [see comment]. Nat Immunol 7:498–506

Smit JJ, Rudd BD, Lukacs NW (2006) Plasmacytoid dendritic cells inhibit pulmonary immunopathology and promote clearance of respiratory syncytial virus. J Exp Med 203:1153–1159

Stary G, Bangert C, Tauber M, Strohal R, Kopp T, Stingl G (2007) Tumoricidal activity of TLR7/8-activated inflammatory dendritic cells. J Exp Med 204:1441–1451

Steidl C, Lee T, Shah SP, Farinha P, Han G, Nayar T, Delaney A, Jones SJ, Iqbal J, Weisenburger DD, Bast MA, Rosenwald A, Muller-Hermelink HK, Rimsza LM, Campo E, Delabie J, Braziel RM, Cook JR, Tubbs RR, Jaffe ES, Lenz G, Connors JM, Staudt LM, Chan WC, Gascoyne RD (2010) Tumor-associated macrophages and survival in classic Hodgkin's lymphoma. N Engl J Med 362:875–885

Steinman RM, Banchereau J (2007) Taking dendritic cells into medicine. Nature 449:419–426

Steinman RM, Hemmi H (2006) Dendritic cells: translating innate to adaptive immunity. Curr Top Microbiol Immunol 311:17–58

Steinman RM, Lustig DS, Cohn ZA (1974) Identification of a novel cell type in peripheral lymphoid organs of mice. 3. Functional properties in vivo. J Exp Med 139:1431–1445

Taniguchi T, Takaoka A (2002) The interferon-alpha/beta system in antiviral responses: a multimodal machinery of gene regulation by the IRF family of transcription factors. Curr Opin Immunol 14:111–116

Theofilopoulos AN, Baccala R, Beutler B, Kono DH (2005) Type I interferons (alpha/beta) in immunity and autoimmunity. Annu Rev Immunol 23:307–336

Tough DF, Borrow P, Sprent J (1996) Induction of bystander T cell proliferation by viruses and type I interferon in vivo [see comment]. Science 272:1947–1950

Treilleux I, Blay JY, Bendriss-Vermare N, Ray-Coquard I, Bachelot T, Guastalla JP, Bremond A, Goddard S, Pin JJ, Barthelemy-Dubois C, Lebecque S (2004) Dendritic cell infiltration and prognosis of early stage breast cancer. Clin Cancer Res 10:7466–7474

Tuma RS (2005) Success of bevacizumab trials raises questions for future studies. J Natl Cancer Inst 97:950–951

Tyagi RK, Mangal S, Garg N, Sharma PK (2009) RNA-based immunotherapy of cancer: role and therapeutic implications of dendritic cells. Expert Rev Anticancer Ther 9:97–114

Uematsu S, Sato S, Yamamoto M, Hirotani T, Kato H, Takeshita F, Matsuda M, Coban C, Ishii KJ, Kawai T, Takeuchi O, Akira S (2005) Interleukin-1 receptor-associated kinase-1 plays an essential role for toll-like receptor (TLR)7- and TLR9-mediated interferon-{alpha} induction. J Exp Med 201:915–923

Urosevic M, Dummer R, Conrad C, Beyeler M, Laine E, Burg G, Gilliet M (2005) Disease-independent skin recruitment and activation of plasmacytoid predendritic cells following imiquimod treatment. J Natl Cancer Inst 97:1143–1153

Valmori D, Dutoit V, Schnuriger V, Quiquerez AL, Pittet MJ, Guillaume P, Rubio-Godoy V, Walker PR, Rimoldi D, Lienard D, Cerottini JC, Romero P, Dietrich PY (2002) Vaccination with a Melan-A peptide selects an oligoclonal T cell population with increased functional avidity and tumor reactivity. J Immunol 168:4231–4240

Vermi W, Bonecchi R, Facchetti F, Bianchi D, Sozzani S, Festa S, Berenzi A, Cella M, Colonna M (2003) Recruitment of immature plasmacytoid dendritic cells (plasmacytoid monocytes) and myeloid dendritic cells in primary cutaneous melanomas. J Pathol 200:255–268

Vicari AP, Chiodoni C, Vaure C, Ait-Yahia S, Dercamp C, Matsos F, Reynard O, Taverne C, Merle P, Colombo MP, O'Garra A, Trinchieri G, Caux C (2002) Reversal of tumor-induced dendritic cell paralysis by CpG immunostimulatory oligonucleotide and anti-interleukin 10 receptor antibody. J Exp Med 196:541–549

Vyas JM, Van der Veen AG, Ploegh HL (2008) The known unknowns of antigen processing and presentation. Nat Rev Immunol 8:607–618

Wagner H (2009) The immunogenicity of CpG-antigen conjugates. Adv Drug Deliv Rev 61:243–247

Wang HY, Wang RF (2007) Regulatory T cells and cancer. Curr Opin Immunol 19:217–223

Wang HY, Lee DA, Peng G, Guo Z, Li Y, Kiniwa Y, Shevach EM, Wang RF (2004) Tumor-specific human CD4+ regulatory T cells and their ligands: implications for immunotherapy. Immunity 20:107–118

Wang B, Kuroiwa JM, He LZ, Charalambous A, Keler T, Steinman RM (2009) The human cancer antigen mesothelin is more efficiently presented to the mouse immune system when targeted to the DEC-205/CD205 receptor on dendritic cells. Ann N Y Acad Sci 1174:6–17

Wei S, Kryczek I, Zou L, Daniel B, Cheng P, Mottram P, Curiel T, Lange A, Zou W (2005) Plasmacytoid dendritic cells induce CD8+ regulatory T cells in human ovarian carcinoma. Cancer Res 65:5020–5026

Wolf AM, Wolf D, Steurer M, Gastl G, Gunsilius E, Grubeck-Loebenstein B (2003) Increase of regulatory T cells in the peripheral blood of cancer patients. Clin Cancer Res 9:606–612

Wong R, Lau R, Chang J, Kuus-Reichel T, Brichard V, Bruck C, Weber J (2004) Immune responses to a class II helper peptide epitope in patients with stage III/IV resected melanoma. Clin Cancer Res 10:5004–5013

Yamazaki S, Steinman RM (2009) Dendritic cells as controllers of antigen-specific Foxp3+ regulatory T cells. J Dermatol Sci 54:69–75

Yamazaki S, Dudziak D, Heidkamp GF, Fiorese C, Bonito AJ, Inaba K, Nussenzweig MC, Steinman RM (2008) CD8+ CD205+ splenic dendritic cells are specialized to induce Foxp3+ regulatory T cells. J Immunol 181:6923–6933

Yewdell JW, Norbury CC, Bennink JR (1999) Mechanisms of exogenous antigen presentation by MHC class I molecules in vitro and in vivo: implications for generating CD8+ T cell responses to infectious agents, tumors, transplants, and vaccines. Adv Immunol 73:1–77

Zea AH, Rodriguez PC, Atkins MB, Hernandez C, Signoretti S, Zabaleta J, McDermott D, Quiceno D, Youmans A, O'Neill A, Mier J, Ochoa AC (2005) Arginase-producing myeloid suppressor cells in renal cell carcinoma patients: a mechanism of tumor evasion. Cancer Res 65:3044–3048

Zou W, Machelon V, Coulomb-L'Hermin A, Borvak J, Nome F, Isaeva T, Wei S, Krzysiek R, Durand-Gasselin I, Gordon A, Pustilnik T, Curiel DT, Galanaud P, Capron F, Emilie D, Curiel TJ (2001) Stromal-derived factor-1 in human tumors recruits and alters the function of plasmacytoid precursor dendritic cells [see comment]. Nat Med 7:1339–1346

Chapter 9
Regulatory T Cells in Cancer

Tyler J. Curiel

1 Introduction

Malignant tumors are immunologically challenging. Although they are pathological, and should thus be subjected to immune destruction, they nonetheless originate from self tissues. Thus, peripheral tolerance and other immune protective measures intervene to prevent autoimmune (antitumor) attack, thereby blunting what could otherwise be meaningful antitumor immunity.

Many T cells with self-reactive potential are deleted in the thymus during fetal development in a process called central tolerance. However, central tolerance is imperfect and does not remove all self-reactive T cells, some of which escape into the periphery, posing a life-long risk of inducing autoimmune disease. Self-reactive T cells that are not eliminated centrally must thus be managed using additional mechanisms, including a system of peripheral immune tolerance. In peripheral immune tolerance, a potential autoimmune attack in development is sensed and subdued usually before significant pathologic consequences ensue. Elegant work by Sakaguchi and others has shown that a key mediator of peripheral tolerance includes a subset of $CD4^+CD25^{hi}$ T cells (Sakaguchi et al. 1995). However, activated effector T cells, including those helping mediate antitumor immunity can also express the $CD4^+CD25^{hi}$ phenotype. Thus, regulatory T cells (Tregs) cannot be distinguished by surface phenotype alone. The forkhead/winged helix nuclear transcription factor FOXP3 regulates a major pathway for Treg differentiation and regulatory function

T.J. Curiel (✉)
Cancer Therapy and Research Center, University of Texas Health
Science Center, San Antonio, TX 78229, USA
e-mail: curielt@uthscsa.edu

(Fontenot et al. 2003, 2005; Hori et al. 2003). Thus, Tregs usually express significant levels of Foxp3, but not all Foxp3-expressing T cells are Tregs (Curiel 2007a, b). This issue of appropriate Treg identification continues to cause confusion in interpreting clinical and experimental data as it relates to potential immunopathogenic roles for Tregs in various settings. This concept is introduced and surveyed in this chapter. Details are found elsewhere in this book.

Much prior work in both small animal models and in human patients has established that Tregs are increased in the blood and solid tumor mass of epithelial carcinomas, lymphomas and sarcomas, and the lymph nodes draining these tumors (Shimizu et al. 1999; Woo et al. 2001, 2002; Liyanage et al. 2002; Shevach 2002; Somasundaram et al. 2002; Bach 2003; Javia and Rosenberg 2003; Sasada et al. 2003; Wolf et al. 2003; Curiel et al. 2004; Kaporis et al. 2007; Loskog et al. 2007; Visser et al. 2007). Initial studies focused on Tregs in blood circulation as the easily accessible compartment. More recent work has attempted to assess whether circulating Tregs accurately predict events in the tumor microenvironment. More recent publications demonstrate that there are increased functional Tregs circulating in blood and infiltrating the tumor in human nasopharyngeal carcinoma (Lau et al. 2007), melanoma (Mourmouras et al. 2007), and colorectal cancer (Ling et al. 2007; Nagorsen et al. 2007). In these colorectal cancer patients, Treg increase is correlated with advanced disease stages. Tregs are also increased in the blood circulation of patients with liquid hematologic malignancies such as acute myelogenous leukemia (Szczepanski et al. 2009). $CD4^+CD25^+FOXP3^+$ T cells infiltrate metastatic brain lesions in human melanoma and non-small cell carcinoma, and in metastatic brain lesions in mouse models of metastatic melanoma, breast, and colon cancer (Sugihara et al. 2009), suggesting that certain immunotherapeutic strategies could also be effective in tumors in the central nervous system. It is now clear that Treg numbers, phenotype and function as suggested from studies of cells in peripheral circulation do not always accurately reflect what is occurring in the local tumor microenvironment. The immunological and clinical significance of these differences remains to be fully established.

2 Categorizing Tregs

Tregs have been categorized using several different schemes. A useful concept is that proposed by Jeff Bluestone (Bluestone and Abbas 2003). In this scheme, Tregs are defined as being of two general types, the natural Treg (nTreg) that arises in thymus under normal homeostatic processes and whose primary function is to mediate peripheral tolerance, and the adaptive Treg that is induced outside the thymus during inflammatory processes, probably to help dampen the inflammation, among other functions. Adaptive Tregs are also called induced Tregs (iTreg), as they will be referred to in this chapter.

3 Properties of Tumor-Associated Tregs

3.1 General Properties

Tumor-associated Tregs are a heterogeneous population of cells arising through distinct pathways of development and mediating disparate functions through a variety of different mechanisms. An excellent review appeared several years ago (Zou 2006). There are no definitive reports to date documenting the relative contributions of specific developmental pathways (such as iTreg vs. nTreg) in a given Treg population in a given tumor, although it has been established in a mouse model that both nTregs and iTregs can contribute to tumor tolerance (Zhou and Levitsky 2007). Such a study in humans has not yet been reported.

Tumor-associated Tregs are generally indistinguishable phenotypically from Tregs identified in other conditions. That is, they are $CD3^+$ T cells that express CD4, CD25, GITR, and CTLA-4 among other features common to most Tregs identified to date. Nrp-1 expression identifies functional Tregs in mice. An $Nrp-1^+$ population with similar functional features was recently described in human cervical cancer (Battaglia et al. 2008). These $Nrp-1^+$ cells appeared preferentially to reside in tumor draining lymph nodes and to be reduced by cytotoxic chemotherapy in proportion to cytoreduction of the tumor mass.

3.2 Tumor-Specific Properties of Tregs

Tumor-associated Tregs also possess characteristics unique and specific to them that are engendered by the tumor microenvironment. For example, $CD4^+CD25^+FOXP3^+$ Tregs in the blood of patients with prostate cancer are more suppressive than those in blood from control individuals, even if total numbers do not differ (Yokokawa et al. 2008). Tumor-associated Tregs in some human cancers could be more prone to induce $CD8^+$ effector T cells through FasL-mediated apoptosis (Strauss et al. 2009). A novel population of tumor-induced $CD4^+CD25^-CD69^+$ Tregs that suppress T cell function through membrane-bound TGF-β was recently described in mouse models of melanoma, hepatocellular carcinoma, and lung cancer (Han et al. 2009). Lack of CD127 (IL-7 receptor α chain) expression predicts functional Tregs in normal human blood (Liu et al. 2006). The functional consequences of CD127 expression are relatively unstudied in tumor Tregs. We have demonstrated that both $CD4^+CD25^+FOXP3^+CD127^+$ and $CD4^+CD25^+FOXP3^+CD127^-$ T cells in blood and ascites of patients with ovarian carcinoma are suppressive Tregs (Interferon-α boosts antitumor immunity through effects on T cells and dendritic cells and augments the clinical efficacy of Treg depletion. Wall et al. 2009). Additional differences are sure to be described over the near term.

3.3 Issues in Identifying *Bona Fide* **Functional Tumor Tregs**

3.3.1 Functional Testing Issues

As discussed further herein, functional testing of putative Treg populations remains the gold standard to confirm their identity. Even so, the specifics of the functional tests used to determine Treg function can lead to different results and conclusions. For example, the strength of the T cell receptor signal in part determines the susceptibility of responder T cells to be suppressed in standard in vitro tests of Treg function. Testing Treg function based on suppressing T cell proliferation in vitro may not be relevant if the Treg primarily functions in vivo to suppress cytokine secretion [as described for Tregs, including tumor-associated Tregs (Visser et al. 2007)] or inhibit dendritic cell function, or exerts its effects on a specific T cell subset not tested, among other considerations. Details of these issues regarding Treg functional testing are found elsewhere in this book.

3.3.2 Surrogates for Functional Testing

Since Treg numbers are limited in human tissues, additional means to corroborate Treg identity in human malignancies have been sought. For example, it has been proposed that FOXP3 expression is adequate to identify functional Tregs in selected human carcinomas (Kryczek et al. 2009). FOXP3 methylation has been proposed as a reliable means to identify functional Tregs using small amounts of precious specimen (Wieczorek et al. 2009). CD39 expression has been proposed to distinguish functional Tregs from other $CD4^+CD25^{hi}$ T cells, including those in cancer patients (Mandapathil et al. 2009). Additional work is required to determine what nonfunctional surrogate tests are adequate for Treg identification in specific conditions. This issue is especially important following immune-based interventions, because treatments can have unexpected and unstudied effects on T cell phenotype that require additional study. Our lab policy is to confirm the functional identity of a potential Treg population in a setting for which such function has not been specifically established, and still to perform confirmatory functional testing in each experimental animal or human subject to the extent possible to continue to understand how reliable the phenotypic descriptors of potentially functional cell populations are. For example, we have found that interferon-α increased the prevalence of Foxp3$^+$ T cells in mice and humans ovarian cancer, although these induced Foxp3$^+$ T cells do not necessarily have Treg function (interferon-α boosts antitumor immunity through effects on T cells and dendritic cells, and augments the clinical efficacy of Treg depletion. Wall et al. 2009).

3.4 Central Questions Regarding the Role of Tregs in Tumor Immunopathology

These include: (1) How do tumor-associated Tregs arise? (2) Why are Tregs elevated in most cancers? (3) What role in tumor immunopathology do Tregs play? (4) How do tumor-associated Tregs mediate their immunopathologic functions? Answers to these overarching questions will provide clues to understanding the immunopathology of cancer and will provide tools to develop effective antitumor immunotherapies, a goal that has generally eluded investigators thus far. This chapter reviews and summarizes our current state of understandings of these questions and poses additional important areas for future research.

4 Origins of Tumor Tregs

Tregs could accumulate in tumors owing to a variety of reasons including: (1) control of autoimmunity, (2) control of inflammation, (3) enhanced de novo differentiation (which entails iTreg generation), (4) recruitment from distant compartments, (5) enhanced local proliferation, and (6) reduced local death. Details of each potential mechanism are described below. Specific mechanisms, however, likely differ depending on the tumor type and perhaps stage, and could differ by anatomic compartment in a given tumor.

4.1 Control of Autoimmunity

Increased Tregs specific for self antigens suggests attempts to control autoimmunity as a mechanism for increased tumor-associated Tregs. Such tumor-associated Tregs specific for normal self antigens that are simultaneously tumor antigens have been described. For example, Tregs specific for the autoantigens gp100, TRP, NY-ESO-1 and survivin have been demonstrated in human melanoma (Vence et al. 2007).

4.2 Control of Inflammation

Most cancers foster a pro-inflammatory environment; chronic inflammation contributes to development of some cancers. Thus, it is likely that some tumor-associated Tregs are increased as a result of local inflammation. Tregs described to date, including those isolated from the tumor microenvironment can inhibit production of inflammatory cytokines in vitro. Nonetheless, Treg accumulation specifically to control tumor-associated inflammation has not yet been formally demonstrated to my knowledge, although in a mouse model of chronic colonic inflammation, Tregs reduced colorectal cancer development by reducing local inflammation (Poutahidis et al. 2007).

4.3 Enhanced De Novo Differentiation

There is experimental data supporting the concept that some tumor environments foster local Treg differentiation. Tumor cells can induce Treg differentiation either by direct action on T cells, or through indirect effects on antigen presenting cells, particularly dendritic cells (Zou 2006) and perhaps on other cell types as well. Both soluble and contact-dependent tumor mechanisms contributing to such Treg generation have been described. An example of a soluble mediator is cyclooxygenase-2, which is associated with (but not yet proved to mediate) Treg increases in human head and neck cancer patients (Bergmann et al. 2007). Tumor TGF-β converts $CD4^+CD25^-$ T cells into Tregs in mouse models for renal cell carcinoma and prostate cancer (Liu et al. 2007b). TGF-β from the human SK-OVCAR3 cell line converts $CD4^+CD25^-$ human cells into Tregs in vitro (Li et al. 2007c). Indoleamine 2,3-dioxygenase from human leukemia cells induces Tregs in vitro. CD70 signals from B cells in non-Hodgkin's lymphoma can augment FOXP3 expression in human $CD4^+CD25^-$ T cells in vitro (Yang et al. 2007b). Gal1 signals in Reed–Sternberg cells in classic Hodgkin's disease can mediate immune suppression and also specifically contribute to generation of Tregs (Juszczynski et al. 2007). We found that tumor B7-H1 signals contribute to iTreg generation in mice with B16 melanoma (Curiel et al. unpublished observations). Additional, yet-to-be-identified tumor-associated factors also participate in Treg generation (Baumgartner et al. 2007; Mittal et al. 2008).

Cells rendered dysfunctional in the tumor microenvironment can induce Tregs or enhance their function. For example, plasmacytoid dendritic cells from mouse tumor draining lymph nodes directly activate existing Tregs via indoleamine 2,3-dioxygenase. The B7-H1/PD-1 suppressive mechanism of these Tregs differs from Tregs activated without indoleamine 2,3-dioxygenase (Sharma et al. 2007). Mouse myeloid dendritic cells and myeloid and plasmacytoid dendritic cells in human cancers also can redirect T cell differentiation to either $FOXP3^+$ Tregs or to $IL-10^+$ Tr1 regulatory cells (Curiel et al. 2003; Wei et al. 2005).

The relative importance of any particular mechanism for local Treg accumulation in cancers remains to be defined and will likely vary in a tumor and compartment-specific manner.

4.4 Enhanced Recruitment

There is ample evidence from different tumor types that tumors secrete factors that preferentially recruit Tregs locally, primarily through CCR4 interactions on Tregs with the chemokines CCL17 or CCL22 in the tumor microenvironment, reviewed in

(Zou 2006). Examples include accumulation of Tregs in ovarian (Curiel et al. 2004) or gastric (Mizukami et al. 2008a, b) carcinoma through CCL17 or CCL22 signals. There is preliminary evidence that CXCR4$^+$ Tregs can be attracted to the tumor microenvironment through local CXCL12 production, as suggested in malignant mesothelioma (Shimizu et al. 2009). Therapeutic IL-2 administration increases Treg CXCR4 expression, boosting accumulation in ovarian cancer patients (Wei et al. 2007), but whether a CXCR4/CXCL12 interaction augments Treg accumulation in untreated ovarian cancer remains to be established. Tumor stromal elements can also help attract Tregs to the tumor microenvironment as do tumor-associated macrophages in ovarian cancer, which secrete CCL22 to attract Tregs into the microenvironment through a CCR4 interaction (Curiel et al. 2004).

4.5 Enhanced Local Proliferation

Tumors can induce local, immature myeloid dendritic cell TGF-β production that promotes Treg proliferation (Ghiringhelli et al. 2005). Adoptive transfer and other techniques have established that tumors secrete factors or express surface molecules that foster local nTreg proliferation (Zhou and Levitsky 2007).

4.6 Reduced Local Treg Death

Reduced local Treg death is a potential mechanism for Treg accumulation in the tumor microenvironment, but remains to be demonstrated. Some therapeutic strategies augment local Treg death in the tumor environment (Hirschhorn-Cymerman et al. 2009).

4.7 Miscellaneous Host Factors

Treg function is reduced under several genetically defined conditions that could have an impact on tumor surveillance or antitumor immunity. Two examples of this type suffice for illustration. IRAK-M is a negative regulator of innate immunity. IRAK-M$^{-/-}$ mice have enhanced antitumor T cell immunity and reduced Tregs (Xie et al. 2007). B7-H1 is a T cell co-signaling molecule with pleiotropic effects on T cells, including the ability to generate IL-10$^+$ Tr1-like Tregs in human ovarian cancer (Curiel et al. 2003) or FOXP3$^+$ iTregs (Krupnick et al. 2005) under certain conditions. Female B7-H1$^{-/-}$ mice have reduced Treg function compared to wild type females (Habicht et al. 2007). We recently demonstrated that female B7-H1$^{-/-}$ mice have augmented antitumor immunity because of their reduced Treg function (Lin et al. 2010).

5 Tumor Treg Content and Clinical Outcomes

5.1 Treg Content and Prognosis

FOXP3 expression has been proposed as a prognostic biomarker for cancer (Schreiber 2007). Nonetheless, for reasons discussed above and those to be discussed below, and because FOXP3 expression can be transient and reversible, thereby altering the functionality of the T cell (Pillai and Karandikar 2007; Zhou et al. 2009), it is unlikely to be a perfect predictive tool in the absence of functional data from FOXP3-expressing cells. Increased tumor Tregs predict reduced survival or treatment response in a number of studies, including in ovarian cancer (Curiel et al. 2004), R0 respected gastric carcinoma (Perrone et al. 2008), hepatocellular carcinoma (Kobayashi et al. 2007; Sasaki et al. 2008), and others reviewed in (Schreiber 2007). Intratumoral Foxp3$^+$ T cells predicted local recurrence in the vertical phase of melanoma (Miracco et al. 2007).

On the other hand, several studies show no prognostic value of Treg content, such as the recent demonstration that tumor-infiltrating FOXP3$^+$CD4$^+$CD25$^+$ T cells did not predict survival in renal cell carcinoma (Siddiqui et al. 2007). A few studies, particularly in hematologic malignancies (Tzankov et al. 2008), suggest that prognosis improves with increased Tregs. CD25$^+$ and FOXP3$^+$ cells were reduced in thymoma vs. normal thymus and thymus of patients with myasthenia gravis, as was *Foxp3* RNA, suggesting reduced Tregs (Scarpino et al. 2007).

Experimental animal models suggest at least one plausible mechanism whereby functional Tregs could be beneficial in cancer. In a mouse model for melanoma, Tregs were shown to augment antitumor immunity, possibly by preventing complete tumor elimination, thereby maintaining sufficient tumor antigen to stimulate antitumor immunity (Kakinuma et al. 2007). Conflicting results in these various reports could arise from a variety of factors, including those discussed below.

5.2 Tumor Treg Content and Response to Therapy

Pretreatment levels of blood Tregs (defined as CD4$^+$CD25^{hi} T lymphocytes) predicted overall survival in response to a dendritic cell vaccine (plus activated T cells in some patients) for human cancer (Wada et al. 2008). Disappearance of tumor infiltrating FOXP3$^+$ cells (and increase in tumor infiltrating CD8$^+$ cells) was correlated with pathologic complete response following neoadjuvant therapy for treating human breast cancer (Ladoire et al. 2008). If such data can be confirmed, particularly by isolating functional cells for testing, they may be useful in predicting long-term efficacy of cytotoxic therapy and also suggest an immune component to successful chemotherapy that bears further investigation. In squamous cell cancers of the head and neck, patients with no evident disease following treatment had more circulating Tregs that were more suppressive vs. those who had not been treated (Strauss et al. 2007), suggesting that treatment somehow expanded suppressive Tregs despite a beneficial outcome.

5.3 Additional Sources of Confusion in Studies of Tregs as Tumor Prognostic Indicators

Demonstrating Treg function can be difficult, particularly in human tissues as sample size is usually limiting. Consequently, prognostic studies often use FOXP3 expression as a surrogate for functional Tregs, but without doing confirmatory functional testing. Studies using immunohistochemistry to detect Foxp3$^+$ cells might not even demonstrate that they are CD3$^+$ T cells. Such approaches could lead to confusion because FOXP3 expression is not an absolute or specific marker for functional Tregs (Curiel 2007a, b). In this regard, it was recently suggested that FOXP3 expression plus cytokine profiling could help distinguish FOXP3$^+$ Tregs from FOXP3$^+$ activated effector cells in certain epithelial carcinomas (Kryczek et al. 2009). Another potential source of conflicting results is that patient populations and factors known to confound survival estimates or treatment response data are not fully defined or identified in some studies.

Aside from their absolute numbers or functional status, Tregs are reported to affect prognosis according to their anatomic location or distribution within an anatomic compartment. For example, in stomach cancer, survival depended on localization patterns but not on total numbers of FOXP3$^+$ cells in the tumor (Mizukami et al. 2008a, b). Tregs could be predictive of survival based on their relative numbers compared to antitumor effector cells. For example, the ratio of FOXP3$^+$ cells to granzyme B$^+$ cells in Hodgkin lymphoma helped predict survival (Kelley et al. 2007). A low CD8$^+$/Treg ratio in tumor infiltrating cells was a poor prognostic marker in a study of cervical cancer (Jordanova et al. 2008). Reduction in FOXP3$^+$ cells simultaneous with increased CD8$^+$ cell infiltration into malignant breast tissue was the best predictor of pathologic complete response to cytotoxic therapy for breast cancer (Ladoire et al. 2008) as in the section "Tumor Treg Content and Response to Therapy." As we come to understand more about these specific aspects of tumor-associated Tregs it is possible that useful and practical means to quantify them will be developed that will further allow accurate algorithms for predicting treatment responses (perhaps including to surgery, radiation and cytotoxic agents) and survival.

6 Tregs in Cancer Prevention

Most work to date on the role of Tregs in cancer has focused on their effects in existing malignancies. Nonetheless, Tregs could also modulate immunoediting or progression of a premalignant lesion to a frankly malignant neoplasm. As one example, in a mouse model of chronic colonic inflammation (mediated by local gut microbes), Tregs reduced the rate of colorectal cancer by dampening inflammation (Poutahidis et al. 2007). In carcinogen-induced sarcoma in mice, resident Tregs inhibited tumor immune surveillance (Betts et al. 2007). Ultraviolet radiation induces skin Tregs that could contribute to skin cancer (Beissert and Loser 2008). In cervical cancer, Tregs might augment malignant progression from nonmalignant cells (Visser et al. 2007). This role for Tregs in affecting malignant progression could be a generic function of Tregs, or could suggest that Tregs in viral-associated cancers play unique roles (Molling et al. 2007), further bolstered by the observation that human papilloma-specific Tregs are found in human cervical cancer (van der Burg et al. 2007). $CD4^+CD25^+$ Tregs are the cells responsible for loss of concomitant immunity (Turk et al. 2004), and thus could be responsible for loss of adequate antitumor immune protection in the preclinical state of cancer progression. Managing Tregs in cancer prevention remains a little explored area worthy of more attention, despite the many obvious difficulties of their management in the absence of an overt malignancy.

7 Tumor Treg Interactions with Other Cells

It is now well established that Treg differentiation and function are affected by interactions with immune and nonimmune cells, including the tumor itself, some of which interactions have been reviewed above. In addition, Tregs can induce tumor-associated macrophages to secrete IL-6 and IL-10, thereby inducing macrophage B7-H4 expression that inhibits effector T cell function (Kryczek et al. 2006). Tumor infiltrating plasmacytoid dendritic cells can alter Treg or Th17 cell differentiation in the draining lymph nodes in B16 melanoma in mice through a process that depends on indoleamine 2,3-dioxygenase produced in the plasmacytoid dendritic cells (Sharma et al. 2009).

8 Tumor Treg Effects on Anticancer Therapies

With the recognition that Tregs can be immunopathogenic in cancer, and with development of adequate techniques to test their function, surprising and unexpected Treg effects of some cancer therapies have been observed. Although these Treg effects have been identified and described, in most instances reviewed below, specific contributions to the mechanisms of these agents of Treg effects are generally unknown.

8.1 Vaccines

Active vaccination induces antigen-specific effector cells that have been extensively studied. Analogous to antigen-specific antitumor effector T cells, Tregs can also be antigen-specific. With this understanding, examinations of vaccine effects on Tregs have recently been undertaken. Such studies have demonstrated that vaccines against tumor antigens can induce tumor-specific Tregs in mouse models for cancer (Zhou et al. 2006). A cervical cancer vaccine-induced CD4$^+$CD25$^+$FOXP3$^+$ cells in humans but their function as Tregs, and their antigen specificity were not demonstrated. A MAGE-A3 peptide vaccine in human melanoma induced circulating MAGE-A3-specific CD4$^+$CD25$^+$FOXP3$^+$ T cells with regulatory properties (Francois et al. 2009). In a dendritic cell vaccine trial for multiple myeloma, the vaccine expanded functionally suppressive blood CD4$^+$CD25$^+$FOXP3$^+$ Tregs (Banerjee et al. 2006). Antitumor vaccination against B cell chronic lymphocytic leukemia lowered blood CD4$^+$CD25$^+$FOXP3$^+$ phenotypic Tregs in another human study (Hus et al. 2008), although the function of these cells was not demonstrated.

Further, it could be possible to design vaccines favoring generation of antigen-specific antitumor effector cells while simultaneously minimizing antigen-specific Treg generation (Palucka et al. 2007). Strategies currently under evaluation include CD40 agonists plus toll-like receptor activation (Ahonen et al. 2008) and a DOTAP vaccine that induces CD8$^+$ T cells while simultaneously reducing Foxp3$^+$ T cells in a mouse cancer vaccine model against human papilloma virus E7 antigen has been developed (Chen et al. 2008). Tumor cells engineered to express CD137 single chain antibody can generate immunity and elicit fewer Tregs than wild type tumor (Yang et al. 2007a). In multiple myeloma, patient dendritic cells inhibited T cell activation, and multiple myeloma tumor cell lysates or idiotype antibodies induced CD4$^+$CD25$^+$FOXP3$^+$ cells in vitro (Han et al. 2008). When these dendritic cells were forced to express calnexin using a lentivirus vector, they augmented generation of tumor antigen-specific effector T cells but FOXP3$^+$ T cell generation was not affected.

8.2 Cytokine Treatments

IL-2 is a standard treatment for selected cases of renal cell carcinoma or malignant melanoma, and was initially selected for its capacity to stimulate effector T cell activation and proliferation. With the recognition that IL-2 is also a critical growth and differentiation factor for Tregs (Malek et al. 2000, 2002), reevaluations of the effects of therapeutic IL-2 on Tregs were undertaken. Systemic IL-2 administration alters Treg trafficking molecules and augments Treg numbers in patients with ovarian cancer (Wei et al. 2007), although clinical and immunologic consequences remain to be defined. IL-2 administration (plus gp100 peptide vaccination) in three phase II melanoma clinical trials variably increased or decreased CD4$^+$CD25$^+$FOXP3$^+$ phenotypic Tregs in circulation, with no clear relationship to clinical response (Sosman et al. 2008). Other cytokines also affect Treg numbers, differentiation, function, or migration. For example, gene therapy-induced IL-12 expression inhibited Treg generation in mice with experimentally induced hepatocellular carcinoma (Zabala et al. 2007).

8.3 Additional Agents

Cyclophosphamide is an alkylating agent originally tested as cytotoxic anticancer therapy. It is now known to deplete Tregs at relatively low doses in mice and humans (Brode and Cooke 2008). Cyclophosphamide boosted dendritic cell vaccine efficacy against melanoma or colon carcinoma in mouse models, in association with reduced phenotypic Treg numbers (Liu et al. 2007a). Nonetheless, at the high doses used as a cytotoxic agent to treat cancer, it is unlikely that specific Treg depleting properties are an essential mechanism of its anticancer effects. Treg numbers and their suppressive function are boosted by histone deacetylase inhibitors (Li et al. 2007a; Tao et al. 2007). IL-2 can enhance this histone deacetylase inhibitor effect (Kato et al. 2007). Retinoids, including all-*trans* retinoic acid, induce Tregs with preferential gut-homing properties (Kang et al. 2007). The aromatase inhibitor, letrozole, may reduce Tregs in breast cancer (Generali et al. 2009). Low dose metronomic temozolamide is reported to reduce phenotypic Tregs in a rat model for glioma, but the function of the phenotypic Tregs was not tested (Banissi et al. 2009). The mTOR inhibitor, rapamycin, which is in clinical trials as an anticancer agent, also modulates Treg numbers and function (Haxhinasto et al. 2008). The thalidomide congeners (known collectively as IMiDs) lenalidomide and pamolidomide reduce Treg numbers and function (Galustian et al. 2009). Effects of lenalidomide and pamolidomide appear not to be through altering IL-10 or TGF-β concentration, but perhaps through altering CD4$^+$ T cell Foxp3 expression. Circulating Treg numbers in blood of selected breast cancer patients receiving the anti-Her2/neu antibody traztuzumab (Herceptin), were reduced concomitant with an increase in Th17 cells, suggesting a disruption of the Th17/Treg balance as a potential mode of therapeutic action (Horlock et al. 2009). The kinase inhibitor imatinib mesylate (Gleevec) enhances vaccine-induced antitumor immunity in mice, at least in part by reducing Treg numbers and function (Larmonier et al. 2008). Imatinib mesylate actions on Tregs appear to be partly through reducing T cell receptor signaling, including reduced expression of the ZAP70 component of the T cell receptor signaling complex (Larmonier et al. 2008). Cyclooxygenase-2 inhibitors have been proposed to reduce colorectal cancer risk in part by reducing Treg function, based on suggestive but not definitive evidence (Yaqub et al. 2008). Cyclooxygenase-2 inhibitors can reduce FOXP3$^+$ cell content in human colorectal cancers (Lonnroth et al. 2008). Unanticipated Treg effects of other drugs used for other indications have been discussed previously (Rüter et al. 2009; Curiel 2008).

The immediately relevant question to be addressed is whether any treatment effects relate to Treg effects, and if so, how this mechanism might be exploited therapeutically. These new data suggest that reassessing the mechanisms of action of certain anticancer drugs, including active vaccines, antiangiogenesis molecules, tyrosine kinase inhibitors, growth factor signaling inhibitors, and many others in addition to those mentioned above could be worthwhile. Such investigations could lead to insights regarding why some agents succeed or fail in individual patients, such as the variable success rate for IL-2 in treating renal cell carcinoma, or provide clues as to how to improve the clinical efficacy of specific agents.

9 Strategies to Manage Tregs

A large body of evidence supports the concept that cancer-associated Tregs are detrimental in many cancers, reviewed in (Zou 2006). The correlative prediction is that reducing Treg function in those cancers in which Tregs are detrimental will be therapeutically beneficial (Curiel 2008). In support, depleting Tregs improved endogenous antitumor immunity (Shimizu et al. 1999), which can be tumor-specific (Tanaka et al. 2002) and which can allow generation of immunity to shared tumor antigens (Golgher et al. 2002). Treg depletion was then shown to improve actively induced antitumor immunity through vaccination or other strategies (Steitz et al. 2001; Sutmuller et al. 2001). Based on the understandings of how Tregs function and accumulate in cancer (Zou 2006; Curiel 2007a, b), possible strategies to reduce Treg function include: depletion or blocking differentiation, trafficking or effector functions; and raising effector cell suppression threshold, or diverting Tregs into a different Th differentiation pathway (Rüter et al. 2009; Curiel 2008). *Depleting* Tregs is the strategy most tested thus far in animal models and human trials (Curiel 2008). However, other potential strategies should be considered for managing Tregs in addition to, or instead of, depleting them. The clinical and immunologic effects of depletion alone could be compromised, as Tregs can regenerate themselves following depletion, and even exceed pre-depletion levels (Colombo and Piconese 2007; Piconese et al. 2008). Specific cancer Treg management strategies include the following.

9.1 Nonspecific Treg Depletion

Based on the high expression of IL-2 receptor α chain (CD25) by Tregs, anti-CD25 antibody (usually PC61) is the modality most commonly employed to deplete Tregs in mice (Sakaguchi et al. 1995). We and others have demonstrated that denileukin diftitox [ONTAK, a recombinant fusion protein consisting of human IL-2 and a portion of diphtheria toxin (Foss 2000)], is also useful to deplete mouse Tregs in naïve and tumor-bearing hosts (Litzinger et al. 2007). The alkylating agent cyclophosphamide (Cytoxan), developed as a traditional cytotoxic agent for cancer therapy (Brode and Cooke 2008), depletes Tregs and boosted the clinical efficacy of dendritic cell vaccines for colon carcinoma or melanoma in tumor-bearing mice (Liu et al. 2007a). In another mouse model, cyclophosphamide depleted ICOS$^+$ and TNFR2$^+$ Tregs, a potentially more suppressive phenotype compared to the total pool of CD4$^+$CD25^{hi} T cells, which include Tregs (van der Most et al. 2009). Cyclophosphamide in selected doses and schedules can deplete functional Tregs in the blood of human cancer patients (Brode and Cooke 2008). Generating anti-Foxp3 immunity with a vaccine increased tumor immunity in mice with experimentally induced renal cell carcinoma (Nair et al. 2007). Anti-Foxp3 vaccine effects potentially could also be through immunity generated against Foxp3 expression in tumor, which has been reported in some cancers (Zuo et al. 2007), but the mechanism was not studied in the renal cell carcinoma vaccine report. Denileukin diftitox, an immunoconjugate of IL-2 genetically fused to diphtheria toxin targeting IL-2 receptor expressing cells (Barnett et al. 2005) and LMB-2, a *Pseudomonas* immunotoxin conjugated to an anti-CD25 antibody Fv fragment that targets $CD25^+$ cells (Powell et al. 2007b), each deplete Tregs in human cancer patients. Autologous mononuclear cells depleted of all $CD25^+$ cells (not just Tregs) in combination with high-dose IL-2 in vivo did not affect prolonged Treg reduction in human subjects (Powell et al. 2007a), although depletion of $CD25^+$ T cells from a hematopoietic stem cell transplant in a mouse model improved antitumor immunity (Jing et al. 2007).

CpG treatment reduces $FOXP3^+$ T cells in lymph nodes of melanoma patients (Molenkamp et al. 2007), although their identity as functional Tregs remains to be established. OX40 ligation can hinder Treg function in tumors, while simultaneously boosting effector T cell function and promoting tumor rejection in mice (Piconese et al. 2008). Adding cyclophosphamide to OX40 ligation further augments antitumor immunity and tumor rejection in a mouse model for melanoma, in part by promoting local Treg apoptosis (Hirschhorn-Cymerman et al. 2009). CpG plus a small molecule STAT3 inhibitor increased tumor infiltration with activated effector T cells and reduced phenotypic Tregs in a mouse model for melanoma (Molavi et al. 2008). Many additional similar examples can also be found. Nonetheless, despite the accumulating data in animal models, the clinical and immunologic efficacy of Treg depletion remains to be definitively determined in any human cancer.

There remain malignancies for which Tregs might not be the principal means of immune dysfunction, and therefore Treg depletion might not be the optimal therapeutic strategy. For example, in a model of lung metastasis using CT26 colon cancer, immune suppression appeared to be mediated primarily by $CD4^+$ NKT cells, and not $CD4^+$ Tregs (Park et al. 2005), although the role of Tregs was not specifically determined in this study. Treg depletion is not always successful in either reversing tumor-specific tolerance or in boosting immune-mediated tumor rejection. For example, depleting Tregs with PC61 antibody did not reverse tumor-specific tolerance or tumor rejection in TRAMP mice at 25–27 weeks of age (Degl'Innocenti et al. 2008).

9.2 Antigen-Specific Treg Targeting

Tumor antigen-specific Tregs arise spontaneously, in the absence of vaccinations or other therapeutic interventions (Wang et al. 2004; Vence et al. 2007), and can also be induced following active vaccination (Zhou et al. 2006). Reducing antigen-specific Treg function rather than global Treg function could mitigate against pathologic autoimmunity as an undesirable treatment side effect, although significant pathologic autoimmunity following human Treg depletion has not been reported, in contrast to the significant autoimmune consequences of other immune strategies such as anti-CTLA-4 antibody treatment (Phan et al. 2003). This lack of significant pathologic autoimmunity induction following Treg depletion is due in part to the fact that Treg depletion alone may be insufficient to generate pathologic autoimmunity

(McHugh and Shevach 2002). No technique that manages antigen-specific Treg function uniquely has yet been described. Tumor Tregs expressing folate receptor 4 are enriched for antigen-specific cells in at least some cancers; reducing the numbers of folate receptor 4+ Tregs augmented immune-driven elimination of tumor in a mouse model (Yamaguchi et al. 2007).

9.3 Raising the Effector Cell Suppression Threshold

Anti-CTLA-4 antibody exerts antitumor immune effects both by reducing Treg function and by increasing the effector cell threshold for Treg-mediated suppression, although raising effector cell suppression threshold may predominate, and anti-CTLA-4 antibody can increase Treg numbers and proliferation in human subjects (Quezada et al. 2008). The relative contributions of these distinct mechanisms of action remain to be fully elucidated and could differ based on tumor type and anatomic compartment. For example, in a recent human clinical trial treatment, anti-CTLA-4 antibody treatment reduced $CD3^+CD4^+FOXP3^+$ cells in the blood that phenotypically resembled Tregs. However, blood $CD8^+$ cytotoxic T cell numbers in that same trial were unaltered. Further, the cells phenotypically resembling Tregs quickly returned to baseline numbers. However, their Treg function was not determined (O'Mahony et al. 2007). Tumor infiltrating T cells that had previously been activated by dendritic cells with genetically silenced A20 (a zinc finger protein) were resistant to Treg-mediated suppression (Song et al. 2008). IL-7 can raise the effector T cell threshold for Treg-mediated suppression in mouse models for autoimmune diseases (Calzascia et al. 2008), but this effect has not been described in tumors. Effector cells that cannot properly activate Notch signaling are resistant to Treg-mediated suppression, at least when the suppressive mechanism involves membrane-bound TGF-β (Ostroukhova et al. 2006).

9.4 Altering Treg Trafficking

IL-2 infusions can alter Treg trafficking, and can increase circulating Treg numbers (van der Vliet et al. 2007; Wei et al. 2007) although in vitro Treg functionality may be reduced (van der Vliet et al. 2007). Preventing Treg ingress into areas where antitumor immunity is primed may be beneficial (Curiel et al. 2004). Cyclophosphamide plus anti-OX40 antibody preferentially boosted effector T cell over Treg trafficking in a mouse melanoma model (Hirschhorn-Cymerman et al. 2009). In immunodeficient mice xenografted with human ovarian carcinoma, anti-CCL22 antibody inhibited Treg ingress into tumor and allowed increased immune-mediated rejection by adoptively transferred $CD8^+$ T cells autologous to the tumor (Zou et al. unpublished data).

9.5 Inhibiting Treg Suppressive Functions

Tumor Tregs exert suppressive activity through a variety of distinct mechanisms (Zou 2006), which can be mitigated by strategies aimed at blocking these mechanisms rather than killing the Treg or diverting its differentiation or its trafficking (Rüter et al. 2009; Curiel 2008). *Escherichia coli* expressing an engineered *listeriolysin-O* gene engender specific cytotoxic T lymphocytes but simultaneously, make local Tregs nonfunctional (Nitcheu-Tefit et al. 2007). STAT3 inhibition lowers Treg suppressive function (Pallandre et al. 2007). OX40 triggering on Tregs infiltrating tumors inhibits their ability to suppress effector T cells and helps mediate immune-mediated tumor rejection (Piconese et al. 2008). Stimulation of GITR by monoclonal antibodies in vitro abrogates the suppressor function of murine Tregs (Shimizu et al. 2002; Kanamaru et al. 2004), but a similar effect has not convincingly been demonstrated in human Tregs (Levings et al. 2002). The importance of Toll-like receptor signaling for tumor immunotherapy is demonstrated by in vitro experiments showing that only virus-based vaccines provide Toll-like receptor signals required for reversing Treg-mediated tolerance. Conversely, dendritic cell-based vaccines that lack Toll-like receptor signaling can break tolerance of CD8$^+$ T cells only after removal of Tregs or with the coadministration of another Toll-like receptor ligand (Yang et al. 2004). These experiments suggest that functional Treg inhibition by Toll-like receptor ligation (such as with TLR9 ligation by CpG oligonucleotides) may be a novel means to boost efficacy of vaccine-based cancer treatments. Sendai virus in CT26 colon cancer inhibited Treg function in mice, possibly through induced IL-6 (Kurooka and Kaneda 2007). Foxp3 must interact with NFAT for development of the suppressive phenotype (Ono et al. 2007), suggesting a novel pathway for therapeutic intervention. Blocking effector cell IL-10 receptor or other strategies might also be useful.

9.6 Blocking Treg Differentiation

Foxp3 mediates Treg differentiation through increasingly understood mechanisms (Li et al. 2007b; Mantel et al. 2007) that could be exploited therapeutically. Tumor factors such as vascular endothelial growth factor inhibit dendritic cell maturation (Gabrilovich et al. 1996). These immature dendritic cells induce defective T cell activation, including induction of Tregs. Means to prevent dysfunctional dendritic cell activation of T cells could thus reduce Treg differentiation. Interferon-α can improve dendritic cell maturation in tumor-bearing mice, which could reduce Treg generation (Interferon-α boosts antitumor immunity through effects on T cells and dendritic cells and augments the clinical efficacy of Treg depletion. Wall et al. 2009).

9.7 Subverting Treg Differentiation

Many tumor-associated Tregs are tumor antigen-specific. If their differentiation could be redirected into a useful pathway, Th1 for example, it might be possible to change a tumor-specific Treg into a tumor-specific effector T cell. This concept is appealing as depleting Tregs could produce a void that refills with Tregs (Colombo and Piconese 2007), and because altering differentiation increases the number of potentially beneficial antitumor effector cells. The recent discovery that a common aryl hydrocarbon receptor controls Th17 vs. Treg differentiation (Quintana et al. 2008) may be usefully exploited in subverting Treg differentiation, provided that the Th17 cells so produced are not detrimental to tumor-specific immunity. In support of such a strategy, in B16 melanoma, indoleamine 2,3-dioxygenase inhibition can direct Tregs to become Th17 cells that could help boost antitumor immunity (Sharma et al. 2009). Dendritic cells conditioned ex vivo with an anti-B7-DC antibody converted antigen-specific Tregs into antitumor Th17 effector cells in a mouse model for melanoma (Radhakrishnan et al. 2008).

9.8 Combining Treg Management with Other Treatment Modalities

The timing of Treg depletion in relationship to other therapeutic interventions greatly affects the immunologic efficacy of combined treatments (Litzinger et al. 2007). Little is known regarding how to use Treg management strategies in combination with other treatment modalities. Depleting effector T cell pools in conjunction with Treg depletion to allow homeostatic effector T cell expansion is an interesting concept, and may partly underlie the mechanism of action of denileukin diftitox. Combining Treg management with cytotoxic agents that induce significant tumor immunogenicity (Obeid et al. 2007) may improve immune responses against cancer, as antigens released by the cytotoxic agent could function as an endogenous vaccination. Critically timed chemotherapy can reverse Treg accumulation (Egilmez et al. 2007).

9.9 Additional Treg Management Considerations

Even following successful Treg depletion, effector cells may nonetheless be incapable of eradicating tumor due to ineffective trafficking, immunoediting, reduced immune effector cell functions, or other reasons. For example, inefficient effector cell trafficking to the appropriate compartment compromised the efficacy of Treg depletion in a mouse model for melanoma (Quezada et al. 2008). When effector cell trafficking was improved following radiation-mediated endothelial cell damage, the immune efficacy of Treg depletion was significantly improved.

It is striking that relatively little has been studied regarding the effects of age or gender on tumor immunity generally, and on the effects of Tregs specifically. The effects of aging on Treg function in naïve mice and humans have led to contradictory results, which are discussed elsewhere. Denileukin diftitox-mediated Treg depletion is ineffective in improving antitumor immunity and slowing tumor growth in a model of B16 melanoma in aged mice, whereas it is highly effective in young mice (Daniel et al. 2009). In our studies of gender differences, we have found that estrogen and B7-H1 co-signaling molecules lead to improved antitumor immunity and resistance to B16 melanoma in young female vs. male mice. These results are in part due to compromised Treg function in naïve female, B7-H1$^{-/-}$ mice (Habicht et al. 2007; Lin et al. 2010). Strikingly, in wild type mice with B16 melanoma, denileukin diftitox-mediated Treg depletion was equally efficacious in either gender, but antibody-mediated B7-H1 blockade was significantly more effective in improving antitumor immunity and slowing tumor growth in females compared to males (Lin et al. 2010). Such data demonstrate the importance of understanding gender-based and age-based differences in tumor-mediated immunopathology for optimal development of immunotherapeutic strategies.

9.10 Other Regulatory Cells

CD8$^+$ T cells, various myeloid cells and NKT cells have previously been described as dysfunctional regulatory cells in cancer (Zou 2005). A recent study demonstrates a population of suppressive CD8$^+$FOXP3$^+$ cells in prostate cancer that function through a contact-dependent mechanism, and whose effects are reduced by TLR8 agonists (Kiniwa et al. 2007). A population of CD8$^+$CD25$^+$Foxp3$^+$ suppressive T cells was reported in blood and tumor tissue of patients with colorectal cancer (Chaput et al. 2009). These colorectal cancer-associated CD8$^+$ Tregs were phenotypically similar to CD4$^+$FOXP3$^+$ Tregs in increased expression of CTLA-4 and GITR, and suppression of proliferation and cytokine secretion of CD4$^+$CD25$^-$ responder T cells in an in vitro assay. In a mouse model for allograft rejection of leukemia, anti-CD3-conditioned mice developed CD8$^+$FOXP3$^+$ suppressor T cells that blocked graft vs. host disease, but not a graft vs. leukemia response (Zhang et al. 2007). Tregs do not account for all of suppression of tumor-specific immunity. For example, in a model for colon cancer in mice a specific NKT cell population and IL-13 were involved in immune suppression (Terabe et al. 2000), which was later suggested not to depend on Tregs (Park et al. 2005). Relative contributions to tumor immunopathology, and therapeutic effects of management of each of these various types of regulatory cells remain to be defined, but represent interesting and important areas for future study.

10 A Potential Malignancy of Tregs

Hematologic neoplasms arising from essentially all elements of the hematopoietic system have been described. Thus, it is not surprising that a neoplasm arising from Tregs might occur as well. For example, FOXP3 expression has been reported in some cutaneous T cell lymphomas. These malignant FOXP3+ T cells also function as typical nonmalignant Tregs in in vitro Treg suppression assays (Yano et al. 2007). Mycosis fungoides cells that acquire FOXP3 expression exhibit aggressive behavior after large cell transformation, which could be due in part to FOXP3-mediated events (Hallermann et al. 2007).

11 Challenges for the Field

It is clear that not all types of malignancies, at selected stages of spread, or in individual hosts, will benefit from specific strategies proposed here. As an example, Tregs could mediate important immunopathology in certain lymphomas. Nonetheless, the steroids often used in lymphoma treatment could vitiate clinically meaningful activation of effector T cells. Appropriate immune monitoring tests that can be used practically have to be developed to monitor the immune consequences of interventions. For example, to study the effects of Treg-mediated T cell suppression, cell sorting capabilities are required as are large numbers of viable immune cells. Such hardware and solutions to logistical issues are not always possible or practical. Development of appropriate proof-of-concept trials can address the unique and specific challenges demanded by these strategies. As an example, if a specific Treg management strategy improves tumor-specific immunity, it will be important to demonstrate that the targeted Treg function was reduced in a specific functional assay and then it will be necessary to develop a method to demonstrate the mechanistic link between the Treg management strategy and improved antitumor immunity. Such assay development entails challenges common to tumor immunology as well as those specific to given strategies. For example, although a specific cytotoxic T lymphocyte epitope is followed in a trial, it is usually unclear whether such an epitope mediates tumor protection, and even if it does, if studying it in blood, as opposed to the local tumor microenvironment, will convey the relevant and useful information required to formulate legitimate conclusions regarding mechanisms of treatment effects. Also, in vaccine strategies, the specific immune response to the vaccinating antigen will be followed despite these limitations. Such a monitoring strategy is generally not applicable to Treg management trials, as no tumor antigen is defined in advance.

Despite our current state of incomplete understandings and outright ignorance, there is much data suggesting that guarded optimism for eventually using Treg management for clinical benefits in our war against cancer is a reasonable and realistic goal.

Acknowledgments I regret not citing many important works from my colleagues due to space limitations. Thanks to Ai-Jie Liu and Sara Ludwig for expert technical assistance. This work was supported by CA105207, FD003118, the Fanny Rippel Foundation, the Voelcker Trust, the Hayes Endowment and UTHSCSA endowments. The Holly Beach Public Library Association, CA54174, Texas STARS, The Hogg Foundation and the Owens Foundation.

References

Ahonen CL, Wasiuk A et al (2008) Enhanced efficacy and reduced toxicity of multifactorial adjuvants compared to unitary adjuvants as cancer vaccines. Blood 111(6):3116–3125

Bach JF (2003) Regulatory T cells under scrutiny. Nat Rev Immunol 3(3):189–198

Banerjee DK, Dhodapkar MV et al (2006) Expansion of FOXP3high regulatory T cells by human dendritic cells (DCs) in vitro and after injection of cytokine-matured DCs in myeloma patients. Blood 108(8):2655–2661

Banissi C, Ghiringhelli F et al (2009) Treg depletion with a low-dose metronomic temozolomide regimen in a rat glioma model. Cancer Immunol Immunother 58(10):1627–1634

Barnett B, Kryczek I et al (2005) Regulatory T cells in ovarian cancer: biology and therapeutic potential. Am J Reprod Immunol 54(6):369–377

Battaglia A, Buzzonetti A et al (2008) Neuropilin-1 expression identifies a subset of regulatory T cells in human lymph nodes that is modulated by preoperative chemoradiation therapy in cervical cancer. Immunology 123(1):129–138

Baumgartner J, Wilson C et al (2007) Melanoma induces immunosuppression by up-regulating FOXP3(+) regulatory T cells. J Surg Res 141(1):72–77

Beissert S, Loser K (2008) Molecular and cellular mechanisms of photocarcinogenesis. Photochem Photobiol 84(1):29–34

Bergmann C, Strauss L et al (2007) Expansion of human T regulatory type 1 cells in the microenvironment of cyclooxygenase 2 overexpressing head and neck squamous cell carcinoma. Cancer Res 67(18):8865–8873

Betts G, Twohig J et al (2007) The impact of regulatory T cells on carcinogen-induced sarcogenesis. Br J Cancer 96(12):1849–1854

Bluestone JA, Abbas AK (2003) Natural versus adaptive regulatory T cells. Nat Rev Immunol 3(3):253–257

Brode S, Cooke A (2008) Immune-potentiating effects of the chemotherapeutic drug cyclophosphamide. Crit Rev Immunol 28(2):109–126

Calzascia T, Pellegrini M et al (2008) CD4 T cells, lymphopenia, and IL-7 in a multistep pathway to autoimmunity. Proc Natl Acad Sci USA 105(8):2999–3004

Chaput N, Louafi S et al (2009) Identification of CD8+CD25+Foxp3+ suppressive T cells in colorectal cancer tissue. Gut 58(4):520–529

Chen W, Yan W et al (2008) A simple but effective cancer vaccine consisting of an antigen and a cationic lipid. Cancer Immunol Immunother 57(4):517–530

Colombo MP, Piconese S (2007) Regulatory-T-cell inhibition versus depletion: the right choice in cancer immunotherapy. Nat Rev Cancer 7(11):880–887

Curiel TJ (2007a) Regulatory T-cell development: is Foxp3 the decider? Nat Med 13(3): 250–253

Curiel TJ (2007b) Tregs and rethinking cancer immunotherapy. J Clin Invest 117(5):1167–1174

Curiel TJ (2008) Regulatory T cells and treatment of cancer. Curr Opin Immunol 20(2): 241–246

Curiel TJ, Wei S et al (2003) Blockade of B7-H1 improves myeloid dendritic cell-mediated antitumor immunity. Nat Med 9(5):562–567

Curiel TJ, Coukos G et al (2004) Specific recruitment of regulatory T cells in ovarian carcinoma fosters immune privilege and predicts reduced survival. Nat Med 10(9):942–949

Daniel BJ, Liu A, Kious MJ et al (2009) Aged mice do not benefit from Treg depletion as melanoma treatment. Paper presented at the Aspen cancer conference, Aspen, CO, 19–22 July 2009

Degl'Innocenti E, Grioni M et al (2008) Peripheral T-cell tolerance associated with prostate cancer is independent from CD4+CD25+ regulatory T cells. Cancer Res 68(1):292–300

Egilmez NK, Kilinc MO et al (2007) Controlled-release particulate cytokine adjuvants for cancer therapy. Endocr Metab Immune Disord Drug Targets 7(4):266–270

Fontenot JD, Gavin MA et al (2003) Foxp3 programs the development and function of CD4+CD25+ regulatory T cells. Nat Immunol 4(4):330–336

Fontenot JD, Rasmussen JP et al (2005) Regulatory T cell lineage specification by the forkhead transcription factor foxp3. Immunity 22(3):329–341

Foss FM (2000) DAB(389)IL-2 (ONTAK): a novel fusion toxin therapy for lymphoma. Clin Lymphoma 1(2):110–116; discussion 117

Francois V, Ottaviani S et al (2009) The CD4(+) T-cell response of melanoma patients to a MAGE-A3 peptide vaccine involves potential regulatory T cells. Cancer Res 69(10):4335–4345

Gabrilovich DI, Chen HL et al (1996) Production of vascular endothelial growth factor by human tumors inhibits the functional maturation of dendritic cells [published erratum appears in Nat Med 1996;2(11):1267]. Nat Med 2(10):1096–1103

Galustian C, Meyer B et al (2009) The anti-cancer agents lenalidomide and pomalidomide inhibit the proliferation and function of T regulatory cells. Cancer Immunol Immunother 58(7):1033–1045

Generali D, Bates G et al (2009) Immunomodulation of FOXP3+ regulatory T cells by the aromatase inhibitor letrozole in breast cancer patients. Clin Cancer Res 15(3):1046–1051

Ghiringhelli F, Puig PE et al (2005) Tumor cells convert immature myeloid dendritic cells into TGF-beta-secreting cells inducing CD4+CD25+ regulatory T cell proliferation. J Exp Med 202(7):919–929

Golgher D, Jones E et al (2002) Depletion of CD25+ regulatory cells uncovers immune responses to shared murine tumor rejection antigens. Eur J Immunol 32(11):3267–3275

Habicht A, Dada S et al (2007) A link between PDL1 and T regulatory cells in fetomaternal tolerance. J Immunol 179(8):5211–5219

Hallermann C, Niermann C et al (2007) Regulatory T-cell phenotype in association with large cell transformation of mycosis fungoides. Eur J Haematol 78(3):260–263

Han S, Wang B et al (2008) Overcoming immune tolerance against multiple myeloma with lentiviral calnexin-engineered dendritic cells. Mol Ther 16(2):269–279

Han Y, Guo Q et al (2009) CD69+ CD4+ CD25- T cells, a new subset of regulatory T cells, suppress T cell proliferation through membrane-bound TGF-beta 1. J Immunol 182(1):111–120

Haxhinasto S, Mathis D et al (2008) The AKT-mTOR axis regulates de novo differentiation of CD4+Foxp3+ cells. J Exp Med 205(3):565–574

Hirschhorn-Cymerman D, Rizzuto GA et al (2009) OX40 engagement and chemotherapy combination provides potent antitumor immunity with concomitant regulatory T cell apoptosis. J Exp Med 206(5):1103–1116

Hori S, Nomura T et al (2003) Control of regulatory T cell development by the transcription factor foxp3. Science 299(5609):1057–1061

Horlock C, Stott B et al (2009) The effects of trastuzumab on the CD4+CD25+FoxP3+ and CD4+IL17A+ T-cell axis in patients with breast cancer. Br J Cancer 100(7):1061–1067

Hus I, Schmitt M et al (2008) Vaccination of B-CLL patients with autologous dendritic cells can change the frequency of leukemia antigen-specific CD8+ T cells as well as CD4+CD25+FoxP3+ regulatory T cells toward an antileukemia response. Leukemia 22(5):1007–1017

Javia LR, Rosenberg SA (2003) CD4+CD25+ suppressor lymphocytes in the circulation of patients immunized against melanoma antigens. J Immunother 26(1):85–93

Jing W, Orentas RJ et al (2007) Induction of immunity to neuroblastoma early after syngeneic hematopoietic stem cell transplantation using a novel mouse tumor vaccine. Biol Blood Marrow Transplant 13(3):277–292

Jordanova ES, Gorter A et al (2008) Human leukocyte antigen class I, MHC class I chain-related molecule A, and CD8+/regulatory T-cell ratio: which variable determines survival of cervical cancer patients? Clin Cancer Res 14(7):2028–2035

Juszczynski P, Ouyang J et al (2007) The AP1-dependent secretion of galectin-1 by Reed Sternberg cells fosters immune privilege in classical Hodgkin lymphoma. Proc Natl Acad Sci USA 104(32):13134–13139

Kakinuma T, Nadiminti H et al (2007) Small numbers of residual tumor cells at the site of primary inoculation are critical for anti-tumor immunity following challenge at a secondary location. Cancer Immunol Immunother 56(7):1119–1131

Kanamaru F, Youngnak P et al (2004) Costimulation via glucocorticoid-induced TNF receptor in both conventional and CD25+ regulatory CD4+ T cells. J Immunol 172(12):7306–7314

Kang SG, Lim HW et al (2007) Vitamin A metabolites induce gut-homing FoxP3+ regulatory T cells. J Immunol 179(6):3724–3733

Kaporis HG, Guttman-Yassky E et al (2007) Human basal cell carcinoma is associated with Foxp3+ T cells in a Th2 dominant microenvironment. J Invest Dermatol 127(10): 2391–2398

Kato Y, Yoshimura K et al (2007) Synergistic in vivo antitumor effect of the histone deacetylase inhibitor MS-275 in combination with interleukin 2 in a murine model of renal cell carcinoma. Clin Cancer Res 13(15 pt 1):4538–4546

Kelley TW, Pohlman B et al (2007) The ratio of FOXP3+ regulatory T cells to granzyme B+ cytotoxic T/NK cells predicts prognosis in classical Hodgkin lymphoma and is independent of bcl-2 and MAL expression. Am J Clin Pathol 128(6):958–965

Kiniwa Y, Miyahara Y et al (2007) CD8+ Foxp3+ regulatory T cells mediate immunosuppression in prostate cancer. Clin Cancer Res 13(23):6947–6958

Kobayashi N, Hiraoka N et al (2007) FOXP3+ regulatory T cells affect the development and progression of hepatocarcinogenesis. Clin Cancer Res 13(3):902–911

Krupnick AS, Gelman AE et al (2005) Murine vascular endothelium activates and induces the generation of allogeneic CD4+25+Foxp3+ regulatory T cells. J Immunol 175(10):6265–6270

Kryczek I, Zou L et al (2006) B7-H4 expression identifies a novel suppressive macrophage population in human ovarian carcinoma. J Exp Med 203(4):871–881

Kryczek I, Liu R et al (2009) FOXP3 defines regulatory T cells in human tumor and autoimmune disease. Cancer Res 69(9):3995–4000

Kurooka M, Kaneda Y (2007) Inactivated Sendai virus particles eradicate tumors by inducing immune responses through blocking regulatory T cells. Cancer Res 67(1):227–236

Ladoire S, Arnould L et al (2008) Pathologic complete response to neoadjuvant chemotherapy of breast carcinoma is associated with the disappearance of tumor-infiltrating foxp3+ regulatory T cells. Clin Cancer Res 14(8):2413–2420

Larmonier N, Janikashvili N et al (2008) Imatinib mesylate inhibits CD4+ CD25+ regulatory T cell activity and enhances active immunotherapy against BCR-ABL- tumors. J Immunol 181(10):6955–6963

Lau KM, Cheng SH et al (2007) Increase in circulating Foxp3+CD4+CD25(high) regulatory T cells in nasopharyngeal carcinoma patients. Br J Cancer 96(4):617–622

Levings MK, Sangregorio R et al (2002) Human CD25+CD4+ T suppressor cell clones produce transforming growth factor beta, but not interleukin 10, and are distinct from type 1 T regulatory cells. J Exp Med 196(10):1335–1346

Li B, Samanta A et al (2007a) FOXP3 interactions with histone acetyltransferase and class II histone deacetylases are required for repression. Proc Natl Acad Sci USA 104(11):4571–4576

Li B, Saouaf SJ et al (2007b) Biochemistry and therapeutic implications of mechanisms involved in FOXP3 activity in immune suppression. Curr Opin Immunol 19(5):583–588

Li X, Ye F et al (2007c) Human ovarian carcinoma cells generate CD4(+)CD25(+) regulatory T cells from peripheral CD4(+)CD25(−) T cells through secreting TGF-beta. Cancer Lett 253(1): 144–153

Lin PY, Sun L, Thibodeaux SR, et al. B7-H1-dependent sex-related differences in tumor immunity and immunotherapy responses. J Immunol 185: 2747–53.

Ling KL, Pratap SE et al (2007) Increased frequency of regulatory T cells in peripheral blood and tumour infiltrating lymphocytes in colorectal cancer patients. Cancer Immun 7:7

Litzinger MT, Fernando R et al (2007) IL-2 immunotoxin denileukin diftitox reduces regulatory T cells and enhances vaccine-mediated T-cell immunity. Blood 110(9):3192–3201

Liu W, Putnam AL et al (2006) CD127 expression inversely correlates with FoxP3 and suppressive function of human CD4+ T reg cells. J Exp Med 203(7):1701–1711

Liu JY, Wu Y et al (2007a) Single administration of low dose cyclophosphamide augments the antitumor effect of dendritic cell vaccine. Cancer Immunol Immunother 56(10):1597–1604

Liu VC, Wong LY et al (2007b) Tumor evasion of the immune system by converting CD4+CD25- T cells into CD4+CD25+ T regulatory cells: role of tumor-derived TGF-beta. J Immunol 178(5):2883–2892

Liyanage UK, Moore TT et al (2002) Prevalence of regulatory T cells is increased in peripheral blood and tumor microenvironment of patients with pancreas or breast adenocarcinoma. J Immunol 169(5):2756–2761

Lonnroth C, Andersson M et al (2008) Preoperative treatment with a non-steroidal anti-inflammatory drug (NSAID) increases tumor tissue infiltration of seemingly activated immune cells in colorectal cancer. Cancer Immun 8:5

Loskog A, Ninalga C et al (2007) Human bladder carcinoma is dominated by T-regulatory cells and Th1 inhibitory cytokines. J Urol 177(1):353–358

Malek TR, Porter BO et al (2000) Normal lymphoid homeostasis and lack of lethal autoimmunity in mice containing mature T cells with severely impaired IL-2 receptors. J Immunol 164(6):2905–2914

Malek TR, Yu A et al (2002) CD4 regulatory T cells prevent lethal autoimmunity in IL-2Rbeta-deficient mice. Implications for the nonredundant function of IL-2. Immunity 17(2):167–178

Mandapathil M, Lang S et al (2009) Isolation of functional human regulatory T cells (Treg) from the peripheral blood based on the CD39 expression. J Immunol Methods 346(1–2):55–63

Mantel PY, Kuipers H et al (2007) GATA3-driven Th2 responses inhibit TGF-beta1-induced FOXP3 expression and the formation of regulatory T cells. PLoS Biol 5(12):e329

McHugh RS, Shevach EM (2002) Cutting edge: depletion of CD4+CD25+ regulatory T cells is necessary, but not sufficient, for induction of organ-specific autoimmune disease. J Immunol 168(12):5979–5983

Miracco C, Mourmouras V et al (2007) Utility of tumour-infiltrating CD25+FOXP3+ regulatory T cell evaluation in predicting local recurrence in vertical growth phase cutaneous melanoma. Oncol Rep 18(5):1115–1122

Mittal S, Marshall NA et al (2008) Local and systemic induction of CD4+CD25+ regulatory T cell population by non-Hodgkin's lymphoma. Blood 111(11):5359–5370

Mizukami Y, Kono K et al (2008a) CCL17 and CCL22 chemokines within tumor microenvironment are related to accumulation of Foxp3+ regulatory T cells in gastric cancer. Int J Cancer 122(10):2286–2293

Mizukami Y, Kono K et al (2008b) Localisation pattern of Foxp3(+) regulatory T cells is associated with clinical behaviour in gastric cancer. Br J Cancer 98(1):148–153

Molavi O, Ma Z et al (2008) Synergistic antitumor effects of CpG oligodeoxynucleotide and STAT3 inhibitory agent JSI-124 in a mouse melanoma tumor model. Immunol Cell Biol 86(6):506–514

Molenkamp BG, van Leeuwen PA et al (2007) Intradermal CpG-B activates both plasmacytoid and myeloid dendritic cells in the sentinel lymph node of melanoma patients. Clin Cancer Res 13(10):2961–2969

Molling JW, de Gruijl TD et al (2007) CD4(+)CD25hi regulatory T-cell frequency correlates with persistence of human papillomavirus type 16 and T helper cell responses in patients with cervical intraepithelial neoplasia. Int J Cancer 121(8):1749–1755

Mourmouras V, Fimiani M et al (2007) Evaluation of tumour-infiltrating CD4+CD25+FOXP3+ regulatory T cells in human cutaneous benign and atypical naevi, melanomas and melanoma metastases. Br J Dermatol 157(3):531–539

Nagorsen D, Voigt S et al (2007) Tumor-infiltrating macrophages and dendritic cells in human colorectal cancer: relation to local regulatory T cells, systemic T-cell response against tumor-associated antigens and survival. J Transl Med 5:62

Nair S, Boczkowski D et al (2007) Vaccination against the forkhead family transcription factor Foxp3 enhances tumor immunity. Cancer Res 67(1):371–380

Nitcheu-Tefit J, Dai MS et al (2007) Listeriolysin O expressed in a bacterial vaccine suppresses CD4+CD25high regulatory T cell function in vivo. J Immunol 179(3):1532–1541

O'Mahony D, Morris JC et al (2007) A pilot study of CTLA-4 blockade after cancer vaccine failure in patients with advanced malignancy. Clin Cancer Res 13(3):958–964

Obeid M, Tesniere A et al (2007) Calreticulin exposure dictates the immunogenicity of cancer cell death. Nat Med 13(1):54–61

Ono M, Yaguchi H et al (2007) Foxp3 controls regulatory T-cell function by interacting with AML1/Runx1. Nature 446(7136):685–689

Ostroukhova M, Qi Z et al (2006) Treg-mediated immunosuppression involves activation of the Notch-HES1 axis by membrane-bound TGF-beta. J Clin Invest 116(4):996–1004

Pallandre JR, Brillard E et al (2007) Role of STAT3 in CD4+CD25+FOXP3+ regulatory lymphocyte generation: implications in graft-versus-host disease and antitumor immunity. J Immunol 179(11):7593–7604

Palucka AK, Ueno H et al (2007) Taming cancer by inducing immunity via dendritic cells. Immunol Rev 220:129–150

Park JM, Terabe M et al (2005) Unmasking immunosurveillance against a syngeneic colon cancer by elimination of CD4+ NKT regulatory cells and IL-13. Int J Cancer 114(1):80–87

Perrone G, Ruffini PA et al (2008) Intratumoural FOXP3-positive regulatory T cells are associated with adverse prognosis in radically resected gastric cancer. Eur J Cancer 44(13): 1875–1882

Phan GQ, Yang JC et al (2003) Cancer regression and autoimmunity induced by cytotoxic T lymphocyte-associated antigen 4 blockade in patients with metastatic melanoma. Proc Natl Acad Sci USA 100(14):8372–8377

Piconese S, Valzasina B et al (2008) OX40 triggering blocks suppression by regulatory T cells and facilitates tumor rejection. J Exp Med 205(4):825–839

Pillai V, Karandikar NJ (2007) Human regulatory T cells: a unique, stable thymic subset or a reversible peripheral state of differentiation? Immunol Lett 114(1):9–15

Poutahidis T, Haigis KM et al (2007) Rapid reversal of interleukin-6-dependent epithelial invasion in a mouse model of microbially induced colon carcinoma. Carcinogenesis 28(12): 2614–2623

Powell DJ Jr, de Vries CR et al (2007a) Inability to mediate prolonged reduction of regulatory T Cells after transfer of autologous CD25-depleted PBMC and interleukin-2 after lymphodepleting chemotherapy. J Immunother 30(4):438–447

Powell DJ Jr, Felipe-Silva A et al (2007b) Administration of a CD25-directed immunotoxin, LMB-2, to patients with metastatic melanoma induces a selective partial reduction in regulatory T cells in vivo. J Immunol 179(7):4919–4928

Quezada SA, Peggs KS et al (2008) Limited tumor infiltration by activated T effector cells restricts the therapeutic activity of regulatory T cell depletion against established melanoma. J Exp Med 205(9):2125–2138

Quintana FJ, Basso AS et al (2008) Control of Treg and TH17 cell differentiation by the aryl hydrocarbon receptor. Nature 453(7191):65–71

Radhakrishnan S, Cabrera R et al (2008) Reprogrammed FoxP3+ T regulatory cells become IL-17+ antigen-specific autoimmune effectors in vitro and in vivo. J Immunol 181(5): 3137–3147

Rüter J, Barnett BG et al (2009) Altering regulatory T cell function in cancer immunotherapy: a novel means to boost efficacy. Front Biosci 14:1761–1770

Sakaguchi S, Sakaguchi N et al (1995) Immunologic self-tolerance maintained by activated T cells expressing IL-2 receptor alpha-chains (CD25). Breakdown of a single mechanism of self-tolerance causes various autoimmune diseases. J Immunol 155(3):1151–1164

Sasada T, Kimura M et al (2003) CD4+CD25+ regulatory T cells in patients with gastrointestinal malignancies: possible involvement of regulatory T cells in disease progression. Cancer 98(5):1089–1099

Sasaki A, Tanaka F et al (2008) Prognostic value of tumor-infiltrating FOXP3+ regulatory T cells in patients with hepatocellular carcinoma. Eur J Surg Oncol 34(2):173–179

Scarpino S, Di Napoli A et al (2007) Expression of autoimmune regulator gene (AIRE) and T regulatory cells in human thymomas. Clin Exp Immunol 149(3):504–512

Schreiber TH (2007) The use of FoxP3 as a biomarker and prognostic factor for malignant human tumors. Cancer Epidemiol Biomarkers Prev 16(10):1931–1934

Sharma MD, Baban B et al (2007) Plasmacytoid dendritic cells from mouse tumor-draining lymph nodes directly activate mature Tregs via indoleamine 2,3-dioxygenase. J Clin Invest 117(9):2570–2582

Sharma MD, Hou DY et al (2009) Indoleamine 2,3-dioxygenase controls conversion of Foxp3+ Tregs to TH17-like cells in tumor-draining lymph nodes. Blood 113(24):6102–6111

Shevach EM (2002) CD4+ CD25+ suppressor T cells: more questions than answers. Nat Rev Immunol 2(6):389–400

Shimizu J, Yamazaki S et al (1999) Induction of tumor immunity by removing CD25+CD4+ T cells: a common basis between tumor immunity and autoimmunity. J Immunol 163(10):5211–5218

Shimizu J, Yamazaki S et al (2002) Stimulation of CD25(+)CD4(+) regulatory T cells through GITR breaks immunological self-tolerance. Nat Immunol 3(2):135–142

Shimizu Y, Dobashi K et al (2009) CXCR4+FOXP3+CD25+ lymphocytes accumulate in CXCL12-expressing malignant pleural mesothelioma. Int J Immunopathol Pharmacol 22(1):43–51

Siddiqui SA, Frigola X et al (2007) Tumor-infiltrating Foxp3-CD4+CD25+ T cells predict poor survival in renal cell carcinoma. Clin Cancer Res 13(7):2075–2081

Somasundaram R, Jacob L et al (2002) Inhibition of cytolytic T lymphocyte proliferation by autologous CD4+/CD25+ regulatory T cells in a colorectal carcinoma patient is mediated by transforming growth factor-beta. Cancer Res 62(18):5267–5272

Song XT, Kabler KE et al (2008) A20 is an antigen presentation attenuator, and its inhibition overcomes regulatory T cell-mediated suppression. Nat Med 14(3):258–265

Sosman JA, Carrillo C et al (2008) Three phase II cytokine working group trials of gp100 (210 M) peptide plus high-dose interleukin-2 in patients with HLA-A2-positive advanced melanoma. J Clin Oncol 26(14):2292–2298

Steitz J, Bruck J et al (2001) Depletion of CD25(+) CD4(+) T cells and treatment with tyrosinase-related protein 2-transduced dendritic cells enhance the interferon alpha-induced, CD8(+) T-cell-dependent immune defense of B16 melanoma. Cancer Res 61(24):8643–8646

Strauss L, Bergmann C et al (2007) The frequency and suppressor function of CD4+CD25highFoxp3+ T cells in the circulation of patients with squamous cell carcinoma of the head and neck. Clin Cancer Res 13(21):6301–6311

Strauss L, Bergmann C et al (2009) Human circulating CD4+CD25highFoxp3+ regulatory T cells kill autologous CD8+ but not CD4+ responder cells by Fas-mediated apoptosis. J Immunol 182(3):1469–1480

Sugihara AQ, Rolle CE et al (2009) Regulatory T cells actively infiltrate metastatic brain tumors. Int J Oncol 34(6):1533–1540

Sutmuller RP, van Duivenvoorde LM et al (2001) Synergism of cytotoxic T lymphocyte-associated antigen 4 blockade and depletion of CD25(+) regulatory T cells in antitumor therapy reveals alternative pathways for suppression of autoreactive cytotoxic T lymphocyte responses. J Exp Med 194(6):823–832

Szczepanski MJ, Szajnik M et al (2009) Increased frequency and suppression by regulatory T cells in patients with acute myelogenous leukemia. Clin Cancer Res 15(10):3325–3332

Tanaka H, Tanaka J et al (2002) Depletion of CD4+ CD25+ regulatory cells augments the generation of specific immune T cells in tumor-draining lymph nodes. J Immunother 25(3):207–217

Tao R, de Zoeten EF et al (2007) Deacetylase inhibition promotes the generation and function of regulatory T cells. Nat Med 13(11):1299–1307

Terabe M, Matsui S et al (2000) NKT cell-mediated repression of tumor immunosurveillance by IL-13 and the IL-4R-STAT6 pathway. Nat Immunol 1(6):515–520

Turk MJ, Guevara-Patino JA et al (2004) Concomitant tumor immunity to a poorly immunogenic melanoma is prevented by regulatory T cells. J Exp Med 200(6):771–782

Tzankov A, Meier C et al (2008) Correlation of high numbers of intratumoral FOXP3+ regulatory T cells with improved survival in germinal center-like diffuse large B-cell lymphoma, follicular lymphoma and classical Hodgkin's lymphoma. Haematologica 93(2):193–200

van der Burg SH, Piersma SJ et al (2007) Association of cervical cancer with the presence of CD4+ regulatory T cells specific for human papillomavirus antigens. Proc Natl Acad Sci USA 104(29):12087–12092

van der Most RG, Currie AJ et al (2009) Tumor eradication after cyclophosphamide depends on concurrent depletion of regulatory T cells: a role for cycling TNFR2-expressing effector-suppressor T cells in limiting effective chemotherapy. Cancer Immunol Immunother 58(8):1219–1228

van der Vliet HJ, Koon HB et al (2007) Effects of the administration of high-dose interleukin-2 on immunoregulatory cell subsets in patients with advanced melanoma and renal cell cancer. Clin Cancer Res 13(7):2100–2108

Vence L, Palucka AK et al (2007) Circulating tumor antigen-specific regulatory T cells in patients with metastatic melanoma. Proc Natl Acad Sci USA 104(52):20884–20889

Visser J, Nijman HW et al (2007) Frequencies and role of regulatory T cells in patients with (pre) malignant cervical neoplasia. Clin Exp Immunol 150(2):199–209

Wada J, Yamasaki A et al (2008) Regulatory T-cells are possible effect prediction markers of immunotherapy for cancer patients. Anticancer Res 28(4C):2401–2408

Wall S, Thibodeaux S, Daniel B et al (2009) International Society for Interferon and Cytokine Research, Lisbon, Portugal, 17–21 Oct 2009

Wang HY, Lee DA et al (2004) Tumor-specific human CD4+ regulatory T cells and their ligands: implications for immunotherapy. Immunity 20(1):107–118

Wei S, Kryczek I et al (2005) Plasmacytoid dendritic cells induce CD8+ regulatory T cells in human ovarian carcinoma. Cancer Res 65(12):5020–5026

Wei S, Kryczek I et al (2007) Interleukin-2 administration alters the CD4+FOXP3+ T-cell pool and tumor trafficking in patients with ovarian carcinoma. Cancer Res 67(15):7487–7494

Wieczorek G, Asemissen A et al (2009) Quantitative DNA methylation analysis of FOXP3 as a new method for counting regulatory T cells in peripheral blood and solid tissue. Cancer Res 69(2):599–608

Wolf AM, Wolf D et al (2003) Increase of regulatory T cells in the peripheral blood of cancer patients. Clin Cancer Res 9(2):606–612

Woo EY, Chu CS et al (2001) Regulatory CD4(+)CD25(+) T cells in tumors from patients with early- stage non-small cell lung cancer and late-stage ovarian cancer. Cancer Res 61(12):4766–4772

Woo EY, Yeh H et al (2002) Regulatory T cells from lung cancer patients directly inhibit autologous T cell proliferation. J Immunol 168(9):4272–4276

Xie Q, Gan L et al (2007) Loss of the innate immunity negative regulator IRAK-M leads to enhanced host immune defense against tumor growth. Mol Immunol 44(14):3453–3461

Yamaguchi T, Hirota K et al (2007) Control of immune responses by antigen-specific regulatory T cells expressing the folate receptor. Immunity 27(1):145–159

Yang Y, Huang CT et al (2004) Persistent toll-like receptor signals are required for reversal of regulatory T cell-mediated CD8 tolerance. Nat Immunol 5(5):508–515

Yang Y, Yang S et al (2007a) Tumor cells expressing anti-CD137 scFv induce a tumor-destructive environment. Cancer Res 67(5):2339–2344

Yang ZZ, Novak AJ et al (2007b) CD70+ non-Hodgkin lymphoma B cells induce Foxp3 expression and regulatory function in intratumoral CD4+CD25 T cells. Blood 110(7):2537–2544

Yano H, Ishida T et al (2007) Regulatory T-cell function of adult T-cell leukemia/lymphoma cells. Int J Cancer 120(9):2052–2057

Yaqub S, Henjum K et al (2008) Regulatory T cells in colorectal cancer patients suppress anti-tumor immune activity in a COX-2 dependent manner. Cancer Immunol Immunother 57(6):813–821

Yokokawa J, Cereda V et al (2008) Enhanced functionality of CD4+CD25highFoxP3+ regulatory T cells in the peripheral blood of patients with prostate cancer. Clin Cancer Res 14(4):1032–1040

Zabala M, Lasarte JJ et al (2007) Induction of immunosuppressive molecules and regulatory T cells counteracts the antitumor effect of interleukin-12-based gene therapy in a transgenic mouse model of liver cancer. J Hepatol 47(6):807–815

Zhang C, Lou J et al (2007) Donor CD8+ T cells mediate graft-versus-leukemia activity without clinical signs of graft-versus-host disease in recipients conditioned with anti-CD3 monoclonal antibody. J Immunol 178(2):838–850

Zhou G, Levitsky HI (2007) Natural regulatory T cells and de novo-induced regulatory T cells contribute independently to tumor-specific tolerance. J Immunol 178(4):2155–2162

Zhou G, Drake CG et al (2006) Amplification of tumor-specific regulatory T cells following therapeutic cancer vaccines. Blood 107(2):628–636

Zhou X, Bailey-Bucktrout SL et al (2009) Instability of the transcription factor Foxp3 leads to the generation of pathogenic memory T cells in vivo. Nat Immunol 10(9):1000–1007

Zou W (2005) Immunosuppressive networks in the tumour environment and their therapeutic relevance. Nat Rev Cancer 5(4):263–274

Zou W (2006) Regulatory T cells, tumour immunity and immunotherapy. Nat Rev Immunol 6(4):295–307

Zuo T, Wang L et al (2007) FOXP3 is an X-linked breast cancer suppressor gene and an important repressor of the HER-2/ErbB2 oncogene. Cell 129(7):1275–1286

Chapter 10
Relationship Between Th17 and Regulatory T Cells in the Tumor Environment

Ilona Kryczek, Ke Wu, Ende Zhao, Guobin Wang, and Weiping Zou

1 Introduction

The importance of an inflammatory milieu in the tumor progression has been recognized for a long time. Inflammatory conditions not only help initiate oncogenic transformation but also support tumor progression (Mantovani et al. 2008). However, anti-inflammatory immune responses established during tumor development, including Treg cells, suppress antitumor immunity, and reduce clinical efficacy of tumor therapy. The balance between the two opposite and exceptive processes, inflammation and tolerance, and ipso facto balance between Th17 cells and Treg cells may play an important role in the tumor progression.

2 Definition of Th17 and Treg Cells

Th17 cells: Th17 cells are a subset of CD4$^+$ T cells, which develop in the presence of TGFβ and IL-6, under the control of RORγt transcriptional factor, into IL-17 producing cells (Ivanov et al. 2006). However, CD8$^+$ T cells can also be differentiated into

---

I. Kryczek • G. Wang • W. Zou (✉)
Department of Surgery, University of Michigan, Ann Arbor, MI 48109, USA
e-mail: wzou@umich.edu

K. Wu
Department of Surgery, Union Hospital, Tongji Medical College, Huazhong University of Science and Technology, Wuhan 430022, China

E. Zhao
Department of Surgery, University of Michigan, Ann Arbor, MI 48109, USA

Department of Surgery, Union Hospital, Tongji Medical College, Huazhong University of Science and Technology, Wuhan 430022, China

IL-17 producing cells. Moreover, several studies have documented that unconventional T cells such as CD4$^-$CD8$^-$ TCR$\gamma\delta^+$ and NKT cells can secrete IL-17 during infection or inflammation or when activated in vitro (Ivanov et al. 2006; Nurieva et al. 2007; Stark et al. 2005; Romani et al. 2008; Roark et al. 2007). IL-17 could be expressed also by non-T cells. It has been demonstrated that human and mouse NK cells, and lymphoid tissue inducers (LTi cells) express IL-17 (Takatori et al. 2009; Michel et al. 2007; Coquet et al. 2008). Therefore, IL-17 is not exclusively attributed to Th17 cells.

Human tumor-associated IL-17 expressing cells are largely CD4$^+$CD3$^+$ (Th17) cells (Kryczek et al. 2007a, 2009a). Mouse tumor-associated IL-17$^+$ cells are basically CD4$^+$ and CD8$^+$ T cells (Kryczek et al. 2007a, 2009b). The IL-17$^+$ NK, NKT, LTi, and TCR$\gamma\delta^+$ T cells are minor populations in tumor-bearing hosts (Kryczek et al. 2007a, 2009a, b). In this chapter, we focus on tumor-associated Th17 cells.

Regulatory T cells (*Tregs*) comprise heterogenic populations of cells capable of negatively regulating immune responses. There are multiple Treg cell subsets, including CD4$^+$ as well as CD8$^+$ T cells, which may exhibit regulatory activity. Here we focus on natural CD4$^+$FOXP3$^+$ T cells (Chen et al. 2003).

3 Distribution of Th17 and Treg Cells in the Tumor Microenvironments

It has been demonstrated that Treg and Th17 cells gradually infiltrate the tumor microenvironment during tumor development (Kryczek et al. 2007a, 2009b). Increased numbers of Tregs and Th17 cells are often observed in patients with cancer (Table 10.1). Although Tregs and Th17 cells infiltrate the same tumor environment, their migratory mechanism and regulation properties seem to be different. Th17 cells are a much smaller fraction of CD4$^+$ T cells than Tregs (Kryczek et al. 2007a, b, 2009b, c). Tregs and Th17 cells are not proportionally increased in the same tumor microenvironments. Tregs are dramatically increased in the tumor tissues whereas the numbers of Th17 cells are limited. Indeed, there exists a reverse correlation between Tregs and Th17 cells in the tumor microenvironments (Kryczek et al. 2009a).

The expansion profile of Tregs and Th17 seems to be distinct. In cancer patients and in tumor-bearing mice, Treg expansion is systemic, while Th17 cells appear to be locally expanded, and limited to the tumor environment. Elevated levels of Tregs have been observed not only in the tumor tissues but also in spleen, peripheral blood, and tumor-draining lymph nodes (TDLN) in tumor-bearing mice (Appay et al. 2006; Meloni et al. 2006; Ormandy et al. 2005; Lau et al. 2007). Interestingly, following tumor development, Th17 cells are increased in the tumor tissues, but not TDLNs (Kryczek et al. 2007a). Similar to tumor-bearing mice, Th17 cells are increased in multiple human tumor types, but rarely in blood and TDLN in patients with cancer (Kryczek et al. 2009a).

Thus, although both Tregs and Th17 cells infiltrate the tumor environment, their profile and kinetic expansion significantly differ. In tumor-bearing hosts, Tregs reveal a systemic expansion and Th17 cells show a local tissue expansion.

Table 10.1 Treg and Th17 cells in the same human tumors

Cancer type	Tregs	Th17
Ovarian cancer	Curiel et al. (2004); Woo et al. (2001); Wolf et al. (2005); Sato et al. (2005)	Kryczek et al. (2009a); Miyahara et al. (2008)
Lung cancer	Woo et al. (2001); Ishibashi et al. (2006)	Koyama et al. (2008)
Breast cancer	Liyanage et al. (2002)	Horlock et al. (2009)
Gastric cancer	Sasada et al. (2003)	Zhang et al. (2008)
Renal cell carcinoma	Attig et al. (2009); Jeron et al. (2009); Siddiqui et al. (2007)	Inozume et al. (2009)

4 Migration of Th17 and Tregs in the Tumor Microenvironments

Both Treg and Th17 cells can traffic into the tumor environment. Tregs express variable levels of peripheral tissue homing molecules including CLA, CCR4, CCR8, $\alpha 4\beta 7$, and $\alpha E\beta 7$ integrins (Curiel et al. 2004; Cavani et al. 2003; Iellem et al. 2001, 2003; Stassen et al. 2004; Allakhverdi et al. 2006; Chen et al. 2006; Hultkrantz et al. 2005). Tregs may traffic into tumor in an organ- or tissue-specific manner (Wei et al. 2005, 2006; Zou 2006; Zou et al. 2004). For example, Tregs migrating to the intestine express integrin $\alpha 4\beta 7$ (CD103) and CCR6, while those destined for the skin express P-selectin, E-selectin, and CCR4. Interestingly, Th17 cells share chemokine receptors with Tregs. In mice IL-17-producing memory cells highly expressed CCR6 and CCR4, whereas IFN-γ^+IL-17$^+$-producing T cells expressed CCR6 and CXCR3 (Kryczek et al. 2008a, 2009a; Acosta-Rodriguez et al. 2007a). Human Th17 cells highly express CCR6 and a variety of integrin molecules (Kryczek et al. 2008a, 2009a). In fact we have observed high levels of Th17 cells in the tumor tissues including lung cancer and colorectal cancer where CCL22 expression is high ((Kryczek et al. 2009c) and unpublished data).

Both Tregs and Th17 cells are sensitive to attractive signaling transmitted by CCR6 and CCR4 receptors. However, different molecules may control Treg and Th17 migration into the tumor. Indeed, human CCR4$^+$ Tregs migrate toward CCL22 produced in the tumor microenvironment, and blockade of CCL22 and CCR4 pathway in vivo reduces Treg cell tumor trafficking (Curiel et al. 2004). Th17 cells express CCR6 which is an example of a chemokine receptor with only one single known specific chemokine ligand, the inflammatory and homeostatic chemokine CCL20. CCL20 is constitutively expressed in liver, lungs, mucosa-associated lymphatic tissue (MALT), and lymphatic tissues – these organs normally contain high levels of Th17 cells (Kryczek et al. 2007a, 2009b). It has been shown that CCL20 is increased in the tumor tissues, and is produced by both cancer cells and TAMs (Kleeff et al. 1999; Thomachot et al. 2004; Bell et al. 1999).

CCL22 and CCL20 are often co-expressed in the same tissues that may explain the presence of both Tregs and Th17 cells in the same environment. It has been reported that a majority of human peripheral blood Tregs (Baecher-Allan et al. 2001; Hoffmann et al. 2004), but not Th17 cells (Kryczek et al. 2009a), express lymphoid homing molecules CD62L and CCR7. This could explain the different distribution of Tregs and Th17 cells in the lymph nodes. Indeed, Tregs but not Th17 cells are accumulated in the tumor-draining lymph nodes (Kryczek et al. 2009a).

As the key chemokines and chemokine receptors controlling tumor trafficking of Tregs and Th17 cells may be different, it is possible that selective manipulation of chemokine and chemokine receptor could control the balance between Th17 and Treg cells in the tumor environment.

5 Environmental Milieu and Treg/Th17 Expansion in the Tumor Environment

Cytokine milieu: Tregs and Th17 cells are generated in the thymus through MHC class II-dependent selection (Sakaguchi 2001; Bensinger et al. 2001; Apostolou et al. 2002). However, both Tregs and Th17 cells can also be induced in the periphery. Foxp3$^+$ Tregs can be generated and expanded outside the thymus in the presence of TGF-β and IL-2 (Chen et al. 2003). Th17 cells require the expression of RORγt, which can be induced by TGF-β. Thus, TGF-β is a molecular link between Tregs and Th17 cells. However, the responsiveness of Tregs and Th17 precursors to TGF-β stimulation is different. High concentrations of TGF-β promote Tregs, and suppress Th17 cell differentiation (Zhou et al. 2008; Acosta-Rodriguez et al. 2007b; Wilson et al. 2007). Further, TGF-β is not required for thymic expression of Foxp3 (Huehn et al. 2009). Although, low and moderate concentrations of TGF-β favors differentiation of naive T cells into Th17 cells, the sole presence of TGF-β is not sufficient. Aside from TGF-β, IL-6 (Bettelli et al. 2006; Mangan et al. 2006; Veldhoen et al. 2006a) or IL-21 (Nurieva et al. 2007; Korn et al. 2007; Zhou et al. 2007; Yang et al. 2008a) or IL-1 (Kryczek et al. 2007b; Chung et al. 2009; Kimura et al. 2007) is requisite to promote the differentiation of Th17 cells. Interestingly, all these cytokines (IL-6, IL-21, and IL-1) have been shown to inhibit Treg differentiation through the STAT3-dependent pathway (Nurieva et al. 2007; Korn et al. 2007; Pasare & Medzhitov 2003; Yang et al. 2008b). IL-23 seems to be an essential survival factor for differentiated Th17 cells (Khader et al. 2005; Yen et al. 2006). Mice lacking IL-23 have almost no Th17 cells, suggesting that even if the cells are generated normally, they fail to expand or survive in the absence of IL-23.

The reciprocal relationship between Treg and Th17 cells is further regulated by IL-2. IL-2 is indispensable for Treg induction and function. However, IL-2 inhibits the generation of Th17 cells directly via STAT5 signaling (Kryczek et al. 2007a, b; Laurence et al. 2007). The opposite effects of IL-2 on Th17 and Treg cell differentiation are observed in tumor-bearing hosts. IL-2 reduces Th17 cells in the tumor, whereas it increases Tregs in the tumor and TDLN (Kryczek et al. 2007a). IL-2 treatment also decreases Th17 cells in ovarian cancer patients (unpublished data). Recently, it has been found that TGF-β with retinoic acid can induce Tregs (Mucida et al. 2007; Sun et al. 2007; Coombes et al. 2007).

Retinoic acid inhibits Th17 through SMAD activation, and IL-6 and IL-23 receptor expression inhibition (Sun et al. 2007; Coombes et al. 2007; Xiao et al. 2008; Kang et al. 2007; Benson et al. 2007). The role of TGFβ in human Th17 cell development remains controversial (Acosta-Rodriguez et al. 2007b; Wilson et al. 2007; Yang et al. 2008a; Manel et al. 2008). Thymic Th17 precursors constitutively express both ROR_c and the IL-23R, but not IL-17 (Cosmi et al. 2008). It has been suggested that induction of IL-17 expression appears in periphery, after secondary stimulation of Th17 precursors in the presence of IL-1β and IL-23 (Cosmi et al. 2008). In accordance with this observation, tumor-associated Th17 expansion is not associated with IL-6 and TGFβ, but with IL-1β (Kryczek et al. 2009a). Blockade of IL-1, but not IL-6 and TGF-β, inhibits tumor-associated Th17 cell induction (Kryczek et al. 2009a).

Both Tregs and Th17 cells can be expanded or differentiated from specific precursors locally in the tumor environment under controlling of pro-inflammatory and regulatory cytokine milieu (Fig. 10.1).

Tregs and Th17 cells crosstalk: Tregs may be converted into Th17 cells in the presence of inflammatory signals and vice versa Th17 into Tregs under regulatory condition (Zhou et al. 2008; Yang et al. 2008b). In vitro reciprocity between the Th17 and Treg developmental programs on the single-cell level has been proposed (Zhou et al. 2008; Yang et al. 2008b). However, there is no evidence whether the conversion is operative in vivo in the tumor environment. Tumor environment is enriched with pro-inflammatory cytokines (especially IL-6), which should theoretically prevent Th17 conversion into Treg cells. Tregs can suppress Th17 cell expansion in the ovarian cancer microenvironment through the adenosinergic pathway (Kryczek et al. 2009a). Tumor-associated Tregs highly express CD39; an ectonucleotidase that cleaves ATP in a rate-limiting step to form AMP, which can then be cleaved by CD73 to form adenosine (Deaglio et al. 2007; Borsellino et al. 2007). It has recently been shown that extracellular ATP can promote Th17 cells in vivo (Atarashi et al. 2008) and induces IL-23 production by APC in vitro (Schnurr et al. 2005a). Furthermore, binding of adenosine to A2A receptor on T cells results in increased the intracellular cAMP and suppression of IL-17 production by Th17 cells (Fletcher et al. 2009).

Tregs may control Th17 cells through Treg-derived IL-10 (Maloy et al. 2003) or Treg-induced APC IL-10 (Misra et al. 2004; Veldhoen et al. 2006b; Kryczek et al. 2006a). Tregs-derived IL-10 can act in an autocrine manner to inhibit APC function (Kryczek et al. 2006a). Importantly, Treg-conditioned monocytes and macrophages are poor producers of pro-inflammatory cytokines including IL-23, IL-6, and IL-1β even after activation with toll-like receptor-ligands like LPS (Tiemessen et al. 2007; Taams et al. 2005; Oehler-Janne et al. 2008). These observations are consistent with the phenotype of IL-10-deficient animals. There are increased levels of IL-17 and Th17 cells in the $IL-10^{-/-}$ mice (Montufar-Solis et al. 2008; Gu et al. 2008). IL-10 can also modulate Th17 function. It has been shown that IL-10 decreases the amount of IL-17 secreted by Th17 cells in mice and human (Oehler-Janne et al. 2008; Kirkham et al. 2006). In summary, Tregs can inhibit Th17 cell expansion in the tumor microenvironment.

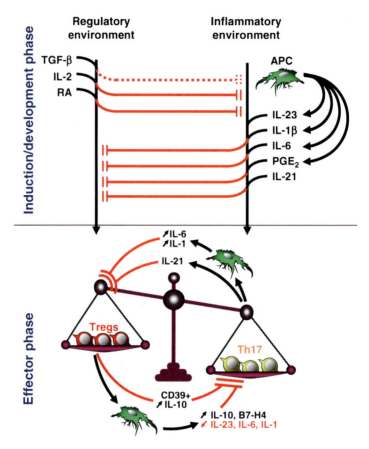

Fig. 10.1 Regulation the balance between Tregs and Th17 cells in the tumor environment. Inflammatory environment induces Th17 cells and inhibits Tregs: induction phase: IL-1, IL-6, PGE_2, and T cells derived-IL-21 promote Th17 development, but inhibit Treg expansion. Effector phase: expanded Th17 cells produce IL-21 and induce IL-6 and IL-1 production by TAMs, stroma, and tumor, and further inhibit Tregs. Regulatory environment induces Tregs and inhibits Th17 cells: induction phase: IL-2 and retinoic acid (RA) induce Tregs and inhibits Th17 differentiation. TGF-β in high concentration stimulates Treg induction and inhibits Th17 development. Effector phase: Tregs inhibit Th17 cells through CD39 and IL-10. IL-10 can further reduce the production of Th17 inducing cytokines, IL-23, IL-6, and IL-1 by APCs

6 Tumor-Associated Macrophages (TAMs) and Th17 Cells in the Tumor Microenvironments

Although Tregs can inhibit Th17 expansion, Th17 and Treg cells are both increased in the tumor microenvironment (Kryczek et al. 2009a, b, 2008b). It suggests that distinct mechanisms may allow Th17 cells to expand in the tumor microenvironment. TAMs are capable of inducing Th17 cell development in ovarian cancer (Kryczek et al. 2009a) and hepatocellular carcinoma (Kuang et al. 2010). This induction is mediated by IL-1β, but not IL-1α, and IL-23 (Kryczek et al. 2009a). In human autoimmune disease, in addition to IL-1β, IL-1α and IL-23 are involved in APC-mediated memory Th17 cell expansion (Kryczek et al. 2008a, b). This suggests the existence of distinct mechanisms in inducing Th17 cells in patients with tumors and autoimmune diseases. In addition to IL-1, TAMs, tumor stroma, and tumor cells can mediate Th17 expansion through prostaglandin E_2 (PGE_2) synthesis (Wang et al. 2007). It is widely accepted that alterations of PGE_2 have key roles in influencing the development multiple cancers (Greenhough et al. 2009). Among prostanoids, PGE_2 has long been known as an immunomodulatory substance that suppresses T_H1 differentiation. However, suppressive PGE_2 activity has been shown mostly in vitro and is rarely seen in vivo, raising the possibility that PGE_2 acts differently in vivo in regulating immune responses. Stimulatory action of PGE_2 on T_H17 expansion was reported in human peripheral blood mononuclear cells (Chizzolini et al. 2008; Boniface et al. 2009). PGE2 acts via receptor EP2- and EP4-mediated signaling and cyclic AMP pathways to upregulate IL-23 and IL-1 receptor expression on T cells (Chizzolini et al. 2008; Boniface et al. 2009), and additionally PGE_2 enhances IL-23 production by APCs. Moreover, the recent work by Yao and colleagues has shown the pathological relevance of PGE_2-EP4 signaling in promotion of immune inflammation through T_H1 differentiation and T_H17 expansion (Yao et al. 2009).

The stimulatory effect of TAMs on Th17 induction is striking. Our group and others have documented potent immune suppressive effects of TAMs (Kryczek et al. 2006a, b, 2007c). It is not clear how Th17 cells escape from TAM-mediated suppressive activity. TAMs express inhibitory B7 family members including B7-H1 and B7-H4 (Zou 2005; Zou & Chen 2008), and mediate their suppressive activity through cell-to-cell-contact manner. The suppressive effect of B7-H1 is transmitted after binding to PD-1 (programmed cell death-1) expressed on activated T cells (Freeman et al. 2000). However, experimental evidence indicates that additional receptor(s) other than PD-1 can mediate the functions of B7-H1. In the absence of PD-1 or if binding to PD-1 is blocked, B7-H1 can have stimulatory effects on T-cell immunity (Zou 2005; Zou & Chen 2008). IFN-γ stimulates B7-H1 expression on APCs and abates the Th1 polarization capacity of APCs through B7-H1. However, IFN-γ enables APCs to induce Th17 cell expansion from memory T cells through IL-1 and IL-23 in a B7-H1-independent manner (Kryczek et al. 2008b; Curiel et al. 2003). Th17 cells in the human ovarian cancer environment do not express PD-1. Th17 cells could be resistant to B7-H1-mediated suppression (Kryczek et al. 2009a). Expansion of human Th17 cells seems to be weakly dependent on co-stimulatory signaling mediated by ICOS (Park et al. 2005), 4-1BB (Liu et al. 2005), and CD40 ligand (Schnurr et al. 2005b). All these observations suggest that Th17 cells in the tumor environment are more dependent on monokines (IL-1 and IL-6), rather than co-inhibitory and stimulatory B7 molecules.

7 Functional Relevance of Th17 and Treg Cells in the Tumor Microenvironment

Tumor initiation: The importance of an inflammatory milieu in the initiation of cancer progression has been well described (Mantovani et al. 2008; Lin & Karin 2007; Coussens & Werb 2002). For instance, the development of carcinomas of colon, stomach, liver, bladder, prostate, and pancreas has been attributed to inflammatory bowel disorders, *Helicobacter pylori*-induced gastric inflammation, chronic hepatitis (often associated with HCV or HBV infection), cholecystitis, inflammatory atrophy of the prostate, and chronic pancreatitis, respectively (reviewed in (Kundu & Surh 2008)). Repeated tissue damage and regeneration of tissue, in the presence of highly reactive nitrogen and oxygen species released from inflammatory cells, interact with DNA in proliferating epithelium resulting in permanent genomic alterations. Indeed, in a mouse model of IBD caused by IL-10 deficiency, the frequency of DNA mutations observed in the colon in the absence of exogenous carcinogens was four to fivefold greater than in IL-10-sufficient mice. Dr. Huppert and colleagues have demonstrated that IL-17 can directly induce NADPH oxidase- or xanthine oxidase-dependent reactive oxygen species (ROS) production (Huppert et al. 2010).

During the past decade, evidence has accumulated regarding the essential roles of Tregs in the control of physiological and pathological immune responses. The major physiological role played by Tregs is a "cooling down" of the immune response to prevent tissue damage and development of autoimmune response. Whereas the suppressive nature of Tregs in inflammation is well established, there are only limited data describing the role of Tregs in immunosurveillance of inflammation-associated cancer. Considering the suppressive nature of Tregs, Tregs should inhibit inflammation and prevent or reduce tumor initiation induced by inflammation. In fact, earlier investigations using the Min mouse model of polyposis revealed a protective role for Tregs in bacterial-induced chronic inflammation and cancer (Erdman et al. 2003) and even hereditary colon cancer (Erdman et al. 2005). The antitumor activity of Tregs was associated with reduced expression of proinflammatory cyclooxygenase-2 (Cox-2). Gounaris et al. proposed that adoptively transferred Tregs protect against colon cancer through suppression of focal mastocytosis in adenomatous polyps (Gounaris et al. 2009). The action of adoptively transferred Tregs was associated with their capacity to produce IL-10. Tregs from recipient mice failed to produce IL-10 and promote rather than suppress mastocytosis. Tregs can also inhibit tumor initiation through TGF-β production. Becker et al. has shown that mice deficient in TGF-β receptor showed increased tumor growth in experimental CAC using AOM/DSS, whereas mice overexpressing TGF-β had significantly reduced tumor development (Becker et al. 2004). Therefore, it is possible that Tregs could be beneficial due to their anti-inflammatory role. However, Tregs can suppress protective antitumor immunity, and potentially enhance tumor initiation. For instance, Tregs accumulated in gastric mucosa of patients with *Helicobacter pylori* to suppress *H. pylori*-specific effector cell responses in vitro, and induce gastric adenocarcinoma. This suggests that Tregs may play a dual role in tumor initiation.

IL-17, a hallmark cytokine of Th17 cells, plays a well-established proinflammatory role in a variety of pathological scenarios (Kolls & Linden 2004). It is possible that tumor initiation is a resultant of kinetic balances between Tregs and Th17 cells. Increased numbers of functional Tregs are reported in the lamina propria and mesenteric lymph nodes of patients with inflammatory bowel disease (IBD) (Kryczek et al. 2009c; Makita et al. 2004; Sitohy et al. 2008; Yu et al. 2007). We observed a similar increased percentage of Tregs in IBD and colon carcinoma; however, the fraction of Th17 cells was significantly higher in IBD (Kryczek et al. 2009c). Thus, the absolute number and the balance between Tregs and Th17 cells may determine the fate of local inflammatory reaction.

Chronic inflammation represents a major pathologic basis for the malignancies. Th17 cells may favor, and Tregs may suppress tumor initiation. However, as antitumor immunity is an important component of inflammation, the net effects of Th17 and Tregs on tumor initiation may be much more complicated than we thought. Nonetheless, limited information is available on the role of Tregs and Th17 in the initiation phase of inflammation-associated cancer. At this stage, it is impossible to distinguish the impact of each population on tumor initiation, growth, and metastasis.

Tumor development: The direct effects of Th17 cells on tumor development remains unknown. As Th17 cells produce IL-17 and many other cytokines, here we discuss the role of IL-17 and its associated cytokine IL-23 in tumor development. Earlier studies have shown that exogenous IL-17 promotes tumor growth in immune deficient mice by inducing tumor vascularization (Tartour et al. 1999; Numasaki et al. 2003, 2005). Apart from a minor direct effect on the proliferation and survival of tumor cells (Zhang et al. 2008), due to limited expression of IL-17 receptor on tumor cells, the major protumor role of IL-7 is related to their impact on surrounding tumor tissues. IL-17 has been known to induce a wide range of angiogenic mediators (Numasaki et al. 2004; Takahashi et al. 2005; Honorati et al. 2006; Kehlen et al. 1999; Fossiez et al. 1996). These mediators may promote tumor vascularization, tumor cell migration, and influence tumor metastasis. IL-23 has been shown to promote tumor growth and prevent immunosurveillance (Langowski et al. 2006). As IL-23 can promote and stabilize Th17 cell development, it is assumed that the protumor activity of IL-17 may be associated with IL-23. However, in multiple human tumors, IL-17 is not associated with IL-23, and IL-23 plays a minor role, if any, in Th17 cell development in the tumor microenvironment (Kryczek et al. 2009a). Furthermore, in patients with ovarian cancer, IL-17 is quantitatively and mechanistically associated with CXCL9 and CXCL10 – two potent antiangiogenic cytokines – but not with the well-defined angiogenic factors IL-8 and VEGF in ovarian cancer (Kryczek et al. 2009a). The results obtained in immune deficient animals do not reflect the impact of Th17 cells and other immune cells on tumor development. For example, monocytes-derived IL-27 stimulates Th17 cells to coexpress IL-10 that can negate the ability of these cells to induce angiogenesis or inflammation (Stumhofer et al. 2007; Awasthi et al. 2007).

Although IL-17 may promote tumor development in immune deficient mice, the overall activity of Th17 cells appears to be beneficial for cancer patients and tumor-bearing immune competent animals. High levels of IL-17 in ovarian cancer positively predict patient survival. In patients with prostate cancer, a significant inverse correlation is found between Th17 skewing and tumor grade (Sfanos et al. 2008). Transgenic T cells polarized with TGF-β and IL-6 can induce tumor eradication in mice. Moreover, these Th17-polarized cells were even more effective than Th1 cells in mediating rejection of large B16 melanomas (Muranski et al. 2008). Hirahara et al. (2001) and Benchetrit et al. (2002) demonstrated that IL-17 inhibits tumor growth in a T-cell-dependent manner. Tumor growth and lung metastasis were enhanced in IL-17-deficient mice. This was associated with decreased tumor-specific effector Th1 and NK cells in the TDLN and tumors. This observation was confirmed by Martin-Orozco and colleagues in a melanoma model (Martin-Orozco et al. 2009). Blocking indoleamine 2,3-dioxygenase (IDO) (Sharma et al. 2009), dendritic cell/tumor cell fusion hybrid vaccination (Yamamoto et al. 2009), immune adjuvant treatments with IL-7 (Pellegrini et al. 2009), and hsp70 (Kottke et al. 2007) result in improved antitumor immunity, which is associated with marked CD8$^+$ T cell activation and enhanced IL-17 expressing cells. Therefore, the effect of Th17 cells on tumor development is influenced by the existence of an adaptive immune system. In the presence of a functional immune system, IL-17 or Th17 cells may promote tumor rejection, whereas in the immune deficient host, IL-17 may favor tumor growth and angiogenesis.

This possibility is further supported by clinical investigations in patients with ovarian cancer. The levels of tumor ascites IL-17 or/and Th17 cells are a significant positive predictor of patient survival (Kryczek et al. 2009a). There is a large body of evidence indicating a negative role for tumor-infiltrating Tregs in clinical outcome of cancer patients (Wei et al. 2006; Zou 2006; Barnett et al. 2005, 2008). These studies provide clinical evidence linking Th17 cells to immune protection and Tregs to immune suppression in patients with cancer.

Similarly, if one analyzes the possible impact of Tregs on tumor growth in the absence of functional immune system, Tregs may inhibit tumor growth through suppressing the production of pro-inflammatory cytokines and tumor vascularization. Tregs can express TGF-β. Treatment with TGF-β enhances tumor invasion in vitro and metastasis in vivo (Welch et al. 1990). TGF-β increases migration and invasion of epithelial cells, while systemic inhibition of TGF-β reduces the number of metastases from MMTV-PyVmT overexpressing tumors (Ueda et al. 2004; Muraoka et al. 2002). TGF-β plasma levels are elevated in patients with breast, pancreatic and prostate cancer, and these levels correlate with advanced stage, metastases, and poorer clinical outcome (reviewed in (Teicher 2007)). Nonetheless, as Tregs may not be the major source of TGF-β in vivo, the direct effect of Treg-derived TGF-β on tumor cell biology may not be pathologically relevant.

On the other hand, the immune regulatory effects of Tregs have been well established and accepted. In the early 80s, Drs. North, Bursuker, and Berendt showed that CD4$^+$ T cells isolated from tumor-bearing mice inhibit tumor rejection (Berendt & North 1980; Bursuker & North 1984; North & Bursuker 1984). Later, a subpopulation of T cells responsible for this tolerance was identified as CD4$^+$CD25$^+$Foxp3$^+$ Tregs (Onizuka et al. 1999; Sakaguchi 2005). Tregs can inhibit antitumor immunity through multiple mechanisms (Wei et al. 2006; Zou 2005, 2006). Although some aspects of Treg activity (e.g., anti-inflammatory effect) may potentially reduce tumor growth, Treg-mediated potent immune suppression outweighs their anti-inflammatory activity, and in turn enhances tumor growth and development.

8 Mechanisms of Action of Th17 and Tregs in the Tumor Microenvironment

Tumor infiltrating Th17 cells highly express effector cytokines (Kryczek et al. 2009a), similar to that observed in polyfunctional effector T cells of patients with infectious diseases (Precopio et al. 2007; Almeida et al. 2007). This phenotype was universally found in six different human cancer types that we examined. In contrast to Th17 cells, Tregs expressed minimal amounts of effector cytokines including IL-2, IL-8, IFNγ, TNFα, and GM-CSF (Kryczek et al. 2009c). The simultaneous production of other than IL-17 cytokines allows Th17 cells to execute the effect on the synergistic way of IL-17 with other factors. IL-17 often has been found to execute their effects through enhancing IFNγ and/or TNF-α activity. The collaborative effects among these cytokines including IL-17 and IFNγ may be decisive in determining the biological activities of Th17 cells in human tumors as demonstrated in this and other human studies (Kryczek et al. 2008a). Moreover, IL-17 was found to induce IL-1β and TNF-α in macrophages, and these cytokines can further synergize with IL-17 to activate chemokines (Aggarwal & Gurney 2002). IL-17 and IFNγ synergistically induce the production of Th1-type chemokines, CXCL9 and CXCL10, but not Th2-type chemokines, CXCL12 and CCL22. Moreover, IL-17 is positively associated with tumor-infiltrating IFNγ+ effector T cells and CXCL9 and CXCL10 levels in the tumor environment. It has been suggested that enhancing tumor-specific antitumor immunity by IL-17 is also related to augmenting the expression of MHC (Hirahara et al. 2001). The association between IL-17 and cytotoxic T cells and NK cells were observed in other tumor models. In mice with melanoma, polarized Th17 cells mediate tumor regression in an IFNγ-dependent manner (Muranski et al. 2008). In addition, IL-17 has been shown to inhibit the growth of hematopoietic tumors such as mastocytoma and plasmocytoma by enhancing CTL activity (Benchetrit et al. 2002). Tumor growth and metastasis are enhanced in IL-17 deficient mice. This effect is accompanied by reduced IFN-gamma levels in tumor-infiltrating NK cells and T cells (Kryczek et al. 2009b). Tumor-associated Th17 cells expressed CXCL20 receptor – CCR6. Interestingly, forced intra-tumoral expression of CCL20 results in tumor-specific cellular immunity and significant growth suppression of established tumors (Fushimi et al. 2000). This effect was related to enhanced cytotoxic T-cell activity which was sufficient to protect naïve mice against a subsequent tumor challenge after transfer of splenocytes from tumor-bearing animals that received in vivo administration of CCL20.

Th17 cells act through a variety of cytokines (IL-2, IL-8, IFNγ, TNFα, IL-21, and IL-22). Tregs produce TGF-β and IL-10, however, Tregs from IL-10 knockout and neonatal TGF-beta1 deficient mice were as suppressive as Tregs from wild-type animals (Kryczek et al. 2006a; Piccirillo et al. 2002). Both anti-IL-10 and anti-TGF-β fail to perturb the suppressive activity of Tregs (Piccirillo et al. 2002; Thornton & Shevach 1998; Nakamura et al. 2001). Tregs suppressor function can occur independently of TGF-β and IL-10 and a significant portion of Tregs actions seems not to be cytokine dependent. It has been proposed that constitutive expression of the high-affinity IL-2 receptor (CD25) on Tregs could provide absorption of IL-2 and deprive the effector T cells of their major survival factor. Furthermore, Tregs-mediated suppression is dependent, at least in vitro, on a cell-to-cell interaction among Tregs and effector T cells. As we discussed before, Tregs can inhibit effector T cells function through expression of cell surface endonucleosidases (Kryczek et al. 2009a; Deaglio et al. 2007; Bopp et al. 2007). They can also directly kill conventional T cells using perforin or granzyme-dependent mechanisms (Gondek et al. 2005). Several studies have proved that Tregs inhibit local immune response through interaction with DC/APC. It has been shown that Tregs can downregulate the expression of co-stimulatory molecules (CD80 and CD86) (Cederbom et al. 2000) and upregulate co-inhibitory molecule B7-H4 (Kryczek et al. 2006a, 2007c). Furthermore, CTLA-4 expressed by Tregs has been shown to trigger the induction of the enzyme IDO when interacting with its ligands on DCs. IDO catalyzes the conversion of tryptophan to immunosuppressive metabolites (Grohmann et al. 2002; Collins et al. 2002).

9 Conclusion

Tumors are localized in an inflammatory and immune suppressive microenvironment and both Th17 and Treg cells are found in the tumor microenvironment. Although IL-17 can promote tumor vascularization, growth, and metastasis in immune deficient mice, there is no direct evidence showing that Th17 cells enhance tumorigenesis in immune competent hosts. On the contrary, Th17 cells can enhance antitumor response by promoting immune cell tumor infiltration and effector cell activation in the tumor microenvironment. Tregs can suppress Th17 cell development in the tumor microenvironment. The ratio between Th17 and Treg cells may importantly determine the fate of local immunity in the tumor microenvironment. Therefore, understanding the underlying mechanisms by which Tregs and Th17 cells migrate, expand, and function may provide new tools to treat patients with cancer.

References

Acosta-Rodriguez EV et al (2007a) Surface phenotype and antigenic specificity of human interleukin 17-producing T helper memory cells. Nat Immunol 8(6):639–646

Acosta-Rodriguez EV et al (2007b) Interleukins 1beta and 6 but not transforming growth factor-beta are essential for the differentiation of interleukin 17-producing human T helper cells. Nat Immunol 8(9):942–949

Aggarwal S, Gurney AL (2002) IL-17: prototype member of an emerging cytokine family. J Leukoc Biol 71(1):1–8
Allakhverdi Z et al (2006) Expression of CD103 identifies human regulatory T-cell subsets. J Allergy Clin Immunol 118(6):1342–1349
Almeida JR et al (2007) Superior control of HIV-1 replication by CD8+ T cells is reflected by their avidity, polyfunctionality, and clonal turnover. J Exp Med 204(10):2473–2485
Apostolou I et al (2002) Origin of regulatory T cells with known specificity for antigen. Nat Immunol 3(8):756–763
Appay V et al (2006) New generation vaccine induces effective melanoma-specific CD8+ T cells in the circulation but not in the tumor site. J Immunol 177(3):1670–1678
Atarashi K et al (2008) ATP drives lamina propria T(H)17 cell differentiation. Nature 455(7214):808–812
Attig S et al (2009) Simultaneous infiltration of polyfunctional effector and suppressor T cells into renal cell carcinomas. Cancer Res 69(21):8412–8419
Awasthi A et al (2007) A dominant function for interleukin 27 in generating interleukin 10-producing anti-inflammatory T cells. Nat Immunol 8(12):1380–1389
Baecher-Allan C et al (2001) CD4+ CD25high regulatory cells in human peripheral blood. J Immunol 167(3):1245–1253
Barnett B et al (2005) Regulatory T cells in ovarian cancer: biology and therapeutic potential. Am J Reprod Immunol 54(6):369–377
Barnett BG et al (2008) Regulatory T cells: a new frontier in cancer immunotherapy. Adv Exp Med Biol 622:255–260
Becker C et al (2004) TGF-beta suppresses tumor progression in colon cancer by inhibition of IL-6 trans-signaling. Immunity 21(4):491–501
Bell D et al (1999) In breast carcinoma tissue, immature dendritic cells reside within the tumor, whereas mature dendritic cells are located in peritumoral areas. J Exp Med 190(10):1417–1426
Benchetrit F et al (2002) Interleukin-17 inhibits tumor cell growth by means of a T-cell-dependent mechanism. Blood 99(6):2114–2121
Bensinger SJ et al (2001) Major histocompatibility complex class II-positive cortical epithelium mediates the selection of CD4(+)25(+) immunoregulatory T cells. J Exp Med 194(4):427–438
Benson MJ et al (2007) All-trans retinoic acid mediates enhanced T reg cell growth, differentiation, and gut homing in the face of high levels of co-stimulation. J Exp Med 204(8):1765–1774
Berendt MJ, North RJ (1980) T-cell-mediated suppression of anti-tumor immunity. An explanation for progressive growth of an immunogenic tumor. J Exp Med 151(1):69–80
Bettelli E et al (2006) Reciprocal developmental pathways for the generation of pathogenic effector TH17 and regulatory T cells. Nature 441(7090):235–238
Boniface K et al (2009) Prostaglandin E2 regulates Th17 cell differentiation and function through cyclic AMP and EP2/EP4 receptor signaling. J Exp Med 206(3):535–548
Bopp T et al (2007) Cyclic adenosine monophosphate is a key component of regulatory T cell-mediated suppression. J Exp Med 204(6):1303–1310
Borsellino G et al (2007) Expression of ectonucleotidase CD39 by Foxp3+ Treg cells: hydrolysis of extracellular ATP and immune suppression. Blood 110(4):1225–1232
Bursuker I, North RJ (1984) Generation and decay of the immune response to a progressive fibrosarcoma. II. Failure to demonstrate postexcision immunity after the onset of T cell-mediated suppression of immunity. J Exp Med 159(5):1312–1321
Cavani A et al (2003) Human CD25+ regulatory T cells maintain immune tolerance to nickel in healthy, nonallergic individuals. J Immunol 171(11):5760–5768
Cederbom L, Hall H, Ivars F (2000) CD4+ CD25+ regulatory T cells down-regulate co-stimulatory molecules on antigen-presenting cells. Eur J Immunol 30(6):1538–1543
Chen W et al (2003) Conversion of peripheral CD4+ CD25- naive T cells to CD4+ CD25+ regulatory T cells by TGF-beta induction of transcription factor Foxp3. J Exp Med 198(12):1875–1886
Chen X et al (2006) Pertussis toxin as an adjuvant suppresses the number and function of CD4+ CD25+ T regulatory cells. Eur J Immunol 36(3):671–680

Chizzolini C et al (2008) Prostaglandin E2 synergistically with interleukin-23 favors human Th17 expansion. Blood 112(9):3696–3703

Chung Y et al (2009) Critical regulation of early Th17 cell differentiation by interleukin-1 signaling. Immunity 30(4):576–587

Collins AV et al (2002) The interaction properties of costimulatory molecules revisited. Immunity 17(2):201–210

Coombes JL et al (2007) A functionally specialized population of mucosal CD103+ DCs induces Foxp3+ regulatory T cells via a TGF-beta and retinoic acid-dependent mechanism. J Exp Med 204(8):1757–1764

Coquet JM et al (2008) Diverse cytokine production by NKT cell subsets and identification of an IL-17-producing CD4-NK1.1- NKT cell population. Proc Natl Acad Sci USA 105(32):11287–11292

Cosmi L et al (2008) Human interleukin 17-producing cells originate from a CD161+ CD4+ T cell precursor. J Exp Med 205(8):1903–1916

Coussens LM, Werb Z (2002) Inflammation and cancer. Nature 420(6917):860–867

Curiel TJ et al (2003) Blockade of B7-H1 improves myeloid dendritic cell-mediated antitumor immunity. Nat Med 9(5):562–567

Curiel TJ et al (2004) Specific recruitment of regulatory T cells in ovarian carcinoma fosters immune privilege and predicts reduced survival. Nat Med 10(9):942–949

Deaglio S et al (2007) Adenosine generation catalyzed by CD39 and CD73 expressed on regulatory T cells mediates immune suppression. J Exp Med 204(6):1257–1265

Erdman SE et al (2003) CD4(+)CD25(+) regulatory lymphocytes require interleukin 10 to interrupt colon carcinogenesis in mice. Cancer Res 63(18):6042–6050

Erdman SE et al (2005) CD4+ CD25+ regulatory lymphocytes induce regression of intestinal tumors in ApcMin/+ mice. Cancer Res 65(10):3998–4004

Fletcher JM et al (2009) CD39+ Foxp3+ regulatory T Cells suppress pathogenic Th17 cells and are impaired in multiple sclerosis. J Immunol 183(11):7602–7610

Fossiez F et al (1996) T cell interleukin-17 induces stromal cells to produce proinflammatory and hematopoietic cytokines. J Exp Med 183(6):2593–2603

Freeman GJ et al (2000) Engagement of the PD-1 immunoinhibitory receptor by a novel B7 family member leads to negative regulation of lymphocyte activation. J Exp Med 192(7):1027–1034

Fushimi T et al (2000) Macrophage inflammatory protein 3alpha transgene attracts dendritic cells to established murine tumors and suppresses tumor growth. J Clin Invest 105(10):1383–1393

Gondek DC et al (2005) Cutting edge: contact-mediated suppression by CD4+ CD25+ regulatory cells involves a granzyme B-dependent, perforin-independent mechanism. J Immunol 174(4):1783–1786

Gounaris E et al (2009) T-regulatory cells shift from a protective anti-inflammatory to a cancer-promoting proinflammatory phenotype in polyposis. Cancer Res 69(13):5490–5497

Greenhough A et al (2009) The COX-2/PGE2 pathway: key roles in the hallmarks of cancer and adaptation to the tumour microenvironment. Carcinogenesis 30(3):377–386

Grohmann U et al (2002) CTLA-4-Ig regulates tryptophan catabolism in vivo. Nat Immunol 3(11):1097–1101

Gu Y et al (2008) Interleukin 10 suppresses Th17 cytokines secreted by macrophages and T cells. Eur J Immunol 38(7):1807–1813

Hirahara N et al (2001) Inoculation of human interleukin-17 gene-transfected Meth-A fibrosarcoma cells induces T cell-dependent tumor-specific immunity in mice. Oncology 61(1):79–89

Hoffmann P et al (2004) Large-scale in vitro expansion of polyclonal human CD4(+)CD25high regulatory T cells. Blood 104(3):895–903

Honorati MC et al (2006) Interleukin-17, a regulator of angiogenic factor release by synovial fibroblasts. Osteoarthr Cartil 14(4):345–352

Horlock C et al (2009) The effects of trastuzumab on the CD4+ CD25+ FoxP3+ and CD4+ IL17A+ T-cell axis in patients with breast cancer. Br J Cancer 100(7):1061–1067

Huehn J, Polansky JK, Hamann A (2009) Epigenetic control of FOXP3 expression: the key to a stable regulatory T-cell lineage? Nat Rev Immunol 9(2):83–89

Hultkrantz S, Ostman S, Telemo E (2005) Induction of antigen-specific regulatory T cells in the liver-draining celiac lymph node following oral antigen administration. Immunology 116(3):362–372

Huppert J et al (2010) Cellular mechanisms of IL-17-induced blood-brain barrier disruption. FASEB J 24(4):1023–1034

Iellem A et al (2001) Unique chemotactic response profile and specific expression of chemokine receptors CCR4 and CCR8 by CD4(+)CD25(+) regulatory T cells. J Exp Med 194(6):847–853

Iellem A, Colantonio L, D'Ambrosio D (2003) Skin-versus gut-skewed homing receptor expression and intrinsic CCR4 expression on human peripheral blood CD4+ CD25+ suppressor T cells. Eur J Immunol 33(6):1488–1496

Inozume T et al (2009) IL-17 secreted by tumor reactive T cells induces IL-8 release by human renal cancer cells. J Immunother 32(2):109–117

Ishibashi Y et al (2006) Expression of Foxp3 in non-small cell lung cancer patients is significantly higher in tumor tissues than in normal tissues, especially in tumors smaller than 30 mm. Oncol Rep 15(5):1315–1319

Ivanov II et al (2006) The orphan nuclear receptor RORgammat directs the differentiation program of proinflammatory IL-17+ T helper cells. Cell 126(6):1121–1133

Jeron A et al (2009) Frequency and gene expression profile of regulatory T cells in renal cell carcinoma. Tumour Biol 30(3):160–170

Kang SG et al (2007) Vitamin A metabolites induce gut-homing FoxP3+ regulatory T cells. J Immunol 179(6):3724–3733

Kehlen A et al (1999) Interleukin-17 stimulates the expression of IkappaB alpha mRNA and the secretion of IL-6 and IL-8 in glioblastoma cell lines. J Neuroimmunol 101(1):1–6

Khader SA et al (2005) IL-23 compensates for the absence of IL-12p70 and is essential for the IL-17 response during tuberculosis but is dispensable for protection and antigen-specific IFN-gamma responses if IL-12p70 is available. J Immunol 175(2):788–795

Kimura A, Naka T, Kishimoto T (2007) IL-6-dependent and -independent pathways in the development of interleukin 17-producing T helper cells. Proc Natl Acad Sci USA 104(29):12099–12104

Kirkham BW et al (2006) Synovial membrane cytokine expression is predictive of joint damage progression in rheumatoid arthritis: a two-year prospective study (the DAMAGE study cohort). Arthritis Rheum 54(4):1122–1131

Kleeff J et al (1999) Detection and localization of Mip-3alpha/LARC/Exodus, a macrophage proinflammatory chemokine, and its CCR6 receptor in human pancreatic cancer. Int J Cancer 81(4):650–657

Kolls JK, Linden A (2004) Interleukin-17 family members and inflammation. Immunity 21(4):467–476

Korn T et al (2007) IL-21 initiates an alternative pathway to induce proinflammatory T(H)17 cells. Nature 448(7152):484–487

Kottke T et al (2007) Induction of hsp70-mediated Th17 autoimmunity can be exploited as immunotherapy for metastatic prostate cancer. Cancer Res 67(24):11970–11979

Koyama K et al (2008) Reciprocal CD4+ T-cell balance of effector CD62Llow CD4+ and CD62LhighCD25+ CD4+ regulatory T cells in small cell lung cancer reflects disease stage. Clin Cancer Res 14(21):6770–6779

Kryczek I et al (2006a) Cutting edge: induction of B7-H4 on APCs through IL-10: novel suppressive mode for regulatory T cells. J Immunol 177(1):40–44

Kryczek I et al (2006b) B7-H4 expression identifies a novel suppressive macrophage population in human ovarian carcinoma. J Exp Med 203(4):871–881

Kryczek I et al (2007a) Cutting edge: Th17 and regulatory T cell dynamics and the regulation by IL-2 in the tumor microenvironment. J Immunol 178(11):6730–6733

Kryczek I et al (2007b) Cutting edge: opposite effects of IL-1 and IL-2 on the regulation of IL-17+ T cell pool IL-1 subverts IL-2-mediated suppression. J Immunol 179(3):1423–1426

Kryczek I et al (2007c) Relationship between B7-H4, regulatory T cells, and patient outcome in human ovarian carcinoma. Cancer Res 67(18):8900–8905

Kryczek I et al (2008a) Induction of IL-17+ T cell trafficking and development by IFN-gamma: mechanism and pathological relevance in psoriasis. J Immunol 181(7):4733–4741

Kryczek I et al (2008b) Cutting edge: IFN-gamma enables APC to promote memory Th17 and abate Th1 cell development. J Immunol 181(9):5842–5846

Kryczek I et al (2009a) Phenotype, distribution, generation, and functional and clinical relevance of Th17 cells in the human tumor environments. Blood 114(6):1141–1149

Kryczek I et al (2009b) Endogenous IL-17 contributes to reduced tumor growth and metastasis. Blood 114(2):357–359

Kryczek I et al (2009c) FOXP3 defines regulatory T cells in human tumor and autoimmune disease. Cancer Res 69(9):3995–4000

Kuang DM et al (2010) Activated monocytes in peritumoral stroma of hepatocellular carcinoma promote expansion of memory T helper 17 cells. Hepatology 51(1):154–164

Kundu JK, Surh YJ (2008) Inflammation: gearing the journey to cancer. Mutat Res 659(1–2):15–30

Langowski JL et al (2006) IL-23 promotes tumour incidence and growth. Nature 442(7101):461–465

Lau KM et al (2007) Increase in circulating Foxp3+ CD4+ CD25(high) regulatory T cells in nasopharyngeal carcinoma patients. Br J Cancer 96(4):617–622

Laurence A et al (2007) Interleukin-2 signaling via STAT5 constrains T helper 17 cell generation. Immunity 26(3):371–381

Lin WW, Karin M (2007) A cytokine-mediated link between innate immunity, inflammation, and cancer. J Clin Invest 117(5):1175–1183

Liu XK, Clements JL, Gaffen SL (2005) Signaling through the murine T cell receptor induces IL-17 production in the absence of costimulation, IL-23 or dendritic cells. Mol Cells 20(3):339–347

Liyanage UK et al (2002) Prevalence of regulatory T cells is increased in peripheral blood and tumor microenvironment of patients with pancreas or breast adenocarcinoma. J Immunol 169(5):2756–2761

Makita S et al (2004) CD4+ CD25bright T cells in human intestinal lamina propria as regulatory cells. J Immunol 173(5):3119–3130

Maloy KJ et al (2003) CD4+ CD25+ T(R) cells suppress innate immune pathology through cytokine-dependent mechanisms. J Exp Med 197(1):111–119

Manel N, Unutmaz D, Littman DR (2008) The differentiation of human T(H)-17 cells requires transforming growth factor-beta and induction of the nuclear receptor RORgammat. Nat Immunol 9(6):641–649

Mangan PR et al (2006) Transforming growth factor-beta induces development of the T(H)17 lineage. Nature 441(7090):231–234

Mantovani A et al (2008) Cancer-related inflammation. Nature 454(7203):436–444

Martin-Orozco N et al (2009) T helper 17 cells promote cytotoxic T cell activation in tumor immunity. Immunity 31(5):787–798

Meloni F et al (2006) Foxp3 expressing CD4+ CD25+ and CD8+ CD28- T regulatory cells in the peripheral blood of patients with lung cancer and pleural mesothelioma. Hum Immunol 67(1–2):1–12

Michel ML et al (2007) Identification of an IL-17-producing NK1.1(neg) iNKT cell population involved in airway neutrophilia. J Exp Med 204(5):995–1001

Misra N et al (2004) Cutting edge: human CD4+ CD25+ T cells restrain the maturation and antigen-presenting function of dendritic cells. J Immunol 172(8):4676–4680

Miyahara Y et al (2008) Generation and regulation of human CD4+ IL-17-producing T cells in ovarian cancer. Proc Natl Acad Sci USA 105(40):15505–15510

Montufar-Solis D et al (2008) Massive but selective cytokine dysregulation in the colon of IL-10-/- mice revealed by multiplex analysis. Int Immunol 20(1):141–154

Mucida D et al (2007) Reciprocal TH17 and regulatory T cell differentiation mediated by retinoic acid. Science 317(5835):256–260

Muranski P et al (2008) Tumor-specific Th17-polarized cells eradicate large established melanoma. Blood 112(2):362–373

Muraoka RS et al (2002) Blockade of TGF-beta inhibits mammary tumor cell viability, migration, and metastases. J Clin Invest 109(12):1551–1559

Nakamura K, Kitani A, Strober W (2001) Cell contact-dependent immunosuppression by CD4(+) CD25(+) regulatory T cells is mediated by cell surface-bound transforming growth factor beta. J Exp Med 194(5):629–644

North RJ, Bursuker I (1984) Generation and decay of the immune response to a progressive fibrosarcoma. I. Ly-1+ 2- suppressor T cells down-regulate the generation of Ly-1-2+ effector T cells. J Exp Med 159(5):1295–1311

Numasaki M et al (2003) Interleukin-17 promotes angiogenesis and tumor growth. Blood 101(7):2620–2627

Numasaki M, Lotze MT, Sasaki H (2004) Interleukin-17 augments tumor necrosis factor-alpha-induced elaboration of proangiogenic factors from fibroblasts. Immunol Lett 93(1):39–43

Numasaki M et al (2005) IL-17 enhances the net angiogenic activity and in vivo growth of human non-small cell lung cancer in SCID mice through promoting CXCR-2-dependent angiogenesis. J Immunol 175(9):6177–6189

Nurieva R et al (2007) Essential autocrine regulation by IL-21 in the generation of inflammatory T cells. Nature 448(7152):480–483

Oehler-Janne C et al (2008) HIV-specific differences in outcome of squamous cell carcinoma of the anal canal: a multicentric cohort study of HIV-positive patients receiving highly active antiretroviral therapy. J Clin Oncol 26(15):2550–2557

Onizuka S et al (1999) Tumor rejection by in vivo administration of anti-CD25 (interleukin-2 receptor alpha) monoclonal antibody. Cancer Res 59(13):3128–3133

Ormandy LA et al (2005) Increased populations of regulatory T cells in peripheral blood of patients with hepatocellular carcinoma. Cancer Res 65(6):2457–2464

Park H et al (2005) A distinct lineage of CD4 T cells regulates tissue inflammation by producing interleukin 17. Nat Immunol 6(11):1133–1141

Pasare C, Medzhitov R (2003) Toll pathway-dependent blockade of CD4+ CD25+ T cell-mediated suppression by dendritic cells. Science 299(5609):1033–1036

Pellegrini M et al (2009) Adjuvant IL-7 antagonizes multiple cellular and molecular inhibitory networks to enhance immunotherapies. Nat Med 15(5):528–536

Piccirillo CA et al (2002) CD4(+)CD25(+) regulatory T cells can mediate suppressor function in the absence of transforming growth factor beta1 production and responsiveness. J Exp Med 196(2):237–246

Precopio ML et al (2007) Immunization with vaccinia virus induces polyfunctional and phenotypically distinctive CD8(+) T cell responses. J Exp Med 204(6):1405–1416

Roark CL et al (2007) Exacerbation of collagen-induced arthritis by oligoclonal, IL-17-producing gamma delta T cells. J Immunol 179(8):5576–5583

Romani L et al (2008) Defective tryptophan catabolism underlies inflammation in mouse chronic granulomatous disease. Nature 451(7175):211–215

Sakaguchi S (2001) Policing the regulators. Nat Immunol 2(4):283–284

Sakaguchi S (2005) Naturally arising Foxp3-expressing CD25+ CD4+ regulatory T cells in immunological tolerance to self and non-self. Nat Immunol 6(4):345–352

Sasada T et al (2003) CD4+ CD25+ regulatory T cells in patients with gastrointestinal malignancies: possible involvement of regulatory T cells in disease progression. Cancer 98(5):1089–1099

Sato E et al (2005) Intraepithelial CD8+ tumor-infiltrating lymphocytes and a high CD8+/regulatory T cell ratio are associated with favorable prognosis in ovarian cancer. Proc Natl Acad Sci USA 102(51):18538–18543

Schnurr M et al (2005a) Extracellular nucleotide signaling by P2 receptors inhibits IL-12 and enhances IL-23 expression in human dendritic cells: a novel role for the cAMP pathway. Blood 105(4):1582–1589

Schnurr M et al (2005b) Tumor antigen processing and presentation depend critically on dendritic cell type and the mode of antigen delivery. Blood 105(6):2465–2472

Sfanos KS et al (2008) Phenotypic analysis of prostate-infiltrating lymphocytes reveals TH17 and Treg skewing. Clin Cancer Res 14(11):3254–3261

Sharma MD et al (2009) Indoleamine 2,3-dioxygenase controls conversion of Foxp3+ Tregs to TH17-like cells in tumor-draining lymph nodes. Blood 113(24):6102–6111

Siddiqui SA et al (2007) Tumor-infiltrating Foxp3-CD4+ CD25+ T cells predict poor survival in renal cell carcinoma. Clin Cancer Res 13(7):2075–2081

Sitohy B et al (2008) Basal lymphoid aggregates in ulcerative colitis colon: a site for regulatory T cell action. Clin Exp Immunol 151(2):326–333

Stark MA et al (2005) Phagocytosis of apoptotic neutrophils regulates granulopoiesis via IL-23 and IL-17. Immunity 22(3):285–294

Stassen M et al (2004) Human CD25+ regulatory T cells: two subsets defined by the integrins alpha 4 beta 7 or alpha 4 beta 1 confer distinct suppressive properties upon CD4+ T helper cells. Eur J Immunol 34(5):1303–1311

Stumhofer JS et al (2007) Interleukins 27 and 6 induce STAT3-mediated T cell production of interleukin 10. Nat Immunol 8(12):1363–1371

Sun CM et al (2007) Small intestine lamina propria dendritic cells promote de novo generation of Foxp3 T reg cells via retinoic acid. J Exp Med 204(8):1775–1785

Taams LS et al (2005) Modulation of monocyte/macrophage function by human CD4+ CD25+ regulatory T cells. Hum Immunol 66(3):222–230

Takahashi H et al (2005) Interleukin-17 enhances bFGF-, HGF- and VEGF-induced growth of vascular endothelial cells. Immunol Lett 98(2):189–193

Takatori H et al (2009) Lymphoid tissue inducer-like cells are an innate source of IL-17 and IL-22. J Exp Med 206(1):35–41

Tartour E et al (1999) Interleukin 17, a T-cell-derived cytokine, promotes tumorigenicity of human cervical tumors in nude mice. Cancer Res 59(15):3698–3704

Teicher BA (2007) Transforming growth factor-beta and the immune response to malignant disease. Clin Cancer Res 13(21):6247–6251

Thomachot MC et al (2004) Breast carcinoma cells promote the differentiation of CD34+ progenitors towards 2 different subpopulations of dendritic cells with CD1a(high)CD86(−)Langerin- and CD1a(+)CD86(+)Langerin+ phenotypes. Int J Cancer 110(5):710–720

Thornton AM, Shevach EM (1998) CD4+ CD25+ immunoregulatory T cells suppress polyclonal T cell activation in vitro by inhibiting interleukin 2 production. J Exp Med 188(2):287–296

Tiemessen MM et al (2007) CD4+ CD25+ Foxp3+ regulatory T cells induce alternative activation of human monocytes/macrophages. Proc Natl Acad Sci USA 104(49):19446–19451

Ueda Y et al (2004) Overexpression of HER2 (erbB2) in human breast epithelial cells unmasks transforming growth factor beta-induced cell motility. J Biol Chem 279(23):24505–24513

Veldhoen M et al (2006a) TGFbeta in the context of an inflammatory cytokine milieu supports de novo differentiation of IL-17-producing T cells. Immunity 24(2):179–189

Veldhoen M et al (2006b) Modulation of dendritic cell function by naive and regulatory CD4+ T cells. J Immunol 176(10):6202–6210

Wang MT, Honn KV, Nie D (2007) Cyclooxygenases, prostanoids, and tumor progression. Cancer Metastasis Rev 26(3–4):525–534

Wei S et al (2005) Plasmacytoid dendritic cells induce CD8+ regulatory T cells in human ovarian carcinoma. Cancer Res 65(12):5020–5026

Wei S, Kryczek I, Zou W (2006) Regulatory T-cell compartmentalization and trafficking. Blood 108(2):426–431

Welch DR, Fabra A, Nakajima M (1990) Transforming growth factor beta stimulates mammary adenocarcinoma cell invasion and metastatic potential. Proc Natl Acad Sci USA 87(19):7678–7682

Wilson NJ et al (2007) Development, cytokine profile and function of human interleukin 17-producing helper T cells. Nat Immunol 8(9):950–957

Wolf D et al (2005) The expression of the regulatory T cell-specific forkhead box transcription factor FoxP3 is associated with poor prognosis in ovarian cancer. Clin Cancer Res 11(23):8326–8331

Woo EY et al (2001) Regulatory CD4(+)CD25(+) T cells in tumors from patients with early-stage non-small cell lung cancer and late-stage ovarian cancer. Cancer Res 61(12):4766–4772

Xiao S et al (2008) Retinoic acid increases Foxp3+ regulatory T cells and inhibits development of Th17 cells by enhancing TGF-beta-driven Smad3 signaling and inhibiting IL-6 and IL-23 receptor expression. J Immunol 181(4):2277–2284

Yamamoto M et al (2009) Enhancement of anti-tumor immunity by high levels of Th1 and Th17 with a combination of dendritic cell fusion hybrids and regulatory T cell depletion in pancreatic cancer. Oncol Rep 22(2):337–343

Yang L et al (2008a) IL-21 and TGF-beta are required for differentiation of human T(H)17 cells. Nature 454(7202):350–352

Yang XO et al (2008b) Molecular antagonism and plasticity of regulatory and inflammatory T cell programs. Immunity 29(1):44–56

Yao C et al (2009) Prostaglandin E2-EP4 signaling promotes immune inflammation through Th1 cell differentiation and Th17 cell expansion. Nat Med 15(6):633–640

Yen D et al (2006) IL-23 is essential for T cell-mediated colitis and promotes inflammation via IL-17 and IL-6. J Clin Invest 116(5):1310–1316

Yu QT et al (2007) Expression and functional characterization of FOXP3+ CD4+ regulatory T cells in ulcerative colitis. Inflamm Bowel Dis 13(2):191–199

Zhang B et al (2008) The prevalence of Th17 cells in patients with gastric cancer. Biochem Biophys Res Commun 374(3):533–537

Zhou L et al (2007) IL-6 programs T(H)-17 cell differentiation by promoting sequential engagement of the IL-21 and IL-23 pathways. Nat Immunol 8(9):967–974

Zhou L et al (2008) TGF-beta-induced Foxp3 inhibits T(H)17 cell differentiation by antagonizing RORgammat function. Nature 453(7192):236–240

Zou W (2005) Immunosuppressive networks in the tumour environment and their therapeutic relevance. Nat Rev Cancer 5(4):263–274

Zou W (2006) Regulatory T cells, tumour immunity and immunotherapy. Nat Rev Immunol 6(4):295–307

Zou W, Chen L (2008) Inhibitory B7-family molecules in the tumour microenvironment. Nat Rev Immunol 8(6):467–477

Zou L et al (2004) Bone marrow is a reservoir for CD4+ CD25+ regulatory T cells that traffic through CXCL12/CXCR4 signals. Cancer Res 64(22):8451–8455

Chapter 11
Mechanisms and Control of Regulatory T Cells in Cancer

Bin Li and Rong-Fu Wang

1 Introduction

CD4$^+$ regulatory T (Treg) cells play an important role in mediating immune suppression to prevent autoimmune diseases. Depletion of Treg cells in normal hosts results in various types of autoimmune diseases because the host immune system is unchecked, and progresses to attack the body's own tissues or organs. Despite the importance of these cells in preventing autoimmune diseases, their accumulation in the tumor microenvironment dampens antitumor immune responses and may, at least in part, explain why current clinical trials with cancer peptides or dendritic cells (DCs) pulsed with antigenic peptides can induce only weak and transient immune responses, and fail to produce therapeutic efficacy of cancer treatment. Besides naturally occurring Treg cells, many subsets of Treg cells have been identified, including inducible CD4$^+$ Treg cells, CD8$^+$ Foxp3$^+$ Treg, and γδ$^+$ TCR Treg cells in cancer patients. Foxp3 is a master regulator of Treg cells; its expression is critically controlled by many factors including TCR signaling, and cytokines such as TGF-β and IL-2. Understanding of the molecular mechanisms and strategies which modulate regulatory function of Treg cells has been an important research area for both basic and clinical application, where the goal is to treat and prevent immune-related diseases and cancer. In this review, we highlight recent advances in our understanding of subsets, immune regulation of Treg cells, Foxp3 expression, and discuss important implications for cancer immunotherapy.

B. Li
Key Laboratory of Molecular Virology and Immunology, Institute Pasteur of Shanghai,
Shanghai Institutes for Biological Sciences, Chinese Academy of Sciences,
Shanghai 200025, P.R. China

R.-F. Wang (✉)
Department of Pathology and Immunology, and Center for Cell and Gene Therapy,
Baylor College of Medicine, Houston, TX 77030, USA
e-mail: rongfuw@bcm.edu

2 Phenotypic Markers and Subsets of Treg Cells

Although expression of CD25, the TNF-family molecule GITR, and cytotoxic T-lymphocyte antigen-4 (CTLA4) has served as useful markers of Treg cells, they are not necessarily only associated with Treg cell function, in that they are also expressed by activated effector lymphocytes (Sakaguchi 2004). Foxp3 is a specific marker identified to date for CD4$^+$ Treg cells in mice (Fontenot et al. 2003; Hori et al. 2003; Khattri et al. 2003) and humans (Walker et al. 2003; Wang et al. 2004). However, human Foxp3 expression is not as restricted as their murine counterpart, as Foxp3 is also expressed in effector T cells at a relatively low level. Human Foxp3 contains two isoforms: one encodes full-length of Foxp3, while the other encodes a short version of the protein lacking exon 2 (amino acids 71–105) (Allan et al. 2005; Ziegler 2006). There is no short isoform of Foxp3 in murine CD4$^+$ Treg cells. More recently, CD127 expression, the alpha chain of the interleukin-7 receptor, was found to inversely correlate with Foxp3 and the suppressive function of CD4$^+$ Treg cells (Liu et al. 2006b; Seddiki et al. 2006). Because CD127 expression on effector T cells is downregulated after T cell activation, the combined use of these markers including CD25$^+$, Foxp3$^+$, and CD127$^-$ allows one to isolate a Treg population with suppressive function.

Besides naturally occurring CD4$^+$ CD25$^+$ Treg cells, several additional subsets of Treg cells have been identified and characterized, leading to the current view of Treg cell heterogeneity, in which subsets of these cells are defined by distinct suppressive mechanisms or phenotypic markers.

(a) *Naturally occurring CD4$^+$ CD25$^+$ Treg (nTreg) cells*: This subset represents a small fraction (5–6%) of the overall CD4$^+$ T cell population and is derived from thymus without specific antigen stimulation. These cells express a high level of GITR and Foxp3 molecules and mediate immune suppression through a cell–cell contact mechanism (Sakaguchi 2004). Recent reports show that TCR-mediated NF-κB activation is critical for the development of nTreg cells (Long et al. 2009; Ruan et al. 2009).

(b) *Adaptively induced CD4$^+$ Treg cells*: Like those naturally occurring counterparts, antigen-specific CD4$^+$ Treg cells express a high level of GITR and Foxp3, and suppress immune responses through a cell contact-dependent or soluble factor-dependent (other than IL-10 and/or TGF-β) mechanisms once they are activated after exposure to a specific antigen (Wang et al. 2004, 2005). Although the origin of adaptively induced CD4$^+$ Treg cells remains largely obscure, they may arise from antigen experienced CD4$^+$CD25$^-$ T cells within the suppressive cytokine milieu of tumor sites or after interaction with naturally occurring CD4$^+$ CD25$^+$ T cells. Recent studies demonstrate the conversion of peripheral naïve CD4$^+$ CD25$^-$ T cells to CD4$^+$ CD25$^+$ Treg cells by activation or TGF-β stimulation of bulk T cell populations (Chen et al. 2003; Walker et al. 2003). Results obtained in transgenic mice models show that the extent of self-peptide stimulation affects the peripheral generation and expansion of CD4$^+$CD25$^+$ Treg cells, and thus directs the selection and accumulation of such cells at sites where self-peptide is expressed (Apostolou et al. 2002; Apostolou and Von Boehmer 2004; Jordan et al. 2001).

(c) *Antigen-induced Tr1 cells*: These Treg cells are induced in peripheral tissues by MHC/peptide stimulation, secret large amounts of IL-10 and/or TGF-β, and suppress immune responses through a cytokine-dependent mechanism (Roncarolo et al. 2006; Weiner 2001). Generation of these Tr1 cells requires IL-10 in the culture medium or IL-10-secreting immature DCs. So far, no specific marker for these cells has been identified. Foxp3 is not constitutively expressed in this population of cells (Roncarolo et al. 2006). Therefore, one unique feature of these cells is their ability to secrete a large amount of IL-10 and/or TGF-β. Although most studies of Tr1 are related to oral tolerance and allergy, one study shows that tumor-infiltrating lymphocytes from gastric cancer patients contains both $CD4^+CD25^{hi}$ Treg and $CD4^+CD25^{int}$ T cells secreting IL-10 but not IFN-γ, characteristic of Tr1 cells (Kawaida et al. 2005).

(d) $CD8^+$ *Treg cells*: Not all Treg cells are $CD4^+$ T cells. Indeed, $CD8^+$ Treg cells have been identified to mediate immune suppression in an antigen-dependent manner (Jiang and Chess 2004). Such cells suppress antigen-activated $CD4^+$ T cells in a TCR-specific manner restricted by the MHC class Ib molecule Qa-1 (Hu et al. 2004). $CD8^+$ $CD28^-$ Treg cells have also been reported to suppress antigen-presenting cells (APC), including DCs that present the same peptide/MHC complexes to which $CD8^+$ Treg cells were primed (Vlad et al. 2005). More recently, $CD8^+$ $CD25^+$ Treg, $CD8^+$ $CD25^+$ Foxp3$^+$ Treg cells, and $CD8^+$ IL-10 producing Treg cells have been identified in humans and mice (Endharti et al. 2005; Shao et al. 2005; Wei et al. 2005). These cells appear to recognize different antigens and are functionally similar to $CD4^+CD25^+$ Treg cells.

(e) *TCR γδ$^+$ Treg cells*: TCR-γδ$^+$ T cells represent a small population of T cells consisting of γ and δ TCR chains with limited TCR usage. They are distinct from αβ T cells and are capable of recognizing antigens without the requirement of MHC molecules. Thus, these cells function as innate lymphocytes and play an important role in immune surveillance against invading pathogens, tumors, and tissue injury. Recent studies also show that they may function as professional APC (Brandes et al. 2005). The role of γδ$^+$ T cells in the induction of tissue tolerance has been suggested, but the direct evidence for γδ$^+$ Treg cells are lacking. We recently identified a dominant population (30–40%) of γδ$^+$ T cells in breast cancer- and prostate cancer-infiltrating T cell populations. These T cells are exclusively γδ1 T cells, possess the potent ability to suppress the proliferation of T cells, and blocked DC maturation and function (Peng et al. 2007).

(f) *NKT regulatory T cells*: While it has been demonstrated that CD1d-dependent NKT cells are critical in mediating antitumor immunity (Fujii et al. 2003; Hayakawa et al. 2003; Liu et al. 2005; Smyth et al. 2002), recent studies show that NKT cells may mediate immune suppression (Moodycliffe et al. 2000; Terabe et al. 2000, 2003). Further studies revealed that CD1d-restricted V{alpha}14 J{alpha}18$^-$ (type II), but not V{alpha}14 J{alpha}18$^+$ (type I), NKT cells are responsible for immune suppression (Terabe et al. 2005).

3   Foxp3 Is a Key Regulator of Treg Cells

It has been firmly proven that the forkhead box transcription factor Foxp3 is a key regulator of Treg cells (Figs. 11.1 and 11.2) (Lu and Rudensky 2009). Foxp3 was originally identified as a gene mutated in human patients with Immune Dysregulation, Polyendocrinopathy, Enteropathy, X-Linked Syndrome (IPEX) (Bennett et al. 2001; Chatila et al. 2000; Wildin et al. 2001), as well as the X-linked recessive mouse mutant with a Scurfy phenotype (Brunkow et al. 2001). Subsequently, Foxp3 was found as an essential and sufficient transcription factor for the development and function of murine natural Treg cells developed in the thymus (Fontenot et al. 2003; Hori et al. 2003; Khattri et al. 2003). Retroviral transduction of Foxp3 into naïve CD4$^+$ T cells converts these cells to adopt a suppressive phenotype (Hori et al. 2003). Knockout of Foxp3 leads to a lack of development and function of CD4$^+$CD25$^+$ Treg cells, and Foxp3 null mice develop serious autoimmune diseases which could be cured by adoptively transferring normal CD4$^+$ CD25$^+$ T cells expressing wild-type Foxp3 (Fontenot et al. 2003). Further genetic studies in transgenic mice confirmed the role of Foxp3 in Treg function; however, the development of Treg cells in the thymus could be initiated before Foxp3 expression is induced (Hill et al. 2007; Lin et al. 2007). Continued Foxp3 expression at high levels is essential to maintain the transcriptional and functional program established during natural Treg cell development (Williams and Rudensky 2007). Understanding the underlying mechanisms of Foxp3-mediated transcriptional regulation in Treg cells will provide therapeutic opportunities in treating human diseases, including autoimmunity, allergy, infection, and cancer (Li et al. 2007c).

4   Expression of Foxp3 Is Regulated by Multiples Factors: TCR, TGF-β, Retinoic Acids, Stat3, IL-2 (NFAT), and mTOR

Foxp3 expression is spatially and temporally controlled in a signal-dependent manner in both natural Treg and inducible Treg (iTreg) cells. It was originally thought that Foxp3 is only expressed in natural CD4$^+$CD25$^+$ Treg cells. Multiple factors, including TCR stimulation and through immunomodulating cytokine signals such as TGF-β and IL-2, could induce Foxp3 expression and convert CD4$^+$ CD25$^-$ T effector cells to CD4$^+$ CD25$^+$ iTreg cells with suppressive activity in vitro and in vivo (Chen et al. 2003; Fantini et al. 2004; Zheng et al. 2004). Moreover, many chemical agents and metabolite-mediated signaling pathways may also regulate Foxp3 expression in Treg cells. For instance, the vitamin A metabolite retinoic acid produced in gut-associated DCs may positively regulate TGF-β-mediated induction of Foxp3 and promote iTreg cell differentiation while repressing RORγt induction and antagonizing Th17 cell differentiation induced by TGF-β plus IL-6 (Benson et al. 2007; Coombes et al. 2007; Mucida et al. 2007; Sun et al. 2007). The underlying

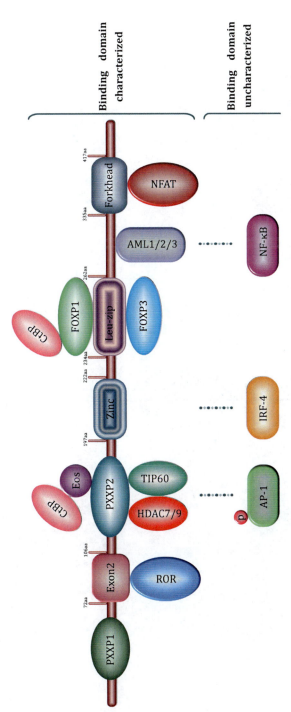

Fig. 11.1 Interactions of transcription factors and transcriptional coregulators with FOXP3. FOXP3 may form more than one high molecular weight nuclear complex in vivo, which is essential for FOXP3-mediated programming of Treg cells. Currently, identified transcription factors and enzymatic cofactors in FOXP3 complex include ROR-α and ROR-γt, RUNX1/2/3, NFATc2, NF-κB, FOXP1, IRF4, AP-1, and Eos, while enzymatic coregulators include TIP60 and HDAC7. ROR-α and ROR-γt specifically interact with the exon2 encoding region of FOXP3, which only present in the larger isoform of human FOXP3a and murine FoxP3, but not the smaller isoform of human FOXP3b. FOXP1 and FOXP3 itself can form homo- or hetero-oligmer with each other via the leucine zipper domain. AML1/AML2/AML3 interacts with FOXP3 at the linker region between the leucine zipper and the forkhead domain. Enzymatic transcriptional coregulators including TIP60 and HDAC7/9 as well as transcription factor Eos may interact with the proline-rich region between the Exon2 encoding region and zinc finger motif. Other transcriptional corepressor, such as CtBP, may indirectly interact with FOXP3 complex via Eos or FOXP1 as an adaptor. Other FOXP3-binding transcription factors include NFκB, IRF-4, GATA3, phosphorylated AP-1, and phosphorylated STAT3 although their detailed interacting domains on FOXP3 remain uncharacterized

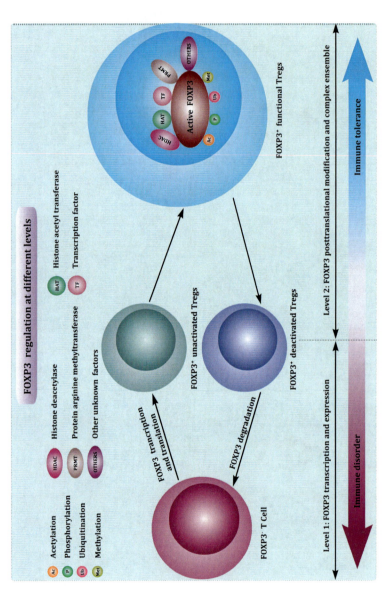

Fig. 11.2 FOXP3 is regulated at both transcriptional and posttranslational levels. *FOXP3* gene transcription is the first step which is essential but not sufficient for Treg function. The posttranslational modifications, including acetylation, methylation, phosphorylation, and ubiquitination, of FOXP3 protein are critical for the regulatory role of activated FOXP3+ Treg cells in immune tolerance. Moreover, the ordered FOXP3 complex ensemble may involve different transcription factors (TF) and enzymatic coregulators including HAT/HDAC/PRMT and others, which control site-specific histone modification and chromatin remodeling at different sites of DNA to either positively or negatively regulate gene transcription in functional Treg cells

mechanism by which retinoic acid promotes iTreg cell production remains largely unclear. Retinoic acid may enhance TGF-β signaling-mediated Smad3 activation, as well as inhibit IL-6 and IL-23 receptor expression (Xiao et al. 2008). Peroxisome proliferator-activated receptor gamma (PPARγ) activation in DCs may positively regulate retinoic acid-mediated DC induction of Treg cells via promoting the synthesis of retinoic acid (Housley et al. 2009).

A variety of cell surface receptors and their downstream pathways regulate Foxp3 transcription and expression in Treg cells (Ohkura and Sakaguchi 2009) (Figs. 11.2 and 11.3). For instance, TCR activation is an essential step for murine natural Treg development and Foxp3 expression (Shevach 2009). The IL-2 signal-activated Jak-STAT pathway in Treg cells is essential for maintaining Foxp3 expression as well as the survival and proliferation of Treg cells in vivo (Fontenot et al. 2005; Yao et al. 2007). In mouse developing thymocytes, CD28 costimulation is essential to induce Foxp3 expression, stabilize Foxp3 mRNA transcripts, and initiate natural Treg differentiation (Nazarov-Stoica et al. 2009; Tai et al. 2005). In human, CD28 costimulation is also essential for Treg cell expansion and function (Golovina et al. 2008). Moreover, TGF-β signaling in the thymus is critical to sustain Foxp3 expression and clonal expansion of nTreg cells (Liu et al. 2008). Different pathogen recognition receptors such as the Toll-like receptor may either positively or negatively regulate the function of Treg cells via modulation of Foxp3 activity (Peng et al. 2005; Sutmuller et al. 2006b). It will be interesting to test whether other pathogen recognition receptors expressed in Foxp3+ Treg cells, such as NLR and RLR, may play a role in regulating Foxp3 activity. The Akt-mTOR pathway may serve as a strong repressor of the development and function of Treg cells both in vitro and in vivo (Cobbold et al. 2009; Delgoffe et al. 2009; Haxhinasto et al. 2008; Sauer et al. 2008). More recently, the S1P1-Akt-mTOR signaling pathway was identified as a negative regulator of Foxp3 levels and the development and function of natural Treg cells (Liu et al. 2009). Many transcriptional factors, including NFAT, AP1, Stat5, Smad3, CREB, and c-Rel, bind to the Foxp3 promoter and conserved noncoding sequences to control Foxp3 expression (Kim and Leonard 2007; Long et al. 2009; Zheng et al. 2010). Other cell surface receptor signals which may regulate Foxp3 levels and Treg cell activity include the Interleukin-6 receptor (Dominitzki et al. 2007; Korn et al. 2008; Samanta et al. 2008), Interleukin-4 receptor (Dardalhon et al. 2008), Interleukin-7 receptor (Mazzucchelli et al. 2008), TNFRSF4/OX40 (Niedbala et al. 2007; So and Croft 2007; Vu et al. 2007), 4-1-BB (Elpek et al. 2007; Zhang et al. 2007), Inducible T cell co-stimulator (ICOS) (Burmeister et al. 2008; Herman et al. 2004; Ito et al. 2008), Programmed cell death 1 (PD-1) (Franceschini et al. 2009; Wang et al. 2008, 2009), Cytotoxic T-lymphocyte-associated antigen 4 (CTLA-4) (Sansom and Walker 2006; Wing et al. 2008; Zheng et al. 2006), Glucocorticoid-induced TNFR-related protein (GITR) (Shevach and Stephens 2006; Wang et al. 2004), Notch signaling pathway (Kared et al. 2006; Ostroukhova et al. 2006; Samon et al. 2008), and the β-catenin/Wnt signaling pathway (Ding et al. 2008).

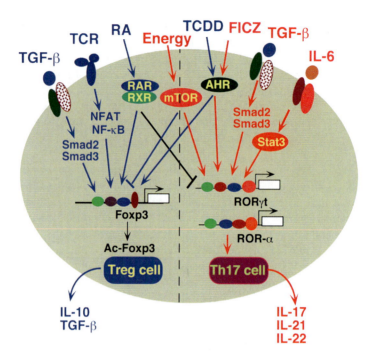

Fig. 11.3 Reciprocal regulation of Treg and Th17 cells by multiple signaling pathways. FOXP3 and RORγt are master regulators for Treg cells producing IL-10 and TGF-β and Th17 cells secreting IL-17, IL-21, and IL-22, respectively. Both TCR stimulation and TGF-β signaling are required for the generation of Treg and Th17 cells. However, TGF-β plus IL-6 promote Th17 cell differentiation and inhibit Treg cell development. Retinoic acid (RA) promotes Treg cell differentiation and inhibits Th17 cells. By contrast, activation of mammalian target of rapamycin (mTOR) by energy metabolism inhibits Treg cell differentiation, but promotes Th17 cell development. The aryl hydrocarbon receptor (AHR) mediated signaling can be activated by different ligands. 6-formylindolo[3,2-b]carbazole (FICZ), a tryptophan-derived photoproduct, favors Th17 cell differentiation, while 2,3,7,8-tetrachlorodibenzo-p-dioxin (TCDD) induced Treg cells. Thus, AHR regulates Treg and TH17 cell differentiation in a ligand-specific manner

5 Posttranslational Modification and the Transcriptional Complex of Foxp3

Foxp3 is an acetylated and phosphorylated protein, where posttranslational modification may regulate its chromatin binding and transcriptional activity (Fig. 11.2) (Li and Greene 2007; Li et al. 2007a). How extracellular signals regulate Foxp3 posttranslational modification and its transcriptional complex ensemble remain unclear. Recently, we found that TGF-β and IL-6 signals modulated Foxp3 acetylation and chromatin binding (Samanta et al. 2008). The IL-6 signal may negatively regulate Foxp3 protein levels in Treg cells via ubiquitination-mediated degradation (Li and Greene, unpublished data).

Foxp3 is a multiple domain containing transcription factor that belongs to the forkhead box P subfamily, including Foxp1, Foxp2, Foxp3, and Foxp4 (Figs. 11.1 and 11.2). Both Foxp1 and Foxp3 are highly expressed well in Treg cells, and Foxp3 may form an oligomer complex with itself or Foxp1 in regulating transcriptional repression (Li et al. 2007b). The N-terminus of Foxp3 consists of two proline-rich motifs separated by an exon-2 encoding region that specifically interacts with, and may antagonize, the function of orphan retinoic acid nuclear receptor (ROR) family transcription factors including RORα and RORγt (Zhou et al. 2008) (Fig. 11.1). The second proline-rich motif is essential for Foxp3-mediated transcriptional repression, by directly recruiting enzymatic transcriptional corepressors such as TIP60 and HDAC7 (Li et al. 2007a), or indirectly by interacting with other transcription factors such as the Ikaros family member Eos which further recruits corepressors such as CtBP1 (Pan et al. 2009). The interaction of Foxp3 and CtBP1 is dependent on the expression of Eos in Treg cells since knockdown of Eos in Treg disrupts the Foxp3–CtBP1 interaction (Pan et al. 2009). Other two Foxp subfamily members, including Treg expressing Foxp1, also contain a CtBP1-binding motif and may repress gene transcription via recruiting the CtBP1 corepressor complex (Li et al. 2004), so it remains to be answered as to why Foxp3 could not recruit CtBP1 indirectly by heterodimerizing with Foxp1 in Treg cells when Eos expression is depleted in Treg. Foxp3 also contains a C2H2 zinc finger motif with an unknown function, followed by a leucine zipper domain, which mediates its homo-oligomerization or heter-oligomerization with other Foxp subfamily members such as Foxp1. The linker region between the leucine zipper domain and C-terminal forkhead domain of Foxp3 may directly interact with transcription factor Runt-related transcription factor 1(RUNX1)/RUNX2/RUNX3, which is critical for Foxp3-mediated suppressive activity in Treg (Ono et al. 2007). Besides DNA binding on site-specific chromatin, the forkhead domain of Foxp3 is also involved in its functional complex ensemble with other transcriptional factors including NFAT (Wu et al. 2006) and NFκB (Bettelli et al. 2005).

6 Target Genes Controlled by Foxp3 and Transcription Factors

Foxp3 directly binds to about 1,000 site-specific gene promoters in Treg cells, and represses gene transcription such as IL-2, IFN-γ, IL-4, while activates others including CTLA4, CD25, and GITR (Zheng et al. 2007). The underlying mechanism by which Foxp3 activates these certain gene transcription targets remains unclear. Interestingly, a couple of Foxp3 targeting genes also encode key modulators of T cell activation and function (Marson et al. 2007). Moreover, Foxp3 may specifically regulate gene transcription of several key transcription factors which are important for Foxp3$^+$ Treg cells-mediated immune suppression on certain types of immune cells (Zheng et al. 2007). For instance, Foxp3 may regulate gene transcription of the T helper 2 (Th2) cell specifying transcription factor IRF4, which is critical for Treg-mediated suppression on Th2 cells (Zheng et al. 2009). Foxp3 may also upregulate gene expression of the T helper 1 (Th1) cell specifying transcription factor T-bet during inflammation, which is essential for Treg-mediated suppression on Th1 cells (Koch et al. 2009). More recently, comparative analysis of gene profiles in wild-type and Foxp3-deficient Treg cells has revealed that the initiation of Treg development may start earlier than Foxp3 induction, which suggests that other transcriptional factors upregulated in Treg cells earlier than Foxp3 may contribute to Treg development (Kuczma et al. 2009; Lin et al. 2007). Foxp3 interacts with a couple of transcription factors, including RORs, RUNXs, FOXP1, NFATc2, NFκB, and Eos, as well as enzymatic corepressors such as TIP60/HDAC7/HDAC9, and many chromatin remodeling factors (Li and Greene 2007). Identifying these enzymatic corepressors associated with Foxp3 provides a unique opportunity to pharmaceutically modulate FOXP3 activity in Treg cells (Li et al. 2007c). For instance, deacetylation inhibitors which target HDACs in the Foxp3 transcriptional complex may have a positive role in promoting Treg-mediated immune suppression to fight autoimmune diseases (Saouaf et al. 2009), and have beneficial effects in transplantation (Tao et al. 2007).

7 Differentiation and Plasticity of Treg Cells

Many signaling pathways control Treg cell differentiation and plasticity, depending upon environmental cues (Fig. 11.3). TGF-β and IL-2 are important factors in the development and conversion of Treg cells. However, TGF-β plus IL-6 inhibit Treg cell differentiation and promote Th17 cell commitment (Bettelli et al. 2006; Mangan et al. 2006; Veldhoen et al. 2006). Moreover, several small molecule compounds such as RA and ligands for the aryl hydrocarbon receptor (AHR) can reciprocally regulate Th17 and Treg cell differentiation (Benson et al. 2007; Mucida et al. 2007; Quintana et al. 2008; Veldhoen et al. 2008). RA promotes Treg cell development and inhibits Th17 cell differentiation (Benson et al. 2007; Mucida et al. 2007), while 6-forylindolo carbazole (FICZ) inhibits Treg cell development and promotes Th17 cell differentiation (Quintana et al. 2008; Veldhoen et al. 2008). Specific deletion of Foxp3 in mature and fully differentiated Treg cells results in the loss of Treg cells and fatal autoimmune response (Kim et al. 2007; Williams and Rudensky 2007), suggesting that continuous expression of Foxp3 is required for the maintenance of Treg cells and their suppressive function. It has been demonstrated that adoptive transfer of Foxp3$^+$ Treg cells into lymphopenic hosts leads to a loss of Foxp3 expression and differentiation into follicular T-helper cells (Tsuji et al. 2009), but not mouse recipients with fully developed lymphoid compartments (Komatsu et al. 2009). Furthermore, Foxp3$^+$ Treg cells can be readily converted into Th1 or Th17 cells in the presence of high amounts of IL-6 or in a Th1 cell polarized environment (Oldenhove et al. 2009; Xu et al. 2007; Yang et al. 2008). Consistent with these observations, a recent study shows an epigenetic mechanism underlying the specificity and plasticity of effector and regulatory T cells (Wei et al. 2009).

8 Suppressive Mechanisms of Treg Cells

CD4+ Treg cells require antigen-specific activation or polyclonal TCR stimulation to exert their suppressive function. Once activated, they can suppress CD4+ and CD8+ T cells in an antigen-nonspecific manner. However, most suppressive assays are based on an in vitro coculture system for inhibiting the proliferation of naïve T cells after anti-CD3 antibody stimulation. The precise suppressive mechanisms for both human and mouse Treg cells remain to be determined, although several mechanisms have been proposed (Sakaguchi et al. 2010; Shevach 2002, 2009; Vignali et al. 2008; von Boehmer 2005). These include cell-contact dependent and cytokine (IL-10 and TGF-β) dependent suppressive mechanisms. Murine Treg cells may also use IL-35 to suppress T cell response, but human Treg cells do not constitutively express IL-35 (Bardel et al. 2008; Collison et al. 2007). It is clear that more than one mechanism of CD4+ Treg cell-mediated suppression appears to operate in vitro and in vivo.

It appears that tumor-specific CD4+ Treg cells suppress immune responses (proliferation and IL-2 secretion of naïve or effector T cells) through a cell-contact mechanism (Wang et al. 2004, 2005). In addition, tumor-specific CD4+ and $\gamma\delta^+$ Treg cells secrete an unidentified soluble factor(s) rather than IL-10 to mediate the suppression of proliferation of both naïve CD4+ T cells and CD8+ T cells (Peng et al. 2007). Recent study shows that CTLA4 is crucial for Treg cell-mediated suppression through downregulation of CD80 and CD86 expression on DCs (Wing et al. 2008). Thus, further studies are needed to define the key molecules that directly mediate immune suppression of naïve T cells by Treg cells.

9 Treg Cells and Their Antigen Specificity in Cancer

Treg cells in cancer may play a significant role in the suppression of antitumor immune responses against cancer cells. The elevated percentages of CD4+CD25+ Treg cells in total T cell populations have been isolated from tumor tissues or peripheral blood in variety of cancers, including lung cancer (Woo et al. 2001), breast cancer (Liyanage et al. 2002), ovarian (Curiel et al. 2004), melanoma (Viguier et al. 2004; Wang et al. 2004, 2005), liver cancer (Ormandy et al. 2005; Unitt et al. 2005), gastric cancer (Kawaida et al. 2005), and lymphoma (Yang et al. 2006). Tumor-derived Treg cells are in general a stable Treg cell population with potent suppressive activity. High percentages of Treg cells in ovarian cancer is associated with the poor prognosis of cancer patients in one study (Curiel et al. 2004), while another study demonstrates that the ratio of CD8+ T cells to Treg cells, but not Treg cells alone, is a better predictor of patient survival (Sato et al. 2005). Therefore, direct correlation or association of a high percentage of Treg cells and clinical prediction of patient survival requires further investigation.

The generation and maintenance of Treg cells have long been speculated to require the presence of target antigen or tissues (Samy et al. 2005; Shevach 2002; Wang et al. 2004), but very little is known about the identity of antigens recognized by Treg cells.

Besides chemokine-mediated attraction of Treg cells to tumor sites (Curiel et al. 2004), ligands/antigens expressed by cancer cells may play a critical role in the recruitment, maintenance, and expansion of Treg cells, leading to elevated percentages of Treg cells at tumor sites (Zhou et al. 2006). To understand antigen specificity of tumor-infiltrating CD4+ T cells, we used tumor-infiltrating CD4+ T cells to screen Ii-fusion cDNA libraries constructed with tumor cell-derived RNA. This has led to successful identification of several ligands recognized by CD4+ T helper or Treg cells. Treg cells specific for LAGE1 (a homolog of NY-ESO-1) and ARTC1 (antigen recognized by Treg cell) share the common characteristics of naturally occurring Treg cells (Wang et al. 2004, 2005). Due to their specific expression pattern of LAGE1 and ARTC1 (i.e., dominantly expressed in cancer and normal testis, but not in other normal tissues tested), these Treg cells are activated only when they encounter tumor cells, thus providing the molecular basis for their specificity in the induction of immune tolerance. However, Treg cells also recognize tissue-specific tumor antigens (Vence et al. 2007). Treg cells specific for tumor-specific antigens as well as tissue-specific self-antigens are present in cancer patients. Using an in vitro system, we recently found that CD4+ T cell clones with the same antigen specificity, but with different T cell functions, can be generated (Voo et al. 2005). Some of CD4+ T cell clones that recognize the same EBNA1-derived peptide are CD4+ T helper cells, while other clones with the same antigen specificity possess suppressive function (Voo et al. 2005). Thus, it is likely that the same antigenic peptides can stimulate CD4+ helper, regulatory T cells, or both, but whether they stimulate CD4+ T cells to differentiate into T-helper or Treg cells may depend on antigen dose, peptide/MHC avidity, costimulatory molecules, and cytokines in the tumor microenvironment.

10 Manipulation of the Suppressive Function of Treg Cells: Implications for Immunotherapy

A key question in cancer immunotherapy is how to overcome the suppressive function of Treg cells. Because the CD25 marker is not specific to Treg cells, depletion with anti-CD25 may eliminate both Treg cells and activated effector cells (Attia et al. 2005; Dannull et al. 2005). Hence, more specific and effective reagents are needed to deplete Treg cells in cancer patients. CTLA-4, GITR, and OX40 are highly expressed in natural and inducible Treg cells (Ndhlovu et al. 2004). However, these molecules are also expressed in effector cells upon activation. More recently, folate receptor 4 has been shown to be highly expressed in Treg cells compared with effector cells (Yamaguchi et al. 2007). Antibodies against these molecules (anti-CTLA-4, anti-CD25, anti-OX40, anti-GITR, and anti-Folate receptor 4) have been used to block Treg cell function or deplete Treg cells in various animal models (Boden et al. 2003; Yamaguchi et al. 2007). Among them, OX40 antibody has been shown to turn off the suppressive function of Treg cells or induce T cell apoptosis (Ito et al. 2006; Piconese et al. 2008; Valzasina et al. 2005; Vu et al. 2007). However, the mechanism by which anti-OX40 mediates inhibition of Treg cell function is not clear because this antibody also stimulates effector cells and DCs. Further studies

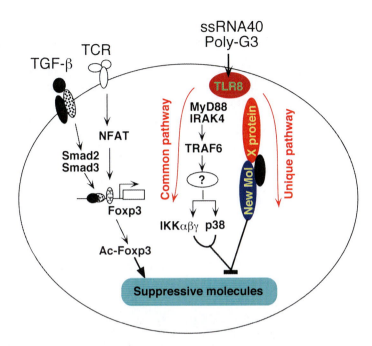

Fig. 11.4 Control of Treg cell suppressive function through Toll-like receptor 8 signaling. Many TLRs can activate NF-κB signaling and type I interferon pathways. However, TLR8, but not TLR7 or TLR9, plays a critical role in the control of Treg cell function. TLR8 may use the common NF-κB and unique but undefined signaling pathways to control Treg cell function

are needed to delineate the molecular mechanisms by which this antibody reduces Treg cell suppression and enhances effector T cell responses.

An alternative approach to antibody blockade of Treg cell function is to reverse the suppressive function of Treg cells. It has been demonstrated that TLR signaling activation on DCs can render naïve T cells refractory to suppression mediated by Treg cells in mice (Pasare and Medzhitov 2003). We recently demonstrated that Poly-G oligonucleotides can directly reverse the suppressive function of Treg cells in the absence of DCs (Peng et al. 2005). The ability of Poly-G oligonucleotides to reverse the suppressive function of Treg cells can be demonstrated in both antigen-specific and naturally occurring CD4$^+$CD25$^+$ Treg cells, and requires signaling from TLR8 to MyD88 pathway as well as unidentified TLR8-specific unique signaling (Fig. 11.4). Importantly, natural ligands for human TLR8, ssRNA40 derived from HIV viral sequences (Heil et al. 2004), completely reversed the suppressive function of Treg cells, while ligands for other TLRs failed to do so. However, Poly-G oligonucleotides could not reverse the suppressive activity of murine Treg cells, because TLR8 is not functional in mice. Activation of human TLR2 and TLR5 may enhance the suppressive function of Treg cells (Chen et al. 2009; Crellin et al. 2005). Recent studies show that activation of TLR2 with its ligand (Pam3Cys) directly increases the proliferation of human and murine Treg cells and temporally reverses their suppressive function (Liu et al. 2006a; Oberg et al. 2010; Sutmuller et al. 2006a).

However, another study shows that TLR2 ligand does not alter the suppressive function of murine Treg cells (Chen et al. 2009). Thus, it is likely that the mechanisms for TLR-mediated regulation of Treg cell suppression in humans are different from those in mice. Clinical trials using TLR8-based drugs will be an important step to test whether blocking Treg cell function can improve the potential of cancer vaccines.

Acknowledgements This work is in part supported by grants from National Institutes of Health and Cancer Research Institute.

References

Allan SE, Passerini L, Bacchetta R, Crellin N, Dai M, Orban PC, Ziegler SF, Roncarolo MG, Levings MK (2005) The role of 2 FOXP3 isoforms in the generation of human CD4+ Tregs. J Clin Invest 115:3276–3284

Apostolou I, Sarukhan A, Klein L, von Boehmer H (2002) Origin of regulatory T cells with known specificity for antigen. Nat Immunol 3:756–763

Apostolou I, Von Boehmer H (2004) In vivo instruction of suppressor commitment in naive T cells. J Exp Med 199:1401–1408

Attia P, Maker AV, Haworth LR, Rogers-Freezer L, Rosenberg SA (2005) Inability of a fusion protein of IL-2 and diphtheria toxin (Denileukin Diftitox, DAB389IL-2, ONTAK) to eliminate regulatory T lymphocytes in patients with melanoma. J Immunother 28:582–592

Bardel E, Larousserie F, Charlot-Rabiega P, Coulomb-L'Hermine A, Devergne O (2008) Human CD4+ CD25+ Foxp3+ regulatory T cells do not constitutively express IL-35. J Immunol 181:6898–6905

Bennett CL, Christie J, Ramsdell F, Brunkow ME, Ferguson PJ, Whitesell L, Kelly TE, Saulsbury FT, Chance PF, Ochs HD (2001) The immune dysregulation, polyendocrinopathy, enteropathy, X-linked syndrome (IPEX) is caused by mutations of FOXP3. Nat Genet 27:20–21

Benson MJ, Pino-Lagos K, Rosemblatt M, Noelle RJ (2007) All-trans retinoic acid mediates enhanced T reg cell growth, differentiation, and gut homing in the face of high levels of co-stimulation. J Exp Med 204:1765–1774

Bettelli E, Carrier Y, Gao W, Korn T, Strom TB, Oukka M, Weiner HL, Kuchroo VK (2006) Reciprocal developmental pathways for the generation of pathogenic effector TH17 and regulatory T cells. Nature 441:235–238

Bettelli E, Dastrange M, Oukka M (2005) Foxp3 interacts with nuclear factor of activated T cells and NF-kappa B to repress cytokine gene expression and effector functions of T helper cells. Proc Natl Acad Sci USA 102:5138–5143

Boden E, Tang Q, Bour-Jordan H, Bluestone JA (2003) The role of CD28 and CTLA4 in the function and homeostasis of CD4+ CD25+ regulatory T cells. Novartis Found Symp 252:55–63; discussion 63–56, 106–114

Brandes M, Willimann K, Moser B (2005) Professional antigen-presentation function by human gammadelta T Cells. Science 309:264–268

Brunkow ME, Jeffery EW, Hjerrild KA, Paeper B, Clark LB, Yasayko SA, Wilkinson JE, Galas D, Ziegler SF, Ramsdell F (2001) Disruption of a new forkhead/winged-helix protein, scurfin, results in the fatal lymphoproliferative disorder of the scurfy mouse. Nat Genet 27:68–73

Burmeister Y, Lischke T, Dahler AC, Mages HW, Lam KP, Coyle AJ, Kroczek RA, Hutloff A (2008) ICOS controls the pool size of effector-memory and regulatory T cells. J Immunol 180:774–782

Chatila TA, Blaeser F, Ho N, Lederman HM, Voulgaropoulos C, Helms C, Bowcock AM (2000) JM2, encoding a fork head-related protein, is mutated in X-linked autoimmunity-allergic disregulation syndrome. J Clin Invest 106:R75–R81

Chen Q, Davidson TS, Huter EN, Shevach EM (2009) Engagement of TLR2 does not reverse the suppressor function of mouse regulatory T cells, but promotes their survival. J Immunol 183:4458–4466

Chen W, Jin W, Hardegen N, Lei KJ, Li L, Marinos N, McGrady G, Wahl SM (2003) Conversion of peripheral CD4+ CD25- naive T cells to CD4+ CD25+ regulatory T cells by TGF-beta induction of transcription factor Foxp3. J Exp Med 198:1875–1886

Cobbold SP, Adams E, Farquhar CA, Nolan KF, Howie D, Lui KO, Fairchild PJ, Mellor AL, Ron D, Waldmann H (2009) Infectious tolerance via the consumption of essential amino acids and mTOR signaling. Proc Natl Acad Sci USA 106:12055–12060

Collison LW, Workman CJ, Kuo TT, Boyd K, Wang Y, Vignali KM, Cross R, Sehy D, Blumberg RS, Vignali DA (2007) The inhibitory cytokine IL-35 contributes to regulatory T-cell function. Nature 450:566–569

Coombes JL, Siddiqui KR, Arancibia-Carcamo CV, Hall J, Sun CM, Belkaid Y, Powrie F (2007) A functionally specialized population of mucosal CD103+ DCs induces Foxp3+ regulatory T cells via a TGF-beta and retinoic acid-dependent mechanism. J Exp Med 204:1757–1764

Crellin NK, Garcia RV, Hadisfar O, Allan SE, Steiner TS, Levings MK (2005) Human CD4+ T cells express TLR5 and its ligand flagellin enhances the suppressive capacity and expression of FOXP3 in CD4+ CD25+ T regulatory cells. J Immunol 175:8051–8059

Curiel TJ, Coukos G, Zou L, Alvarez X, Cheng P, Mottram P, Evdemon-Hogan M, Conejo-Garcia JR, Zhang L, Burow M et al (2004) Specific recruitment of regulatory T cells in ovarian carcinoma fosters immune privilege and predicts reduced survival. Nat Med 10:942–949

Dannull J, Su Z, Rizzieri D, Yang BK, Coleman D, Yancey D, Zhang A, Dahm P, Chao N, Gilboa E et al (2005) Enhancement of vaccine-mediated antitumor immunity in cancer patients after depletion of regulatory T cells. J Clin Invest 115:3623–3633

Dardalhon V, Awasthi A, Kwon H, Galileos G, Gao W, Sobel RA, Mitsdoerffer M, Strom TB, Elyaman W, Ho IC et al (2008) IL-4 inhibits TGF-beta-induced Foxp3+ T cells and, together with TGF-beta, generates IL-9+ IL-10+ Foxp3(–) effector T cells. Nat Immunol 9:1347–1355

Delgoffe GM, Kole TP, Zheng Y, Zarek PE, Matthews KL, Xiao B, Worley PF, Kozma SC, Powell JD (2009) The mTOR kinase differentially regulates effector and regulatory T cell lineage commitment. Immunity 30:832–844

Ding Y, Shen S, Lino AC, Curotto de Lafaille MA, Lafaille JJ (2008) Beta-catenin stabilization extends regulatory T cell survival and induces anergy in nonregulatory T cells. Nat Med 14:162–169

Dominitzki S, Fantini MC, Neufert C, Nikolaev A, Galle PR, Scheller J, Monteleone G, Rose-John S, Neurath MF, Becker C (2007) Cutting edge: trans-signaling via the soluble IL-6R abrogates the induction of FoxP3 in naive CD4+ CD25 T cells. J Immunol 179:2041–2045

Elpek KG, Yolcu ES, Franke DD, Lacelle C, Schabowsky RH, Shirwan H (2007) Ex vivo expansion of CD4+ CD25+ FoxP3+ T regulatory cells based on synergy between IL-2 and 4-1BB signaling. J Immunol 179:7295–7304

Endharti AT, Rifa M, Shi Z, Fukuoka Y, Nakahara Y, Kawamoto Y, Takeda K, Isobe K, Suzuki H (2005) Cutting edge: CD8+CD122+ regulatory T cells produce IL-10 to suppress IFN-gamma production and proliferation of CD8+ T cells. J Immunol 175:7093–7097

Fantini MC, Becker C, Monteleone G, Pallone F, Galle PR, Neurath MF (2004) Cutting edge: TGF-beta induces a regulatory phenotype in CD4+ CD25- T cells through Foxp3 induction and down-regulation of Smad7. J Immunol 172:5149–5153

Fontenot JD, Gavin MA, Rudensky AY (2003) Foxp3 programs the development and function of CD4(+)CD25(+) regulatory T cells. Nat Immunol 4:330–336

Fontenot JD, Rasmussen JP, Gavin MA, Rudensky AY (2005) A function for interleukin 2 in Foxp3-expressing regulatory T cells. Nat Immunol 6:1142–1151

Franceschini D, Paroli M, Francavilla V, Videtta M, Morrone S, Labbadia G, Cerino A, Mondelli MU, Barnaba V (2009) PD-L1 negatively regulates CD4+ CD25+ Foxp3+ Tregs by limiting STAT-5 phosphorylation in patients chronically infected with HCV. J Clin Invest 119:551–564

Fujii S, Shimizu K, Smith C, Bonifaz L, Steinman RM (2003) Activation of natural killer T cells by alpha-galactosylceramide rapidly induces the full maturation of dendritic cells in vivo and thereby acts as an adjuvant for combined CD4 and CD8 T cell immunity to a coadministered protein. J Exp Med 198:267–279

Golovina TN, Mikheeva T, Suhoski MM, Aqui NA, Tai VC, Shan X, Liu R, Balcarcel RR, Fisher N, Levine BL et al (2008) CD28 costimulation is essential for human T regulatory expansion and function. J Immunol 181:2855–2868

Haxhinasto S, Mathis D, Benoist C (2008) The AKT-mTOR axis regulates de novo differentiation of CD4+ Foxp3+ cells. J Exp Med 205:565–574

Hayakawa Y, Rovero S, Forni G, Smyth MJ (2003) Alpha-galactosylceramide (KRN7000) suppression of chemical- and oncogene-dependent carcinogenesis. Proc Natl Acad Sci USA 100:9464–9469

Heil F, Hemmi H, Hochrein H, Ampenberger F, Kirschning C, Akira S, Lipford G, Wagner H, Bauer S (2004) Species-specific recognition of single-stranded RNA via toll-like receptor 7 and 8. Science 303:1526–1529

Herman AE, Freeman GJ, Mathis D, Benoist C (2004) CD4+ CD25+ T regulatory cells dependent on ICOS promote regulation of effector cells in the prediabetic lesion. J Exp Med 199:1479–1489

Hill JA, Feuerer M, Tash K, Haxhinasto S, Perez J, Melamed R, Mathis D, Benoist C (2007) Foxp3 transcription-factor-dependent and -independent regulation of the regulatory T cell transcriptional signature. Immunity 27:786–800

Hori S, Nomura T, Sakaguchi S (2003) Control of regulatory T cell development by the transcription factor foxp3. Science 299:1057–1061

Housley WJ, O'Conor CA, Nichols F, Puddington L, Lingenheld EG, Zhu L, Clark RB (2009) PPARgamma regulates retinoic acid-mediated DC induction of Tregs. J Leukoc Biol 86:293–301

Hu D, Ikizawa K, Lu L, Sanchirico ME, Shinohara ML, Cantor H (2004) Analysis of regulatory CD8 T cells in Qa-1-deficient mice. Nat Immunol 5:516–523

Ito T, Hanabuchi S, Wang YH, Park WR, Arima K, Bover L, Qin FX, Gilliet M, Liu YJ (2008) Two functional subsets of FOXP3+ regulatory T cells in human thymus and periphery. Immunity 28:870–880

Ito T, Wang YH, Duramad O, Hanabuchi S, Perng OA, Gilliet M, Qin FX, Liu YJ (2006) OX40 ligand shuts down IL-10-producing regulatory T cells. Proc Natl Acad Sci USA 103:13138–13143

Jiang H, Chess L (2004) An integrated view of suppressor T cell subsets in immunoregulation. J Clin Invest 114:1198–1208

Jordan MS, Boesteanu A, Reed AJ, Petrone AL, Holenbeck AE, Lerman MA, Naji A, Caton AJ (2001) Thymic selection of CD4+ CD25+ regulatory T cells induced by an agonist self-peptide. Nat Immunol 2:301–306

Kared H, Adle-Biassette H, Fois E, Masson A, Bach JF, Chatenoud L, Schneider E, Zavala F (2006) Jagged2-expressing hematopoietic progenitors promote regulatory T cell expansion in the periphery through notch signaling. Immunity 25:823–834

Kawaida H, Kono K, Takahashi A, Sugai H, Mimura K, Miyagawa N, Omata H, Ooi A, Fujii H (2005) Distribution of CD4+ CD25high regulatory T-cells in tumor-draining lymph nodes in patients with gastric cancer. J Surg Res 124:151–157

Khattri R, Cox T, Yasayko SA, Ramsdell F (2003) An essential role for Scurfin in CD4(+)CD25(+) T regulatory cells. Nat Immunol 4:337–342

Kim HP, Leonard WJ (2007) CREB/ATF-dependent T cell receptor-induced FoxP3 gene expression: a role for DNA methylation. J Exp Med 204:1543–1551

Kim JM, Rasmussen JP, Rudensky AY (2007) Regulatory T cells prevent catastrophic autoimmunity throughout the lifespan of mice. Nat Immunol 8:191–197

Koch MA, Tucker-Heard G, Perdue NR, Killebrew JR, Urdahl KB, Campbell DJ (2009) The transcription factor T-bet controls regulatory T cell homeostasis and function during type 1 inflammation. Nat Immunol 10:595–602

Komatsu N, Mariotti-Ferrandiz ME, Wang Y, Malissen B, Waldmann H, Hori S (2009) Heterogeneity of natural Foxp3+ T cells: a committed regulatory T-cell lineage and an uncommitted minor population retaining plasticity. Proc Natl Acad Sci USA 106:1903–1908

Korn T, Mitsdoerffer M, Croxford AL, Awasthi A, Dardalhon VA, Galileos G, Vollmar P, Stritesky GL, Kaplan MH, Waisman A et al (2008) IL-6 controls Th17 immunity in vivo by inhibiting the conversion of conventional T cells into Foxp3+ regulatory T cells. Proc Natl Acad Sci USA 105:18460–18465

Kuczma M, Podolsky R, Garge N, Daniely D, Pacholczyk R, Ignatowicz L, Kraj P (2009) Foxp3-deficient regulatory T cells do not revert into conventional effector CD4+ T cells but constitute a unique cell subset. J Immunol 183(6):3731–3741

Li B, Greene MI (2007) FOXP3 actively represses transcription by recruiting the HAT/HDAC complex. Cell Cycle 6:1432–1436

Li B, Samanta A, Song X, Iacono KT, Bembas K, Tao R, Basu S, Riley JL, Hancock WW, Shen Y et al (2007a) FOXP3 interactions with histone acetyltransferase and class II histone deacetylases are required for repression. Proc Natl Acad Sci USA 104:4571–4576

Li B, Samanta A, Song X, Iacono KT, Brennan P, Chatila TA, Roncador G, Banham AH, Riley JL, Wang Q et al (2007b) FOXP3 is a homo-oligomer and a component of a supramolecular regulatory complex disabled in the human XLAAD/IPEX autoimmune disease. Int Immunol 19:825–835

Li B, Saouaf SJ, Samanta A, Shen Y, Hancock WW, Greene MI (2007c) Biochemistry and therapeutic implications of mechanisms involved in FOXP3 activity in immune suppression. Curr Opin Immunol 19:583–588

Li S, Weidenfeld J, Morrisey EE (2004) Transcriptional and DNA binding activity of the Foxp1/2/4 family is modulated by heterotypic and homotypic protein interactions. Mol Cell Biol 24:809–822

Lin W, Haribhai D, Relland LM, Truong N, Carlson MR, Williams CB, Chatila TA (2007) Regulatory T cell development in the absence of functional Foxp3. Nat Immunol 8:359–368

Liu G, Burns S, Huang G, Boyd K, Proia RL, Flavell RA, Chi H (2009) The receptor S1P1 overrides regulatory T cell-mediated immune suppression through Akt-mTOR. Nat Immunol 10:769–777

Liu H, Komai-Koma M, Xu D, Liew FY (2006a) Toll-like receptor 2 signaling modulates the functions of CD4+ CD25+ regulatory T cells. Proc Natl Acad Sci USA 103:7048–7053

Liu K, Idoyaga J, Charalambous A, Fujii S, Bonito A, Mordoh J, Wainstok R, Bai XF, Liu Y, Steinman RM (2005) Innate NKT lymphocytes confer superior adaptive immunity via tumor-capturing dendritic cells. J Exp Med 202:1507–1516

Liu W, Putnam AL, Xu-Yu Z, Szot GL, Lee MR, Zhu S, Gottlieb PA, Kapranov P, Gingeras TR, de St Groth BF et al (2006b) CD127 expression inversely correlates with FoxP3 and suppressive function of human CD4+ T reg cells. J Exp Med 203:1701–1711

Liu Y, Zhang P, Li J, Kulkarni AB, Perruche S, Chen W (2008) A critical function for TGF-beta signaling in the development of natural CD4+ CD25+ Foxp3+ regulatory T cells. Nat Immunol 9:632–640

Liyanage UK, Moore TT, Joo HG, Tanaka Y, Herrmann V, Doherty G, Drebin JA, Strasberg SM, Eberlein TJ, Goedegebuure PS et al (2002) Prevalence of regulatory T cells is increased in peripheral blood and tumor microenvironment of patients with pancreas or breast adenocarcinoma. J Immunol 169:2756–2761

Long M, Park SG, Strickland I, Hayden MS, Ghosh S (2009) Nuclear factor-kappaB modulates regulatory T cell development by directly regulating expression of Foxp3 transcription factor. Immunity 31:921–931

Lu LF, Rudensky A (2009) Molecular orchestration of differentiation and function of regulatory T cells. Genes Dev 23:1270–1282

Mangan PR, Harrington LE, O'Quinn DB, Helms WS, Bullard DC, Elson CO, Hatton RD, Wahl SM, Schoeb TR, Weaver CT (2006) Transforming growth factor-beta induces development of the T(H)17 lineage. Nature 441:231–234

Marson A, Kretschmer K, Frampton GM, Jacobsen ES, Polansky JK, MacIsaac KD, Levine SS, Fraenkel E, von Boehmer H, Young RA (2007) Foxp3 occupancy and regulation of key target genes during T-cell stimulation. Nature 445:931–935

Mazzucchelli R, Hixon JA, Spolski R, Chen X, Li WQ, Hall VL, Willette-Brown J, Hurwitz AA, Leonard WJ, Durum SK (2008) Development of regulatory T cells requires IL-7Ralpha stimulation by IL-7 or TSLP. Blood 112:3283–3292

Moodycliffe AM, Nghiem D, Clydesdale G, Ullrich SE (2000) Immune suppression and skin cancer development: regulation by NKT cells. Nat Immunol 1:521–525

Mucida D, Park Y, Kim G, Turovskaya O, Scott I, Kronenberg M, Cheroutre H (2007) Reciprocal TH17 and regulatory T cell differentiation mediated by retinoic acid. Science 317:256–260

Nazarov-Stoica C, Surls J, Bona C, Casares S, Brumeanu TD (2009) CD28 signaling in T regulatory precursors requires p56lck and rafts integrity to stabilize the Foxp3 message. J Immunol 182:102–110

Ndhlovu LC, Takeda I, Sugamura K, Ishii N (2004) Expanding role of T-cell costimulators in regulatory T-cell function: recent advances in accessory molecules expressed on both regulatory and nonregulatory T cells. Crit Rev Immunol 24:251–266

Niedbala W, Cai B, Liu H, Pitman N, Chang L, Liew FY (2007) Nitric oxide induces CD4+ CD25+ Foxp3 regulatory T cells from CD4+ CD25 T cells via p53, IL-2, and OX40. Proc Natl Acad Sci USA 104:15478–15483

Oberg HH, Ly TT, Ussat S, Meyer T, Kabelitz D, Wesch D (2010) Differential but direct abolishment of human regulatory T cell suppressive capacity by various TLR2 ligands. J Immunol 184:4733–4740

Ohkura N, Sakaguchi S (2009) A novel modifier of regulatory T cells. Nat Immunol 10:685–686

Oldenhove G, Bouladoux N, Wohlfert EA, Hall JA, Chou D, Dos Santos L, O'Brien S, Blank R, Lamb E, Natarajan S et al (2009) Decrease of Foxp3+ Treg cell number and acquisition of effector cell phenotype during lethal infection. Immunity 31:772–786

Ono M, Yaguchi H, Ohkura N, Kitabayashi I, Nagamura Y, Nomura T, Miyachi Y, Tsukada T, Sakaguchi S (2007) Foxp3 controls regulatory T-cell function by interacting with AML1/Runx1. Nature 446:685–689

Ormandy LA, Hillemann T, Wedemeyer H, Manns MP, Greten TF, Korangy F (2005) Increased populations of regulatory T cells in peripheral blood of patients with hepatocellular carcinoma. Cancer Res 65:2457–2464

Ostroukhova M, Qi Z, Oriss TB, Dixon-McCarthy B, Ray P, Ray A (2006) Treg-mediated immunosuppression involves activation of the Notch-HES1 axis by membrane-bound TGF-beta. J Clin Invest 116:996–1004

Pan F, Yu H, Dang EV, Barbi J, Pan X, Grosso JF, Jinasena D, Sharma SM, McCadden EM, Getnet D et al (2009) Eos mediates Foxp3-dependent gene silencing in CD4+ regulatory T cells. Science 325:1142–1146

Pasare C, Medzhitov R (2003) Toll pathway-dependent blockade of CD4+ CD25+ T cell-mediated suppression by dendritic cells. Science 299:1033–1036

Peng G, Guo Z, Kiniwa Y, Voo KS, Peng W, Fu T, Wang DY, Li Y, Wang HY, Wang R-F (2005) Toll-like receptor 8 mediated-reversal of CD4+ regulatory T cell function. Science 309:1380–1384

Peng G, Wang HY, Peng W, Kiniwa Y, Seo K, Wang R-F (2007) Tumor-infiltrating gamma-delta T cells suppress T and dendritic cell function via mechanisms controlled by a unique Toll-like receptor signaling pathway. Immunity 27:334–348

Piconese S, Valzasina B, Colombo MP (2008) OX40 triggering blocks suppression by regulatory T cells and facilitates tumor rejection. J Exp Med 205:825–839

Quintana FJ, Basso AS, Iglesias AH, Korn T, Farez MF, Bettelli E, Caccamo M, Oukka M, Weiner HL (2008) Control of T(reg) and T(H)17 cell differentiation by the aryl hydrocarbon receptor. Nature 453:65–71

Roncarolo MG, Gregori S, Battaglia M, Bacchetta R, Fleischhauer K, Levings MK (2006) Interleukin-10-secreting type 1 regulatory T cells in rodents and humans. Immunol Rev 212:28–50

Ruan Q, Kameswaran V, Tone Y, Li L, Liou HC, Greene MI, Tone M, Chen YH (2009) Development of Foxp3(+) regulatory t cells is driven by the c-Rel enhanceosome. Immunity 31:932–940

Sakaguchi S (2004) Naturally arising CD4+ regulatory T cells for immunologic self-tolerance and negative control of immune responses. Annu Rev Immunol 22:531–562

Sakaguchi S, Miyara M, Costantino CM, Hafler DA (2010) FOXP3+ regulatory T cells in the human immune system. Nat Rev Immunol 10:490–500

Samanta A, Li B, Song X, Bembas K, Zhang G, Katsumata M, Saouaf SJ, Wang Q, Hancock WW, Shen Y et al (2008) TGF-beta and IL-6 signals modulate chromatin binding and promoter occupancy by acetylated FOXP3. Proc Natl Acad Sci USA 105:14023–14027

Samon JB, Champhekar A, Minter LM, Telfer JC, Miele L, Fauq A, Das P, Golde TE, Osborne BA (2008) Notch1 and TGFbeta1 cooperatively regulate Foxp3 expression and the maintenance of peripheral regulatory T cells. Blood 112:1813–1821

Samy ET, Parker LA, Sharp CP, Tung KS (2005) Continuous control of autoimmune disease by antigen-dependent polyclonal CD4+ CD25+ regulatory T cells in the regional lymph node. J Exp Med 202:771–781

Sansom DM, Walker LS (2006) The role of CD28 and cytotoxic T-lymphocyte antigen-4 (CTLA-4) in regulatory T-cell biology. Immunol Rev 212:131–148

Saouaf SJ, Li B, Zhang G, Shen Y, Furuuchi N, Hancock WW, Greene MI (2009) Deacetylase inhibition increases regulatory T cell function and decreases incidence and severity of collagen-induced arthritis. Exp Mol Pathol 87(2):99–104

Sato E, Olson SH, Ahn J, Bundy B, Nishikawa H, Qian F, Jungbluth AA, Frosina D, Gnjatic S, Ambrosone C et al (2005) Intraepithelial CD8+ tumor-infiltrating lymphocytes and a high CD8+/regulatory T cell ratio are associated with favorable prognosis in ovarian cancer. Proc Natl Acad Sci USA 102:18538–18543

Sauer S, Bruno L, Hertweck A, Finlay D, Leleu M, Spivakov M, Knight ZA, Cobb BS, Cantrell D, O'Connor E et al (2008) T cell receptor signaling controls Foxp3 expression via PI3K, Akt, and mTOR. Proc Natl Acad Sci USA 105:7797–7802

Seddiki N, Santner-Nanan B, Martinson J, Zaunders J, Sasson S, Landay A, Solomon M, Selby W, Alexander SI, Nanan R et al (2006) Expression of interleukin (IL)-2 and IL-7 receptors discriminates between human regulatory and activated T cells. J Exp Med 203:1693–1700

Shao L, Jacobs AR, Johnson VV, Mayer L (2005) Activation of CD8+ regulatory T cells by human placental trophoblasts. J Immunol 174:7539–7547

Shevach EM (2002) CD4+ CD25+ suppressor T cells: more questions than answers. Nat Rev Immunol 2:389–400

Shevach EM (2009) Mechanisms of foxp3+ T regulatory cell-mediated suppression. Immunity 30:636–645

Shevach EM, Stephens GL (2006) The GITR-GITRL interaction: co-stimulation or contrasuppression of regulatory activity? Nat Rev Immunol 6:613–618

Smyth MJ, Crowe NY, Hayakawa Y, Takeda K, Yagita H, Godfrey DI (2002) NKT cells – conductors of tumor immunity? Curr Opin Immunol 14:165–171

So T, Croft M (2007) Cutting edge: OX40 inhibits TGF-beta- and antigen-driven conversion of naive CD4 T cells into CD25+ Foxp3+ T cells. J Immunol 179:1427–1430

Sun CM, Hall JA, Blank RB, Bouladoux N, Oukka M, Mora JR, Belkaid Y (2007) Small intestine lamina propria dendritic cells promote de novo generation of Foxp3 T reg cells via retinoic acid. J Exp Med 204:1775–1785

Sutmuller RP, den Brok MH, Kramer M, Bennink EJ, Toonen LW, Kullberg BJ, Joosten LA, Akira S, Netea MG, Adema GJ (2006a) Toll-like receptor 2 controls expansion and function of regulatory T cells. J Clin Invest 116:485–494

Sutmuller RP, Morgan ME, Netea MG, Grauer O, Adema GJ (2006b) Toll-like receptors on regulatory T cells: expanding immune regulation. Trends Immunol 27:387–393

Tai X, Cowan M, Feigenbaum L, Singer A (2005) CD28 costimulation of developing thymocytes induces Foxp3 expression and regulatory T cell differentiation independently of interleukin 2. Nat Immunol 6:152–162

Tao R, de Zoeten EF, Ozkaynak E, Chen C, Wang L, Porrett PM, Li B, Turka LA, Olson EN, Greene MI et al (2007) Deacetylase inhibition promotes the generation and function of regulatory T cells. Nat Med 13:1299–1307

Terabe M, Matsui S, Noben-Trauth N, Chen H, Watson C, Donaldson DD, Carbone DP, Paul WE, Berzofsky JA (2000) NKT cell-mediated repression of tumor immunosurveillance by IL-13 and the IL-4R-STAT6 pathway. Nat Immunol 1:515–520

Terabe M, Matsui S, Park JM, Mamura M, Noben-Trauth N, Donaldson DD, Chen W, Wahl SM, Ledbetter S, Pratt B et al (2003) Transforming growth factor-beta production and myeloid cells are an effector mechanism through which CD1d-restricted T cells block cytotoxic T lymphocyte-mediated tumor immunosurveillance: abrogation prevents tumor recurrence. J Exp Med 198:1741–1752

Terabe M, Swann J, Ambrosino E, Sinha P, Takaku S, Hayakawa Y, Godfrey DI, Ostrand-Rosenberg S, Smyth MJ, Berzofsky JA (2005) A nonclassical non-Valpha14Jalpha18 CD1d-restricted (type II) NKT cell is sufficient for down-regulation of tumor immunosurveillance. J Exp Med 202:1627–1633

Tsuji M, Komatsu N, Kawamoto S, Suzuki K, Kanagawa O, Honjo T, Hori S, Fagarasan S (2009) Preferential generation of follicular B helper T cells from Foxp3+ T cells in gut Peyer's patches. Science 323:1488–1492

Unitt E, Rushbrook SM, Marshall A, Davies S, Gibbs P, Morris LS, Coleman N, Alexander GJ (2005) Compromised lymphocytes infiltrate hepatocellular carcinoma: the role of T-regulatory cells. Hepatology 41:722–730

Valzasina B, Guiducci C, Dislich H, Killeen N, Weinberg AD, Colombo MP (2005) Triggering of OX40 (CD134) on CD4(+)CD25+ T cells blocks their inhibitory activity: a novel regulatory role for OX40 and its comparison with GITR. Blood 105:2845–2851

Veldhoen M, Hirota K, Westendorf AM, Buer J, Dumoutier L, Renauld JC, Stockinger B (2008) The aryl hydrocarbon receptor links TH17-cell-mediated autoimmunity to environmental toxins. Nature 453:106–109

Veldhoen M, Hocking RJ, Atkins CJ, Locksley RM, Stockinger B (2006) TGFbeta in the context of an inflammatory cytokine milieu supports de novo differentiation of IL-17-producing T cells. Immunity 24:179–189

Vence L, Palucka AK, Fay JW, Ito T, Liu YJ, Banchereau J, Ueno H (2007) Circulating tumor antigen-specific regulatory T cells in patients with metastatic melanoma. Proc Natl Acad Sci USA 104:20884–20889

Vignali DA, Collison LW, Workman CJ (2008) How regulatory T cells work. Nat Rev Immunol 8:523–532

Viguier M, Lemaitre F, Verola O, Cho MS, Gorochov G, Dubertret L, Bachelez H, Kourilsky P, Ferradini L (2004) Foxp3 expressing CD4(+)CD25(high) regulatory T cells are overrepresented in human metastatic melanoma lymph nodes and inhibit the function of infiltrating T cells. J Immunol 173:1444–1453

Vlad G, Cortesini R, Suciu-Foca N (2005) License to heal: bidirectional interaction of antigen-specific regulatory T cells and tolerogenic APC. J Immunol 174:5907–5914

von Boehmer H (2005) Mechanisms of suppression by suppressor T cells. Nat Immunol 6:338–344

Voo KS, Peng G, Guo Z, Fu T, Li Y, Frappier L, Wang RF (2005) Functional characterization of EBV-encoded nuclear antigen 1-specific CD4+ helper and regulatory T cells elicited by in vitro peptide stimulation. Cancer Res 65:1577–1586

Vu MD, Xiao X, Gao W, Degauque N, Chen M, Kroemer A, Killeen N, Ishii N, Chang Li X (2007) OX40 costimulation turns off Foxp3+ Tregs. Blood 110:2501–2510

Walker MR, Kasprowicz DJ, Gersuk VH, Benard A, Van Landeghen M, Buckner JH, Ziegler SF (2003) Induction of FoxP3 and acquisition of T regulatory activity by stimulated human CD4+ CD25- T cells. J Clin Invest 112:1437–1443

Wang HY, Lee DA, Peng G, Guo Z, Li Y, Kiniwa Y, Shevach EM, Wang RF (2004) Tumor-specific human CD4+ regulatory T cells and their ligands: implication for immunotherapy. Immunity 20:107–118

Wang HY, Peng G, Guo Z, Shevach EM, Wang R-F (2005) Recognition of a new ARTC1 peptide ligand uniquely expressed in tumor cells by antigen-specific CD4+ gegulatory T cells. J Immunol 174:2661–2670

Wang L, Pino-Lagos K, de Vries VC, Guleria I, Sayegh MH, Noelle RJ (2008) Programmed death 1 ligand signaling regulates the generation of adaptive Foxp3+ CD4+ regulatory T cells. Proc Natl Acad Sci USA 105:9331–9336

Wang W, Lau R, Yu D, Zhu W, Korman A, Weber J (2009) PD1 blockade reverses the suppression of melanoma antigen-specific CTL by CD4+ CD25(Hi) regulatory T cells. Int Immunol 21:1065–1077

Wei G, Wei L, Zhu J, Zang C, Hu-Li J, Yao Z, Cui K, Kanno Y, Roh TY, Watford WT et al (2009) Global mapping of H3K4me3 and H3K27me3 reveals specificity and plasticity in lineage fate determination of differentiating CD4+ T cells. Immunity 30:155–167

Wei S, Kryczek I, Zou L, Daniel B, Cheng P, Mottram P, Curiel T, Lange A, Zou W (2005) Plasmacytoid dendritic cells induce CD8+ regulatory T cells in human ovarian carcinoma. Cancer Res 65:5020–5026

Weiner HL (2001) Induction and mechanism of action of transforming growth factor-beta-secreting Th3 regulatory cells. Immunol Rev 182:207–214

Wildin RS, Ramsdell F, Peake J, Faravelli F, Casanova JL, Buist N, Levy-Lahad E, Mazzella M, Goulet O, Perroni L et al (2001) X-linked neonatal diabetes mellitus, enteropathy and endocrinopathy syndrome is the human equivalent of mouse scurfy. Nat Genet 27:18–20

Williams LM, Rudensky AY (2007) Maintenance of the Foxp3-dependent developmental program in mature regulatory T cells requires continued expression of Foxp3. Nat Immunol 8:277–284

Wing K, Onishi Y, Prieto-Martin P, Yamaguchi T, Miyara M, Fehervari Z, Nomura T, Sakaguchi S (2008) CTLA-4 control over Foxp3+ regulatory T cell function. Science 322:271–275

Woo EY, Chu CS, Goletz TJ, Schlienger K, Yeh H, Coukos G, Rubin SC, Kaiser LR, June CH (2001) Regulatory CD4(+)CD25(+) T cells in tumors from patients with early-stage non-small cell lung cancer and late-stage ovarian cancer. Cancer Res 61:4766–4772

Wu Y, Borde M, Heissmeyer V, Feuerer M, Lapan AD, Stroud JC, Bates DL, Guo L, Han A, Ziegler SF et al (2006) FOXP3 controls regulatory T cell function through cooperation with NFAT. Cell 126:375–387

Xiao S, Jin H, Korn T, Liu SM, Oukka M, Lim B, Kuchroo VK (2008) Retinoic acid increases Foxp3+ regulatory T cells and inhibits development of Th17 cells by enhancing TGF-beta-driven Smad3 signaling and inhibiting IL-6 and IL-23 receptor expression. J Immunol 181:2277–2284

Xu L, Kitani A, Fuss I, Strober W (2007) Cutting edge: regulatory T cells induce CD4+ CD25-Foxp3- T cells or are self-induced to become Th17 cells in the absence of exogenous TGF-beta. J Immunol 178:6725–6729

Yamaguchi T, Hirota K, Nagahama K, Ohkawa K, Takahashi T, Nomura T, Sakaguchi S (2007) Control of immune responses by antigen-specific regulatory T cells expressing the folate receptor. Immunity 27:145–159

Yang XO, Nurieva R, Martinez GJ, Kang HS, Chung Y, Pappu BP, Shah B, Chang SH, Schluns KS, Watowich SS et al (2008) Molecular antagonism and plasticity of regulatory and inflammatory T cell programs. Immunity 29:44–56

Yang ZZ, Novak AJ, Stenson MJ, Witzig TE, Ansell SM (2006) Intratumoral CD4+ CD25+ regulatory T-cell-mediated suppression of infiltrating CD4+ T cells in B-cell non-Hodgkin lymphoma. Blood 107:3639–3646

Yao Z, Kanno Y, Kerenyi M, Stephens G, Durant L, Watford WT, Laurence A, Robinson GW, Shevach EM, Moriggl R et al (2007) Nonredundant roles for Stat5a/b in directly regulating Foxp3. Blood 109:4368–4375

Zhang P, Gao F, Wang Q, Wang X, Zhu F, Ma C, Sun W, Zhang L (2007) Agonistic anti-4-1BB antibody promotes the expansion of natural regulatory T cells while maintaining Foxp3 expression. Scand J Immunol 66:435–440

Zheng SG, Wang JH, Gray JD, Soucier H, Horwitz DA (2004) Natural and induced CD4+ CD25+ cells educate CD4+ CD25- cells to develop suppressive activity: the role of IL-2, TGF-beta, and IL-10. J Immunol 172:5213–5221

Zheng SG, Wang JH, Stohl W, Kim KS, Gray JD, Horwitz DA (2006) TGF-beta requires CTLA-4 early after T cell activation to induce FoxP3 and generate adaptive CD4+ CD25+ regulatory cells. J Immunol 176:3321–3329

Zheng Y, Chaudhry A, Kas A, deRoos P, Kim JM, Chu TT, Corcoran L, Treuting P, Klein U, Rudensky AY (2009) Regulatory T-cell suppressor program co-opts transcription factor IRF4 to control T(H)2 responses. Nature 458:351–356

Zheng Y, Josefowicz S, Chaudhry A, Peng XP, Forbush K, Rudensky AY (2010) Role of conserved non-coding DNA elements in the Foxp3 gene in regulatory T-cell fate. Nature 463:808–812

Zheng Y, Josefowicz SZ, Kas A, Chu TT, Gavin MA, Rudensky AY (2007) Genome-wide analysis of Foxp3 target genes in developing and mature regulatory T cells. Nature 445:936–940

Zhou G, Drake CG, Levitsky HI (2006) Amplification of tumor-specific regulatory T cells following therapeutic cancer vaccines. Blood 107:628–636

Zhou L, Lopes JE, Chong MM, Ivanov II, Min R, Victora GD, Shen Y, Du J, Rubtsov YP, Rudensky AY et al (2008) TGF-beta-induced Foxp3 inhibits T(H)17 cell differentiation by antagonizing RORgammat function. Nature 453:236–240

Ziegler SF (2006) FOXP3: of mice and men. Annu Rev Immunol 24:209–226

Chapter 12
Myeloid-Derived Suppressor Cells in Cancer

Wiaam Badn and Vincenzo Bronte

1 Introduction

Cancer patients and animals with experimental tumors develop immune dysfunctions associated with the presence of progressively growing tumors, which might explain the often disappointing results obtained in different immunotherapeutic trials. Several immunosuppressive mechanisms have been identified during the last 20 years (Zou 2005; Bronte and Mocellin 2009), and the inability of T cells to mount efficient antitumor immune responses has been demonstrated to depend, at least in part, on the suppressive action of myeloid-derived suppressor cells (MDSCs) accumulated at the tumor site, as well as in the peripheral lymphoid organs (Serafini et al. 2006; Dolcetti et al. 2008). This accumulation is directly correlated to increased tumor burden and inversely to T-cell proliferation and cytokine production (Li et al. 2004; Diaz-Montero et al. 2009; Donkor et al. 2009). During normal, steady-state hematopoiesis, immature myeloid precursors differentiate to granulocytes, monocytes/macrophages, and dendritic cells (DCs), which lack suppressive influence on the immune response and can prime antigen-specific T lymphocytes. On the other hand, during different pathological conditions including cancer, heightened myelopoiesis occurs in association with an arrest in the differentiation program, leading to the expansion and accumulation of myeloid cells at different maturation stages. These cells, referred as MDSCs, exert negative influence on antigen-primed T lymphocytes.

In addition to MDSCs, other cells from both the innate and adaptive arms of the immune system can regulate antitumor immunity, such as a subpopulation of cells with NK and T-cell surface markers called NKT cells (Terabe et al. 2000, 2003), and regulatory T (Treg) cells (Wang and Wang 2007). Emerging evidence suggests that crosstalk between different suppressive cells and regulatory mechanisms are

W. Badn • V. Bronte(✉)
Istituto Oncologico Veneto, Via Gattamelata 64, 35128 Padova, Italy
e-mail: enzo.bronte@unipd.it

required to maintain a firm suppressive network in cancer. Since MDSCs interfere with such interplay at various levels, in this chapter we will focus mostly on the origin, phenotype, and action of such cells.

2 Origin and Characterization

According to the current view about steady-state hematopoiesis, MDSCs are thought to originate in the bone marrow (or other myelogenous compartments such as the spleen in mice), from the common myeloid progenitor (CMP) and the granulocyte/macrophage progenitor (GMP), through a procedure including several commitment steps and intermediate progenitor stages (Fig. 12.1) (Iwasaki and Akashi 2007). The main problem in MDSCs field is that there is not a single marker, either a surface molecule or transcription factor, which can uniquely identify these cells. The markers originally identified in mice are the αM integrin CD11b and the molecule Gr-1 (Ly6G/Ly6C) (Bronte et al. 1998, 2000). Under normal conditions, CD11b$^+$Gr-1$^+$ cells constitute about 20–30% of the bone marrow cells and a small proportion of the

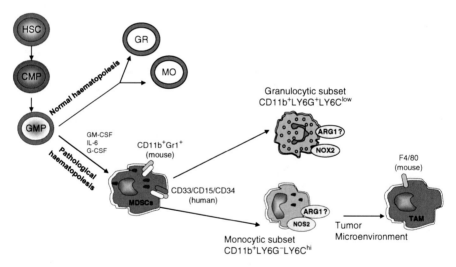

Fig. 12.1 MDSCs origin and differentiation. MDSCs are believed to originate from the common myeloid progenitor (CMP) and the granulocyte/monocytes progenitor (GMP) in the bone marrow as well as in the spleen in mice. During normal myelopoiesis, the GMP further differentiates to generate the distinct cell types, granulocytes and monocytes. However, during pathological myelopoiesis, such as inflammatory conditions including tumor progression, abnormal myelopoiesis occur, where increased levels of granulocyte-macrophage-CSF (GM-CSF) and interleukine 6 (IL-6) lead to the generation and expansion of MDSCs. Two different subset were identified, the granulocytic and the monocytic subset of MDSCs, when activated they seemed to use different mechanisms of suppression. The less suppressive granulocytic subset seemed to overproduce reactive oxygen species (ROS) following the upregulation of NADPH oxidase (NOX2). Interestingly, in our recent paper, we showed that in this population, upregulation of both ARG2 and NOS3 occurred. On the other hand the monocytic subset seemed to utilize the NOS2 and ARG1 in their suppressive activity

splenocytes (2–3%). However, during pathological conditions such as tumor growth, there is an expansion of CD11b$^+$Gr-1$^+$ cells in blood, lymph nodes, spleen, bone marrow, and tumor site. In the spleen, CD11b$^+$Gr-1$^+$ cells can expand to represent greater than 20% of total cells (Serafini et al. 2006; Gabrilovich and Nagaraj 2009). MDSCs encompass a large heterogeneous population including immature cells but also elements closer to mature leukocytes such as granulocytes and monocytes, sharing features such as the common myeloid origin and the suppressive activity on T cells.

3 MDSC Phenotype and Subsets

Recent data indicate that simple characterization of MDSCs as Gr-1$^+$CD11b$^+$ cells is not sufficient and does not correlate fully with their functional activity; therefore, different groups including ours put some efforts to exploit and characterize different MDSC subsets. Based on the expression of the epitopes recognized by anti-Gr-1 antibody (Ly6G and Ly6C), two MDSC subsets were identified: granulocytic and monocytic MDSCs (Gallina et al. 2006; Movahedi et al. 2008; Sawanobori et al. 2008; Youn et al. 2008).

3.1 Granulocytic MDSCs

The granulocytic subset of MDSCs possesses a CD11b$^+$Ly6G$^+$Ly6C^{low} phenotype. In different mouse tumor models, expansion of the granulocytic subset was shown to be greater than the monocytic fraction (Youn et al. 2008). The two MDSC subsets used different mechanisms to suppress T-cell functions. In one study, the activity of the granulocytic subset was dependent on the generation of reactive oxygen species (ROS) (Youn et al. 2008), which was triggered by increased expression of phagocytic NADPH oxidase NOX2, under the control of the STAT3 transcription factor (Corzo et al. 2009). However, in another study, the activity of this subset seemed to be independent of ROS production, since ROS-scavenging enzymes did not reverse the suppression (Movahedi et al. 2008). Although the suppressive mechanism was not identified, the suppressive activity required the production of IFN-γ by activated T cells, but was independent of STAT1 transcription factor and the enzyme inducible nitric oxide (NO) synthase (NOS2, further discussed below). Granulocytic MDSCs might also comprise cells supporting tumor neoangiogenesis by releasing the prokineticin 2 protein, also known as BV8 (Shojaei et al. 2007).

3.2 Monocytic MDSCs

The monocytic subset of MDSCs consists of mononuclear cells with CD11b$^+$Ly6G$^-$Ly6C^{hi} phenotype and was reported to be more suppressive than the granulocytic subset, mediating immunosuppressive activity via the NOS2-dependent pathway (Movahedi et al. 2008; Youn et al. 2008). We originally found that monocytic-like cells expressing higher levels of the alpha chain of the IL-4 receptor (IL-4Rα, CD124) compared with the granulocytic-like MDSCs and were responsible for suppression by integrating signals provided by both IFN-γ and IL-13 (Gallina et al. 2006). These cytokines regulated the activity of the inducible forms of L-arginine metabolizing enzymes, NOS2 and arginase 1 (ARG1). However, IL-4Rα is not a suitable marker for MDSC subset separation because of its weak intensity; moreover, in some tumor models, granulocytic-like MDSCs can express IL-4Rα at high levels (Youn et al. 2008). More recently, based on immunomagnetic sorting techniques, our group identified three subpopulations of MDSCs in the spleen of tumor-bearing hosts: CD11b$^+$/Gr-1^{high}, CD11b$^+$/Gr-1^{int}, and the CD11b$^+$/Gr-1^{low}. These populations exhibited different suppressive properties, with CD11b$^+$/Gr-1$^{int/low}$ being the most suppressive and the granulocytic CD11b$^+$/Gr-1^{high} the less suppressive population (Dolcetti et al. 2010). Again, the suppressive activity of these populations seemed to depend on NOS2 and ARG1 interplay.

Monocytic MDSCs give rise to immunosuppressive macrophages when cultured in vitro and it is likely that this subsets might represent a pool of circulating precursors that, after reaching the tumor microenvironment attracted by CCL2 chemokine, can differentiate and generate tumor-associated macrophages, which represent the prevalent infiltrating cells of tumor stroma (Sica and Bronte 2007; Movahedi et al. 2008; Sawanobori et al. 2008).

3.3 Human MDSCs

In humans, MDSCs were originally characterized as CD11b$^+$ cells expressing the common marker CD33 but lacking mature leukocyte markers and HLA-DR expression (Almand et al. 2001). However, in renal cell cancer patients, a population of activated CD15$^+$CD66b$^+$ granulocytes was shown to possess immune suppressive properties mostly dependent on ARG1 activity (Rodriguez et al. 2009); moreover, CD14$^+$HLA-DR$^{-/low}$ cells in peripheral blood mononuclear cells from hepatocellular carcinoma patients were shown to activate Treg lymphocytes in vitro (Hoechst et al. 2008). It appears that in humans and mice both granulocytic (CD15$^+$) and monocytic (CD14$^+$) cells circulating in blood of cancer patients can contain elements with distinct immunoregulatory properties, as we recently observed in patients with melanoma and colon cancer (Mandruzzato et al. 2009). Interestingly, similar to mouse studies, IL-4Rα/CD124 expression was increased in both populations.

4 Expansion and Activation

The expansion and activation of MDSCs are controlled by two main groups of factors. Tumor-derived factors (TDFs) produced by tumor cells themselves support the expansion of MDSCs through the stimulation of myelopoiesis

(Dolcetti et al. 2008). The second group of factors is produced mainly by activated T cells and tumor-associated stroma, and promotes the activation of the MDSC inhibitory program. TDF family consists of PGE2 prostaglandin, a product of the enzyme cyclooxygenase 2 (COX2), stem-cell factor (SCF), M-CSF, IL-6, granulocyte/macrophage colony-stimulating factor (GM-CSF), and vascular endothelial growth factor (VEGF) (Serafini et al. 2006; Sica and Bronte 2007; Talmadge 2007; Gabrilovich and Nagaraj 2009). These factors trigger several different signaling pathways in MDSCs that involve the signal transducer and activator of transcription (STAT) family of transcription factors. In particular, STAT3 was reported to regulate the expansion of MDSCs by stimulating myelopoiesis and inhibiting myeloid-cell differentiation, and by regulating MDSC survival by inducing the expression of Bcl-xl and cyclin D1 (Kortylewski et al. 2005; Kujawski et al. 2008). It is difficult to replicate entirely the effects of various TDFs in vitro and define the common denominator among TDFs that might induce MDSCs from bone marrow precursors. However, we recently found that GM-CSF in combination with either IL-6 or G-CSF promoted the rapid generation of highly immunosuppressive MDSCs from whole bone marrow. The effect of these cytokine combination was dependent on the upregulation of the transcription factor C/EBPβ. Indeed, the genetic knock out of C/EBPβ gene completely ablated the suppressive activity of MDSCs, both in vitro and in vivo (Marigo et al. 2010). Interestingly, G-CSF alone promoted the prevalent expansion of the less suppressive granulocytic subset Dolcetti et al. 2010.

The factors activating MDSCs involve production of cytokines such as IFN-γ, IL-4, IL-13, IL-10, and transforming growth factor-β (TGF-β), which activate distinct signaling pathways in MDSCs, mainly involving STAT1 and STAT6. STAT1 is the main transcription factor activated by IFN-γ and is involved in upregulation of NOS2 expression by MDSCs. Indeed, blockade of IFN-γ abolishes MDSC-mediated T-cell suppression (Movahedi et al. 2008). The effect of IFN γ was further confirmed in MDSCs isolated from $Stat1^{-/-}$ mice, which failed to inhibit T-cell activation, because they were not able to upregulate the expression of NOS2 (Movahedi et al. 2008). On the other hand, the binding of either IL-4 or IL-13 to IL-4Rα activates STAT6 signaling pathway (Rutschman et al. 2001), and the ligation of IL-4Rα results in the induction and upregulation of ARG1 in MDSCs (Bronte et al. 2003; Gallina et al. 2006; Junttila et al. 2008). The important role of IL-4Rα in inducing immunosuppressive activity on T cells was clearly demonstrated by analyzing the function of MDSCs in IL-4Rα knockout mice (Gallina et al. 2006). In agreement with these results, $STAT6^{-/-}$ mice immunologically rejected spontaneous metastatic mammary carcinoma and survived indefinitely when their primary tumors are removed, in part by preventing signaling through IL-4Rα and blocking the production of ARG1 by MDSCs (Sinha et al. 2005). Moreover, STAT6 pathway was also found to be involved in the IL-13-induced production of TGF-β by MDSCs in mice with sarcoma. Interestingly, in this model IL-13 was produced by type II NKT cells conditioned by tumor microenvironmental signals (Terabe et al. 2003), thus serving as one example of an immunosuppressive network in cancer.

5 Mechanisms of Suppressive Activity

5.1 ARG1

As mentioned above, high expression of the two enzymes metabolizing the amino acid L-arginine, NOS2 and ARG1, has been detected in MDSC subsets and causally related to their suppressive activity on T cells (Bronte and Zanovello 2005). ARG converts L-arg to urea and L-ornithine. Two distinct isoforms of ARG have been identified: ARG1 and ARG2. Besides its high expression in the liver as a component of the urea cycle, ARG1 expression is induced in mice myeloid cells in response to Th2-type cytokines and inflammatory signals, including IL-4, IL-13, TGF-β, and GM-CSF (Rodriguez and Ochoa 2008). Therefore, ARG1 has been implicated in promoting different immunological responses, with large effects on the induction of immune suppression (Fig. 12.2). High expression of ARG1 by MDSCs deplete L-arginine from the microenvironment, thereby inhibiting T-cell proliferation. Although the exact pathway by which ARG1 induces immune dysfunctions is still unclear, one mechanism has been suggested and involves decreased expression of the CD3ζ chain of the T-cell receptor on T cells, thereby impeding the function of these cells (Rodriguez et al. 2004). These observations were further confirmed in patients with renal cell carcinoma, suggesting a relevance of ARG1-mediated suppression in the clinical setting (Rodriguez et al. 2009). Increased ARG activation was also associated with H_2O_2 production, which in turn negatively regulated CD3ζ chain expression (Otsuji et al. 1996; Kusmartsev et al. 2004). In addition to its activity on the CD3ζ chain of T cells, the increased expression of ARG1 in MDSCs was shown to induce the development of naturally occurring, antigen-specific Treg cells in a B cell lymphoma model (Serafini et al. 2008). This is another feature employed by MDSCs to indirectly induce prolonged suppression. The presence of ARG1 in various MDSC subsets was recently demonstrated (Gabrilovich and Nagaraj 2009). However, our preliminary observations in ARG1-YFP reporter mice indicate its appearance in the Gr-1$^{int/low}$ subpopulations (Badn, unpublished data).

5.2 NOS2

In addition to ARG1, NOS2 also utilizes L-arginine, but generates NO and L-citrulline. Increased NOS2 activity in MDSCs from tumor-bearing hosts resulted in T-cell suppression, by modulating several features of T cell and antigen-presenting cells (APC) interplay, such as activation, proliferation, cytokine production, and induction of T-cell apoptosis (Fig. 12.2). The suppressive action of NO on T cells was clearly demonstrated using NOS2 inhibitors both in vitro and in vivo (De Santo et al. 2005; Badn et al. 2007a) in different tumor models. This effect was confirmed using MDSCs, isolated from NOS2 null mice, which lost their suppressive activity and did not inhibit T-cell proliferation (Mazzoni et al. 2002; Movahedi

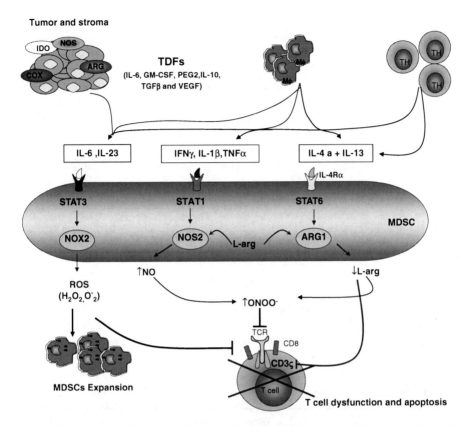

Fig. 12.2 Pathways regulating expansion and activation of MDSCs. Tumor-derived factors (TDFs) produced by tumor cells themselves support the expansion of MDSCs. PGE2 prostaglandin, a product of the enzyme cyclooxygenase 2 (COX2), interleukin 6, and 23 (IL-6, IL-23) trigger several different signaling pathways in MDSCs that involve the signal transducer and activator of transcription (STAT) family of transcription factors in particular STAT3. Activation of STAT3 induces the expression of NADPH oxidase (NOX2), which starts to generate high levels of ROS, that are both immunosuppressive for T cells as well as inhibit MDSCs maturation to functional antigen-presenting cells (APCs). On the other hand, activated T cells and tumor-associated stroma via production of cytokines such as IFNγ, IL-4, IL-13, and IL-10 (TGFα) promote the activation of MDSC, which activate signaling pathways mainly involving STAT1 and STAT6. STAT1 is the main transcription factor activated by IFNγ and is involved in the upregulation of NOS2 expression by MDSCs and production of NO. NO reacts with other oxidants such as super oxide and forms peroxynitrite (ONOO−). ONOO− causes nitration of tyrosine residues, which inhibit the activation-induced protein phosphorylation in T cells, resulting in T cell apoptosis. STAT6 on the other hand is activated following the binding of either IL-4 or IL-13 to IL-4R, which induces upregulation of ARG1 in MDSCs. High expression of ARG1 by MDSCs depletes L-arginine from the microenvironment, thereby decreasing the expression of the CD3 chain of the T-cell receptor on T cells, which blocks the function and proliferation of T cells. PGE2 in addition to its effect on MDSCs expansion has been reported to induce Treg, which might be an indirect effect mediated by ARG1 upregulation via PGE2

et al. 2008). NOS2 expression is triggered by Th1- and inflammatory cytokines such as interferons (IFN-γ in particular), IL-1, and tumor necrosis factor-α (TNF-α) produced by activated T cells. NO-mediated suppression requires cell–cell contact, is partly regulated by T-cell protein tyrosine phosphatase in myeloid cells, and blocks early events of IL-2 receptor signaling cascade in T cells, through a process requiring phosphorylation blockade of intracellular signaling proteins JAK3, STAT5, AKT, and ERK (Mazzoni et al. 2002; Dupuis et al. 2003). Interestingly, while ARG1 expression was detected in both granulocytic and monocytic MDSCs (at least considering as a whole findings in both mouse and human cells), NOS2-mediated suppressive pathway seems to be restricted to mouse monocytic MDSCs (Mazzoni et al. 2002; Bronte et al. 2003; Movahedi et al. 2008). Evidence of NO involvement in human MDSC-dependent suppression is still lacking.

It is still unclear why T cells are so vulnerable to NO-mediated cytotoxicity/cytostasis. One possible explanation is that NO has a high affinity for thiol compounds and reacts readily with glutathione (GSH) and forms S-nitrosoglutathione (GSNO), which serves later on as an NO donor. Interestingly, T cells express the enzyme gamma-glutamyl-transpeptidase on their surface. This enzyme breaks down extracellular GSNO to release NO (Henson et al. 1999). In addition to the direct inhibitory effects, NO can react with other oxidants such as super oxide, and generate reactive nitrogen species such as peroxynitrite. Peroxynitrites are powerful oxidants, and act by inducing posttranslational protein modifications, involving nitration and nitrosylation of tyrosine, cysteine, tryptophan, and methionine residues in the down-stream cascade of the T-cell receptor, which can ultimately result in T-cell apoptosis (Brito et al. 1999; Szabo et al. 2007). High levels of peroxynitrite was detected at sites of MDSC accumulation and associated with increased tumor burden (Bentz et al. 2000; Ekmekcioglu et al. 2000). The peroxynitrite activity on T cells was further highlighted very recently: nitration of the T-cell receptor and CD8 molecules was shown to cause altered recognition of the MHC-peptide complex by T cells and rendered them unresponsive to antigen-specific stimulation (Nagaraj et al. 2007).

5.3 NOX2

NOX2 is the catalytic subunit (also known as gp91phox) of NADPH oxidase, which generates high levels of ROS, following association with the cytosolic subunits (p47phox, p67phox, p40phox, and Rac) in the activated enzyme (Lambeth 2004). Increased levels of ROS (mostly H_2O_2) were detected at sites where MDSCs accumulated, both in cancer patients and in rodent tumor models (Mantovani et al. 2003; Szuster-Ciesielska et al. 2004; Corzo et al. 2009). NOX2 controls the increased ROS production in MDSCs (Kusmartsev et al. 2004; Corzo et al. 2009), a suppressive pathway apparently restricted to granulocytic MDSCs. This pathway is involved in a signaling cascade regulated by the STAT3 transcription factor (Corzo et al.

2009). ROS-mediated immunosuppression seems to be two-sided, relying on both T-cell inhibition as well as impairment of MDSC maturation to functional DCs or macrophages (Kusmartsev et al. 2004; Nefedova et al. 2004).

5.4 COX2

The metabolism of arachidonic acid is central during infection and inflammation as well as tumor progression. COX2, which catalyzes the production of PGE2, was shown to be overexpressed in several tumor types, and its expression correlated with poor prognosis (Gasparini et al. 2003). PGE2 affects various processes during tumor development including angiogenesis, invasiveness, inflammation, and immunosuppression (Dannenberg et al. 2001). The suppressive role of COX2 seems to be partly dependent on the inhibition of Th1-type and the stimulation of Th2-type responses. Indeed, treatment with COX2 inhibitor was reported to increase lymphocyte infiltration, IL-12, and IFN-γ levels, as well as to decrease IL-10 (Stolina et al. 2000). The role of COX2 in MDSCs seems to be indirect, and via induction of ARG1 in MDSC (Rodriguez et al. 2005). This mechanism might also be responsible for the observed role of COX2 in the induction of Treg cells via ARG1 upregulation (see below). In addition to its role via ARG1, it might synergize with NOS2 to induce immunosuppression. Indeed, in a glioma tumor model using a simultaneous COX and NOS2 inhibitor, enhanced immune responses were observed with increased survival in treated animals (Badn et al. 2007b).

6 Treg Cells and MDSC Interplay

The induction of Treg cells by MDSCs is a rather novel finding and might constitute an indirect mechanism by which MDSCs ensure a persistent tolerance in tumor-bearing hosts. Although, the exact mechanism mediating the induction of Treg cells is still not clear, both NOS2 and ARG1 have been implicated. In a colon carcinoma model, MDSCs were found to induce the expansion of CD4$^+$CD25$^+$Foxp3$^+$ Treg cells and suppress the expansion of effector CD4$^+$ T cells through a NOS-dependent pathway (Huang et al. 2006). On the other hand, in a B cell lymphoma model, MDSCs-induced proliferation of naturally occurring, antigen-specific CD4$^+$CD25$^+$Foxp3$^+$ Treg cells was blocked only by ARG inhibitors (Serafini et al. 2008). Moreover, COX2 activity and PGE2 production from MDSCs might contribute to generation and expansion of Treg cells in tumor-bearing hosts (Sharma et al. 2005a). This effect was mediated by PGE2 signaling through its receptors, EP2 and EP4, as the induction of Treg cells was reduced in EP4- and completely ablated in EP2-null mice. Furthermore, COX2 inhibition reduced the intra-tumoral levels of CD4$^+$CD25$^+$Foxp3$^+$ Treg cells and correlated with increased Th1-type cytokines

(Sharma et al. 2005b). However, since PGE2 controls the expression of ARG1, it might be possible that induction of Treg cells by PGE2 is indirectly mediated by ARG activity.

7 Conclusions: Therapeutic Targeting of MDSCs

The suppressive action of MDSCs, both in experimental models and in human cancers, can represent an obstacle to cancer immunotherapy. Thus, to achieve successful immunotherapy, approaches either converting or eliminating the suppressive features of MDSCs are needed. These strategies include inhibition of MDSC expansion, induction of their differentiation to mature cells, and inhibition of their suppressive activity, via targeting the factors involved in their suppressive machinery. Our group has focused on the inhibition of NOS2 and ARG1 enzyme activity, since these two enzymes, alone or in combination, mediate immune dysfunctions in several experimental tumor models. We found that nitroaspirin (NCX-4016) administration restored T-cell responsiveness in tumor-bearing mice by reducing both ARG and NOS activity in CD11b$^+$ suppressor cells and enhanced the efficacy of cancer vaccination (De Santo et al. 2005). Interestingly, nitroaspirin and novel compounds we have developed to control L-arginine metabolism also cause a dramatic reduction of peroxynitrite generation within the tumor microenvironment (De Santo et al. 2005 and unpublished results). Other groups have instead exploited the possibility of forcing MDSC differentiation toward more mature myeloid cells. Indeed administration of all-trans retinoic acid (ATRA, a variant of vitamin A metabolites) was shown to induce differentiation of MDSCs, which resulted in decreased numbers of MDSCs, and was correlated with increased T-cell responses and improved the efficacy of antitumor vaccine therapy (Kusmartsev et al. 2003). The mechanism by which ATRA induced the differentiation of MDSCs involved inhibition of ROS production in these cells. Studies with ATRA or nitroaspirin confirm the complexity of MDSC biology and suggest that a combination of different approaches might more effectively tackle their negative influence on the immune system against cancer.

Acknowledgments This work was supported by grants from the Italian Ministry of Health, Fondazione Cassa di Risparmio di Padova e Rovigo, Italian Association for Cancer Research (AIRC), Progetto Locale SUN 2008, Istituto Superiore Sanità -Alleanza Contro il Cancro (project no. ACC8), and Swedish Research Council (Vetenskapsrådet, VR).

References

Almand B, Clark JI et al (2001) Increased production of immature myeloid cells in cancer patients: a mechanism of immunosuppression in cancer. J Immunol 166(1):678–689

Badn W, Hegardt P et al (2007a) Inhibition of inducible nitric oxide synthase enhances anti-tumour immune responses in rats immunized with IFN-gamma-secreting glioma cells. Scand J Immunol 65(3):289–297

Badn W, Visse E et al (2007b) Postimmunization with IFN-gamma-secreting glioma cells combined with the inducible nitric oxide synthase inhibitor mercaptoethylguanidine prolongs survival of rats with intracerebral tumors. J Immunol 179(6):4231–4238

Bentz BG, Haines GK 3rd et al (2000) Increased protein nitrosylation in head and neck squamous cell carcinogenesis. Head Neck 22(1):64–70

Brito C, Naviliat M et al (1999) Peroxynitrite inhibits T lymphocyte activation and proliferation by promoting impairment of tyrosine phosphorylation and peroxynitrite-driven apoptotic death. J Immunol 162(6):3356–3366

Bronte V, Apolloni E et al (2000) Identification of a CD11b(+)/Gr-1(+)/CD31(+) myeloid progenitor capable of activating or suppressing CD8(+) T cells. Blood 96(12):3838–3846

Bronte V, Mocellin S (2009) Suppressive influences in the immune response to cancer. J Immunother 32(1):1–11

Bronte V, Serafini P et al (2003) IL-4-induced arginase 1 suppresses alloreactive T cells in tumor-bearing mice. J Immunol 170(1):270–278

Bronte V, Wang M et al (1998) Apoptotic death of CD8+ T lymphocytes after immunization: induction of a suppressive population of Mac-1+/Gr-1+ cells. J Immunol 161(10):5313–5320

Bronte V, Zanovello P (2005) Regulation of immune responses by L-arginine metabolism. Nat Rev Immunol 5(8):641–654

Corzo CA, Cotter MJ et al (2009) Mechanism regulating reactive oxygen species in tumor-induced myeloid-derived suppressor cells. J Immunol 182(9):5693–5701

Dannenberg AJ, Altorki NK et al (2001) Cyclo-oxygenase 2: a pharmacological target for the prevention of cancer. Lancet Oncol 2(9):544–551

De Santo C, Serafini P et al (2005) Nitroaspirin corrects immune dysfunction in tumor-bearing hosts and promotes tumor eradication by cancer vaccination. Proc Natl Acad Sci U S A 102(11):4185–4190

Diaz-Montero CM, Salem ML et al (2009) Increased circulating myeloid-derived suppressor cells correlate with clinical cancer stage, metastatic tumor burden, and doxorubicin-cyclophosphamide chemotherapy. Cancer Immunol Immunother 58(1):49–59

Dolcetti L, Marigo I et al (2008) Myeloid-derived suppressor cell role in tumor-related inflammation. Cancer Lett 267(2):216–225

Dolcetti L, Peranzoni E et al (2010) Hierarchy of immunosuppressive strength among myeloid-derived suppressor cell subsets is determined by GM-CSF. Eur J Immunol 40(1):22–35

Donkor MK, Lahue E et al (2009) Mammary tumor heterogeneity in the expansion of myeloid-derived suppressor cells. Int Immunopharmacol 9(7–8):937–948

Dupuis M, De Jesus Ibarra-Sanchez M et al (2003) Gr-1+ myeloid cells lacking T cell protein tyrosine phosphatase inhibit lymphocyte proliferation by an IFN-gamma- and nitric oxide-dependent mechanism. J Immunol 171(2):726–732

Ekmekcioglu S, Ellerhorst J et al (2000) Inducible nitric oxide synthase and nitrotyrosine in human metastatic melanoma tumors correlate with poor survival. Clin Cancer Res 6(12):4768–4775

Gabrilovich DI, Nagaraj S (2009) Myeloid-derived suppressor cells as regulators of the immune system. Nat Rev Immunol 9(3):162–174

Gallina G, Dolcetti L et al (2006) Tumors induce a subset of inflammatory monocytes with immunosuppressive activity on CD8+ T cells. J Clin Invest 116(10):2777–2790

Gasparini G, Longo R et al (2003) Inhibitors of cyclo-oxygenase 2: a new class of anticancer agents? Lancet Oncol 4(10):605–615

Henson SE, Nichols TC et al (1999) The ectoenzyme gamma-glutamyl transpeptidase regulates antiproliferative effects of S-nitrosoglutathione on human T and B lymphocytes. J Immunol 163(4):1845–1852

Hoechst B, Ormandy LA et al (2008) A new population of myeloid-derived suppressor cells in hepatocellular carcinoma patients induces CD4(+)CD25(+)Foxp3(+) T cells. Gastroenterology 135(1):234–243

Huang B, Pan PY et al (2006) Gr-1+ CD115+ immature myeloid suppressor cells mediate the development of tumor-induced T regulatory cells and T-cell anergy in tumor-bearing host. Cancer Res 66:1123–1131

Iwasaki H, Akashi K (2007) Myeloid lineage commitment from the hematopoietic stem cell. Immunity 26(6):726–740

Junttila IS, Mizukami K et al (2008) Tuning sensitivity to IL-4 and IL-13: differential expression of IL-4Ralpha, IL-13Ralpha1, and gammac regulates relative cytokine sensitivity. J Exp Med 205(11):2595–2608

Kortylewski M, Kujawski M et al (2005) Inhibiting Stat3 signaling in the hematopoietic system elicits multicomponent antitumor immunity. Nat Med 11(12):1314–1321

Kujawski M, Kortylewski M et al (2008) Stat3 mediates myeloid cell-dependent tumor angiogenesis in mice. J Clin Invest 118(10):3367–3377

Kusmartsev S, Cheng F et al (2003) All-trans-retinoic acid eliminates immature myeloid cells from tumor-bearing mice and improves the effect of vaccination. Cancer Res 63(15):4441–4449

Kusmartsev S, Nefedova Y et al (2004) Antigen-specific inhibition of CD8+ T cell response by immature myeloid cells in cancer is mediated by reactive oxygen species. J Immunol 172(2):989–999

Lambeth JD (2004) NOX enzymes and the biology of reactive oxygen. Nat Rev Immunol 4(3):181–189

Li Q, Pan PY et al (2004) Role of immature myeloid Gr-1+ cells in the development of antitumor immunity. Cancer Res 64(3):1130–1139

Mandruzzato S, Solito S et al (2009) IL4Ralpha+ myeloid-derived suppressor cell expansion in cancer patients. J Immunol 182(10):6562–6568

Mantovani G, Maccio A et al (2003) Antioxidant agents are effective in inducing lymphocyte progression through cell cycle in advanced cancer patients: assessment of the most important laboratory indexes of cachexia and oxidative stress. J Mol Med 81(10):664–673

Marigo I, Bosio E et al (2010) Tumor-induced tolerance and immune suppression depend on the C/EBPbeta transcription factor. Immunity 32(6):790–802

Mazzoni A, Bronte V et al (2002) Myeloid suppressor lines inhibit T cell responses by an NO-dependent mechanism. J Immunol 168(2):689–695

Movahedi K, Guilliams M et al (2008) Identification of discrete tumor-induced myeloid-derived suppressor cell subpopulations with distinct T cell-suppressive activity. Blood 111(8):4233–4244

Nagaraj S, Gupta K et al (2007) Altered recognition of antigen is a mechanism of CD8+ T cell tolerance in cancer. Nat Med 13(7):828–835

Nefedova Y, Huang M et al (2004) Hyperactivation of STAT3 is involved in abnormal differentiation of dendritic cells in cancer. J Immunol 172(1):464–474

Otsuji M, Kimura Y et al (1996) Oxidative stress by tumor-derived macrophages suppresses the expression of CD3 zeta chain of T-cell receptor complex and antigen-specific T-cell responses. Proc Natl Acad Sci U S A 93(23):13119–13124

Rodriguez PC, Ernstoff MS et al (2009) Arginase I-producing myeloid-derived suppressor cells in renal cell carcinoma are a subpopulation of activated granulocytes. Cancer Res 69(4):1553–1560

Rodriguez PC, Hernandez CP et al (2005) Arginase I in myeloid suppressor cells is induced by COX-2 in lung carcinoma. J Exp Med 202(7):931–939

Rodriguez PC, Ochoa AC (2008) Arginine regulation by myeloid derived suppressor cells and tolerance in cancer: mechanisms and therapeutic perspectives. Immunol Rev 222:180–191

Rodriguez PC, Quiceno DG et al (2004) Arginase I production in the tumor microenvironment by mature myeloid cells inhibits T-cell receptor expression and antigen-specific T-cell responses. Cancer Res 64(16):5839–5849

Rutschman R, Lang R et al (2001) Cutting edge: Stat6-dependent substrate depletion regulates nitric oxide production. J Immunol 166(4):2173–2177

Sawanobori Y, Ueha S et al (2008) Chemokine-mediated rapid turnover of myeloid-derived suppressor cells in tumor-bearing mice. Blood 111(12):5457–5466

Serafini P, Borrello I et al (2006) Myeloid suppressor cells in cancer: recruitment, phenotype, properties, and mechanisms of immune suppression. Semin Cancer Biol 16(1):53–65

Serafini P, Mgebroff S et al (2008) Myeloid-derived suppressor cells promote cross-tolerance in B-cell lymphoma by expanding regulatory T cells. Cancer Res 68(13):5439–5449

Sharma S, Yang SC et al (2005a) Tumor cyclooxygenase-2/prostaglandin E2-dependent promotion of FOXP3 expression and CD4+ CD25+ T regulatory cell activities in lung cancer. Cancer Res 65(12):5211–5220

Sharma S, Zhu L et al (2005b) Cyclooxygenase 2 inhibition promotes IFN-gamma-dependent enhancement of antitumor responses. J Immunol 175(2):813–819

Shojaei F, Wu X et al (2007) Bv8 regulates myeloid-cell-dependent tumour angiogenesis. Nature 450(7171):825–831

Sica A, Bronte V (2007) Altered macrophage differentiation and immune dysfunction in tumor development. J Clin Invest 117(5):1155–1166

Sinha P, Clements VK et al (2005) Interleukin-13-regulated M2 macrophages in combination with myeloid suppressor cells block immune surveillance against metastasis. Cancer Res 65(24):11743–11751

Stolina M, Sharma S et al (2000) Specific inhibition of cyclooxygenase 2 restores antitumor reactivity by altering the balance of IL-10 and IL-12 synthesis. J Immunol 164(1):361–370

Szabo C, Ischiropoulos H et al (2007) Peroxynitrite: biochemistry, pathophysiology and development of therapeutics. Nat Rev Drug Discov 6(8):662–680

Szuster-Ciesielska A, Hryciuk-Umer E et al (2004) Reactive oxygen species production by blood neutrophils of patients with laryngeal carcinoma and antioxidative enzyme activity in their blood. Acta Oncol 43(3):252–258

Talmadge JE (2007) Pathways mediating the expansion and immunosuppressive activity of myeloid-derived suppressor cells and their relevance to cancer therapy. Clin Cancer Res 13(18 Pt 1):5243–5248

Terabe M, Matsui S et al (2000) NKT cell-mediated repression of tumor immunosurveillance by IL-13 and the IL-4R-STAT6 pathway. Nat Immunol 1(6):515–520

Terabe M, Matsui S et al (2003) Transforming growth factor-beta production and myeloid cells are an effector mechanism through which CD1d-restricted T cells block cytotoxic T lymphocyte-mediated tumor immunosurveillance: abrogation prevents tumor recurrence. J Exp Med 198(11):1741–1752

Wang HY, Wang RF (2007) Regulatory T cells and cancer. Curr Opin Immunol 19(2):217–223

Youn JI, Nagaraj S et al (2008) Subsets of myeloid-derived suppressor cells in tumor-bearing mice. J Immunol 181(8):5791–5802

Zou W (2005) Immunosuppressive networks in the tumour environment and their therapeutic relevance. Nat Rev Cancer 5(4):263–274

Chapter 13
Myeloid-Derived Suppressive Cells and Their Regulatory Mechanisms in Cancer

Ge Ma, Ping-Ying Pan, and Shu-Hsia Chen

1 Introduction

1.1 Identification of MDSC

Myeloid-derived suppressor cells (MDSCs) were first described over 20 years ago in patients with cancer. Their functional importance in tumor progression and immune suppression has not been recognized until recently. In general, MDSCs are a heterogeneous population of immature myeloid cells (IMCs) that comprises myeloid progenitor cells, immature macrophages, immature granulocytes, and immature dendritic cells (DCs). They are present in an activated state that is characterized by increased production of reactive oxygen and nitrogen species (ROS and RNS), and arginase 1 (Arg1) (Corzo et al. 2009; Gabrilovich and Nagaraj 2009; Pan et al. 2008b). They are also potent suppressors of various T-cell functions (Huang et al. 2006).

1.2 Surface Makers and Subsets of MDSC

Because of their myeloid origin, MDSCs bear various markers of the myeloid lineage. In mice, the phenotype of MDSCs is $CD11b^+Gr-1^+$, which can be further

---

Ge Ma • P.-Y. Pan (✉)
Department of Gene and Cell Medicine, Mount Sinai School of Medicine,
1425 Madison Avenue, Room 13-02, New York, NY 10029-6574, USA
e-mail: ping-ying.pan@mssm.edu

S.-H. Chen
Department of Gene and Cell Medicine, Mount Sinai School of Medicine,
1425 Madison Avenue, Room 13-02, New York, NY 10029-6574, USA

Department of Surgery, Mount Sinai School of Medicine, 1425 Madison Avenue,
Room 13-02, New York, NY 10029-6574, USA

divided into two major subsets based on the differential expression of Ly6C and CD115: CD11b⁺Ly6G⁺Ly6C^{low}CD115⁻ granulocytic MDSCs and CD11b⁺Ly6G⁻Ly6C^{hi}CD115⁺ monocytic MDSCs (Huang et al. 2006; Movahedi et al. 2008). Unlike mouse MDSC, the human counterpart does not have a universal marker. Depending on the type of cancer, the reported phenotypes of human MDSCs include Lin⁻HLA-DR⁻CD33⁺ in renal cancer, neck and head cancer, breast cancer (Zea et al. 2005), CD11b⁺CD14⁻CD33⁺ in lung cancer (Mirza et al. 2006), and CD14⁺HLA-DR$^{-/low}$ in melanoma and hepatocellular carcinoma patients (Filipazzi et al. 2007; Hoechst et al. 2008). Additionally, a population of CD15⁺ cells of cancer patients has been described in the peripheral blood (Youn et al. 2008).

1.3 Expansion and Activation of MDSC

In healthy individuals, IMCs lack suppressive activity and are present in the bone marrow, but rarely found in secondary lymphoid organs. IMCs that are generated in the bone marrow quickly differentiate into mature granulocytes, monocytes/macrophages, or DCs upon entry into the periphery. Many pathological conditions, such as malignancy, infectious diseases, trauma, bone marrow transplantation, and some autoimmune diseases, can partially block the differentiation of IMCs into mature myeloid cells that can result in the expansion of the MDSC population. In cancer patients, accumulation of MDSCs in lymphoid organs and in tumors in response to various growth factors and cytokines is predominant.

Several cytokines and growth factors have been shown to be involved in MDSC expansion and activation in the cancer microenvironment. Factors that induce MDSC expansion include cyclooxygenase 2 (COX2), prostaglandins, stem-cell factor (SCF), M-CSF, IL-6, granulocyte/macrophage CSF (GM-CSF), and vascular endothelial growth factor (VEGF) (Table 13.1) (Bunt et al. 2007; Gabrilovich et al. 1998; Pan et al. 2008b; Serafini et al. 2004; Sinha et al. 2007b). Most of these factors trigger signaling pathways in MDSCs that converge on members of Janus kinase (JAK) family and signal transducer and activator of transcription 3 (STAT3). These signaling molecules are mainly involved in cell survival, proliferation, differentiation, and apoptosis. It has become clear that the suppressive activity of MDSCs requires not only factors that promote their expansion, but also factors that activate MDSCs. These factors include IFNγ, ligands of Toll-like receptors (TLRs), IL-4, IL-13, and transforming growth factor-β (TGF-β), which are produced mainly by activated T cells and tumor stromal cells, or as a result of tumor-cell death (Bronte et al. 2003; Gallina et al. 2006; Kusmartsev and Gabrilovich 2005; Movahedi et al. 2008; Sinha et al. 2005; Terabe et al. 2003). Activation of MDSCs by these factors leads to signaling of various pathways in MDSCs that involve STAT6, STAT1, and nuclear factor-κB (NF-κB) (Table 13.1).

Table 13.1 Cytokines and growth factors involved in MDSC expression and activation

Factor	Function	Signal
VEGF	Expansion	STAT3
GM-CSF	Expansion	STAT3
G-CSF	Expansion	STAT3
M-CSF	Expansion	STAT3
Pristaglandinns	Expansion	STAT3
IFNγ	Activation	STAT1
C5a	Activation	
SCF	Expansion	STAT3
S100A8 and S100A9	Expansion	NF-κB
TLRs	Activation	NF-κB
TGFβ	Activation	Smad
IL-1β	Activation	NF-kB
IL-6	Expansion	STAT3
IL-10	Expansion	STAT3
IL-12	Activation	STAT1

1.4 MDSC Accumulation, Chronic Inflammation, and Cancer

Accumulating evidence indicates that chronic inflammation is associated with tumor formation. The inflammatory response persists in the tumor microenvironment during tumor progression, which begins with ischemia followed by interstitial and cellular edema, appearance of immune cells and finally, growth of blood vessels and tissue repair. Various immune cells are present in the tumor including those mediating adaptive immunity, T lymphocytes, DC, and occasional B cells, as well as effectors of innate immunity, e.g., macrophages, polymorphonuclear leukocytes (PMN) and, rare occasion, natural killer (NK) cells (Whiteside 2008). These host immune cells as well as tumor cells produce a myriad of cytokines and growth factors, the combined effect of which mediates MDSC accumulation and activation. Early studies demonstrated that the inflammation-associated molecules VEGF and SCF were associated with the accumulation of MDSC and suggested that inflammation might facilitate immune suppression. Furthermore, proinflammatory cytokines IL-1β and IL-6 and the bioactive lipid PGE2 were shown to induce MDSC accumulation and activation. These studies suggest that an indirect mechanism by which inflammation promotes tumor progression is through the induction of MDSCs that suppress immune surveillance and antitumor immunity, thereby removing the barrier that impedes tumor growth.

2 Tumor Environment Factors for MDSC Expansion

2.1 Vascular Endothelial Growth Factor

VEGF, a secreted growth factor produced by many tumors, is crucial in the formation and maintenance of blood vessels and blood cells. In addition to its well-characterized role in angiogenesis, VEGF inhibits DC differentiation, inhibits T-cell formation, and most importantly, leads to the accumulation of functional MDSCs in naïve mice with chronic infusion of VEGF (Gabrilovich 2004; Gabrilovich et al. 1998; Melani et al. 2003; Yang et al. 2004). MDSC accumulation was shown to be dependent on signaling through VEGFR2, but not VEGFR1 (Huang et al. 2007). Further studies revealed that the accumulation of MDSCs in response to VEGFR2 signaling depends on VEGFR2-induced increases in GM-CSF production (Larrivee et al. 2005).

2.2 Stem Cell Factor

SCF is a growth factor important for the survival, proliferation, and differentiation of hematopoietic stem cells and other hematopoietic progenitor cells. It binds to the c-kit receptor (CD117) to induce signaling; thus it is also known as kit ligand. Studies have shown that SCF is highly expressed in several human and murine tumors. Mice bearing SCF knockdown tumors or tumor-bearing mice treated with anti-c-kit blocking antibodies exhibited a significant reduction in MDSC expansion. Interestingly, the blockade of SCF also led to a reduction in the suppressive function of MDSCs (Pan et al. 2008b).

2.3 IL-1β

IL-1β induced accumulation of MDSC, increased levels of ROS and enhanced suppressive activity against $CD4^+$ and $CD8^+$ T cells. IL-1β induced MDSC had also longer life in vivo than MDSC induced in less inflammatory environments (Bunt et al. 2006; Song et al. 2005; Voronov et al. 2003). In addition to increasing the levels of MDSC, IL-1β is important in the crosstalk between MDSC and macrophages through the LPS-TLR4 pathway and MyD88 pathway, which increases secretion of IL-10 and IL-12 in the tumor environment and further activates macrophage function (Delano et al. 2007). Therefore, TLRs differentially regulate MDSC accumulation, and activation through TLR4 is critical for MDSC-mediated exacerbation of a tumor-promoting type 2 phenotype that favors tumor progression (Bunt et al. 2009).

2.4 Cyclooxygenase (COX)-2-Dependent PGE2

Cyclooxygenase (COX) 2 is the inducible isoform of rate-limiting enzymes involved in the synthesis of PGE2. COX2-dependent PGE2 (COX2/PGE2) is abundantly produced by inflammatory cells and increased in numerous disease states. PGE2 and COX-2 are mainly produced by many tumors and they are major contributors to the inflammatory tumor milieu (Alleva et al. 1993; Taketo 1998a, b). Tumor-infiltrating macrophages also produce PGE2, further amplifying inflammation at the tumor site. In addition to its direct tumor promoting effect, PGE2 was identified as an inducer of MDSC. Co-culture of E prostanoid agonists induced mouse c-kit$^+$ bone marrow precursor cells to be differentiated into suppressive Gr-1$^+$CD11b$^+$ MDSC. Mouse MDSC expresses all of the four PGE2 receptors (EP1–4). Moreover, tumor-bearing mice, deficient in EP-2, displayed reduced tumor growth and their MDSCs were less suppressive, compared with MDSC from wild-type mice. Therefore, elevated levels of PGE2 promote tumor progression through nonimmune mechanisms and through the induction of MDSC expansion that inhibits antitumor immunity (Sinha et al. 2007b; Rodriguez et al. 2005).

2.5 S100A8 and S100A9

The S100A8 and S100A9 proteins are members of a large family of proteins that includes inflammatory and noninflammatory molecules. Heterodimeric S100A8/A9 complexes are calcium-binding proteins that are released by neutrophils and activated monocytes. Several lines of evidence demonstrate that S100A9 proteins regulate the accumulation and suppressive functions of MDSC (Foell et al. 2007; Hiratsuka et al. 2006). S100A9 mediates these effects via at least two mechanisms: (1) they block the differentiation of myeloid precursors into DC and macrophages through a STAT3-dependent mechanism; and (2) they chemoattract MDSC to tumor sites through a NF-κB-dependent pathway. Unlike the other mediators, MDSCs also produce S100A8/A9 proteins, providing an autocrine feedback loop that sustains the accumulation and retention of MDSC while concomitantly chemoattracting additional proinflammatory mediators (Cheng et al. 2008; Sinha et al. 2008).

2.6 C5a

In addition to its classical role in antibody-mediated cell lysis, the complement system is a key player in innate immunity against infection and in inflammatory reactions. C5a, also known as anaphylatoxin, and C3a have inherent inflammatory activity, are chemoattractants, and localize to endothelial cells within solid tumors.

Recent studies using C5a receptor-deficient mice revealed that C5a also facilitated tumor progression and that it mediated its effects by binding to C5a receptors on MDSC. C5a increased the migration of granulocytic/neutrophil-like MDSC, but not monocytic MDSC, into solid tumors and peripheral lymphoid organs. It also increased the expression of ROS and RNS in monocytic, but not granulocytic/neutrophil-like, MDSC. Both of these activities resulted in MDSCs that were more immunosuppressive (Guo and Ward 2005; Markiewski et al. 2008; Markiewski and Lambris 2007).

3 Role of Myeloid-Derived Suppressor Cells in Promotion of Tumor Growth and in Immune Suppression Associated with Tumor

MDSCs, a major suppressor cell type in the tumor microenvironment, can suppress antitumor responses through multiple mechanisms (Fig. 13.1) and promote tumor progression directly. These include induction of T-cell anergy, Treg induction, modulation of the tumor environment, and promotion of tumor angiogenesis. Many factors produced by MDSC are involved in MDSC-mediated immune suppression. Moreover, through crosstalk with other immune cells, such as T cells, NK cells, Treg cells, and macrophages, MDSCs play a critical role in maintaining the suppressive and tumor-promoting characteristics of the tumor microenvironment.

3.1 Arg1 and iNOS

Arg1 and inducible nitric oxide (NO) synthase (iNOS) were the first identified effectors produced by MDSC in cancer. Further studies have demonstrated the suppressive activity of MDSCs is associated with the metabolism of L-arginine. L-Arginine serves as a substrate of iNOS (which generates NO) and Arg1 (which converts L-arginine into urea and L-ornithine) (Bronte and Zanovello 2005; Rodriguez and Ochoa 2008). MDSCs express high levels of both Arg1 and iNOS upon stimulation with IL-4/IL-13 and IFNγ, respectively. A direct role of both enzymes in the inhibition of T-cell function is well established. Recent data suggests that there is a close correlation between the availability of L-arginine and the capacity of T-cell proliferation (Ochoa et al. 2007; Rodriguez et al. 2005). The increased activity of Arg1 in MDSCs leads to enhanced arginine catabolism, which depletes this nonessential amino acid from the microenvironment. The shortage of L-arginine inhibits T-cell proliferation through several mechanisms, including decreasing the expression of CD3 δ-chain and preventing the upregulation of expression of the cell cycle regulators cyclin D3 and cyclin-dependent kinase (Bingisser et al. 1998; Harari and Liao 2004; Rodriguez et al. 2002, 2007; Taheri et al. 2001). NO suppresses T-cell function through a number of mechanisms that involve the

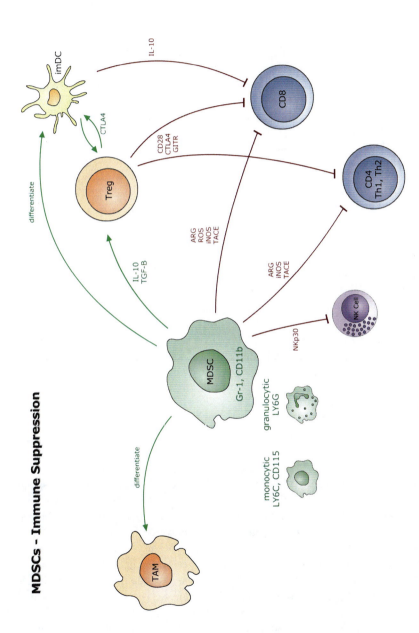

Fig. 13.1 Immune suppression mechanisms mediated by MDSC. MDSCs can suppress immune responses directly through expressions of suppressive cytokines (e.g., IL-10, and TGF-β) and enzymes (e.g., iNOS, Arg1, and TACE) as well as indirectly through Treg expansion and crosstalk with macrophages

inhibition of JAK3 and STAT5 function in T cells, the inhibition of MHC class II expression and the induction of T-cell apoptosis (Rivoltini et al. 2002).

3.2 ROS

ROS is another important factor that contributes to the suppressive activity of MDSCs. Increased production of ROS has emerged to be one of the main characteristics of MDSCs from both tumor-bearing mice and patients with cancer (Agostinelli and Seiler 2006; Kusmartsev et al. 2004, 2005; Mantovani et al. 2003; Schmielau and Finn 2001; Szuster-Ciesielska et al. 2004; Waris and Ahsan 2006; Youn et al. 2008). Inhibition of ROS production by MDSCs isolated from tumor-bearing mice and cancer patients completely abrogated the suppressive effect of these cells *in vitro*. Interestingly, the ligation of integrins that were expressed on the surface of MDSCs was shown to contribute to the increased ROS production following the interaction of MDSCs with T cells. In addition, several known tumor-derived factors, such as TGF-β, IL-3, IL-6, IL-10, platelet-derived growth factor (PDGF), and GM-CSF, can induce the production of ROS by MDSC (Sauer et al. 2001).

Recent findings indicate that different subsets of MDSCs might use different mechanisms to suppress T-cell proliferation. As described earlier, two main subsets of MDSCs have been identified, granulocytic and monocytic subsets. Granulocytic MDSCs were found to express high levels of ROS and low levels of NO, whereas the monocytic subset expressed low levels of ROS and high levels of NO; both subsets expressed Arg1. Interestingly, both MDSC subsets suppressed antigen-specific T-cell proliferation to an equal extent despite having different mechanisms of action (Youn et al. 2008).

3.3 *Peroxynitrite*

More recently, peroxynitrite has been shown to be a crucial mediator for suppression of T-cell function by MDSC. Peroxynitrite is a product of a chemical reaction between NO and superoxide anion, and is one of the most powerful oxidants produced in the body. It induces the nitration and nitrosylation of the amino acids cysteine, methionine, tryptophan, and tyrosine (Vickers et al. 1999). Increased levels of peroxynitrite are present at sites where MDSCs and inflammatory cells accumulate, including sites of ongoing immune reactions. In addition, high levels of peroxynitrite are associated with tumor progression in many types of cancer (Bentz et al. 2000; Cobbs et al. 2003; Ekmekcioglu et al. 2000; Kinnula et al. 2004; Nakamura et al. 2006), an effect that has been linked with T-cell unresponsiveness. Peroxynitrite production by MDSCs during direct contact with T cells results in nitration of the T-cell receptor and CD8 molecules, which alters the specific peptide binding of the T cells and rendered them unresponsive to antigen-specific stimulation (Nagaraj et al. 2007).

3.4 MDSC Crosstalk with Macrophages

Crosstalk between MDSCs and macrophages is one of the mechanisms by which MDSCs facilitate tumor progression (Sinha et al. 2007a). The consequence of crosstalk is a decrease in production of IL-12 by macrophages, leading to a preferential development of the tumor-promoting type 2 macrophage (M2) phenotype. MDSC-mediated down-regulation of macrophage production of IL-12 is dependent on IL-10 expression by MDSC. More recently, it was shown that IL-1β induced inflammation enhanced the suppressive phenotype of MDSC and crosstalk between MDSC and macrophages by signaling through the TLR4 pathway (Bunt et al. 2009). MDSCs from mice bearing 4T1 tumors expressing IL-1β (4T1/IL-1β) produced a significantly higher level of IL-10 upon co-culture with classically activated macrophages when compared to those isolated from mice bearing parental tumors. Moreover, MDSCs from heightened inflammatory environments (i.e., those from BALB/c mice with 4T1/IL-1β tumors) and activated with LPS and IFNγ in the absence of macrophages produced significantly more IL-10 than MDSCs from less inflammatory environments (i.e., those from BALB/c mice with 4T1 tumors). Treatment with LPS and IFNγ increased CD14 expression on MDSC, but did not induce MDSC differentiation to macrophages or DC. Interestingly, inflammation (treatment with LPS and IFNγ) increased CD14 expression on MDSC and enhanced the ability of MDSC to secrete IL-10 and down-regulate IL-12 production by macrophages through a LPS/TLR4-dependent pathway in MDSC. Therefore, in addition to the direct effect of TLR4 activation in MDSC, which enhances suppression of antitumor immunity, the increase in CD14 expression on MDSC enables crosstalk with TLR4 on macrophages, thereby skewing them toward the pro-angiogenic and tumor-promoting M2 phenotype.

3.5 Treg Induction

Considerable evidence exists in support of a link between MDSCs and Tregs. MDSC-mediated Treg induction has been demonstrated *in vitro* and in tumor-bearing mice (Huang et al. 2006). Further supporting evidence comes from the correlation of decreased Treg population with decreased MDSCs in tumor-bearing mice treated with anti-c-kit blocking antibody or sunitinib malate, a inhibitor of c-kit (Ozao-Choy et al. 2009), and in mice bearing SCF knockdown tumors (Pan et al. 2008b). MDSC-mediated Treg induction requires the activation of tumor-specific T cells, the presence of IFNγ and IL-10 (Huang et al. 2006), the expression of cytotoxic lymphocyte antigen 4 (CTLA4) and Arg1 by MDSCs (Serafini et al. 2008; Yang et al. 2006). MDSCs may induce Treg expansion through the production of cytokines, direct cell–cell interaction, or both. Increasing evidence supports that Treg induction by MDSCs requires direct cell–cell contact and antigen-presentation. MDSCs isolated from mice bearing A20 B-cell lymphoma transfected with influenza hemagglutinin (HA) as surrogate tumor antigen were able to present antigen to HA-specific Treg, thereby expanding tumor-specific Treg (Serafini et al. 2008).

Furthermore, the expression of co-stimulatory molecule CD40 on MDSC, which is significantly enhanced upon IFNγ stimulation, is required for MDSC mediated T-cell suppression and activation of tumor-specific Tregs. MDSCs derived from CD40 deficient mice, lost the capacity to induce T-cell tolerance and Treg expansion *in vivo* (Pan et al. 2010). Taken together, these studies support the notion that MDSC-mediated Treg expansion requires antigen-presentation by MDSC and engagement of CD40 on MDSCs with CD40L on Treg.

3.6 Angiogenesis

MDSC is also an important regulator of tumor angiogenesis. They are able to promote tumor angiogenesis not only by releasing matrix metalloproteinase 9 (MMP9), known to promote tumor angiogenesis by regulating the bioavailability of VEGF, but also by directly differentiating into endothelial cells and incorporating into tumor blood vessels (Yang et al. 2004). Furthermore, anti-VEGF refractoriness is associated with the ability of tumor cells to recruit $CD11b^+Gr-1^+$ MDSCs. Recruitment of these myeloid cells is also sufficient to confer resistance to anti-VEGF treatment (Shojaei et al. 2007). Taken together, these findings point to a role played by MDSCs in tumor angiogenesis, apart from their role in maintaining T-cell tolerance in the tumor-bearing host, as a tumor escape mechanism (Noonan et al. 2008).

3.7 TNF-α Converting Enzyme (TACE)

TNF-α converting enzyme (TACE), also known as a disintegrin and a metalloproteinase domain 17 (ADAM17), is a metalloproteinase that plays a pivotal role in the cleavage and activation of membrane-anchored receptor ligands. A recent study provides evidence that MDSCs likely down-regulate L-selectin through expression of TACE on their plasma membrane (Hanson et al. 2009). Therefore, MDSCs may down-regulate L-selectin expression on naïve T cells, thereby decreasing their ability to home to sites where they would be activated.

4 Strategies of Prevention of Immune Suppression Associated with Myeloid-Derived Suppressor Cells in Cancer Immunotherapy

4.1 MDSCs Limit Immunotherapy Outcome in Cancer

The immune system can recognize and eliminate transformed tumor cells. In addition to preventing clinically apparent cancer through immune surveillance, the immune system has the capacity to eradicate established tumors. This is the basic concept of immunotherapy. Various methods to enhancing antitumor immunity have been utilized in cancer immunotherapy. T cells and NK cells are recognized as the major antitumor effector cells. Therefore, tremendous efforts have been devoted to determine ways to enhance their tumor killing activity. Adoptive T cell transfer has been used in treatment of metastatic melanomas. Furthermore, immune-enhancing approaches, such as the use of IL-2, IFNα, IFNγ, IL-12, and 41BBL, and blockade of negative co-stimulator molecules, such as CTLA-4 and PD1, have been attempted (Ozao-Choy et al. 2009; Finke et al. 2008; Ko et al. 2009; Rabinovich et al. 2007; Wang and Wang 2007). However, the success of immune-based cancer therapies has been limited due to immune tolerance associated with malignancy. Tumor tissue is an immune suppressive environment. Several tumor-produced molecules, including tumor-derived gangliosides, TGFβ, COX2, and PGE2, are implicated in T-cell suppression. Importantly, tumors also promote the accumulation of immune cells that are suppressive to effector T cells. The most common of these include Tregs and MDSCs, which are suppressor cells that reduce the efficacy of cancer immune therapy.

Antiangiogenesis is another major strategy in cancer immune therapy. Although antiangiogenesis agents bevacizumab, sunitinib, and sorafenib have achieved relative success in the setting of aggressive metastatic tumors such as renal cell carcinoma (RCC), the clinical responses produced are short-lived in many patients (Shojaei and Ferrara 2007). Antiangiogenesis drugs stabilize tumor growth in most patients and shrink tumors in some; however, all patients eventually have disease progression after treatment, usually within months (Miller et al. 2005). This eventual disease progression is thought to reflect an adaptive response to drugs by tumors, which allows for "evasive resistance" to angiogenesis inhibitors (Kerbel 2005). Experimental evidence in humans and mice supports the theory that, in the presence of angiogenesis inhibitors, tumors up-regulate alternative proangiogenic signaling pathways, recruit MDSC that negate the need for VEGF signaling, increase pericyte coverage of vasculature, and finally, activate invasive and metastatic activities that provide access to normal tissue vasculature.

4.2 Effectors Involved in MDSC Metabolite as a Target in Immunotherapy

As described previously, the tumor microenvironment contains multiple cytokines and growth factors that are involved in MDSC expansion and activation. At the same time, MDSC produces Arg1, iNOS, ROS, NOS, and suppressive cytokines that further inhibit antitumor immune response and promote tumor growth. These pathways might offer potential targets for therapeutic interventions (Bronte and Mocellin 2009).

The inducible isoform of the cyclooxygenase enzyme, COX2, which is overexpressed in multiple tumor types and, also through synthesis of the arachidonic acid derivative prostaglandin-E2 (PGE2), affects various processes that are relevant to tumorigenesis and malignant progression, such as apoptosis, angiogenesis, and invasiveness. PGE2 also plays an important role in MDSC expansion and activation. Several selective COX2 inhibitors (e.g., celecoxib and rofecoxib) are already available for clinical use. These drugs have been tested in phase 2 clinical trials in combination with chemotherapeutic agents in patients with different carcinomas and, for the most part, have shown additional clinical benefit beyond what has been observed with chemotherapy alone (Csiki et al. 2005; Ferrari et al. 2006). However, the mechanisms of action responsible for the effect remain undetermined. Targeting the family of prostaglandin receptors serves as an alternative means to block the PGE2 pathway in cancer. Several small-molecule antagonists of EP2 and/or EP4 are currently in development for various indications.

MDSCs and tumor-associated macrophages (TAMs), rather than the tumor cells themselves, are an important primary source of tumor-associated Arg activity. In addition to its direct effects on tumor proliferation, Arg activity has also been shown to be associated with MDSC-mediated immune suppression. Treatment with the Arg inhibitor N-hydroxynor-L-Arg (nor-NOHA) impairs subcutaneous tumor formation by Lewis lung carcinoma cells in syngeneic animals but not in severe combined immunodeficient mice, which is indicative of an immune-mediated effect (Rodriguez et al. 2004). MDSCs were shown to up-regulate both Arg1 and NOS2 pathways simultaneously and use them in conjunction to suppress antigen-activated T cells. Gr-1$^+$CD11b$^+$ MDSCs that are isolated from NOS2-null mice do not inhibit T-cell proliferation, suggesting that NO is also an essential component of MDSC-mediated immune suppression. Combination of the Arg inhibitor N-hydroxyl-Arg with the NOS inhibitor NG-monomethyl-arginine (L-NMMA) can restore the expansion and cytolytic function of T cells infiltrating human prostate cancer in an organ culture model (Bronte et al. 2005). Treatment of tumor-bearing animals with nitroaspirin increased the number of tumor-specific CTLs and prolonged patient survival when combined with a tumor vaccine (De Santo et al. 2005).

Given the ability of phosphodiesterase 5 (PDE5) inhibitors to inhibit Arg1 and NOS2 activity in MDSCs, these compounds have been tested as potential adjuvants for immunotherapy. PDE5 inhibition reverted tumor induced immunosuppressive mechanisms, restored immune surveillance in mice, and allowed the spontaneous generation of a measurable antitumor immune response that significantly delayed tumor progression in the absence of any immunotherapeutic intervention. Moreover, by removing MDSC-mediated suppression, PDE5 inhibitors also enhanced intratumoral T-cell infiltration and activation, and synergized with the antitumor efficacy of adoptive T-cell therapy (Serafini et al. 2006). These results have significant clinical implications, since PDE5 inhibitors are safe and effective agents already used in the clinic.

4.3 MDSC-Mediated T-Cell Tolerance as a Target in Immunotherapy

MDSCs are accumulated in tumor-bearing mice and patients and can induce Treg cells in tumor-bearing mice and cancer patients. Several strategies have been employed to block the suppressive functions and Treg expansion mediated by MDSC.

One strategy has been to deplete MDSC *in vivo*; however, no specific marker for MDSC depletion is currently available. Although Gr-1 has been used as a marker to deplete this population in mice, this strategy cannot be used in the clinic due to the lack of an equivalent marker for human MDSC (Pekarek et al. 1995). Nonetheless, various groups have shown that depletion of MDSC can improve tumor killing and decrease immune tolerance in animal models (Seung et al. 1995).

Other strategies include attempts to limit the accumulation of MDSC in the tumor-bearing host. Researchers have found that tumor-derived SCF appears to be critical in promoting MDSC expansion and accumulation. Mice with SCF-silenced tumor cells have a significantly decreased number of MDSCs and a less tolerogenic tumor microenvironment is associated with SCF silencing in tumor cells. In addition, treatment of tumor-bearing mice with anti-c-kit (SCF receptor) blocking monoclonal antibodies in conjunction with immune-based therapy can significantly improve the long-term survival rate of large tumor-bearing mice (Pan et al. 2008b). Small molecule inhibitors that block c-kit signaling are currently available for the treatment of gastrointestinal stromal tumors and might be useful for the purpose of reversing MDSC mediated immune suppression (Rubin et al. 2007; von Mehren 2006).

Other pharmaceutical small molecule drugs also provide an important strategy to block the function of MDSC. Treatment of sildenafil reduces the MDSC-mediated suppressive machinery of Arg1 and NO, enhances intratumoral T cell infiltration and activation, and reduces tumor outgrowth in tumor-bearing mice. Other studies show that aspirin derivatives may also reduce the suppressive activities of MDSC (De Santo et al. 2005).

Since MDSCs exhibit an immature phenotype of the myeloid lineage, strategies to promote differentiation of this cell population may also prevent Treg development and MDSC suppressive functions. MDSCs can differentiate into monocyte/macrophages and DCs under specific culture conditions (Bronte et al. 2000; Li et al. 2004). MDSCs can also differentiate into $CD11c^+$ cells that express CD80 and I-A/I-E (MHC class II) in the presence of recombinant murine granulocyte macrophage colony-stimulating factor (GM-CSF). Furthermore, intratumoral gene delivery of GM-CSF not only promoted the differentiation of carboxyfluoroscein succinimidyl ester (CFSE)-labeled MDSCs into $CD11c^+$ cells with the characteristics of mature DCs ($CD80^+$, $I-A/I-E^+$), but also enhanced innate NK and adaptive cytolytic T-cell activities in mice treated with interleukin (IL)-12 and anti-4-1BB combination therapy (Pan et al. 2004). More importantly, intratumoral delivery of GM-CSF and IL-12 genes in combination with 4-1BB costimulation greatly improved the long-term survival rate of mice bearing large tumors and eradicated the untreated existing hepatic tumor (Li et al. 2004).

All-trans retinoic acid (ATRA) as well as other cytokine regimens including treatment with IFNγ plus TNF (tumor necrosis factor) has also been used to induce the differentiation of MDSCs (Kusmartsev et al. 2003; Young et al. 1990). These strategies appear to be promising in animal models; however, further translation and proof of their ability to overcome immune tolerance and thus improve the immune therapeutic outcome in cancer patients needs to be thoroughly investigated (Pan et al. 2008a).

4.4 Tregs as a Major Target in Immunotherapy

Blockade of MDSC induced Treg expansion in tumor hosts can also be used to disrupt tumor-induced immune tolerance. The peripheral inducible Treg is the major subtype of Treg found at tumor sites and plays a key role in immune suppression in cancer, in contrast to the natural Treg that controls autoimmune disease. Studies have found suppression of tumor growth, enhancement of antitumor vaccine activity, and increased immune response in Treg depleted mice and in humans (Onizuka et al. 1999; Shimizu et al. 1999; Steitz et al. 2001). Therefore, one strategy to decrease immune tolerance has been to eliminate Tregs in patients.

An IL-2 diphtheria toxin fusion protein, ONTAK, has been developed that can deplete Tregs. In addition, depletion of $CD25^+$ Treg by specific antibodies has been explored. Mahnke et al. have tested ONTAK in patients and have found that treatment with ONTAK depletes Treg cells in the peripheral blood (while maintaining other cell populations), is well tolerated, and increases circulating peptide-specific $CD8^+$ cells in about 90% of vaccinated melanoma patients (Mahnke et al. 2007). Another group has studied the effects of ONTAK combined with a recombinant poxviral vaccine in a murine model. The results showed that injection of ONTAK 1 day prior to vaccination enhanced antigen-specific T-cell responses above the levels induced by vaccination alone, thus showing an advantage in combination therapy (Mahnke et al. 2007). It remains to be seen whether this treatment will have similar and long-term effects in humans. Other innovative strategies to decrease the Treg population have been to target the suppressive functions of Treg. Poly G oligonucleotides has been used to reverse the suppression mediated by Treg via TLR8 and MyD88 pathways (Peng et al. 2005). However, the length of time that poly G needs to be used so that Treg suppressive functions can be continuously blocked remains a critical issue and requires further investigation and development.

5 Conclusion

MDSCs are a heterogeneous population of myeloid cells that comprises myeloid progenitor cells, immature macrophages, immature granulocytes, and immature DCs, which bear common markers and are identified as $Gr-1^+CD11b^+$ cells in mice. But human MDSCs express various myeloid markers, depending on the tumor type and currently cannot be identified by a universal marker. Tumor inflammatory environment and growth factors maintain MDSC expansion and activation characterized by the increased production of ROS, NOS, and Arg1. MDSCs not only employ various mechanisms to directly and indirectly suppress antitumor responses, but also promote tumor angiogenesis that further facilitates tumor growth. All of these tumor-promoting mechanisms mediated by MDSCs are potential targets for intervention. However, intervention with MDSC-associated pro-tumor activity alone may not achieve satisfactory therapeutic outcome and should be used with other immune-based therapies.

References

Agostinelli E, Seiler N (2006) Non-irradiation-derived reactive oxygen species (ROS) and cancer: therapeutic implications. Amino Acids 31:341–355

Alleva DG, Burger CJ, Elgert KD (1993) Tumor growth increases Ia- macrophage synthesis of tumor necrosis factor-alpha and prostaglandin E2: changes in macrophage suppressor activity. J Leukoc Biol 53:550–558

Bentz BG, Haines GK 3rd, Radosevich JA (2000) Increased protein nitrosylation in head and neck squamous cell carcinogenesis. Head Neck 22:64–70

Bingisser RM, Tilbrook PA, Holt PG, Kees UR (1998) Macrophage-derived nitric oxide regulates T cell activation via reversible disruption of the Jak3/STAT5 signaling pathway. J Immunol 160:5729–5734

Bronte V, Mocellin S (2009) Suppressive influences in the immune response to cancer. J Immunother 32:1–11

Bronte V, Zanovello P (2005) Regulation of immune responses by L-arginine metabolism. Nat Rev Immunol 5:641–654

Bronte V, Apolloni E, Cabrelle A, Ronca R, Serafini P, Zamboni P, Restifo NP, Zanovello P (2000) Identification of a CD11b(+)/Gr-1(+)/CD31(+) myeloid progenitor capable of activating or suppressing CD8(+) T cells. Blood 96:3838–3846

Bronte V, Serafini P, De Santo C, Marigo I, Tosello V, Mazzoni A, Segal DM, Staib C, Lowel M, Sutter G et al (2003) IL-4-induced arginase 1 suppresses alloreactive T cells in tumor-bearing mice. J Immunol 170:270–278

Bronte V, Kasic T, Gri G, Gallana K, Borsellino G, Marigo I, Battistini L, Iafrate M, Prayer-Galetti T, Pagano F et al (2005) Boosting antitumor responses of T lymphocytes infiltrating human prostate cancers. J Exp Med 201:1257–1268

Bunt SK, Sinha P, Clements VK, Leips J, Ostrand-Rosenberg S (2006) Inflammation induces myeloid-derived suppressor cells that facilitate tumor progression. J Immunol 176:284–290

Bunt SK, Yang L, Sinha P, Clements VK, Leips J, Ostrand-Rosenberg S (2007) Reduced inflammation in the tumor microenvironment delays the accumulation of myeloid-derived suppressor cells and limits tumor progression. Cancer Res 67:10019–10026

Bunt SK, Clements VK, Hanson EM, Sinha P, Ostrand-Rosenberg S (2009) Inflammation enhances myeloid-derived suppressor cell cross-talk by signaling through Toll-like receptor 4. J Leukoc Biol 85:996–1004

Cheng P, Corzo CA, Luetteke N, Yu B, Nagaraj S, Bui MM, Ortiz M, Nacken W, Sorg C, Vogl T et al (2008) Inhibition of dendritic cell differentiation and accumulation of myeloid-derived suppressor cells in cancer is regulated by S100A9 protein. J Exp Med 205:2235–2249

Cobbs CS, Whisenhunt TR, Wesemann DR, Harkins LE, Van Meir EG, Samanta M (2003) Inactivation of wild-type p53 protein function by reactive oxygen and nitrogen species in malignant glioma cells. Cancer Res 63:8670–8673

Corzo CA, Cotter MJ, Cheng P, Cheng F, Kusmartsev S, Sotomayor E, Padhya T, McCaffrey TV, McCaffrey JC, Gabrilovich DI (2009) Mechanism regulating reactive oxygen species in tumor-induced myeloid-derived suppressor cells. J Immunol 182:5693–5701

Csiki I, Morrow JD, Sandler A, Shyr Y, Oates J, Williams MK, Dang T, Carbone DP, Johnson DH (2005) Targeting cyclooxygenase-2 in recurrent non-small cell lung cancer: a phase II trial of celecoxib and docetaxel. Clin Cancer Res 11:6634–6640

De Santo C, Serafini P, Marigo I, Dolcetti L, Bolla M, Del Soldato P, Melani C, Guiducci C, Colombo MP, Iezzi M et al (2005) Nitroaspirin corrects immune dysfunction in tumor-bearing hosts and promotes tumor eradication by cancer vaccination. Proc Natl Acad Sci U S A 102:4185–4190

Delano MJ, Scumpia PO, Weinstein JS, Coco D, Nagaraj S, Kelly-Scumpia KM, O'Malley KA, Wynn JL, Antonenko S, Al-Quran SZ et al (2007) MyD88-dependent expansion of an immature GR-1(+)CD11b(+) population induces T cell suppression and Th2 polarization in sepsis. J Exp Med 204:1463–1474

Ekmekcioglu S, Ellerhorst J, Smid CM, Prieto VG, Munsell M, Buzaid AC, Grimm EA (2000) Inducible nitric oxide synthase and nitrotyrosine in human metastatic melanoma tumors correlate with poor survival. Clin Cancer Res 6:4768–4775

Ferrari V, Valcamonico F, Amoroso V, Simoncini E, Vassalli L, Marpicati P, Rangoni G, Grisanti S, Tiberio GA, Nodari F et al (2006) Gemcitabine plus celecoxib (GECO) in advanced pancreatic cancer: a phase II trial. Cancer Chemother Pharmacol 57:185–190

Filipazzi P, Valenti R, Huber V, Pilla L, Canese P, Iero M, Castelli C, Mariani L, Parmiani G, Rivoltini L (2007) Identification of a new subset of myeloid suppressor cells in peripheral blood of melanoma patients with modulation by a granulocyte-macrophage colony-stimulation factor-based antitumor vaccine. J Clin Oncol 25:2546–2553

Finke JH, Rini B, Ireland J, Rayman P, Richmond A, Golshayan A, Wood L, Elson P, Garcia J, Dreicer R et al (2008) Sunitinib reverses type-1 immune suppression and decreases T-regulatory cells in renal cell carcinoma patients. Clin Cancer Res 14:6674–6682

Foell D, Wittkowski H, Vogl T, Roth J (2007) S100 proteins expressed in phagocytes: a novel group of damage-associated molecular pattern molecules. J Leukoc Biol 81:28–37

Gabrilovich D (2004) Mechanisms and functional significance of tumour-induced dendritic-cell defects. Nat Rev Immunol 4:941–952

Gabrilovich DI, Nagaraj S (2009) Myeloid-derived suppressor cells as regulators of the immune system. Nat Rev Immunol 9:162–174

Gabrilovich D, Ishida T, Oyama T, Ran S, Kravtsov V, Nadaf S, Carbone DP (1998) Vascular endothelial growth factor inhibits the development of dendritic cells and dramatically affects the differentiation of multiple hematopoietic lineages in vivo. Blood 92:4150–4166

Gallina G, Dolcetti L, Serafini P, De Santo C, Marigo I, Colombo MP, Basso G, Brombacher F, Borrello I, Zanovello P et al (2006) Tumors induce a subset of inflammatory monocytes with immunosuppressive activity on CD8+ T cells. J Clin Invest 116:2777–2790

Guo RF, Ward PA (2005) Role of C5a in inflammatory responses. Annu Rev Immunol 23:821–852

Hanson EM, Clements VK, Sinha P, Ilkovitch D, Ostrand-Rosenberg S (2009) Myeloid-derived suppressor cells down-regulate L-selectin expression on CD4+ and CD8+ T cells. J Immunol 183:937–944

Harari O, Liao JK (2004) Inhibition of MHC II gene transcription by nitric oxide and antioxidants. Curr Pharm Des 10:893–898

Hiratsuka S, Watanabe A, Aburatani H, Maru Y (2006) Tumour-mediated upregulation of chemoattractants and recruitment of myeloid cells predetermines lung metastasis. Nat Cell Biol 8:1369–1375

Hoechst B, Ormandy LA, Ballmaier M, Lehner F, Kruger C, Manns MP, Greten TF, Korangy F (2008) A new population of myeloid-derived suppressor cells in hepatocellular carcinoma patients induces CD4(+)CD25(+)Foxp3(+) T cells. Gastroenterology 135:234–243

Huang B, Pan PY, Li Q, Sato AI, Levy DE, Bromberg J, Divino CM, Chen SH (2006) Gr-1+ CD115+ immature myeloid suppressor cells mediate the development of tumor-induced T regulatory cells and T-cell anergy in tumor-bearing host. Cancer Res 66:1123–1131

Huang Y, Chen X, Dikov MM, Novitskiy SV, Mosse CA, Yang L, Carbone DP (2007) Distinct roles of VEGFR-1 and VEGFR-2 in the aberrant hematopoiesis associated with elevated levels of VEGF. Blood 110:624–631

Kerbel RS (2005) Therapeutic implications of intrinsic or induced angiogenic growth factor redundancy in tumors revealed. Cancer Cell 8:269–271

Kinnula VL, Torkkeli T, Kristo P, Sormunen R, Soini Y, Paakko P, Ollikainen T, Kahlos K, Hirvonen A, Knuutila S (2004) Ultrastructural and chromosomal studies on manganese superoxide dismutase in malignant mesothelioma. Am J Respir Cell Mol Biol 31:147–153

Ko JS, Bukowski RM, Fincke JH (2009) Myeloid-derived suppressor cells: a novel therapeutic target. Curr Oncol Rep 11:87–93

Kusmartsev S, Gabrilovich DI (2005) STAT1 signaling regulates tumor-associated macrophage-mediated T cell deletion. J Immunol 174:4880–4891

Kusmartsev S, Cheng F, Yu B, Nefedova Y, Sotomayor E, Lush R, Gabrilovich D (2003) All-trans-retinoic acid eliminates immature myeloid cells from tumor-bearing mice and improves the effect of vaccination. Cancer Res 63:4441–4449

Kusmartsev S, Nefedova Y, Yoder D, Gabrilovich DI (2004) Antigen-specific inhibition of CD8+ T cell response by immature myeloid cells in cancer is mediated by reactive oxygen species. J Immunol 172:989–999

Kusmartsev S, Nagaraj S, Gabrilovich DI (2005) Tumor-associated CD8+ T cell tolerance induced by bone marrow-derived immature myeloid cells. J Immunol 175:4583–4592

Larrivee B, Pollet I, Karsan A (2005) Activation of vascular endothelial growth factor receptor-2 in bone marrow leads to accumulation of myeloid cells: role of granulocyte-macrophage colony-stimulating factor. J Immunol 175:3015–3024

Li Q, Pan PY, Gu P, Xu D, Chen SH (2004) Role of immature myeloid Gr-1+ cells in the development of antitumor immunity. Cancer Res 64:1130–1139

Mahnke K, Schonfeld K, Fondel S, Ring S, Karakhanova S, Wiedemeyer K, Bedke T, Johnson TS, Storn V, Schallenberg S et al (2007) Depletion of CD4+ CD25+ human regulatory T cells in vivo: kinetics of Treg depletion and alterations in immune functions in vivo and in vitro. Int J Cancer 120:2723–2733

Mantovani G, Maccio A, Madeddu C, Mura L, Gramignano G, Lusso MR, Massa E, Mocci M, Serpe R (2003) Antioxidant agents are effective in inducing lymphocyte progression through cell cycle in advanced cancer patients: assessment of the most important laboratory indexes of cachexia and oxidative stress. J Mol Med 81:664–673

Markiewski MM, Lambris JD (2007) The role of complement in inflammatory diseases from behind the scenes into the spotlight. Am J Pathol 171:715–727

Markiewski MM, DeAngelis RA, Benencia F, Ricklin-Lichtsteiner SK, Koutoulaki A, Gerard C, Coukos G, Lambris JD (2008) Modulation of the antitumor immune response by complement. Nat Immunol 9:1225–1235

Melani C, Chiodoni C, Forni G, Colombo MP (2003) Myeloid cell expansion elicited by the progression of spontaneous mammary carcinomas in c-erbB-2 transgenic BALB/c mice suppresses immune reactivity. Blood 102:2138–2145

Miller KD, Sweeney CJ, Sledge GW Jr (2005) Can tumor angiogenesis be inhibited without resistance? EXS (94):95–112

Mirza N, Fishman M, Fricke I, Dunn M, Neuger AM, Frost TJ, Lush RM, Antonia S, Gabrilovich DI (2006) All-trans-retinoic acid improves differentiation of myeloid cells and immune response in cancer patients. Cancer Res 66:9299–9307

Movahedi K, Guilliams M, Van den Bossche J, Van den Bergh R, Gysemans C, Beschin A, De Baetselier P, Van Ginderachter JA (2008) Identification of discrete tumor-induced myeloid-derived suppressor cell subpopulations with distinct T cell-suppressive activity. Blood 111:4233–4244

Nagaraj S, Gupta K, Pisarev V, Kinarsky L, Sherman S, Kang L, Herber DL, Schneck J, Gabrilovich DI (2007) Altered recognition of antigen is a mechanism of CD8+ T cell tolerance in cancer. Nat Med 13:828–835

Nakamura Y, Yasuoka H, Tsujimoto M, Yoshidome K, Nakahara M, Nakao K, Nakamura M, Kakudo K (2006) Nitric oxide in breast cancer: induction of vascular endothelial growth factor-C and correlation with metastasis and poor prognosis. Clin Cancer Res 12:1201–1207

Noonan DM, De Lerma Barbaro A, Vannini N, Mortara L, Albini A (2008) Inflammation, inflammatory cells and angiogenesis: decisions and indecisions. Cancer Metastasis Rev 27:31–40

Ochoa AC, Zea AH, Hernandez C, Rodriguez PC (2007) Arginase, prostaglandins, and myeloid-derived suppressor cells in renal cell carcinoma. Clin Cancer Res 13:721s–726s

Onizuka S, Tawara I, Shimizu J, Sakaguchi S, Fujita T, Nakayama E (1999) Tumor rejection by in vivo administration of anti-CD25 (interleukin-2 receptor alpha) monoclonal antibody. Cancer Res 59:3128–3133

Ozao-Choy J, Ma G, Kao J, Wang GX, Meseck M, Sung M, Schwartz M, Divino CM, Pan PY, Chen SH (2009) The novel role of tyrosine kinase inhibitor in the reversal of immune suppression and modulation of tumor microenvironment for immune-based cancer therapies. Cancer Res 69:2514–2522

Pan PY, Li Y, Li Q, Gu P, Martinet O, Thung S, Chen SH (2004) In situ recruitment of antigen-presenting cells by intratumoral GM-CSF gene delivery. Cancer Immunol Immunother 53:17–25

Pan PY, Ozao J, Zhou Z, Chen SH (2008a) Advancements in immune tolerance. Adv Drug Deliv Rev 60:91–105

Pan PY, Wang GX, Yin B, Ozao J, Ku T, Divino CM, Chen SH (2008b) Reversion of immune tolerance in advanced malignancy: modulation of myeloid-derived suppressor cell development by blockade of stem-cell factor function. Blood 111:219–228

Pan PY, Ma G, Weber KJ, Ozao-Choy J, Wang G, Yin B, Divino CM, Chen SH (2010) Immune stimulatory receptor CD40 is required for T-cell suppression and T regulatory cell activation mediated by myeloid-derived suppressor cells in cancer. Cancer Res. 70:99–108

Pekarek LA, Starr BA, Toledano AY, Schreiber H (1995) Inhibition of tumor growth by elimination of granulocytes. J Exp Med 181:435–440

Peng G, Guo Z, Kiniwa Y, Voo KS, Peng W, Fu T, Wang DY, Li Y, Wang HY, Wang RF (2005) Toll-like receptor 8-mediated reversal of CD4+ regulatory T cell function. Science 309:1380–1384

Rabinovich GA, Gabrilovich D, Sotomayor EM (2007) Immunosuppressive strategies that are mediated by tumor cells. Annu Rev Immunol 25:267–296

Rivoltini L, Carrabba M, Huber V, Castelli C, Novellino L, Dalerba P, Mortarini R, Arancia G, Anichini A, Fais S et al (2002) Immunity to cancer: attack and escape in T lymphocyte-tumor cell interaction. Immunol Rev 188:97–113

Rodriguez PC, Ochoa AC (2008) Arginine regulation by myeloid derived suppressor cells and tolerance in cancer: mechanisms and therapeutic perspectives. Immunol Rev 222:180–191

Rodriguez PC, Zea AH, Culotta KS, Zabaleta J, Ochoa JB, Ochoa AC (2002) Regulation of T cell receptor CD3zeta chain expression by L-arginine. J Biol Chem 277:21123–21129

Rodriguez PC, Quiceno DG, Zabaleta J, Ortiz B, Zea AH, Piazuelo MB, Delgado A, Correa P, Brayer J, Sotomayor EM et al (2004) Arginase I production in the tumor microenvironment by mature myeloid cells inhibits T-cell receptor expression and antigen-specific T-cell responses. Cancer Res 64:5839–5849

Rodriguez PC, Hernandez CP, Quiceno D, Dubinett SM, Zabaleta J, Ochoa JB, Gilbert J, Ochoa AC (2005) Arginase I in myeloid suppressor cells is induced by COX-2 in lung carcinoma. J Exp Med 202:931–939

Rodriguez PC, Quiceno DG, Ochoa AC (2007) L-arginine availability regulates T-lymphocyte cell-cycle progression. Blood 109:1568–1573

Rubin BP, Heinrich MC, Corless CL (2007) Gastrointestinal stromal tumour. Lancet 369:1731–1741

Sauer H, Wartenberg M, Hescheler J (2001) Reactive oxygen species as intracellular messengers during cell growth and differentiation. Cell Physiol Biochem 11:173–186

Schmielau J, Finn OJ (2001) Activated granulocytes and granulocyte-derived hydrogen peroxide are the underlying mechanism of suppression of t-cell function in advanced cancer patients. Cancer Res 61:4756–4760

Serafini P, Carbley R, Noonan KA, Tan G, Bronte V, Borrello I (2004) High-dose granulocyte-macrophage colony-stimulating factor-producing vaccines impair the immune response through the recruitment of myeloid suppressor cells. Cancer Res 64:6337–6343

Serafini P, Meckel K, Kelso M, Noonan K, Califano J, Koch W, Dolcetti L, Bronte V, Borrello I (2006) Phosphodiesterase-5 inhibition augments endogenous antitumor immunity by reducing myeloid-derived suppressor cell function. J Exp Med 203:2691–2702

Serafini P, Mgebroff S, Noonan K, Borrello I (2008) Myeloid-derived suppressor cells promote cross-tolerance in B-cell lymphoma by expanding regulatory T cells. Cancer Res 68:5439–5449

Seung LP, Rowley DA, Dubey P, Schreiber H (1995) Synergy between T-cell immunity and inhibition of paracrine stimulation causes tumor rejection. Proc Natl Acad Sci USA 92:6254–6258

Shimizu J, Yamazaki S, Sakaguchi S (1999) Induction of tumor immunity by removing CD25+ CD4+ T cells: a common basis between tumor immunity and autoimmunity. J Immunol 163:5211–5218

Shojaei F, Ferrara N (2007) Antiangiogenic therapy for cancer: an update. Cancer J 13:345–348

Shojaei F, Wu X, Malik AK, Zhong C, Baldwin ME, Schanz S, Fuh G, Gerber HP, Ferrara N (2007) Tumor refractoriness to anti-VEGF treatment is mediated by CD11b+ Gr1+ myeloid cells. Nat Biotechnol 25:911–920

Sinha P, Clements VK, Ostrand-Rosenberg S (2005) Interleukin-13-regulated M2 macrophages in combination with myeloid suppressor cells block immune surveillance against metastasis. Cancer Res 65:11743–11751

Sinha P, Clements VK, Bunt SK, Albelda SM, Ostrand-Rosenberg S (2007a) Cross-talk between myeloid-derived suppressor cells and macrophages subverts tumor immunity toward a type 2 response. J Immunol 179:977–983

Sinha P, Clements VK, Fulton AM, Ostrand-Rosenberg S (2007b) Prostaglandin E2 promotes tumor progression by inducing myeloid-derived suppressor cells. Cancer Res 67:4507–4513

Sinha P, Okoro C, Foell D, Freeze HH, Ostrand-Rosenberg S, Srikrishna G (2008) Proinflammatory S100 proteins regulate the accumulation of myeloid-derived suppressor cells. J Immunol 181:4666–4675

Song X, Krelin Y, Dvorkin T, Bjorkdahl O, Segal S, Dinarello CA, Voronov E, Apte RN (2005) CD11b+/Gr-1+ immature myeloid cells mediate suppression of T cells in mice bearing tumors of IL-1beta-secreting cells. J Immunol 175:8200–8208

Steitz J, Bruck J, Lenz J, Knop J, Tuting T (2001) Depletion of CD25(+) CD4(+) T cells and treatment with tyrosinase-related protein 2-transduced dendritic cells enhance the interferon alpha-induced, CD8(+) T-cell-dependent immune defense of B16 melanoma. Cancer Res 61:8643–8646

Szuster-Ciesielska A, Hryciuk-Umer E, Stepulak A, Kupisz K, Kandefer-Szerszen M (2004) Reactive oxygen species production by blood neutrophils of patients with laryngeal carcinoma and antioxidative enzyme activity in their blood. Acta Oncol 43:252–258

Taheri F, Ochoa JB, Faghiri Z, Culotta K, Park HJ, Lan MS, Zea AH, Ochoa AC (2001) L-Arginine regulates the expression of the T-cell receptor zeta chain (CD3zeta) in Jurkat cells. Clin Cancer Res 7:958s–965s

Taketo MM (1998a) Cyclooxygenase-2 inhibitors in tumorigenesis (part I). J Natl Cancer Inst 90:1529–1536

Taketo MM (1998b) Cyclooxygenase-2 inhibitors in tumorigenesis (Part II). J Natl Cancer Inst 90:1609–1620

Terabe M, Matsui S, Park JM, Mamura M, Noben-Trauth N, Donaldson DD, Chen W, Wahl SM, Ledbetter S, Pratt B et al (2003) Transforming growth factor-beta production and myeloid cells are an effector mechanism through which CD1d-restricted T cells block cytotoxic T lymphocyte-mediated tumor immunosurveillance: abrogation prevents tumor recurrence. J Exp Med 198:1741–1752

Vickers SM, MacMillan-Crow LA, Green M, Ellis C, Thompson JA (1999) Association of increased immunostaining for inducible nitric oxide synthase and nitrotyrosine with fibroblast growth factor transformation in pancreatic cancer. Arch Surg 134:245–251

von Mehren M (2006) Beyond imatinib: second generation c-KIT inhibitors for the management of gastrointestinal stromal tumors. Clin Colorectal Cancer 6(Suppl 1):S30–S34

Voronov E, Shouval DS, Krelin Y, Cagnano E, Benharroch D, Iwakura Y, Dinarello CA, Apte RN (2003) IL-1 is required for tumor invasiveness and angiogenesis. Proc Natl Acad Sci U S A 100:2645–2650

Wang HY, Wang RF (2007) Regulatory T cells and cancer. Curr Opin Immunol 19:217–223

Waris G, Ahsan H (2006) Reactive oxygen species: role in the development of cancer and various chronic conditions. J Carcinog 5:14

Whiteside TL (2008) The tumor microenvironment and its role in promoting tumor growth. Oncogene 27:5904–5912

Yang L, DeBusk LM, Fukuda K, Fingleton B, Green-Jarvis B, Shyr Y, Matrisian LM, Carbone DP, Lin PC (2004) Expansion of myeloid immune suppressor Gr+ CD11b+ cells in tumor-bearing host directly promotes tumor angiogenesis. Cancer Cell 6:409–421

Yang R, Cai Z, Zhang Y, Yutzy WH 4th, Roby KF, Roden RB (2006) CD80 in immune suppression by mouse ovarian carcinoma-associated Gr-1+CD11b+ myeloid cells. Cancer Res 66:6807–6815

Youn JI, Nagaraj S, Collazo M, Gabrilovich DI (2008) Subsets of myeloid-derived suppressor cells in tumor-bearing mice. J Immunol 181:5791–5802

Young MR, Young ME, Wright MA (1990) Myelopoiesis-associated suppressor-cell activity in mice with Lewis lung carcinoma tumors: interferon-gamma plus tumor necrosis factor-alpha synergistically reduce suppressor cell activity. Int J Cancer 46:245–250

Zea AH, Rodriguez PC, Atkins MB, Hernandez C, Signoretti S, Zabaleta J, McDermott D, Quiceno D, Youmans A, O'Neill A et al (2005) Arginase-producing myeloid suppressor cells in renal cell carcinoma patients: a mechanism of tumor evasion. Cancer Res 65:3044–3048

Chapter 14
Cell Surface Co-signaling Molecules in the Control of Innate and Adaptive Cancer Immunity

Stasya Zarling and Lieping Chen

Recent advances in cancer immunotherapy have focused on manipulating co-signaling pathways to direct or fine-tune antitumor immune responses. This is based on the findings that co-signaling pathways are pivotal in positive and negative regulation of innate and adaptive immunity to antigens. Importantly, cancer cells as well as cells in cancer microenvironments often aberrantly express co-signaling molecules to evade tumor immunity. We will focus our discussion on two co-signaling pathways including CD137/CD137L and B7-H1/PD-1. The data from animal models and clinical trials indicate that monoclonal antibodies and recombinant proteins targeting these co-signaling molecules are able to stimulate antitumor immune responses or ablate immune suppression. Co-signaling molecules thus add a new modality for mechanism-based design of combined immunotherapy in the future.

1 Co-signal in Shaping the Immune Response

The immune system has the spectacular ability to recognize foreign pathogens and discriminate them from self. This ensures attack only on potentially dangerous microbes or infected cells, keeping normal tissue healthy while carefully avoiding autoimmune disease. The innate immune system plays a crucial role in the early detection of pathogenic agents and helps to guide the adaptive immune response. Neutrophils, monocytes/macrophages, dendritic cells (DCs), and natural killer (NK) cells all participate in the early detection of pathogens. Over the past decade, there has been increased knowledge of receptors required during innate immune recognition. Toll-like receptors (TLRs) bind pathogen-associated molecular patterns (PAMPS)

S. Zarling • L. Chen (✉)
Department of Oncology and the Sidney Kimmel Comprehensive Cancer Center,
Johns Hopkins University School of Medicine, Baltimore, MD, USA
e-mail: lchen42@jhmi.edu

on the pathogen cell surface or intracellular-associated molecules (i.e. nucleic acid structures) (Kumar et al. 2009).

During a normal immune response antigen presenting cells (APCs), such as DCs and macrophages, patrol the peripheral tissues for pathogens or infected cells. Immature DCs pick up antigen in the periphery and then migrate to secondary lymphoid organs, such as the spleen and lymph nodes, to interact with cells of the adaptive immune system. Functionally, DCs are over 100 times more potent APCs than macrophages at presenting antigens (Tseng et al. 2001). Within the T cell zones, DCs will mature and upregulate co-signaling (costimulatory or coinhibitory) molecules while decreasing their phagocytic activity, effectively changing their role to stimulation of adaptive immunity. These co-signaling molecules are extremely important in directing and fine-tuning the immune response. The modified two-signal hypothesis shows that in order to obtain a productive immune response to antigens, the T cell receptor (TCR) must encounter antigen in the context of peptide-MHC complexes (signal 1) as well as interact with a positive co-signaling or costimulatory molecules (signal 2). If either signal is given alone, there may be no response resulting in either anergy or ignorance (Baxter and Hodgkin 2002). On the other hand, a T cell response is controlled or even prevented by negative co-signaling or coinhibitory molecules against potential damages. The types of co-signaling molecules are expressed can be regulated by innate immune signals such as chemokines present within the microenvironment or TLR activation on the APC (Lee and Iwasaki 2007). While DCs play a central role in the direct activation of T cells, NK cells may also directly kill infected or transformed cells in addition to secreting cytokines during an innate immune response that can direct the adaptive response (Wilcox et al. 2002d).

Co-signaling molecules fall into two major gene families: B7-CD28 family and the tumor necrosis factor (TNF) superfamily. The B7 family currently consists of eight members, B7-1, B7-2, B7-H1, B7-H2, B7-H3, B7-H4, B7-H6, and B7-DC. The most well-studied molecules are B7-1 and B7-2 that interact with costimulatory CD28 and coinhibitory CTLA-4. B7-1 (CD80) and B7-2 (B70, CD86) were the first two members of the B7 family identified and although they show only about 25% identity, they contain similar tertiary structures and utilize the same receptors (Sansom 2000). The family was first expanded within the last decade with the discovery of B7-H1, a homologue to B7-1 with implicated suppressive functions for T cell responses in vitro (Dong et al. 1999). With the discovery of PD-1 (programmed death-1) as a counter-receptor for B7-H1, its coinhibitory function was confirmed and renamed as PD-1 ligand one (PD-L1) (Freeman et al. 2000). This nomenclature, however, fails to recognize additional receptor(s) for B7-H1 (Butte et al. 2007) as well as the fact that B7-H1 could serve as a receptor with PD-1 as its ligand (Dong et al. 2003; Chen 2004). To make this issue more complicated, B7-H1 is also found to have T cell stimulatory function in some experimental models in vitro and in vivo (Chen 2004). PD-1 also has a second ligand called B7-DC (with the similar reason, it was also renamed as PD-L2). B7-DC is only found on macrophages and DCs, although an early study claims its broad expression pattern (Latchman et al. 2001). The functions of B7-DC are more controversial as both costimulatory and coinhibitory functions were identified in vitro and in vivo (Chen 2004). A lesson learned from these studies is that the functions of co-signaling molecules are complex and they are determined in the context of interacting ligand–receptor, target cells, and the types of immune responses. In this chapter, we focus our discussion on their interaction with PD-1 as coinhibitory ligands.

The TNF family has also been a hot topic for discussion in cancer immunotherapy due mostly to the costimulatory receptor 4-1BB (CD137) and its ligand 4-1BBL (CD137L). Although 4-1BB has been well studied over the past 2 decades, there is still a great deal that is not well understood. Classically, signaling through 4-1BB induces proliferation, enhances survival, and increases cytolytic activity of $CD8^+$ T cells (Wang et al. 2009a). Interestingly, although 4-1BB is considered a stimulatory receptor, treatment with anti-4-1BB agonistic antibodies has been used to also to treat autoimmune diseases in several mouse models such as experimental autoimmune encephalomyelitis (EAE) (Sun et al. 2002b), systemic lupus erythematosus (SLE) (Sun et al. 2002a; Foell et al. 2003), and arthritis (Foell et al. 2004; Seo et al. 2004). Thus, agonistic antibodies against 4-1BB have been promising in their unique ability to treat cancer without inducing autoimmune disease, which can be a common drawback to immune stimulation.

2 Co-signal and Cancer Immunotherapy

Foreign pathogens are not the only danger to healthy tissue. Genetic changes can result in transformation of normal cells leading to uncontrolled growth and tissue invasion properties of cancer. Because these cells originate from self, the immune system does not always recognize the danger. This can be due to either immunological ignorance mediated through coinhibitory ligands on APCs or the direct expression of coinhibitory ligands on the tumor cells. For example, B7-H1 expression has been reported in many human cancers and can negatively regulate cytolytic T cell (CTL) response (Dong and Chen 2003). To study its possible role in tumor-mediated immune suppression, human 624 melanoma tumor cells were transfected with B7-H1 resulting in increased apoptosis of $C8^+$ CTL clones. This phenomenon could be inhibited by the addition of anti-B7-H1 blocking antibody. Additionally, B7-H1 positive tumors were more resistant to killing by CTL (Dong et al. 2002). Cancer immunotherapy hopes to utilize the power of the immune system in order to regress or suppress tumor growth through enhancing the existing immune response or overcoming immune evasion strategies employed by tumors (Sharma et al. 2009).

Recently, there has been much research into the use of monoclonal antibodies against co-signaling molecules as a way to manipulate the immune response. Monoclonal antibodies are then able to either promote direct killing or indirectly target growth and pro-angiogenic mediators of tumor cells (Melero et al. 2007). However, challenges can exist with the use of monoclonal antibodies. In order to avoid host immune responses against the antibody, fully human or humanized antibodies need to be genetically engineered, resulting in a human antibody that contains a distinct idiotype, antigenic binding site, from the endogenous repertoire

(Melero et al. 2007). Agonistic antibodies against costimulatory molecules are able to enhance the CTL response against tumor cells, whereas blocking antibodies specific for coinhibitory molecules are able to stop the suppression of the immune response. Careful considerations need to be taken with the use of agonistic antibodies, as there can be drawbacks to generating broad stimulation of the immune system. In 2006, a superagonist antibody against CD28 (TGN1412) demonstrated the dangers involved when six normal volunteers from a phase I clinical trial were all hospitalized with cytokine-release syndrome. Four of the six cases resulted in severe multiorgan failure, although no deaths were reported (Melero et al. 2007).

Due to the risk of toxicity associated with the use of monoclonal antibodies, some research has begun to focus on stimulating or blocking the target molecule with the use of soluble ligands. Monoclonal antibodies have a unique high affinity for their target molecule whereas soluble ligands would rely on the natural affinity for the target. Ligands have been studied both in a soluble form (Xiao et al. 2007; Muller et al. 2008; Schabowsky et al. 2009; Sharma et al. 2009) as well as in the context of artificial APCs (Zhang et al. 2007).

Tumor antigen-based vaccines have been extensively tested in clinical trials with limited success. A possible reason is the generation of immunosuppressive microenvironment around cancer tissues by either lack of costimulatory molecules or increase of coinhibitory molecules (Chen 2004; Kryczek et al. 2007). Thus, tumor vaccines in the context of other immunostimulatory methods described above would be ideal, where the tumor vaccine can provide antigen specificity, while monoclonal antibodies can enhance and protect ongoing immune responses, especially those in the cancer microenvironment.

Yet another immunotherapy utilizing co-signaling molecules under investigation is adoptive immunotherapy. Adoptive cell transfer utilizes autologous or allogeneic lymphocytes with antitumor activity to enhance tumor immunity. Furthermore, T cell clones with the best effector response and low expression of inhibitory molecules can be chosen and expanded ex vivo before transfer (Rosenberg et al. 2008). Lymphodepletion with chemotherapy can enhance the efficacy of adoptive transfer through creating space for further expansion of transferred cells in vivo as well as removal of regulatory T cells. Adoptive transfer in combination with lymphodepletion showed substantial results with ~50% regression in patients with metastatic melanoma (Dudley et al. 2005). Ex vivo expansion of autologous T cell clones with unique recognition specificity would reduce the risk for graft vs. host disease, and currently using co-signaling molecules for expansion is being explored clinically (June 2007; Paulos et al. 2008). It is also possible to combine adoptive transfer of T cells with therapeutic antibodies to co-signaling molecules to overcome potential problems associated with adoptive transfer such as programmed cell death.

Although each cancer immunotherapy strategy discussed here has shown promising advancements, it is most likely the case that these strategies will be most effective in combination either with each other or with current methods of cancer treatment such as chemotherapy and/or radiation. The focus of this chapter is to explore the current immunotherapies being investigated for each of the two main co-signaling families, B7-H1/PD-1 from the B7-CD28 family and 4-1BB/4-1BBL of the TNF superfamily.

3 Utilizing the TNF Superfamily Co-signaling Molecules in Immunotherapy

In the last century, many attempts have been made at the treatment of cancer including the injection of live or killed bacteria. It was then discovered in 1975 that the effectiveness of this therapy was through induction of TNF (Old 1988; Lynch 2008). The TNF superfamily now consists of TNF, OX40L, CD70, LIGHT, CD30L, and 4-1BBL as well as others. The cloning of 4-1BBL led to the formation of the superfamily in 1993 (Goodwin et al. 1993; Lynch 2008) and has expanded since. 4-1BB (CD137), the receptor for 4-1BBL, was previously identified in 1989 from a cDNA screen of T cell genes (Kwon and Weissman 1989). The TNF family is responsible for a wide array of activities ranging from apoptosis (such as TRAIL, Fas, etc) to maturation and regulation of B cell (CD40) and T cell (4-1BB, OX40) immune responses (Lynch 2008). TNF family molecules can be expressed on the cell surface either as monomers or as higher order complexes, but interact with their cognate receptors in trimeric complexes (Croft 2003). TNF molecules usually associate as homotrimers, but the formation of heteromultimers has been reported although the function of these complexes are still not well known (Melero et al. 2008). Although some family members, such as Fas, are able to directly trigger caspases through death domains (DD), signaling for all other TNF family members utilizes TNF-associated factor (TRAF) molecules with TRAF2 common to all costimulatory TNF family member signaling pathways (Watts 2005; Kober et al. 2008; Melero et al. 2008). TRAF2 acts as a ubiquitin ligase; however, instead of resulting in degradation, polyubiqutination at Lys63 establishes a docking site for TANK-binding kinase (TBK)-1 (Melero et al. 2008). 4-1BB is one of the most well-studied molecules of this superfamily and it is well established that downstream signaling leads to the activation of NFκB and AP-1 (Watts 2005; Melero et al. 2008).

3.1 CD137/4-1BB as a Co-signaling Receptor

4-1BB is inducible on many cell types including activated $CD4^+$ and $CD8^+$ cells, as well as NK cells, DCs, follicular DCs (FDCs), monocytes, and neutrophils. In contrast to CD28, which is constitutively expressed on naïve cells, 4-1BB is upregulated upon activation peaking at 24–48 h (Kober et al. 2008). 4-1BB is a 256aa, 27.5 kDa Type I transmembrane protein, which upon engaging its ligand (4-1BBL) has been shown to increase proliferation, inhibit apoptosis, and increase cytotoxicity of $CD8^+$ T cells (Cheuk et al. 2004; Myers and Vella 2005). Inhibition of apoptosis is due to increased levels of the antiapoptotic factors $Bcl\text{-}X_L$ and Bfl-1 (Lynch 2008). 4-1BB and 4-1BBL deficient mice develop normally, implying they are not essential to the immune response but may be involved in increasing the efficacy of weak immune responses (Kwon et al. 2002; Lynch 2008). However, one interesting observation was found in a 4-1BBL transgenic (4-1BBLTg) mouse, where a progressive loss of B cells along with decreased circulating antibody and humoral responses in response to antigen challenge was seen (Zhu et al. 2001). In another study, similar results were also found with repeated injections of anti-4-1BB monoclonal antibody (mAb), where the increased number of CD8$^+$ cells and increased IFNγ led to decreased B cell development in the bone marrow and increased apoptosis in the preB cell stage through downregulation of Bcl-X_L and Bcl-2 (Lee et al. 2009b). Potentially, this decreased B cell response is the reason why treatment of autoimmune disease is also possible with anti-4-1BB antibody.

There has been a great deal learned about the function of 4-1BB through the use of agonistic mAb, which mimics the role of 4-1BBL. For example, IFNγ and NK cells are absolutely required for the antitumor effects of anti-4-1BB mAb. IFNγ knock-out mice were still able to mount full CD8$^+$ CTL responses in the lymph node, however tumor growth still progressed. IFNγ has been suggested to regulate T cell migration into the tumor site through the suppression of angiogenesis (Wilcox et al. 2002b). Additionally, removal of NK cells through depleting antibodies completely abrogates antitumor effects in several tumor models (Murillo et al. 2008).

Although the expression of 4-1BB has been demonstrated in both CD4$^+$ and CD8$^+$ cells, there is some evidence for preferential stimulation of CD8$^+$ cells while a second TNFR molecule, OX40, plays a similar role in CD4$^+$ cells. In vitro studies have shown that 4-1BB is able to stimulate both CD8$^+$ and CD4$^+$ cells; however, in vivo analyses support the idea that its major role is in the CD8$^+$ subset (Dawicki and Watts 2004). Blockade of the 4-1BB pathway showed greater effects on CD8$^+$ cells and knock-out studies determined that OX40 and 4-1BB are expressed at different time points on T cells and act independently of each other in the CD4$^+$ or CD8$^+$ subsets (Dawicki et al. 2004).

4-1BB mAb has also contributed some insight into the role of 4-1BB on memory T cells. Several studies of viral infection such as LCMV (Tan et al. 1999) and influenza virus (Bertram et al. 2002) have shown that although 4-1BB deficient mice are able to mount an effective primary response, the recall response to secondary challenge is impaired suggesting that 4-1BB signal is necessary during the priming of T cell responses to produce an effective memory response. However, when 4-1BB signal was provided to memory phenotype cells in the absence of antigen-MHC complex through the use of mAb, a significant increase in proliferation was observed (Zhu et al. 2007). Also, this antigen-independent growth signal was observed in the absence of IL-15 and depended on the direct binding of antibody to 4-1BB present on memory T cells (Zhu et al. 2007). Since this effect is antigen-independent, stimulation of existing memory T cells early in a response may then be able to trigger the release of cytokines that are able to further enhance the innate immune response.

The broad expression pattern of 4-1BB allows for it to function in innate immune cells as well as adaptive cells. In a *Listeria monocytogenes* infection model, where the innate immune response is essential to control of bacterial spreading in the early stage, 4-1BB KO mice are more susceptible to infection. Also, when agonistic anti-4-1BB antibody is used for treatment of *L. monocytogenes* infection, there is increased infiltration of neutrophils and monocytes in infected livers, promoting survival (Lee et al. 2009a). Additionally, these infiltrating cells show increased expression of activation markers, phagocytic activity, and reactive oxygen species

(Lee et al. 2009a). DCs provide a crucial link between innate and adaptive immunity by picking up antigen within the tissues and trafficking back to the secondary lymphoid organs to present antigen to T cells in the context of MHC molecules. DCs express 4-1BB and can be stimulated by agonistic antibody. 4-1BB on DCs may be able to stimulate them to enhance uptake of antigen and expression of other costimulatory molecules thereby stimulating the primary T cell response, maintaining memory as well as helping effector T cells to overcome regulation by Tregs (Sharma et al. 2009). 4-1BB signaling on DCs also can induce production of IL-6 and IL-12 as well as increase their ability to stimulate T cells (Wilcox et al. 2002a). In fact, it is possible that antigen presentation is the limiting factor to the efficacy of anti-4-1BB antibody (Melero et al. 2008). Finally, NK cells have also been shown to play a crucial role in anti-4-1BB activity. Similar to co-signaling in T cells, NK cell activation is also dependent on an elaborate network of stimulatory and inhibitory receptors. Inhibition occurs through the binding of MHC class I molecules, thus NK cells are activated when encountering a cell that has "missing self." Stimulation occurs through NKG2D binding MICA/MICB (human) or H-60 and RaeI (mouse) that are preferentially expressed on tumors (Wilcox et al. 2002d). The pathway leading to direct or indirect activation of NK cells is still unclear; however, they may be playing a role in increased IFNγ production and increased $CD8^+$ cell responses (Wilcox et al. 2002d; Murillo et al. 2008).

3.2 Stimulation of 4-1BB by Agonistic Antibody for Cancer Immunotherapy

Owing to selective expression on antigen-experienced T cells, 4-1BB makes a great candidate for cancer immunotherapy without the global stimulation that is achieved with anti-CD28 antibody (Schabowsky et al. 2009). Furthermore, 4-1BB treatment may be superior to anti-CD28 since CD28 is downregulated shortly after activation, leading to $CD8^+CD28^-$ cells that can play a suppressive role (Xiao et al. 2007). Additionally, it has been suggested that upon antibody binding, surface 4-1BB is internalized into an endosomal compartment thereby desensitizing the cell to further stimulation (Melero et al. 2008). Anti-4-1BB monoclonal antibodies have been shown to eradicate tumors in many mouse models (Wilcox et al. 2002c). The antitumor activity of anti-4-1BB appears to be dependent on the presence of $CD8^+$ cells and NK cells (Wilcox et al. 2002d; Melero et al. 2007; Murillo et al. 2008). Interestingly CD4 help does not appear to be crucial in mediating these antitumor effects, as depletion of $CD4^+$ cells actually works synergistically with 4-1BB in eradication of tumors (Melero et al. 2007; Lynch 2008) and it appears that this is due to depletion of Treg (Houot et al. 2009).Since anti-4-1BB is not expressed on naïve cells, its primary action in immunotherapy is to stimulate the effector and memory cell compartment (Melero et al. 2007). In fact, after tumor resection and treatment with anti-4-1BB in a melanoma model, 60% of mice were protected from tumor rechallenge. Anti-4-1BB was able to stimulate and expand antigen-specific memory T cells without the use of an antigen-specific vaccine. However, the effect on the memory compartment was only partially required for this effect. Bone marrow chimeras were able to establish that the effect of anti-4-1BB is dependent on the expression on both hematopoetic and nonhematopoetic cells (Narazaki et al. 2010). One of the risks associated with immune stimulation for cancer therapy is the risk of triggering autoimmune disease (Melero et al. 2007). However, anti-4-1BB monoclonal antibodies are unique in their ability to treat both tumor and autoimmune models in mice. This phenomenon may be attributed to the suppressive effects of 4-1BB on the $CD4^+$ cell and B cell compartments. The reduced risks makes 4-1BB a great target for use in immunotherapy while avoiding some of the usual disastrous side effects associated with immune stimulation.

Agonistic anti-4-1BB antibody has been studied for treatment of a mouse model of multiple myeloma. In this model, NK cell numbers were increased in the tumor-draining lymph node and $CD8^+$ cells predominated the tumor infiltrating lymphocyte population (Murillo et al. 2008). The pathways involved in NK cell accumulation are still unclear, but NK cell activation may be a contributing factor to increased IFNγ production (Murillo et al. 2008), which is required for the antitumor effect of the monoclonal antibody. NK cells may also be playing a helper role in developing CTLs, evidenced by the requirement of NK cells for the regression of P815. P815 is resistant to direct NK cell lysis yet the effect of anti-4-1BB treatment was completely eliminated by $NK1.1^+$ cell depletion (Wilcox et al. 2002d).

In addition to increased CD8 proliferation, anti-4-1BB antibodies enhance cytotoxicity primarily through the increased production of IFNγ. IFNγ is essential for stimulatory function of 4-1BB and antitumor effects (Wilcox et al. 2002b). However, the increased IFNγ expression from anti-4-1BB treatment can result in increased expression of B7-H1 on T cells or tumor cells (Dong et al. 2002; Xiao et al. 2007). To combat the immunosuppressive effects of B7-H1 expression, the use of soluble PD-1 has been studied in combination with 4-1BBL treatment resulting in a synergistic antitumor effect (Xiao et al. 2007).

Monoclonal antibodies are not the only form of cancer immunotherapy employing the use of TNF family molecules. Agonistic antibodies can be associated with severe toxicities, and although anti-4-1BB monoclonal antibodies do not appear to induce autoimmune disease, other toxicity risks have been reported (Sharma et al. 2009). Schabowsky et al. (2009) demonstrated that multiple injections of anti-4-1BB at therapeutic doses in naïve mice resulted in transient toxicity and immunological abnormalities demonstrated by enlargement of spleen and lymph nodes. A novel form of 4-1BBL conjugated to a modified form of core streptavidin (SA-4-1BBL) was able to elicit similar or enhanced cytolytic activity compared to antibody treatment without associated toxicity (Schabowsky et al. 2009).

Rationale-based design of combination therapy utilizing anti-4-1BB or 4-1BBL and other mechanistically nonredundant approaches has been tested including tumor vaccine, chemotherapy, and radiation therapy. Combining the use of a tumor vaccine with a costimulatory ligand, such as 4-1BBL, can help boost this weak response. For example, transfection of tumor cells with 4-1BBL has been combined with intratumor injections of the IL-12 gene in mice with some regression, but unfortunately no complete eradication (Lynch 2008). The efficacy of anti-4-1BB antibody in the treatment of mouse lung or breast cancer was also studied in combination with single-dose radiation therapy. It was shown that although antibody treatment alone was not able to completely regress either tumor, a significant increase in antitumor immunity was seen when combined with radiation therapy (Shi and Siemann 2006). Cyclophosphamide, a popular chemotherapeutic agent, is known to be effective at removing Treg cells, a specialized subset of $CD4^+$ cells that inhibit immune responses, directly kill tumors as well as deplete peripheral $CD4^+$ and $CD8^+$ cells. Lymphopenia then creates space within the lymphoid compartment and stimulates homeostatic proliferation. Anti-4-1BB antibody, when combined with cyclophosphamide, protected and amplified peripheral cells that survived chemotherapy treatment while Tregs were still depleted (Kim et al. 2009). In support of this data, anti-4-1BB combined with $CD4^+$ cell depletion showed synergistic effects in the treatment of the weak immunogenic tumor B16 melanoma in mice. B16 melanoma is surprisingly resistant to anti-4-1BB treatment regardless of an increase in $CD8^+$ cell numbers and increased IFNγ production. Depletion of $CD4^+$ cells acted synergistically with anti-4-1BB through facilitating infiltration into tumor site as well as removing immunosuppressive barriers such as Tregs and IDO^+ DCs (Choi et al. 2007). This data supports the idea that 4-1BB preferentially signals to $CD8^+$ cells and allows them to bypass the need for $CD4^+$ help. Additionally, anti-4-1BB has been combined with a wide array of other monoclonal antibodies such as anti-DR5 and anti-CD40 (TriMab) (Uno et al. 2006) or anti-DR5 and anti-CD1d (Teng et al. 2009) as well as anti-OX40 (Gray et al. 2008) to name a few.

4 B7/CD28 Family of Co-signaling Molecules

The molecules of the B7/CD28 family belong to the immunoglobulin superfamily and include B7-1, B7-2, B7-H1, B7-H2, B7-H3, B7-H4, B7-DC, B7-H6, CD28, CTLA-4, ICOS, and PD-1. The family contains both costimulatory and coinhibitory receptor-ligand pairs (Melero et al. 2007). B7-H1 (PD-L1) and B7-DC (PD-L2) provide inhibitory signals through their common receptor PD-1 (Dong et al. 1999; Tseng et al. 2001; Freeman 2008). Common to other B7 family molecules, both B7-H1 and B7-DC contain an IgV domain and an IgC domain in the extracellular region of the molecule (Tamura et al. 2003). They exist as monomers on the cell surface and contain 8 of 14 amino acids in common within their binding sites for PD-1 (Freeman 2008). PD-1 was originally cloned in 1992 from apoptotic cells and is expressed only on activated B and T cells and myeloid cells (Ishida et al. 1992; Freeman 2008; Riley 2009). PD-1 is a 288aa type I transmembrane protein that contains only a single N-terminal extracellular IgV domain with a 20aa stalk followed by a transmembrane domain and cytoplasmic tail (Riley 2009). Upregulation of PD-1 on chronically activated T cells can maintain them in a partially reversible inactive state termed "exhausted" T cells (Goldberg et al. 2007).

4.1 B7-H1/PD-1 Pathways in the Inhibition of T Cell Activation

The discovery of B7-H1 was achieved through searching for homologues to B7-1/B7-2 (Dong et al. 1999). B7-H1 is broadly expressed on all nucleated cells tested so far, as mRNA transcripts were found in a wide variety of tissues (Dong and Chen 2006). However, the expression of its protein was only identified in a subset of human macrophages but can be quickly upregulated by the introduction of IFNγ (Chen 2004). Moreover, tumor-associated IL-10, attributed to either tumor cells or associated macrophages, has been shown to increase B7-H1 expression in an in vitro coculture system using human hepatocellular carcinoma (HCC) (Wu et al. 2009). B7-H1 ordinarily functions as a ligand to PD-1; however, reverse signaling on B7-H1$^+$CD4$^+$ cells with monoclonal antibody or immobilized PD-1 has shown costimulation of growth and cytokine secretion (Chen 2004), indicating that B7-H1 could serve as a receptor. B7-H1 expressed on tumor cells acts as an antiapoptotic factor shielding the tumor cells from death (Azuma et al. 2008). Interestingly, PD-1 is not the only receptor for B7-H1, it has been recently established that B7-H1 is also able to bind B7-1 with an affinity similar to CD28 and CTLA-4 (Wang et al. 2003; Butte et al. 2007). These additional receptors and reverse signaling events may explain some contradictory roles for B7-H1 in different contexts.

PD-1 was originally identified in two cell lines undergoing apoptosis (Ishida et al. 1992). PD-1 is considered a member of the CD28 family; however, upon closer review there are many differences especially in the realm of signaling (Riley 2009). The PD-1 cytoplasmic domain contains an immunoreceptor tyrosine-based inhibition motif (ITIM) followed by an immunoreceptor tyrosine-based switch motif (ITSM) (Riley 2009). It was suggested in early studies that ITIM motif is responsible for PD-1-mediated suppression (Freeman et al. 2000). However, it appears as though the ITISM, not ITIM, is required for the suppressive effects of PD-1 as mutation of the ITIM motif had a negligible effect on its signaling. Upon engagement and phosphorylation of the ITSM, phosphatases SHP-1 and SHP-2 are recruited (Chemnitz et al. 2004). It has been suggested that these events may lead to dephosphorylation of TCR signaling molecules; however, it has also been shown that PD-1 engagement blocks PI3K activation induced by CD3/CD28 costimulation, which denies the cell of necessary resources for cell division or effector function (Riley 2009). Unlike CTLA4 deficient mice that die early due to lymphoproliferative disease, PD-1 knock-out mice show species-specific autoimmune disease later in life, suggesting a role for regulation of immune tolerance (Riley 2009). Expression of PD-1 is upregulated upon activation, but quickly downregulated upon removal of antigen. However, in the case of chronic viral infection or cancer, where antigen is persistent, T cells maintain PD-1 expression (Freeman 2008). During an acute lymphocytic choriomeningitis virus (LCMV) infection model, PD-1 is rapidly downregulated upon resolution of infection. However upon infection with clone 13 LCMV, which establishes a chronic infection, T cells become "exhausted" displaying decreased proliferation effector functions (Barber et al. 2006). Interestingly, the exhausted phenotype of these T cells can be reversed with treatment of a blocking antibody against B7-H1 (Barber et al. 2006). However, although B7-H1 knock-out mice infected with LCMV are able to clear infection, they succumb to other immune pathologies, suggesting that immune tolerance induced by the B7-H1/PD-1 interaction is still important (Riley 2009). Although B7-DC shows slightly higher affinity, most of the inhibitory functions associated with PD-1 are attributed to its interaction with B7-H1 (Goldberg et al. 2007).

4.2 Blocking B7-H1/PD-1 Inhibition for Cancer Immunotherapy

The detection of B7-H1 on human tumor cells has been correlated with a poor prognosis due to increased tolerance (Dong and Chen 2003). Several animal models have explored the role of B7-H1/PD-1 signaling and blockade for tumor treatment. In a metastatic melanoma model, tumor-associated myeloid cells showed increased expression of B7-H1. Also, tumor infiltrating lymphocytes expressed greater numbers of PD-1⁺ T cells as well as higher levels of PD-1 on a per cell basis when compared to normal tissue. These PD-1⁺ infiltrates were also shown to express CTLA4, HLA-DR, and lacked expression of CD127 (Ahmadzadeh et al. 2009). Furthermore, infiltrating T cells specific for the tumor antigen MART-1 expressed higher levels of PD-1 than antigen-specific cells in the peripheral blood, and blockade of B7-H1 with monoclonal antibody was able to restore effector functions in exhausted T cells (Ahmadzadeh et al. 2009). These results demonstrate that the tumor microenvironment plays a crucial role in the expression of PD-1 leading to the exhaustion and inactivation of the immune response (Ahmadzadeh et al. 2009). Okudaira (2009) explored B7-H1/PD-1 in a mouse model of pancreatic cancer, which also supports the role of blocking B7-H1 to stimulate tumor immunity. Blocking antibody against B7-H1 alone was able to reduce the growth of a pancreatic cancer model. It was suggested that an increase in the number of tumor-infiltrating lymphocytes led to an increase in IFNγ expression but also an increase in FoxP3. Whereas anti-B7-DC increased IFNγ and decreased FoxP3, combining anti-B7-H1 with anti-B7-DC effectively induced regression by an increase in IFNγ and decrease in IL-10 (Okudaira et al. 2009).

Blocking antibodies specific for PD-1 have also been employed in cancer immunotherapy. Immune regulation can also be obtained through activation of CD4⁺CD25⁺FoxP3⁺ Treg cells, and antibodies against PD-1 are able to block Treg-mediated suppression (Wang et al. 2009b). Anti-PD-1 antibody reverses inhibition through stimulation of CTL proliferation, evidenced by increased production of IFNγ and TNFα on a per cell basis, as well as blocking their ability to be suppressed by Tregs (Wang et al. 2009b). In the liver, B7-H1 expression on hepatocytes and liver residential APCs contributes to deletion of intrahepatic T cells preventing autoimmunity. However, in HCC Kuppfer cells are the primary cell expressing B7-H1 and mediating decreased effector functions through PD-1 (Wu et al. 2009). Although blocking the B7-H1/PD-1 interaction is able to increase the antitumor immune response and slow tumor growth, individual antibodies have not shown significant tumor regression in most models. Thus, the most effective use of anti-B7-H1 or anti-PD-1 antibodies may be in combination with other treatments or antibodies.

5 Combining 4-1BB and B7-H1/PD-1 Immunotherapies

As mentioned above, anti-4-1BB antibodies are effective at enhancing CTL effector function, particularly through increasing production of IFNγ. However, B7-H1 expression can be increased by IFNγ, which could then lead to suppression of the immune response or even protection of tumor cells (Hirano et al. 2005; Melero et al. 2009). To combat this feedback, it would be beneficial to use an agonistic anti-4-1BB antibody in combination with a blocking antibody aimed at the B7-H1/PD-1 interaction. Hirano et al. 2005 showed that addition of anti-B7-H1 increased the efficacy of anti-4-1BB in a P815 mastocytoma model. P815 confers resistance to anti-4-1BB treatment alone through the upregulation of B7-H1, thus addition of a blocking antibody was able to further increase the frequency of antigen-specific CTLs within the tumor site (Hirano et al. 2005). Additionally, 4-1BBL in combination with soluble PD-1 worked synergistically to effectively treat mouse hepatocarcinoma in vivo. Where 4-1BBL was able to stimulate the immune response, it also led to upregulation of B7-H1 and was not able to decrease the levels of immunosuppressive cytokines IL-10 and TGF-β (Xiao et al. 2007). The addition of soluble PD-1 was able to compensate for these shortcomings (Xiao et al. 2007). Also in a separate mouse model, autologous tumor cells transfected with GM-CSF combined with antibodies against OX-40, CTLA4, or 4-1BB to provide synergistic results (Melero et al. 2009). There is a large potential for a molecule to show little activity on its own, but work synergistically with others. However, unfortunately due to the complex nature of all these signaling pathways and regulatory issues, some molecules that could prove beneficial may be overlooked (Melero et al. 2009). To ensure the safety of treatment, a new therapy can only be combined with another that has been already proven.

6 Current Clinical Trials Targeting Co-signaling Molecules

As mentioned earlier, the clinical trial for the superagonist anti-CD28 monoclonal antibody (TGN1412) has been suspended due to unforeseen severe toxicity. However, there are many other monoclonal antibodies to other co-signaling molecules currently in phase I or phase II clinical trials that are showing promise. CTLA4 is another molecule that has a large number of studies underway or completed and can now be used in combination with other treatments. Fully humanized agonistic anti-4-1BB antibodies (BMS663513) have been generated and are currently under study by Bristol-Myers Squibb. Currently, a phase II study for the use of anti-4-1BB as a monotherapy in stage III or stage IV melanoma is underway (NCT00612664). Additionally, another study utilizing anti-4-1BB in combination with anti-CTLA4 (Ipilimumab, BMS734016) is scheduled to begin phase I in November 2010 (NCT00803374) also for patients with stage III or stage IV melanoma. In addition, Medarex, in combination with Ono Pharmaceuticals in Japan, has developed an anti-PD-1 blocking antibody (MDX-1106/ONO4835) which is being tested in phase I dose escalation studies in patients with advanced malignant solid tumors, recurrent malignancies, or relapsed malignancies (NCT00836888, NCT00730639, NCT00441337).

Tumor immunity plays a very important role in regulating the growth and recurrence of many cancers. An effective T cell response is central to the establishment of effective tumor immunity. However, disrupting the delicate balance maintained by the immune system can be detrimental. The field of cancer immunotherapy has been trying to utilize the immune system's natural ability to recognize and ward off harmful agents while maintaining tolerance to healthy normal tissues. While stimulating immune functions appears at first glance to be a promising treatment, it has been shown that global stimulation of the immune system can have disastrous effects. Therefore, it is prudent to understand the complex network of costimulatory and coinhibitory molecules in order to effectively mimic the natural balance of immune activation and suppression necessary to eradicate tumor cells while limiting autoimmune pathologies.

References

Ahmadzadeh M et al (2009) Tumor antigen-specific CD8 T cells infiltrating the tumor express high levels of PD-1 and are functionally impaired. Blood 114(8):1537–1544

Azuma T et al (2008) B7-H1 is a ubiquitous antiapoptotic receptor on cancer cells. Blood 111(7):3635–3643

Barber DL et al (2006) Restoring function in exhausted CD8 T cells during chronic viral infection. Nature 439(7077):682–687

Baxter AG, Hodgkin PD (2002) Activation rules: the two-signal theories of immune activation. Nat Rev Immunol 2(6):439–446

Bertram EM et al (2002) Temporal segregation of 4-1BB versus CD28-mediated costimulation: 4-1BB ligand influences T cell numbers late in the primary response and regulates the size of the T cell memory response following influenza infection. J Immunol 168(8):3777–3785

Butte MJ et al (2007) Programmed death-1 ligand 1 interacts specifically with the B7-1 costimulatory molecule to inhibit T cell responses. Immunity 27(1):111–122

Chemnitz JM et al (2004) SHP-1 and SHP-2 associate with immunoreceptor tyrosine-based switch motif of programmed death 1 upon primary human T cell stimulation, but only receptor ligation prevents T cell activation. J Immunol 173(2):945–954

Chen L (2004) Co-inhibitory molecules of the B7-CD28 family in the control of T-cell immunity. Nat Rev Immunol 4(5):336–347

Cheuk AT et al (2004) Role of 4-1BB:4-1BB ligand in cancer immunotherapy. Cancer Gene Ther 11(3):215–226

Choi BK et al (2007) Mechanisms involved in synergistic anticancer immunity of anti-4-1BB and anti-CD4 therapy. Cancer Res 67(18):8891–8899

Croft M (2003) Co-stimulatory members of the TNFR family: keys to effective T-cell immunity? Nat Rev Immunol 3(8):609–620

Dawicki W, Watts TH (2004) Expression and function of 4-1BB during CD4 versus CD8 T cell responses in vivo. Eur J Immunol 34(3):743–751

Dawicki W et al (2004) 4-1BB and OX40 act independently to facilitate robust CD8 and CD4 recall responses. J Immunol 173(10):5944–5951

Dong H, Chen L (2003) B7-H1 pathway and its role in the evasion of tumor immunity. J Mol Med 81(5):281–287

Dong H, Chen X (2006) Immunoregulatory role of B7-H1 in chronicity of inflammatory responses. Cell Mol Immunol 3(3):179–187

Dong H et al (1999) B7-H1, a third member of the B7 family, co-stimulates T-cell proliferation and interleukin-10 secretion. Nat Med 5(12):1365–1369

Dong H et al (2002) Tumor-associated B7-H1 promotes T-cell apoptosis: a potential mechanism of immune evasion. Nat Med 8(8):793–800

Dong H et al (2003) Costimulating aberrant T cell responses by B7-H1 autoantibodies in rheumatoid arthritis. J Clin Invest 111(3):363–370

Dudley ME et al (2005) Adoptive cell transfer therapy following non-myeloablative but lymphodepleting chemotherapy for the treatment of patients with refractory metastatic melanoma. J Clin Oncol 23(10):2346–2357

Foell J et al (2003) CD137 costimulatory T cell receptor engagement reverses acute disease in lupus-prone NZB x NZW F1 mice. J Clin Invest 111(10):1505–1518

Foell JL et al (2004) Engagement of the CD137 (4-1BB) costimulatory molecule inhibits and reverses the autoimmune process in collagen-induced arthritis and establishes lasting disease resistance. Immunology 113(1):89–98

Freeman GJ (2008) Structures of PD-1 with its ligands: sideways and dancing cheek to cheek. Proc Natl Acad Sci USA 105(30):10275–10276

Freeman GJ et al (2000) Engagement of the PD-1 immunoinhibitory receptor by a novel B7 family member leads to negative regulation of lymphocyte activation. J Exp Med 192(7):1027–1034

Goldberg MV et al (2007) Role of PD-1 and its ligand, B7-H1, in early fate decisions of CD8 T cells. Blood 110(1):186–192

Goodwin RG et al (1993) Molecular cloning of a ligand for the inducible T cell gene 4-1BB: a member of an emerging family of cytokines with homology to tumor necrosis factor. Eur J Immunol 23(10):2631–2641

Gray JC et al (2008) Optimising anti-tumour CD8 T-cell responses using combinations of immunomodulatory antibodies. Eur J Immunol 38(9):2499–2511

Hirano F et al (2005) Blockade of B7-H1 and PD-1 by monoclonal antibodies potaentiates cancer therapeutic immunity. Cancer Res 65(3):1089–1096

Houot R et al (2009) Therapeutic effect of CD137 immunomodulation in lymphoma and its enhancement by Treg depletion. Blood 114(16):3431–3438

Ishida Y et al (1992) Induced expression of PD-1, a novel member of the immunoglobulin gene superfamily, upon programmed cell death. EMBO J 11(11):3887–3895

June CH (2007) Adoptive T cell therapy for cancer in the clinic. J Clin Invest 117(6):1466–1476

Kim YH et al (2009) Mechanisms involved in synergistic anticancer effects of anti-4-1BB and cyclophosphamide therapy. Mol Cancer Ther 8(2):469–478

Kober J et al (2008) The capacity of the TNF family members 4-1BBL, OX40L, CD70, GITRL, CD30L and LIGHT to costimulate human T cells. Eur J Immunol 38(10):2678–2688

Kryczek I et al (2007) Relationship between B7-H4, regulatory T cells, and patient outcome in human ovarian carcinoma. Cancer Res 67(18):8900–8905

Kumar H et al (2009) Toll-like receptors and innate immunity. Biochem Biophys Res Commun 388(4):621–625

Kwon BS, Weissman SM (1989) cDNA sequences of two inducible T-cell genes. Proc Natl Acad Sci USA 86(6):1963–1967

Kwon BS et al (2002) Immune responses in 4-1BB (CD137)-deficient mice. J Immunol 168(11):5483–5490

Latchman Y et al (2001) PD-L2 is a second ligand for PD-1 and inhibits T cell activation. Nat Immunol 2(3):261–268

Lee HK, Iwasaki A (2007) Innate control of adaptive immunity: dendritic cells and beyond. Semin Immunol 19(1):48–55

Lee SC et al (2009a) Stimulation of the molecule 4-1BB enhances host defense against Listeria monocytogenes infection in mice by inducing rapid infiltration and activation of neutrophils and monocytes. Infect Immun 77(5):2168–2176

Lee SW et al (2009b) Hypercostimulation through 4-1BB distorts homeostasis of immune cells. J Immunol 182(11):6753–6762

Lynch DH (2008) The promise of 4-1BB (CD137)-mediated immunomodulation and the immunotherapy of cancer. Immunol Rev 222:277–286

Melero I et al (2007) Immunostimulatory monoclonal antibodies for cancer therapy. Nat Rev Cancer 7(2):95–106

Melero I et al (2008) Multi-layered action mechanisms of CD137 (4-1BB)-targeted immunotherapies. Trends Pharmacol Sci 29(8):383–390

Melero I et al (2009) Palettes of vaccines and immunostimulatory monoclonal antibodies for combination. Clin Cancer Res 15(5):1507–1509

Muller D et al (2008) A novel antibody-4-1BBL fusion protein for targeted costimulation in cancer immunotherapy. J Immunother 31(8):714–722

Murillo O et al (2008) Therapeutic antitumor efficacy of anti-CD137 agonistic monoclonal antibody in mouse models of myeloma. Clin Cancer Res 14(21):6895–6906

Myers LM, Vella AT (2005) Interfacing T-cell effector and regulatory function through CD137 (4-1BB) co-stimulation. Trends Immunol 26(8):440–446

Narazaki H et al (2010) CD137 anonist antibody prevents cancer recurrence: Contribution of CD137 on both hematopoietic and non-hematopoietic cells. Blood 115(10):1941–1948

Okudaira K et al (2009) Blockade of B7-H1 or B7-DC induces an anti-tumor effect in a mouse pancreatic cancer model. Int J Oncol 35(4):741–749

Old LJ (1988) Tumor necrosis factor. Sci Am 258(5):59–60; 69–75

Paulos CM et al (2008) Adoptive immunotherapy: good habits instilled at youth have long-term benefits. Immunol Res 42(1–3):182–196

Riley JL (2009) PD-1 signaling in primary T cells. Immunol Rev 229(1):114–125

Rosenberg SA et al (2008) Adoptive cell transfer: a clinical path to effective cancer immunotherapy. Nat Rev Cancer 8(4):299–308

Sansom DM (2000) CD28, CTLA-4 and their ligands: who does what and to whom? Immunology 101(2):169–177

Schabowsky RH et al (2009). A novel form of 4-1BBL has better immunomodulatory activity than an agonistic anti-4-1BB Ab-associated severe toxicity. Vaccine 28(2):512–22

Seo SK et al (2004) 4-1BB-mediated immunotherapy of rheumatoid arthritis. Nat Med 10(10):1088–1094

Sharma RK et al (2009) Costimulation as a platform for the development of vaccines: a peptide-based vaccine containing a novel form of 4-1BB ligand eradicates established tumors. Cancer Res 69(10):4319–4326

Shi W, Siemann DW (2006) Augmented antitumor effects of radiation therapy by 4-1BB antibody (BMS-469492) treatment. Anticancer Res 26(5A):3445–3453

Sun Y et al (2002a) Costimulatory molecule-targeted antibody therapy of a spontaneous autoimmune disease. Nat Med 8(12).1405–1413

Sun Y et al (2002b) Administration of agonistic anti-4-1BB monoclonal antibody leads to the amelioration of experimental autoimmune encephalomyelitis. J Immunol 168(3):1457–1465

Tamura H et al (2003) Immunology of B7-H1 and its roles in human diseases. Int J Hematol 78(4):321–328

Tan JT et al (1999) 4-1BB ligand, a member of the TNF family, is important for the generation of antiviral CD8 T cell responses. J Immunol 163(9):4859–4868

Teng MW et al (2009) CD1d-based combination therapy eradicates established tumors in mice. J Immunol 183(3):1911–1920

Tseng SY et al (2001) B7-DC, a new dendritic cell molecule with potent costimulatory properties for T cells. J Exp Med 193(7):839–846

Uno T et al (2006) Eradication of established tumors in mice by a combination antibody-based therapy. Nat Med 12(6):693–698

Wang S et al (2003) Molecular modeling and functional mapping of B7-H1 and B7-DC uncouple costimulatory function from PD-1 interaction. J Exp Med 197(9):1083–1091

Wang C et al (2009a) Immune regulation by 4-1BB and 4-1BBL: complexities and challenges. Immunol Rev 229(1):192–215

Wang W et al (2009b) PD1 blockade reverses the suppression of melanoma antigen-specific CTL by CD4+ CD25(Hi) regulatory T cells. Int Immunol 21(9):1065–1077

Watts TH (2005) TNF/TNFR family members in costimulation of T cell responses. Annu Rev Immunol 23:23–68

Wilcox RA et al (2002a) Cutting edge: expression of functional CD137 receptor by dendritic cells. J Immunol 168(9):4262–4267

Wilcox RA et al (2002b) Impaired infiltration of tumor-specific cytolytic T cells in the absence of interferon-gamma despite their normal maturation in lymphoid organs during CD137 monoclonal antibody therapy. Cancer Res 62(15):4413–4418

Wilcox RA et al (2002c) Provision of antigen and CD137 signaling breaks immunological ignorance, promoting regression of poorly immunogenic tumors. J Clin Invest 109(5):651–659

Wilcox RA et al (2002d) Signaling through NK cell-associated CD137 promotes both helper function for CD8+ cytolytic T cells and responsiveness to IL-2 but not cytolytic activity. J Immunol 169(8):4230–4236

Wu K et al (2009) Kupffer cell suppression of CD8+ T cells in human hepatocellular carcinoma is mediated by B7-H1/programmed death-1 interactions. Cancer Res 69(20):8067–8075

Xiao H et al (2007) Soluble PD-1 facilitates 4-1BBL-triggered antitumor immunity against murine H22 hepatocarcinoma in vivo. Clin Cancer Res 13(6):1823–1830

Zhang H et al (2007) 4-1BB is superior to CD28 costimulation for generating CD8+ cytotoxic lymphocytes for adoptive immunotherapy. J Immunol 179(7):4910–4918

Zhu G et al (2001) Progressive depletion of peripheral B lymphocytes in 4-1BB (CD137) ligand/I-Ealpha)-transgenic mice. J Immunol 167(5):2671–2676

Zhu Y et al (2007) CD137 stimulation delivers an antigen-independent growth signal for T lymphocytes with memory phenotype. Blood 109(11):4882–4889

Chapter 15
Negative Regulators of NF-κB Activation and Type I Interferon Pathways

Caroline Murphy and Luke A.J. O'Neill

1 Introduction

The transcription factor nuclear factor-kappaB (NF-κB) and type I interferons are both important modulators of the innate immune system. NF-κB plays a key role in the up-regulation of pro-inflammatory cytokines, adhesion molecules and chemokines (Hayden et al. 2006), whereas type I IFN is essential for the initiation of an antiviral state in cells, and for the detection of malignant cells (Garcia-Sastre 2002).

The body relies on the presence of innate immune receptors to recognize invading pathogens. Pattern recognition receptors (PRRs) such as Toll-like receptors (TLRs), NOD-like receptors (NLRs) (Kanneganti et al. 2007), Retinoic acid inducible gene I (RIG-I) and melanoma differentiation-associated gene-5 (Mda-5) recognize the presence of invading pathogens by their distinguishing pathogen associated molecular patterns (PAMPs) (Kawai and Akira 2008). PRRs recognize the PAMPs as these are essential components of the invading pathogen and have not been changed through evolution as they are essential to the pathogen's survival. When activated by the presence of their ligand, the PRR signals downstream to initiate an inflammatory response and to activate the antiviral state of the cells. Initiation of the inflammatory response occurs through NF-κB. IFN inducible genes encode for proteins that influence cellular growth arrest, protein synthesis and apoptosis, thus acting to minimize replication action of the virus. Type 1 IFN also acts to increase dendritic cell (DC), natural killer (NK) cell and cytotoxic T cell (CTL) maturation. They also enhance antibody production, a combination of which, helps to clear virally infected and malignant cells.

Interferon was first described by Isaacs and Lindenman in 1957 (Isaacs and Lindenmann 1957). They found a macro-molecular particle which interfered with the virus's ability to replicate and it was termed interferon.

C. Murphy (✉) • L.A.J. O'Neill
School of Biochemistry and Immunology, Trinity College Dublin, Dublin, Ireland
e-mail: murphc25@tcd.ie

The interferon family is divided into three types based on their amino acid sequence homology and their receptor specificity. Type I interferon can be divided into 13 subtypes of IFN-α and a single subtype of IFN-β. IFN-α and IFN-β can be induced in most cell types (Liu 2005).

In this chapter we will summarize the inhibitory mechanisms, both endogenous and from pathogens, that target NF-κB and the type I interferon system – production of both type I interferons and their signalling pathways. The regulation of both is important since if over-active, inflammatory diseases can result. Pathogens also have to manipulate both systems in order to survive.

2 Signals That Lead to Type I IFN Production

The detection of viruses can be largely attributed to Toll-like receptors (TLRs) and RIG-I-like receptors (RLRs) (Kawai and Akira 2008). These activated signalling pathways are shown in Fig. 15.1. TLRs which detect the presence of viral particles are located on early endosomal membranes. TLR3 recognizes double stranded RNA (dsRNA), TLR7 and TLR8 recognize single stranded RNA (ssRNA) while TLR9 recognizes unmethylated CpG DNA. TLRs detect the presence of their ligand through leucine-rich repeat (LRR) motifs on the extracellular portion of the protein. They then signal downstream to adaptor molecules via their Toll/Interleukin-1 receptor (TIR) domain. Further signalling downstream up-regulates NF-κB and interferon regulatory factors (IRFs), which in turn function to promote the production of pro-inflammatory cytokines and type I IFN. Both TLR7 and TLR9 are highly expressed on plasmacytoid DCs (pDCs). Upon viral infection, pDCs produce vast quantities of type I IFN, indicating that TLR7 and TLR9 play major roles in the recognition of viral nucleic acids (Liu 2005).

RLRs such as RIG-I and Mda-5 are cytoplasmic helicases and are localized to the cytoplasm. RIG-I and Mda-5 are composed of an ATPase containing DExD/H box RNA helicase, two CARD (caspase activation and recruitment domain) and a C-terminal domain involved in autoregulation (Kawai and Akira 2008). They recognize viral RNA and upon recognition of their ligands they signal downstream to NF-κB, mitogen-activated protein (MAP) kinases and IRFs which transcribe genes encoding type I IFN and pro-inflammatory cytokines. RIG-I specifically recognizes 5′triphosphate containing viral RNA and up-regulates a downstream signalling pathway which causes the phosphorylation and dimerization of IRF3 by TANK-binding kinase 1 (TBK1) and IKKε (IκB [inhibitor of NF-κB] kinase) complex. Activation of the IRF3 complex causes the translocation of the complex into the cell nucleus to up-regulate transcription of IFN-β, protecting the host from viral infection through the innate immune system.

Downstream of RIG-I and Mda5 is an adaptor molecule known as mitochondiral antiviral signalling adapter (MAVS) also known as IFNβ promoter stimulator 1 (IPS-1). MAVS has an amino-terminal CARD domain and a C-terminal transmembrane domain that localizes it to the mitochondrial membrane. MAVS functions to activate IFN-α, IFN-β and NF-κB promoters in a TBK1-dependent manner (Seth et al. 2005).

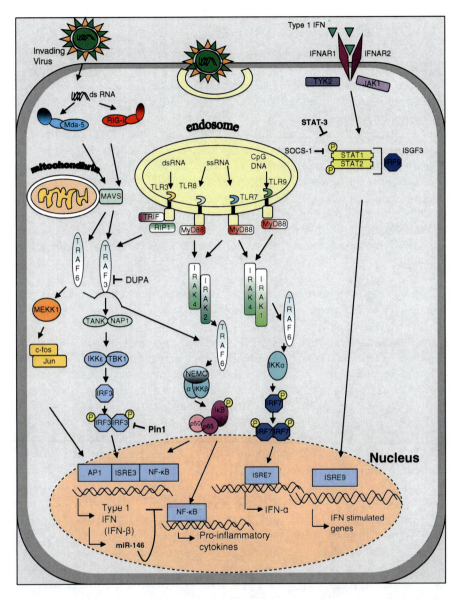

Fig. 15.1 Inhibitors of type I IFN pathway. Invading viruses are endocytosed into the cell at the plasma membrane or they inject their nucleic acids into the cytosol. Cytosolic receptors Mda-5 and RIG-I recognise the presence of viral nucleic acids where they signal downstream via their CARD domains to adaptor IPS-1/MAVS. MAVS found on the mitochondrial membrane signals to TRAF6 and TRAF3. TRAF6 signals to MEKK1, Cfos/Jun and activates transcription factor AP1. TRAF3 signals downstream to up-regulate IRF3 phosphorylation which activates ISRE3, where upon type I IFN is transcribed. DUPA inhibits this pathway at TRAF3 and Pin1 negatively regulates IRF3 activation. Endocytosed viruses are detectded by endosomally located TLRs 3, 7, 8 and 9. TLR3 signals downstream to activate IRF3. TLR7 and 8 function to up-regulate IRAK 4 and 2 and signal downstream to degrade IκB releasing the NF-κB dimer p50/p65 into the nucleus. NF-κB functions to up-regulate transcription of pro-inflammatory cytokines. TLR7 and 9 activate the IRAK4/IRAK1 pathway leading to IRF7 activation and IFN-α transctiption. Released type I IFN activates interferon receptor (IFNAR1/2). Activated IFNAR recruits the JAKs and STATS which form the ISGF3 complex upon IRF9 recruitment. ISGF3 signals to ISRE9 which transcribes type I IFN. STAT3 and SOCS-1 negatively regulate this pathway at STAT1.

Both TLRs and RLRs signal downstream to up-regulate phosphorylation and homodimerization of constitutively expressed IRF-3, triggering translation of type I IFN (IFN-β) and establishing the antiviral innate immune response. IRF-3 is present in cells in an inactive state. Activation of IRF-3 requires the phosphorylation of multiple serine/threonine residues at its carboxy terminus (Lin et al. 1998). Phosphorylation of IRF3 on serine clusters is carried out by TBK-1 and IKK-ε. This allows dimerization of IRF3 to occur followed by its accumulation in the nucleus. The IRF3 dimer forms a complex with transcription factors ATF-2/c-Jun(AP-1) and NF-κB (p65 and p50 heterodimer) and coactivators CBP/p300 allowing it to bind to DNA in a sequence-specific manner (Lin et al. 1998, 1999; Qin et al. 2003; Yoneyama et al. 1998).

IRF7 is expressed at low levels in un-stimulated cells. Upon stimulation of cells with IFN-β, IFN-α is rapidly produced. Signalling through TLR7 and TLR9 causes the pDCs to robustly produce IFN-α. IRAK1 and IKKα are critical for the activation of IRF7, IRAK-1 and IKKα bind and phosphorylate IRF7 (Honda et al. 2004). There is emerging evidence that chronic activation of pDCs through TLR7 and TLR9 by viral RNA complexes may be an important mechanism in driving auto immunity. There are currently significant efforts underway to develop antagonists of TLR7 and TLR9 (Guiducci et al. 2008).

Following the production of type I IFN, the molecules leave the cells to stimulate interferon receptors (IFNAR1 and IFNAR2), promoting the transition from innate to adaptive immunity (Fig. 15.1). The IFNAR heterodimer recruits JAK tyrosine kinases Tyk2 (tyrosine kinase 2) and JAK1 (Janus kinase 1), respectively. In myeloid cells, IFN-α predominantly activates signal transducer and activator of transcription 1 (STAT1), STAT2 and STAT3 (Caraglia et al. 2005; Takaoka and Taniguchi 2003; Katakura et al. 2005; Brierley et al. 2002). JAK1 and Tyk2 tyrosine phosphorylate STAT1 and STAT2 and in combination with IRF9 assemble to form the heterotrimeric IFN-stimulated gene factor 3 (ISGF-3) complex. The ISGF-3 complex moves to the nucleus where it binds to the IFN-stimulated response element (ISRE). Here IFN induces transcription of antiviral mediators and STAT1-dependent inflammatory genes such as CXCL9 and CLCL10. It has been established that STAT1 and STAT2 function to mediate the IFN-α and IFN-β antiviral and inflammatory effects.

3 Negative Regulation of Type 1 IFN: Viral Counter Attack

Several viruses have evolved multiple mechanisms to prevent the production of type I IFN-mediated antiviral response (Table 15.1). Different stages of the interferon pathway are targeted.

Viruses have developed mechanisms to subvert the host immune defence by:

- Allowing virus to exist undetected
- Suppressing IFN synthesis
- Binding and neutralizing secreted IFN molecules
- Blocking IFN signalling
- Inhibiting the action of IFN-induced antiviral proteins

Table 15.1 Viral proteins that target the type I IFN pathway

Target molecule	Virus	Protein	Target interferon	Evading technique	References
ssRNA, dsRNA	Influenza A	NS1	IFN-β	Binds dsRNA, preventing its access to RNA sensors	Wang et al. (2000); de Vries et al. (2009)
	Ebola	VP35	IFN-α/β	Prevents dsRNA from presenting to RIG-I	Cardenas et al. (2006)
RIG-I	Influenza A	NS1	IFN-β	Impairs RIG-I mediated IFN-β	Mibayashi et al. (2007)
Mda-5	Paramyxovirus PIV5	V protein	IFN-β	Inhibits downstream activation of IFN-β	Andrejeva et al. (2004); Childs et al. (2007)
MAVS/Cardiff/Visa/IPS-1	HCV and flavivirus	NS3-4A	IFN-β	Cleaves MAVS at Cys508	Meylan et al. (2005)
PKR	HCV	NS54	IFN-α	Interacts with and inhibits PKR	Gale et al. (1998)
TBK-1	Rabies virus	Phosphoprotein P	IFN-β	Prevents the phosphorylation of IRF3 by targeting TBK1	Brzozka et al. (2005)
	Hanta virus	G1 cytoplasmic tail	IFN-β	Targets TBK1 rendering RIG-I responses inactive	Peter et al. (2006)
IRF3	Classical swine fever virus (CSFV)	Npro	IFN-β	Targets IRF3 for degradation via proteasome	Rumenapf et al. (1998); Bauhofer et al. (2005); La Rocca et al. (2005); Ruggli et al. (2005)
	Bovine respiratory syncytial virus	NS1, NS2	IFN-β	Blocks phosphorylation of IRF3 and IRF3 driven plasmid	Bossert et al. (2003)
	Influenza A	NS1	IFN-β	Blocks IRF3 activity	Talon et al. (2000)
	Ebola	VP35	IFN-β	Blocks IRF3 phosphorylation	Basler et al. (2003)
	HPV	E6	IFN-α/β	Inhibits IRF3 transactivation	Ronco et al. (1998); Li et al. (1999)
Tyk2	HPV	E6	IFN-α	Targets Tyk2, preventing binding to cytoplasmic portion of IFN receptor, inhibits Tyk2 phosphorylation	Ruggli et al. (2005)
IRF9	HPV	E7	IFN-α	Binds and inhibits IRF9, prevents its nuclear translocation, inhibiting ISGF-3	Park et al. (2000)
	HPV		IFN-β	IRF-1 mediated activation of IFN-β	Park et al. (2000)

3.1 Targeting of dsRNA, ssRNA by Viral Proteins

Influenza A virus is a negative-stranded RNA virus. It belongs to the *Orthomyxoviridae* family. Non-structural protein 1 (NS1) is expressed at high levels in virally infected cells and was found to bind dsRNA of Sendai virus and Newcastle disease virus (NDV) preventing the RNA sensor machinery of PKR recognizing their agonists (Hatada and Fukuda 1992). Downstream NF-κB is not activated which is a critical transcription factor required for IFN-β transcription (Wang et al. 2000). Viral protein 35 (VP35) of Ebola binds dsRNA and inhibits type I IFN production induced by RIG-I signalling (Cardenas et al. 2006).

3.2 Viral Targeting of Recognition Machinery

The viral non-structural protein 1 (NS1) of Influenza A virus binds RIG-I in infected cells and impairs the RIG-I-mediated induction of IFN-β (Mibayashi et al. 2007). The viral subversion properties of NS1 have all been mapped to its N-terminal domain (Garcia-Sastre 2002; Hatada and Fukuda 1992). A second viral protein which binds RNA sensors is a V protein from paramyxovirus PIV5. The viral V protein targets the RNA helicase Mda-5 via their highly conserved cysteine-rich C terminal domains. The V protein inhibits the downstream activation of the IFN-β promoter (Andrejeva et al. 2004; Childs et al. 2007).

A further viral protein which binds the RNA recognition machinery is a serine protease from hepatitis C virus (HCV) and flavivirus, known as NS3-4A. NS3-4A binds to the RIG-I and Mda-5 adaptor protein MAVS. This adaptor protein connects the RNA sensors with the downstream complex of TRAF3/TANK/NAP1. NS3-4A specifically cleaves MAVS at Cys 508 (Meylan et al. 2005). The MAVS protein was differentially localized to the cytoplasm in patients with HCV. It has also been found that a series of strains of HCV that were resistant to IFN-α were found to contain NS5A protein which interacted with and inhibited PKR (Gale et al. 1998).

3.3 Targeting Proteins Upstream of Type I IFN

Brzózka and colleagues found that the rabies virus (RV) of the *Rhabdoviridae* family is capable of growing in IFN-competent cells. They identified a viral phosphoprotein P which is an IFN antagonist which prevents the phosporylation of IRF3 by TBK1. So far, the molecular mechanism of action is unclear as co-immunoprecipitation assays have been unsuccessful and co-localization of the phosphoprotein P and TBK1 has not been observed. This suggests that the phopshoprotein P employs an indirect mechanism of action (Brzozka et al. 2005).

The constitutive expression of TBK1 within cells and the severe effect on IFN release in TBK1 knockout cells give an indication of the integral part TBK1 plays in the elimination of viruses from the cells. Consequently TBK1 becomes an important target for the virus to render inactive, to allow viral multiplication within cells. The Hantavirus has developed a strategy to evade the immune response. The viral expression of a G1 cytoplasmic tail from the Hantavirus NY-1V renders it pathogenic. The G1 cytoplasmic tail targets TBK1 inhibiting interferon-mediated responses (Peter et al. 2006).

3.4 Viral Targeting of IRF3

The transcription factor IRF3 is targeted by many viral proteins. Blocking IRF3 prevents its phosphorylation, dimerization and subsequent translocation to the nucleus to induce transcription of IFN-β. IRF3 is targeted by Npro proteins; Npro is a cysteine-like auto-protease (Rumenapf et al. 1998). Npro is found in pestiviruses some of which include classical swine fever virus (CSFV) and bovine diarrhoea virus. The Npro proteins target the IRF3 protein for degradation via the proteasomal pathway (Bauhofer et al. 2005; La Rocca et al. 2005; Ruggli et al. 2005).

Bovine respiratory syncytial virus non-structural proteins NS1 and NS2 can block the activity of IRF3-driven plasmid and phosphorylation of IRF3 (Bossert et al. 2003). The NS1 protein from Influenza A also blocks the activity of IRF3 (Talon et al. 2000). The VP35 protein of Ebola virus acts as an antagonist and inhibits transcriptional activation of IRF3 mammalian promoters. In this case, dimerization of IRF3 is inhibited by suppressing phosphorylation and nuclear translocation (Basler et al. 2003). The VP protein of Ebola blocks the action of the ISG54 and ISG56 promoter and prevents IRF3 dependent activation.

The human papilloma viruses (HPV) are small double-stranded DNA viruses. The HPV 16 E6 and E7 proteins interact directly with components of the IFN signalling pathways (Lin et al. 2001; Ronco et al. 1998). The E6 protein of HPV binds to and inhibits the transcription activation function of IRF3, thereby inhibiting the transcription of IFN-β (Ronco et al. 1998).

3.5 Viral Targeting of IRF9 and IRF1 and Tyk2

The human papilloma virus 16 E7 protein (HPV16 E7) inhibits IFN-α-mediated signalling by binding to IRF9. This prevents its translocation to the nucleus, inhibiting the formation of the ISGF-3 (interferon stimulated gene factor 3) transcription complex that binds IFN-specific response element (ISRE) in the nucleus. E7 also inhibits the IRF1-mediated activation of the IFN-β promoter, recruiting histone deacetylase to the promoter and preventing transcription (Park et al. 2000). The resulting inhibition of IRF-1 target gene transcription results in the decreased expression of IFN-β, TAP1 (transproter associated with antigen processing 1) and MCP-1 (monocyte chemotactic protein 1).

The E6 protein of HPV binds to Tyk2 preventing binding to the cytoplasmic portion of the IFN receptor, thus inhibiting the phosphorylation of Tyk2, STAT1 and STAT2 (Li et al. 1999).

3.6 RNA Silencing Suppressor (RSS) Activity of Viruses

Plants, insects and nematodes have long been known to contain RNA interference (RNAi) molecules to protect against invading viruses. RNAi mechanism is activated by the production of virus-specific double-stranded RNAs (dsRNAs). The RNAi machinery processes the dsRNAs into small interfering RNAs (siRNAs-21 nucleotide dsRNA dublex) by RNAse III-like endonuclease Dicer. Following this, one strand of the siRNA dublex is incorporated into the RNA-induced silencing complex (RISC). The RISC complex then targets viral mRNAs for destruction and as ever the virus has evolved a counter-attack mechanism. RNA silencing suppressors (RSS) were described in plants, the best known is the tombusvirus-encoded P19 protein which acts as a pathogenicity factor. P19 acts to suppress RNAi by blocking the RNAi machinery of the cell from binding siRNAs (Haasnoot et al. 2007). The VP35 protein of Ebola acts as an inhibitor of IFN but it has also recently been shown to act as a RSS.

4 Host Mechanisms to Regulate Type I IFN

Multiple host mechanisms have been found to target the type I IFN system and these will now be described.

4.1 Micro RNA-146a Is a Negative Regulator of the IFN Pathway

Much work has been done on microRNA (miRNA) as regulators of the innate immune system. miRNAs target mRNA and block at the translational level. It has been previously established that many individuals with systemic lupus erythematosus (SLE) have elevated levels of serum IFN-α (Hooks et al. 1979). In 2009 Chen and colleagues identified miRNA-146a to be under-represented in patients with SLE (Tang et al. 2009). The low expression of miR-146a negatively correlated with disease pathogenicity and with the production of interferon. In the SLE patients, inhibition of endogenous miR-146a caused the increased induction of type I interferon in peripheral blood mononuclear cells (PBMCs). TLR7 has been found to be mainly responsible for the excessive induction of type I IFN in the manifestation of both human and murine lupus. Expression profiling of miRNA in lupus patients found six miRNAs at lower levels than healthy controls. As miRNA 146a was previously known to target IRAK1 and TRAF6, they chose to focus on this particular miRNA

(Taganov et al. 2006). Mature miR-146a can be induced by imiquimod R837 a TLR7 ligand, type A CpG a TLR9 ligand, LPS a TLR4 ligand and type I IFN (Tang et al. 2009). It was also discovered that overexpression of miR-146a greatly reduced the induction of IFN-α and IFN-β in PBMCs and that silencing endogenous miR-146a using inhibitory oligonucleotides increased IFN production.

After IFN stimulation, IFN receptors (IFNAR) recruit Tyk2 and JAK1 which in turn recruit STAT1 and STAT2 together with IRF9 to form the IFN-stimulated transcription factor 3 (ISGF-3) transcriptional complex. The transient transfection of miR-146a into HEK 293T/ISRE cells substantially inhibited ISRE gene reporter activity after stimulation with type I IFN. To understand further how miR-146a targeted the type 1 IFN pathway bioinformatics tools were used, two novel targets of miR-146a were identified to be IRF5 and STAT1. Western blotting experiments showed that the presence of miR-146a in 293T cells reduced the expression of IRF5 and STAT1.

4.2 Suppressor of Cytokine Signalling-1 (SOCS-1) Inhibits Type I IFN Signalling

It has been previously established that suppressor of cytokine signalling (SOCS) proteins acts as negative feedback inhibitors for various cytokines which signal through the JAK/STAT pathway (Alexander and Hilton 2004). It has been found that the simplest means of attenuating a response is through a negative feedback loop. The SOCS proteins have a central SH2 domain and a conserved C-terminal motif termed the SOCS box. It was found that SOCS-1 inhibited type I IFN signalling by inhibiting the phosphorylation of STAT1 (Baetz et al. 2004).

4.3 STAT3: Negative Regulator of Type I IFN

Research has now established a role for STAT3 in IFN signalling. Over-expression and RNA interference assays have determined the downstream signalling effects of STAT3. STAT3 is strongly up-regulated after IFN-α stimulated gene transcription. STAT3 inhibits STAT1-mediated IFN signalling by sequestering STAT1 and hindering the formation of DNA-binding STAT1 homodimers (Ho and Ivashkiv 2006).

4.4 Prolyl Isomerase (Pin1) Negatively Regulates the IRF-3-Mediated Antiviral Response

The cytoplasmic peptidyl prolyl-isomerase Pin1 negatively regulates the IRF3-dependent antiviral immune response (Saitoh et al. 2006). Pin1 has a WW domain, which consists of two tryptophan residues. The WW domain specifically recognizes phosphorylated serine or threonine residues followed by a proline causing a conformational change (Wulf et al. 2005; Lu et al. 1996). Pin1 catalyzes cis-trans isomerization of peptide bonds located N-terminally to proline. Pin1 binds serine 399 phosphorylated IRF3, promoting ubiquitination and proteasomal degradation. This suppresses IRF3-dependent transcriptional activation. Using a reporter gene assay with a yeast transcription factor Gal4-IRF3 fusion construct, they found that upon stimulation of TLR3, RIG-I and TLR4 with poly(I)·poly(C), Newcastle disease virus (NDV) and lipopolysaccharide (LPS) respectively that exogenous expression of wild-type Pin1 inhibited IRF3-dependent transcriptional activation in a dose-dependent manner. A mutant form of the WW domain (W34A) does not block IRF3 transcriptional activation. A short hairpin RNA (shRNA) was generated to "knock down" Pin1 expression. It was found that the suppression of endogenous Pin1 expression greatly increased IRF3 dimerization induced by poly(I)·poly(C) and LPS at later time points 3–9 h but not after 1 h. These results indicate that Pin1 preferentially promotes proteasome-dependent degradation of dimeric IRF3. Polyubiquitination is an essential prerequisite for proteasome-dependent degradation and the S339A IRF3 mutant was less susceptible to polyubiquitination than the wild-type protein. These results lead to the conclusion that Pin1 plays a role in regulating ubiquitination and proteasome-mediated proteolysis of IRF3. Although it had by now been found that Pin1 was capable of suppressing IRF3 transcriptional activity, a real-time reporter gene assay showed that suppression of endogenous Pin1 using shRNA substantially prolonged both IRF3-dependent transcription and IFN-β promoter after TLR3 stimulation.

These results show that Pin1 is involved in terminating IRF3 after activation and that Pin1 regulates the expression of IRF3-dependent genes such as IFN-β; however, the expression of Pin1 is not altered during the antiviral response differentiating it from other negative regulators of the immune system.

The Pin1 protein has been previously implicated in breast cancer. Increased expression of Pin1 has been shown to be involved in the malignant transformation of cancer cells. The increased expression of Pin1 suppresses the innate immune system making it more vulnerable to infectious viral entities and could partly explain why cancer cells are more susceptible to lytic infection by Vesicular stomatitis virus (VSV) (Stojdl et al. 2003). Switching off IRF3 allows more viral replication to occur transforming cells into tumour cells.

4.5 DUBA Negatively Regulates TLR, RIG-I and Mda-5 Induced Type I IFN

Deubiquitinating enzyme A (DUBA) is an ovarian tumour (OTU)-type deubiquitinating enzyme. Type-1 IFN induced by TLRs, RIG-I and Mda-5 is negatively regulated in the presence of DUBA (Kayagaki et al. 2007). DUBA cleaves K63 linked polyubiquitin chains from TRAF3, a signalling pathway member upstream of IRF3. This down regulates the signalling to interferon responsive genes.

5 Negative Regulators of NF-κB Pathway

NF-κB pathways are classified into two. These are shown in Fig. 15.2 and the inhibitory mechanisms that target these pathways are also shown and will be described below.

A canonical pathway leads to the degradation of inhibitor of NF-κB (IκB). The canonical pathway is mainly activated by pro-inflammatory cytokines such as TNFα, , interleukin-1 (IL-1) and bacterial derived ligands such as LPS. TNF binds two different receptors TNF-R1 and TNF-R2 and it exerts most of its effects through TNF-R1. TNF binding to TNF-R1 initiates the receptor to recruit the cytoplasmic protein TNF-receptor-associated death domain (TRADD). TRADD operates as a platform for the recruitment of three proteins: FAS-associated death domain (FADD), receptor-interacting protein 1 (RIP1) and TNF-receptor-associated factor 2 (TRAF2). RIP1 and TRAF2 signal to IκB kinase (IKK) complex to activate NF-κB. LPS signals to TLR4 which recruits adaptor molecules MyD88 adaptor like (Mal) and MyD88 through their common Toll/interleukin-1 receptor (TIR) domain (Yamamoto et al. 2004) signalling downstream to up-regulate pro-inflammatory cytokines. TLR4 also recruits adaptor proteins TRAM-TRIF through their TIR domains, TLR4/TRAM/TRIF complex moves into early endosomes where it signals downstream to TRAF3/TBK1/IKKε where IRF3 and IRF7 are up-regulated to produce IFNβ and IFNα (Kagan et al. 2008). TLR4/TRIF/TRAM complex also signals to TRAF6 to signal downstream to NF-κB (Sheedy and O'Neill 2007).

The non-canonical pathway involing p100 processing to a mature p52 subunit is activated by B cell receptors.

The termination of the NF-κB signal is generally carried out by IκB proteins which are generated in response to NF-κB signals and through a negative feedback loop. IκB shuttles the NF-κB heterodimers back to the cytoplasm where they lie dormant awaiting the next round of activation. The deregulation of NF-κB can result in the uncontrolled secretion of these inflammatory factors ultimately leading to damaged host tissues, inflammatory diseases and cancer. To prevent the excessive NF-κB activation the NF-κB signal must be terminated at appropriate time points. Switching off the NF-κB signal at the promoter is necessary to prevent over production of NF-κB-induced genes.

5.1 *The NF-κB Family*

The NF-κB family consists of five members, p50/NF-κB1, p52/NF-κB2, p65/RELA, REL and RELB. Members of the NF-κB family can form 15 possible combinations of homodimers or heterodimers (Ghosh and Hayden 2008). The hetero- or homodimers are confined to the cytoplasm by their binding partners inhibitor of NF-κB (IκB) family members. Upon ligand stimulation IκB family members are phosphorylated by inhibitor of NF-κB kinases (IKKs) complex and are targeted for proteasomal degradation.

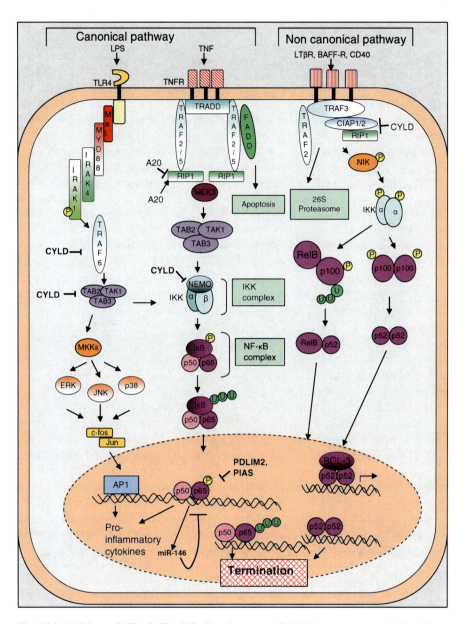

Fig. 15.2 Inhibitors of NF-κB. The NF-κB pathways are divided into two, a canonical pathway utilized by TLRs, TNFR and IL-1R and a non-canonical pathway used by LTβR, B Cell receptor and CD40. Upon activation by their ligands the TLRs form dimeric structures which allow their adaptor proteins to bind via their TIR domains. Mal and MyD88 recruit the IRAK proteins which signal through a series of phosphorylation events to activate transcription factors AP1 and NF-κB. These transcription factors up-regulate the production of pro-inflammatory cytokines. TNF signals through TNFR1 and TNFR2, activating TRADD, FADD and TRAF2/5. This complex recruits RIP1 which signals to activate IKK kinase complex to phosphorylate IκB and removing it for degradation and allowing the release of NF-κB p50/p65 into the nucleus. The negative regulator CYLD suppresses NF-κB activation along the pathway by cleaving K63 linked polyubiquitin chains on specific proteins. A20 acts as a negative feed back inhibitor at RIP1. PDLIM2 terminates NF-κB signal by sequestering it in the nucleus and targeting it for degradation. PIAS1 directly inhibit p65 dimers from binding DNA. miR-146 decreases NF-κB activity by targeting IRAK1 and TRAF6 at the translational level

The NF-κB dimers translocate to the nucleus where they bind to κB sites in promoters or enhancers of target genes. Each member of the NF-κB family shares an amino-terminal REL homology domain (RHD), and is sequestered in an inactive state in the cytoplasm by inhibitors of NF-κB (IκB) family members. Transcriptional activation of p65, REL and RELB is mediated by their C-terminal transactivation domains (TAD) whereas p50 and p52 lack TADs and act as repressors of transcription.

NF-κB signalling is regulated by members of the IκB family. The IκB family consists of three cytoplasmic proteins, IκBα, IκBβ and IκBε and three nuclear proteins, BCL-3, IκBNS and IκBζ. By using knockout cell lines it was found that IκBα is responsible for a strong negative feedback mechanism that turns off NF-κB activation and that IκBβ and IκBε stabilize the NF-κB response during longer stimulations (Hoffman et al. 2002). Upon stimulation by TNF, IL-1β or bacterial derivatives, the IκB proteins are rapidly phosphorylated, ubiquitinated and degraded by the 26S proteasome (Chen et al. 1995).

5.2 Atypical IκB Proteins (Nuclear IκB Proteins BCL-3, IκBNS and IκBζ)

The atypical IκB proteins, BCL-3, IκBζ and IκBNS can regulate NF-κB by either activation or inhibition. The IκB protein BCL-3 was originally identified in B-cell lymphocytic leukaemias. It has a well-described transactivation domain (TAD) and is found in the nucleus of cells. BCL-3 can function as both an initiator of κB transcription by binding to p50 and p52 and activating transcription through its TAD or can function as a transctiptional repressor. It is partly post-translational modification which determines the activational outcome of BCL-3. Activation of transcription by BCL-3 depends on phosphorylation and ubiquitination. It is thought that ubiquitinated but not phosphorylated BCL 3 may act as a negative regulator of NF-κB activity by stabilizing repressive p52 and p50 homodimers in a DNA-bound state, preventing the binding of transcriptionally active dimers to NF-κB promoter sites. This has been proposed to be a method for attaining LPS tolerance (Wessells et al. 2004; Carmody et al. 2007). BCL-3-p50-p50 complexes have been shown to negatively regulate the expression of the pro-inflammatory cytokine IL-23 and have been shown to positively regulate the expression of anti-inflammatory cytokine IL-10. Hence BCL-3 can act as a repressor of inflammation by suppressing pro-inflammatory gene expression and inducing the expression of anti-inflammatory cytokines (Muhlbauer et al. 2008).

IκBNS is a nuclear member of the IκB family. It is induced upon NF-κB up-regulation. The studies carried out in IκBNS deficient mice showed that after the stimulation by LPS the secondary immune response genes such as IL-6 and IL-12 p40 were up-regulated and NF-κB DNA promoter binding activity was prolonged, suggesting that IκBNS plays a role in the negative regulation of NF-κB in response to TLR ligands (Kuwata et al. 2006).

The third nuclear IκB protein IκBζ plays a positive role in the regulation of NF-κB. Although IκBζ lacks a TAD, overexpression experiments have suggested that it has transactivating activity when bound to p50 (Motoyama et al. 2005).

5.3 Controlling NF-κB Signalling by Ubiquitination

The controlled activation of NF-κB is very important to prevent the progression of inflammatory diseases and cancer. Many proteins have been discovered to act as negative regulators of the NF-κB pathway, A20 a zinc finger protein, deubiquitinating enzyme cylindromatosis (CYLD) and protein domain LIM (PDLIM) are all ubiquitin ligases. Ubiquitination plays a major role in both targeting proteins for degradation and also for biological functions. Ubiquitination is carried out by the ubiquitin complex which is composed of three enzymes which operate sequentially: the ubiquitin-activating enzyme (E1), the ubiquitin-conjugating enzyme (E2) and the ubiquitin ligase (E3). Ubiquitination involves the covalent linkage of ubiquitin molecules to a target protein as monomers (monoubiquitination) or polymers (polyubiquitination). Polyubiquitination occurs when ubiquitin chains are linked by the carboxy-terminal glycine of one ubiquitin to an internal lysine of another ubiquitin. Polyubiquintin chains can be linked through lysine 48 (K48) or lysine 63 (K63). Polyubiquitination through K48 targets a protein to proteasomal degradation by the 26S proteasome. Polyubiquitination through K63 facilitates various biological processes such as kinase activity, protein trafficking involving endocytosis and lysosomal targeting. Monoubiquitination of proteins can also occur and leads to vesicle trafficking and chromatin remodelling. Deubiquitinases (DUBs) reverse this reaction by hydrolyzing the ubiquitin chains, switching off the process. The NF-κB pathway utilizes K63 linked ubiquitinated proteins to facilitate protein–protein interactions. By acting as DUB, proteins such as A20, CYLD and PDLIM2 can hydrolyze the K63 linked ubiquitin chains thus negatively regulating the NF-κB signalling pathway.

5.4 A20 Inhibits NF-κB Activation by Dual Editing on the TNF Pathway

The zinc finger protein A20 tightly regulates the activation of NF-κB and its dependent gene expression (Bayert et al. 2000). The induction of A20 serves as a negative feedback mechanism of NF-κB activation. A20 is described as acting in two opposing ways, firstly by the sequential deubiquitination of TNF-receptor interacting protein 1 (RIP1) and secondly, by the ubiquitination of RIP1. RIP1 is then targeted for proteasomal degradation.

A20 is a cytoplasmic protein consisting of an N-terminal OTU domain, and seven novel zinc finger structures with a characteristic Cys-Xaa$_{2-4}$-Cys-Xaa$_{11}$-Cys-Xaa$_{2}$-Cys motif in its C terminal domain (Makarova et al. 2000; Opipari et al. 1990). Studies carried out in A20 deficient mice have shown that the mice developed severe multi-organ inflammation and were extremely susceptible to sub-lethal doses of TNF (Lee et al. 2000). These mice were unable to down regulate NF-κB transcriptional activity due to a constitutively active IKK complex. The mechanism by which

A20 regulates this has remained illusive for some time but it was recently shown that A20 possess two opposite enzymatic activities, first a deubiquitinating activity mediated by it OTU domain and second, a ubiquitin ligase activity mediated by its zinc finger (Evans et al. 2004; Wertz et al. 2004; Boone et al. 2004).

In 2004 Wertz and colleagues identified RIP1 as the crucial target for A20. Following stimulation by TNF, the TNF-R1 recruits RIP1 where it becomes K63 polyubiquitinated by TRAF2, from here the RIP1 mediates downstream signalling to the IKK complex to up-regulate NF-κB. Meanwhile RIP1 becomes deubiquitinated by the N-terminal OTU domain of A20. RIP1 then becomes polyubiquitinated again this time by polyubiquitin chains linked through Lys48, this polyubiquitination is mediated by the fourth finger in the C-terminal zinc finger domain of A20. The Lys48 linked ubiquitination then targets RIP1 for proteasomal degradation terminating the NF-κB activation signal (Heyninck and Beyaert 2005).

5.5 CYLD: A Suppressor of NF-κB Activation

The protein CYLD was originally identified as a mutated gene in a condition called familial cylindromatosis (FC) (Bignell et al. 2000). Recently CYLD mutations have been shown to be involved in many types of cancer including B-cell malignancy which involves the deregulation of NF-κB (Annunziata et al. 2007; Keats et al. 2007). Using RNAi-based functional screening CYLD was found to negatively regulate NF-κB activation (Brummelkamp et al. 2003). CYLD was found to interact with IKKγ(NEMO), TRAF2 and TRAF6 and specifically cleaves K63-linked polyubiquitin chains on these proteins, these proteins are all found on the NF-κB signalling pathway. Cleaving the K63 linked polyubiquitin chains inhibits IKK activation as the K63 linked chains mediate protein–protein interactions with upstream proteins such as Tak1, TRAF2, TRAF6 and RIP1 (Brummelkamp et al. 2003; Kovalenko et al. 2003; Trompouki et al. 2003; Yoshida et al. 2005). CYLD is though to bind TRAF6 via an adaptor protein p62 (Jin et al. 2008; Wooten et al. 2008). IKKγ/NEMO can also bind CYLD and associates with various IKK regulators such as RIP1 and TRAF2. Both IKKγ/NEMO and p62 contain ubiquitin binding domains which mediate protein interaction in an ubiquitin dependent way.

It has been suggested that CYLD and A20 operate at different stages of NF-κB activation. It is thought that CYLD is constitutively active preventing ubiquitination and hence activation of the NF-κB signalling pathway. CYLD knockdown experiments using RNAi have shown that TRAF2 is constitutively active (Reiley et al. 2005). Then, upon stimulation of the NF-κB pathway CYLD is phosphorylated by IKK and no longer possesses its de-ubiquitination activity, thereby allowing ubiquitination followed by activation of components of the NF-κB pathway to occur. In contrast to CYLD, A20 is up-regulated upon NF-κB activation whereas CYLD is constitutively present inhibiting NF-κB.

5.6 PDLIM2-Termination of NF-κB by Intranuclear Sequestration and Degradation of p65 Subunit

It has been found that NF-κB can be down regulated in the absence of IκB, indicating that a second mechanism for down regulating NF-κB must exist. A nuclear protein PDLIM2 functions to sequester NF-κB in the nucleus and targets it for degradation (Tanaka et al. 2007).

PDLIM2 is a nuclear ubiquitin ligase which targets nuclear p65. PDLIM2 has been shown to exert its ubiquitin E3 ligase activity through its LIM domain, as a PDLIM2 mutant lacking the LIM domain was unable to ubiquitinate p65 (Capili et al. 2001). It is found in both T cells and innate immune cells such as DCs and macrophages where NF-κB signalling is mediated by TLRs. It was found using co-immunoprecipitation assays in HEK 293 cells that PDLIM2 selectively binds to p65 and not p50 NF-κB subunits. Using NF-κB luciferase assays they found that the expression of PDLIM2 suppressed p65-dependent luciferase activity in a dose- dependent manner. PDLIM2 carries out its nuclear trafficking by its PDZ domain. The findings indicated that PDLIM2 sequesters p65 and prevents it from up-regulating transcriptional activation. Following TLR stimulation p65 is polyubiquitinated and is targeted to distinct subnuclear domains where p65 is ultimately degraded by the 26S proteaseasome.

5.7 SOCS1 and COMMD1-Terminating NF-κB Transcriptional Activity

SOCS1 acts in a negative feedback loop to inhibit NF-κB transcriptional activity and to target upstream IRAK1 in a dose-dependent manner (Nakagawa et al. 2002). SOCS1 and IRAK1 can form a complex through the SH2 domain of SOCS1 and lead to the possibility that SOCS1 targets IRAK1 for proteasomal degradation. In addition, SOCS1 directly targets p65 subunit of NF-κB with the aid of COMMD1 (copper metabolism (Murr1) domain containing 1) protein by forming an ECS ubiquitin ligase complex. COMMD1 promotes the association between p65 and SOCS1 and between SOCS1 and cullin-1 all of which facilitates the ubiquitination by the ECS complex (Maine et al. 2007). The targeting of p65 to SOCS1-containing ubiquitin ligase complex by COMMD1 is a major contributor to the termination of p65 mediated signalling.

5.8 PIAS Negatively Regulates NF-κB at Early Time Points

Protein inhibitor of activated STAT1 (PIAS) belongs to a family of small ubiquitin-like modifier (SUMO) E3 ligases. They can inhibit signal transducer and activator of transcription (STAT) and NF-κB transcriptional responses. PIAS1 directly inhibits p65 dimers from binding DNA at early time points. PIAS1 deficient cells show an increase in the level of NF-κB dependent genes such as IκBα at 30 min and levels return to normal at 1 h (Lu et al. 2005).

5.9 ABIN-1,2 and 3: Negative Inhibitors of NF-κB Pathway

Yeast two-hybrid studies were carried out to find proteins that bind to the zinc finger protein A20. Two novel proteins were identified named A20-binding inhibitor of NF-κB activation (ABIN-1) and ABIN-2. Overexpression of both ABIN proteins mimicked the NF-κB inhibiting effect of A20 (Heyninck et al. 1999; Van Huffel et al. 2001). Recently a third ABIN protein was identified as an A20-binding inhibitor of NF-κB activation (ABIN) (Wullaert et al. 2007). This protein has now been termed ABIN-3. In response to TNF, IL-1, LPS and 12-O-tetradecanoylphorbol-13-acetate ABIN-3 was shown to inhibit NF-κB activation. The inhibition of NF-κB activation by ABIN-3 is not thought to be related to its ability to bind A20. It is understood that ABIN-3 can inhibit NF-κB independently of A20. The treatment of human monocytic cells with TLR4 ligand LPS strongly induces the expression of ABIN-3. Overexpressed ABIN-3 inhibits NF-κB activation downstream of TRAF6 and upstream of IKKγ. From this, ABIN-3 has been identified as a new player in the negative feedback regulator of LPS-induced NF-κB activation.

5.10 Inhibition of NF-κB Pathway by Micro-RNA 146

NF-κB has long been known as an anti-apoptotic molecule promoting cell survival. A constitutively active NF-κB molecule would be regarded as beneficial to cancer cells where it would promote cell survival, proliferation, angiogenesis and metastasis (Karin 2006). Therefore it is crucial for cells to have mechanisms in place to curb any out-of-control NF-κB activation. Recently it has been shown that when expressed in a human breast cancer cell line MDA-MB-231, miR-146a/b could negatively regulate NF-κB. The decrease in NF-κB activity was shown by the reduction in NF-κB target genes such as IL-8, IL-6 and matrix metalloproteinase-9. Reduced phosphorylation of the NF-κB inhibitor (IκB) was also shown. When miR-146a/b was transfected into these cells, their invasion and migration capacity was impaired compared to control cells. It is thought that when stimulated by IL-1 or the TLRs NF-κB is up-regulated and miR-146 is induced. miR-146 then targets IRAK1 and TRAF6 at a translational level, both of which are part of the NF-κB activation pathway. miR146 targets them as part of a negative feedback loop (Taganov et al. 2006, 2007; Karin 2006).

6 Concluding Remarks

In the past 3 years, multiple mechanisms have been found which control the NF-κB system and the type I IFN system, attesting to the importance of these pathways for host defence and inflammation. The increasing complexity of this regulation represents a major challenge in our efforts to determine the roles of these proteins in disease. Further work should aim to validate these processes *in vivo* and begin the process of manipulating these systems therapeutically. It is likely that new vaccines and anti-inflammatory therapies will emerge from all these insights into the control of innate immunity.

References

Alexander WS, Hilton DJ (2004) The role of suppressors of cytokine signaling (SOCS) proteins in regulation of the immune response. Annu Rev Immunol 22:503–529

Andrejeva J et al (2004) The V proteins of paramyzoviruses bind the IFN-inducible RNA helicase, mda-5 and inhibit its activation of the IFN-beta promoter. Proc Natl Acad Sci USA 101:17264–17269

Annunziata CM et al (2007) Frequent engagement of the classical and alternative NF-kappaB pathways by diverse genetic abnormalities in multiple myeloma. Cancer Cell 12:115–130

Baetz A et al (2004) Suppressor of cytokine signaling (SOCS) proteins indirectly regulate Toll-like receptor signalling in innate immune cells. J Biol Chem 279(52):54708–54715

Basler CF et al (2003) The Ebola virus vp35 protein inhibits activation of interferon regulatory factor 3. J Virol 77:7945–7956

Bauhofer O et al (2005) Role of double-stranded RNA and Npro of classical swine fever virus in the activation of monocyter-derived dendritic cells. Virology 343:93–105

Bayert R et al (2000) A20 and A20-binding proteins as cellular inhibitors of nuclear factor-kappaB dependent gene expression and apoptosis. Biochem Pharmacol 60:1143–1151

Bignell GR et al (2000) Identification of the familial cylindromatosis tumour-suppressor gene. Nat Genet 25:160–165

Boone DL et al (2004) The ubiquitin-modifying enzyme A20 is required for termination of Toll-like receptor responses. Nat Immunol 5:1052–1060

Bossert B et al (2003) Nonstructural protein NS1 and NS2 of bovine respiratory syncytial virus blocks activation of interferon regulatory factor 3. J Virol 77:8661–8668

Brierley MM et al (2002) Review: IFN-alpha/beta receptor interactions to biologic outcomes: understanding the circuitry. J Interferon Cytokine Res 22:835–845

Brummelkamp TR et al (2003) Loss of the cylindromatosis tumour suppressor inhibits apoptosis by activating NF-kappaB. Nature 424:797–801

Brzozka K, Finke S, Conzelmann KK (2005) Identification of rabies virus alpha/beta interferon antagonist: phosphoprotein P interferes with phosphorylation of interferon regulator factor 3. J Virol 79(12):7613–7681

Capili AD et al (2001) Solution structure of the PHD domain from the KAP-1 corepressor: structural determinants for PHD, RING and LIM zinc-binding domains. EMBO J 20:165–177

Caraglia M et al (2005) Alpha-interferon and its effects on signal transduction pathways. J Cell Physiol 202:323–335

Cardenas WB, Loo YM et al (2006) Ebola virus VP35 protein binds double stranded RNA and inhibits alpha/beta interferon production induced by RIG-I signalling. J Virol 80(11): 5168–5178

Carmody RJ et al (2007) Negative regulation of toll-like receptor signalling by NF-κB p50 ubiquitination blockade. Science 317:657–678

Chen Z et al (1995) Signal-induced site-specific phosphorylation targets I kappa B alpha to the ubiquitin-proteasome pathway. Genes Dev 9:1586

Childs K et al (2007) Mda-5, but not RIG-I, is a common target for paramyxovirus V proteins. Virology 359:190–200

de Vries W, Haasnoot J et al (2009) Differential RNA silencing suppression activity of NS1 proteins from different influenza A strains. J Gen Virol 90:1916–1922

Evans PC et al (2004) Zinc-finger protein A20, a regulator of inflammation and cell survival, has de-ubiquitinating activity. Biochem J 378:727–734

Gale M Jr, Blakely CM et al (1998) Control of PKR protein kinase by hepatitis C virus nonstructural 5A protein: molecular mechanisms in kinase regulation. Mol Cell Biol 18:5208–5218

Garcia-Sastre A (2002) Mechanisms of inhibition of the host interferon alpha/beta-mediated antiviral responses by viruses. Microbes Infect 4(6):647–655

Ghosh S, Hayden MS (2008) New regulators of NF-kappaB in inflammation. Nat Rev Immunol 8:837–848

Guiducci C et al (2008) Signalling pathways leading to IFN-alpha production in human plasmacytoid dendritic cell and the possible use of agonists or antagonists of TLR7 and TLR9 in clinical indications. J Intern Med 265:43–57

Haasnoot J et al (2007) The Ebola virus VP35 protein is a suppressor of RNA silencing. PLoS Pathog 3(6 e86):0794–0803

Hatada E, Fukuda R (1992) Binding of influenza A virus NS1 protein to dsRNA in vitro. J Gen Virol 73:3325–3329

Hayden MS, West AP et al (2006) NF-kappaB and the immune response. Oncogene 25:6758–6780

Heyninck K, Beyaert R (2005) A20 inhibits NF-kappaB activation by dual ubiquitin-editing functions. Trends Biochem Sci 30(1):1–4

Heyninck K et al (1999) The zinc finger protein A20 inhibits TNF-induced NF-kappaB-dependent gene expression by interfering with an RIP- or TRAF2-mediated transactivation signal and directly binds to a novel NF-kappaB-inhibiting protein ABIN. J Cell Biol 135:1471–1482

Ho HH, Ivashkiv LB (2006) Role of STAT3 in type I interferon responses – negative regulation of STAT1-dependent inflammatory gene activation. J Biol Chem 281(30):14111–14118

Hoffman A et al (2002) The IκB-NF-κB signaling module: temporal control and selective gene activation. Science 298:1241–1245

Honda K et al (2004) Role of transductional transcriptional processor complex involving MyD88 and IRF-7 in Toll-like receptor signaling. Proc Natl Acad Sci USA 101:15416–15421

Hooks JJ et al (1979) Immune interferon in the circulation of patients with autoimmune disease. N Engl J Med 301:5–8

Isaacs A, Lindenmann J (1957) Virus interference. I. The interferon. Proc R Soc Lond B Biol Sci 147(927):258–267

Jin W et al (2008) Deubiquitinating enzyme CYLD regulates RANK signaling and osteoclastogenesis. J Clin Investig 118:1858–1866

Kagan JCS et al (2008) TRAM couples endocytosis of Toll-like receptor 4 to the induction of interferon-beta. Nat Immunol 9(4):361–368

Kanneganti TD et al (2007) Intracellular NOD-like receptors in host defense and disease. Immun Rev 27:549–559

Karin M (2006) Nuclear factor-kappaB in cancer development and progression. Nature 441:431–436

Katakura K et al (2005) Toll-like receptor 9-induced type I IFN protects mice from experimental colitis. J Clin Investig 115:695–702

Kawai T, Akira S (2008) Toll-like receptor and RIG-I like receptor signalling. Ann NY Acad Sci 1143:1–20

Kayagaki NP et al (2007) DUBA: a deubiquitinase that regulates type I interferon production. Science 318:1628

Keats JJ et al (2007) Promiscuous mutations activate the noncanonical NF-kappaB pathway in multiple myeloma. Cancer Cell 12:131–144

Kovalenko A et al (2003) The tumour suppressor CYLD negatively regulates NF-kappaB signalling by deubiquitination. Nature 424:801–805

Kuwata H et al (2006) IκBNS inhibits induction of a subset of Toll-like receptor-dependent genes and limits inflammation. Immunity 24:41–51

La Rocca SA et al (2005) Loss of interferon regulator factor 3 in cells infected with classical swine fever virus involves the N-terminal protease, Npro. J Virol 79:7127–7147

Lee EG et al (2000) Failure to regulate TNF-induced NF-kappaB and cell death responses in A20 deficient mice. Science 289:2350–2354

Li S et al (1999) The human papilloma virus (HPV)-18 E6 oncoprotein physically associates with Tyk2 and impairs Jak-STAT activation by interferon-alpha. Oncogene 18:5727–5737

Lin RH et al (1998) Virus-dependent phosphorylation of the IRF-3 transcription factor regulates nuclear translocation, transactivation potential, and proteasome-mediated degradation. Mol Cell Biol 18:2986–2996

Lin RM et al (1999) Structural and functional analysis of interferon regulatory factor 3: localisation of the transactivation and autoinhibitory domains. Mol Cell Biol 19:2465–2474

Lin R et al (2001) HHV-8 encoded vIRF-1 represses the interferon antiviral response by blocking IRF-3 recruitment of the CBP/p300 coactivators. Oncogene 20:800–811

Liu YJ (2005) IPC: professional type 1 interferon-producing cells and plasmacytoid dendritic cell precursors. Annu Rev Immunol 23:275–306

Lu KP et al (1996) A human peptidyl-prolyl isomerase essential for regulation of mitosis. Nature 380(6574):544–547

Lu B et al (2005) Negative regulation of NF-κB signalling by PIAS1. Mol Cell Biol 25:1113–1125

Maine G et al (2007) COMMD1 promotes the ubiquitination of NF-κB subunits through a cullin-containing ubiquitin ligase. EMBO J 26:436–447

Makarova KS et al (2000) A novel superfamily of predicted cysteine proteases from eukaryotes, viruses and *Chlamydia pheumoniae*. Trends Biochem Sci 25:50–52

Meylan E et al (2005) Cardif is an adaptor protein in the RIG-I antiviral pathway and is targeted by hepatitis C virus. Nature 437:1167–1172

Mibayashi M et al (2007) Inhibition of retinoic acid-inducible gene -I- mediated induction of interferon-{beta} by the NS1 protein of influenza A virus. J Virol 81:514–524

Motoyama Y et al (2005) Positive and negative regulation of nuclear factor-κB mediated transcription by IκBζ, an inducible nuclear protein. J Biol Chem 280:7444–7451

Muhlbauer M et al (2008) Impaired Bcl3 up-regulation leads to enhanced lipopolysaccharide-induced interleukin (IL)-23-p19 gene expression in IL-10 −/− mice. J Biol Chem 283:14182–14189

Nakagawa R et al (2002) SOCS-1 participates in negative regulation of LPS response. Immunity 17:677–687

Opipari AW Jr et al (1990) The A20 CDNA induced by tumor necrosis factor alpha encodes a novel type of zinc finger protein. J Biol Chem 265:14705–14708

Park J et al (2000) Inactivation of interferon regulatory factor-1 tumor suppressor protein by HPV E7 oncoprotein. Implication for the E7-mediated immune evasion mechanism in cervical carcinogenesis. 275:6764–6769

Peter J et al (2006) The pathogenic NY-1 Hantavirus G1 cytoplasmic tail inhibits RIG-I- and TBK-1- directed interferon responses. J Virol 80(19):9676–9686

Qin BY, Liu C et al (2003) Crystal structure of IRF-3 reveals mechanism of autoinhibition and virus-induced phosphoactivation. Nat Struct Biol 10:913–921

Reiley W et al (2005) Regulation of the deubiquitinating enzyme CYLD by IkappaB kinase gamma-dependent phosphorylation. Mol Cell Biol 25:3886–3895

Ronco LV et al (1998) Human papilloma 16 E6 oncoprotein binds to interferon regulatory factor-3 and inhibits its transcriptional activity. Genes Dev 12:2061–2072

Ruggli N et al (2005) N(pro) of classical swine fever virus is an antagonist of double stranded RNA-mediated apoptosis and IFN-alpha/beta induction. Virology 340:265–276

Rumenapf T et al (1998) N-terminal protease of pestiviruses: identification of putative catalytic residues by site directed mutagenesis. J Virol 72:2544–2547

Saitoh T et al (2006) Negative regulation of interferon-regulatory factor 3- dependent innate antiviral response by the prolyl isomerase Pin1. Nat Immunol 7(6):598–605

Seth RB et al (2005) Identification and characterization of MAVS, a mitochondrial antiviral signaling protein that activates NF-kappaB and IRF 3. Cell 122(5):669–682

Sheedy FJ, O'Neill LA (2007) The Troll in Toll: Mal and Tram as bridges for TLR2 and TLR4 signaling. J Leukocyte Biol 82:196–203

Stojdl DF et al (2003) VSV strains with defects in their ability to shutdown innate immunity are potent systemic anti-cancer agents. Cancer Cell 4(4):263–275

Taganov KD et al (2006) NF-kappaB dependent induction of microRNA miR146, an inhibitor targeted to signaling proteins of innate immune responses. Proc Natl Acad Sci USA 103:12481–12486

Taganov KD et al (2007) MicroRNAs and immunity: tiny players in a big field. Immunity 26:133–137

Takaoka A, Taniguchi T (2003) New aspects of IFN-alpha/beta signalling in immunity, oncogenesis and bone metabolism. Cancer Sci 94:405–411

Talon J et al (2000) Activation of interferon regulatory factor 3 is inhibited by the influenza A virus NS1 protein. J Virol 74:7989–7996

Tanaka T et al (2007) PDLIM2-mediated termination of transcription factor NF-κB activation by intranuclear sequestration and degradation of the p65 subunit. Nat Immunol 8(6):584–591

Tang Y et al (2009) MicroRNA-146a contributes to abnormal activation of type I interferon pathway in human lupus by targeting the key signaling proteins. Arthritis Rheum 60(4):1065–1075

Trompouki E et al (2003) CYLD is a deubiquitinating enzyme that negatively regulates NF-kappaB activation by TNFR family members. Nature 424:793–796

Van Huffel S et al (2001) Identification of a novel A20-binding inhibitor of nuclear factor-kappa B activation termed ABIN-2. J Biol Chem 276:30216–30223

Wang X et al (2000) Influenza A virus NS1 protein prevents activation of NF-kappaB and induction of alpha/beta interferon. J Virol 74(24):11566–11573

Wertz IE et al (2004) De-ubiquitination and ubiquitin ligase domains of A20 downregulate NF-kappaB signalling. Nature 430:694–699

Wessells J et al (2004) BCL-3 and NF κB p50 attenuate lipopolysaccharide-induced inflammatory responses in macrophages. J Biol Chem 279:49995–50003

Wooten MW et al (2008) Essential role of sequestosome 1/p62 in regulating accumulation of Lys63-ubiquitinated proteins. J Biol Chem 283:6783–6789

Wulf G et al (2005) Phosphorylation-specific prolyl isomerization: is there an underlying theme? Nat Cell Biol 7(5):435–441

Wullaert A et al (2007) LIND/ABIN-3 is a novel lipopolysaccharide-inducible inhibitor of NF-κB activation. J Biol Chem 282(1):81–90

Yamamoto M, Takeda K, Akira S (2004) TIR domain containing adaptors define specificity of TLR signalling. Mol Immunol 40(12):861–868

Yoneyama MS et al (1998) Direct triggering of type I interferon system by virus infection: activation of a transcription factor complex containing IRF3 and CBP/p300. EMBO 17:1087–1095

Yoshida H et al (2005) The tumor suppressor CYLD acts as a negative regulator for toll-like receptor 2 signalling via negative cross-talk with TRAF6 and TRAF7. J Biol Chem 280: 41111–41121

Chapter 16
Role of TGF-β in Immune Suppression and Inflammation

Joanne E. Konkel and WanJun Chen

1 Introduction

A delicate balance exists between immune activation (immunity) and immune non-responsiveness (tolerance), which prevents inappropriate responses to self yet also protects against invading pathogens. Transforming growth factor-β (TGF-β) is a key mediator of this balance. First discovered as a growth factor for non-immune cells, TGF-β has gradually been recognized as a critical cytokine in the regulation of immune responses. There are at least three major TGF-β homologs in mammals, TGF-β1-3, with TGF-β1 being the dominant isoform in the immune system. Due to the varied effects of TGF-β and the vast number of cell types it can affect, its activation is a highly regulated process; TGF-β is produced as prepro-TGF-β, and mature TGF-β is bound to a protein called latency associated protein (LAP). TGF-β-LAP can be secreted, but TGF-β is unable to bind its receptors when complexed to LAP and must be liberated in order to mediate its signal.

TGF-β initiates intracellular signaling following binding of type-I and type-II transmembrane serine/threonine kinase receptors to form a heteromeric complex at the cell surface. TGF-β predominately interacts with the type-I receptor ALK5 and the type-II receptor TGF-β receptor-II (TGF-βRII). TGF-β first binds to TGF-βRII which contains a constitutively active serine/theonine kinase (Dennler et al. 2002). TGF-β displays a high affinity for TGF-βRII but fails to interact with isolated ALK5 molecules (Shi and Massague 2003). However, the type I receptor ALK5 can bind the TGF-β:TGF-βRII complex and is phosphorylated by the active kinase of TGF-βRII. This phosphorylation event activates the kinase domain of ALK5 which then propagates the TGF-β signal intracellularly by activating signaling intermediates and Smad proteins.

J.E. Konkel • W. Chen (✉)
Mucosal Immunology Section, Oral Infection and Immunity Branch,
National Institute of Dental and Craniofacial Research, National Institutes
of Health, Bethesda, MD 20892, USA
e-mail: wchen@dir.nidcr.nih.gov

There are five Smad proteins involved in TGF-β signaling, which can be divided into three groups; (1) the receptor-activated Smads (Smad2/3) which are activated by type-I receptors, (2) the common Smad, Smad4, and (3) inhibitory Smads (Smad6/7) which antagonize TGF-β-signaling. The canonical signaling pathway for TGF-β would therefore involve the ALK5 mediated phosphorylation of Smad2 and 3. Generally, Smad2 and 3 then form heteromeric complexes with Smad4 which can then be translocated into the nucleus and regulate the transcription of target genes. However, Smad4 is not required for Smad2 and 3 nuclear translocation; both Smad2 and 3 have a nuclear localization sequence (NLS) (Derynck and Zhang 2003). Activated Smad complexes actually have a low affinity for DNA but manage to bind DNA strongly by first binding to, and forming complexes with, other transcription factors (Dennler et al. 2002). Depending on the interaction partner, transcription can be either positively or negatively affected.

TGF-β can also signal via Smad-independent pathways, specifically phosphorylation-transfer kinase cascades. TGF-β has been shown to activate Rac-Cdc42-dependent signaling, phosphatidylinositol 3-kinase (PI3K) and the mitogen-activated protein kinases (MAPKs) JNK, ERK, and p38 (Derynck and Zhang 2003).

2 Effects of TGF-β on the Immune System

TGF-β affects cells of both the innate and adaptive immune systems, playing a critical role in controlling immune responsiveness. This was clearly demonstrated in mice which lack TGF-β1 (Kulkarni et al. 1993; Shull et al. 1992). These mice succumbed to massive immunopathology with multiorgan inflammation and died within 3–4 weeks of birth. Although generally recognized as an immuno-modulatory cytokine, the function of TGF-β in immune responses is dependent on the cell type and microenvironment. Subsequently, TGF-β has been shown to be required for the development of certain immune cell types and importantly can affect the function of most immune cells. Here we discuss these data.

2.1 Macrophages

Macrophages are not only phagocytes, but also produce cytokines and can present antigen (Ag) to T cells. Treatment of macrophages with TGF-β decreases cytokine production upon LPS stimulation and can inhibit nitric oxide production (Bogdan et al. 1992; Tsunawaki et al. 1988; Vodovotz et al. 1993). Moreover, TGF-β alters the antigen-presenting capacity of macrophages through the inhibition of IFNγ-induced MHC class-II gene expression (Nandan and Reiner 1997) and through reduced expression of the costimulatory molecule CD40 (Takeuchi et al. 1998).

Macrophages play an important role in preventing immune responsiveness to apoptotic cells; rapid clearance of apoptotic cells by macrophages inhibits inflammatory and autoimmune responses to intracellular Ags. TGF-β is a key mediator in this immune suppression. Although apoptotic cells have been shown to secrete TGF-β (Chen et al. 2001a), macrophages also produce TGF-β upon encounter with apoptotic cells (Fadok et al. 1998; Perruche et al. 2008). Incubation of macrophages with apoptotic cells inhibits macrophage LPS-induced responses, and treatment with anti-TGF-β restored LPS responses. Therefore phagocytosis of apoptotic cells is accompanied by active suppression of inflammatory responses, an effect mediated by TGFb.

2.2 Natural Killer Cells

Natural killer (NK) cells are a vital component of the innate immune system but also play key roles in the activation of adaptive immune responses. NK cells mediate these roles through the killing of infected cells and the rapid production of cytokines upon stimulation. TGF-β inhibits cytokine production by NK cells, even in the presence of NK activating cytokines (Bellone et al. 1995). TGF-β can also inhibit the cytolytic ability of NK cells; short-term culture of NK cells in the presence of TGF-β reduces the ability of NK cells to kill target cells (Rook et al. 1986). Mechanistically, TGF-β alters the expression of the NK triggering receptors NKG2D and NKp30, important for cytolytic function (Castriconi et al. 2003). Due to their cytolytic function NK cells also play a vital role in anti-tumor immunity, and reduced NK cell expression of NKG2D has been reported to correlate with increased plasma levels of TGF-β in cancer patients (Lee et al. 2004).

2.3 Dendritic Cells

DC are considered the professional antigen-presenting cells (APCs), and signals derived from DC are vital in determining T cell activation and differentiation. TGF-β is required for the differentiation of Langerhan cells (LC) (Strobl et al. 1997), a population of DC found in the epidermis of the skin, TGF-β$1^{-/-}$ mice lack this population of cells (Borkowski et al. 1996). In vitro, TGF-β can promote the differentiation of DC with an "immature" phenotype; low levels of surface MHC-II, and costimulatory molecules (Geissmann et al. 1999; Yamagata et al. 2004). TGF-β has also been reported to modulate the function of mature DC, reducing their stimulatory capacity (Geissmann et al. 1999). Thus TGF-β could promote immune unresponsiveness through the generation of immature DC and/or by inhibiting DC maturation. Either way it is interesting to note that the administration of TGF-β-treated DC can modulate ongoing (auto)immune responses (Faunce et al. 2004). In addition, TGF-β can be secreted by immature DC (Morelli et al. 2001), which can be triggered by exposure to and digestion of apoptotic cells (Perruche et al. 2008). Collectively, it appears TGF-β can modulate adaptive immune responses by acting on DC, and affecting how DC orchestrate ongoing immune responses.

2.4 B Cells

The effects of TGF-β on B cells are primarily immunosuppressive, inhibiting the proliferation of B cell progenitors (Kee et al. 2001) and mature B cells, and inhibiting antibody production (with the clear exception of IgA) (Kehrl et al. 1986a). Examination of mice with a conditional deletion of TGF-βRII on B cells showed B cells to be hyper-responsive, leading to increased serum Ig levels of most isotypes except IgA (Cazac and Roes 2000). Importantly, increased titers of anti-DNA antibodies were also noted. Examination of the TGF-β-induced transcriptome has been performed by comparative gene expression profiling in wild-type and TGF-βRII specific knockout B cells (Roes et al. 2003). This study demonstrated that TGF-βRII stimulation attenuated B cell receptor (BCR) signaling through the induction of inositol-polyphosphate phosphatase Ship-1, which antagonized PI3K, and CD72, which recruited an inhibitory phosphatase to the BCR complex. IL-4 signaling, important for B cell proliferation and survival, was also inhibited by TGF-βRII-signaling. Thus, TGF-β can affect the activation, differentiation, and homeostasis of B cells.

3 T Cells

TGF-β affects many aspects of T cell biology, and it is on this cell type which this review will primarily focus. TGF-β1$^{-/-}$ mice rapidly develop a progressive inflammatory syndrome affecting multiple organs, but to what extent does T cell dysfunction contribute to disease? The autoimmune phenotype of TGF-β1$^{-/-}$ mice is prevented by crossing these mice with SCID or Rag$^{-/-}$ mice; moreover, elimination of T cells, but not B cells, also reverses the disease phenotype (Bommireddy et al. 2004). Subsequently it was demonstrated that mice, in which TGF-β-signaling was specifically ablated in T cells (by specific deletion of TGF-βRII or TGF-βRI) recapitulated the multiorgan disease seen in TGF-β1$^{-/-}$ (Li et al. 2006; Liu et al. 2008; Marie et al. 2006). Thus, these data highlight that TGF-β mediates critical control over T cells.

3.1 TGF-β in T Cell Development

TGF-β-signaling plays a vital role in the differentiation of invariant natural killer T cells (iNKT cells). Mice with a T cell specific deletion of TGF-βRII have reduced numbers of canonical CD1d-restricted NKT cells in both the thymus and periphery (Li et al. 2006; Marie et al. 2006). TGF-β has been shown to control iNKT precursor differentiation, with different branches of TGF-β-signaling effecting iNKT precursors at different points during maturation (Doisne et al. 2009).

Recent data have shown that TGF-β is required for the development of natural, CD4$^+$CD25$^+$Foxp3$^+$ regulatory T cells (nTreg) (Liu et al. 2008). Genetic ablation of

TGF-β receptor-I specifically in T cells prevented nTreg development in neonate mice (3–5 days old) but allowed for nTreg expansion in mice 7 days and older. This late expansion of nTregs was attributed to overproduction of, and greater sensitivity to, IL-2, as deletion of IL-2 in TGF-βRI conditional knockout mice resulted in the complete absence of nTregs.

3.2 TGF-β Effects on T Cell Function

It has long been known that TGF-β has an antiproliferative effect on T cells in vitro (Kehrl et al. 1986b). How does TGF-β inhibit T cell proliferation? TGF-β likely inhibits IL-2 production, as TGF-β can inhibit IL-2 transcription via a Smad3-dependent mechanism (Brabletz et al. 1993; McKarns et al. 2004). TGF-β treatment has also been shown to alter the expression of a number of regulators of the cell cycle. Levels of c-myc, cyclin D2, and cyclin E, all targets of IL-2-induced transcription, were reduced in TGF-β-treated T cells lines (Nelson et al. 2003). Cyclin-dependent kinase 4 (cdk4) expression was also decreased in primary T cells treated with TGF-β (Wolfraim et al. 2004).

As already stated, mice in which TGF-βRII or TGF-βRI is genetically ablated in T cells showed massive immunopathology. Examination of T cells from these conditional knockout mice showed peripheral $CD4^+$ and $CD8^+$ T cells expanded more upon stimulation than wild-type (WT) T cells. Peripheral TGF-βRII$^{-/-}$ T cells also showed a more activated phenotype and increased cytokine production (Li et al. 2006; Liu et al. 2008; Marie et al. 2006). The activated phenotype and T cell mediated pathology in mice in which TGF-βR is specifically deleted in T cells could be due to: (1) spontaneous/incorrect activation of the T cells due to lack of TGF-β control (2) expansion of self-reactive TGF-βR deficient T cells which mediate the inflammatory disease, (3) inability of TGF-βR deficient Tregs to control effector T cells. Current data would suggest a T cell intrinsic role for TGF-β-signaling in controlling the activation of pathogenic self-reactive T cells. Mixed bone marrow (bm) chimeras of wild type (WT) mice and mice with the T cell specific deletion of TGF-βRII had normal numbers of Tregs yet developed multiorgan inflammatory disease, highlighting that WT Tregs were unable to control TGF-βRII$^{-/-}$ T cells (Li et al. 2006; Marie et al. 2006). Moreover, transfer of WT Tregs into mice with the T cell specific deletion of TGF-βRII failed to prevent the lethal inflammatory disease. These data demonstrate WT Tregs, like TGF-βRII$^{-/-}$ Tregs, cannot control TGF-βRII$^{-/-}$ T cells; therefore, disease phenotype was not specifically due to Treg malfunction.

The question remained as to whether the activated T cells found in mice lacking TGF-β-signaling were activated in an antigen-specific manner or via bystander mechanisms not involving the TCR. Even prior to the use of the T cell specific TGF-βRII$^{-/-}$ mice, data suggested the former to be correct. Two groups crossed TGF-β1$^{-/-}$ mice to DO11.10 and DO11.10xRag1$^{-/-}$ mice and demonstrated that restriction of the $CD4^+$ T cell repertoire reduced immune-mediated pathology in the TGF-β1$^{-/-}$ mice

(Bommireddy et al. 2006; Robinson et al. 2006). Data from mice which have TGF-βRII deleted specifically on T cells have confirmed these observations. Li et al crossed the T cell specific TGF-βRII$^{-/-}$ mice with OT-IIxRag1$^{-/-}$ mice and showed that unlike TGFβRII$^{-/-}$ T cells, the majority of TGF-βRII$^{-/-}$ OT-IIxRag1$^{-/-}$ cells did not differentiate into Th1 or Th2 cells. Thus, in the absence of their cognate ligand, TGF-βRII$^{-/-}$ OT-II cells do not differentiate into effector cells and hence the mice show reduced immunopathology.

A compounding factor in determining the cause of heightened TGF-βRII$^{-/-}$ T cell activation is the suggestion that TGF-β promotes the survival of naïve T cells. In OT-IIxRag1$^{-/-}$ mice crossed with the T cell specific TGF-βRII$^{-/-}$, reduced numbers of OT-II cells in the spleen, lymph nodes, and blood were seen. As previously stated, these TGF-βRII$^{-/-}$ OT-IIxRag1$^{-/-}$ fail to differentiate into T helper cells, and the authors suggest that in the absence of TGF-β-responsiveness, naïve T cells which fail to become T helper cells, undergo apoptosis. This is in line with an earlier study which showed increased thymocyte and peripheral T cell apoptosis in TGF-β1$^{-/-}$ mice (Chen et al. 2001b).

4 TGF-β and Tregs

TGF-β plays vital roles in the maintenance of peripheral tolerance mediated by Tregs. First, TGF-β is essential for the generation of Foxp3$^+$ Treg cells from peripheral naïve CD4$^+$ T cells (Chen et al. 2003). As previously discussed, TGF-β is also required for the generation of nTregs in neonatal mice. TGF-β has been shown to be important for the survival/maintenance of peripheral nTregs; evidence supporting this there were reduced numbers of peripheral nTregs in mice with a T cell specific deletion of TGF-βRI/II (Li et al. 2006; Liu et al. 2008). TGF-βRII$^{-/-}$ nTregs proliferated more upon stimulation, therefore reduced nTreg numbers were suggested to be due to reduced nTreg survival.

4.1 TGF-β and Naïve T Cell Differentiation

Perhaps the most striking role of TGF-β relating to Tregs came with the demonstration that TGF-β-signaling, in the context of TCR stimulation, induces Foxp3 expression in naïve CD4$^+$CD25$^-$Foxp3$^-$ T cells and converts them into Foxp3$^+$ Tregs (termed "induced" Tregs) with potent suppressive capabilities (Chen et al. 2003). This conversion has been shown to occur in mouse (Chen et al. 2003) and human (Fantini et al. 2004). T cells in vitro and importantly has been shown to occur in vivo in a variety of settings in mice. Systemic increases in TGF-β were shown to substantially increase Foxp3$^+$ Treg cell numbers (Perruche et al. 2008). Induction of Foxp3 in naive T cells following administration of Ag coupled to DC-targeting antibodies (Kretschmer et al. 2005) and administration of low doses of soluble peptide (Apostolou and von Boehmer 2004) were both shown to be TGF-β-dependent.

It has long been known that TGF-β is a powerful inhibitor of Th1 and Th2 differentiation (Fiorentino et al. 1989; Sad and Mosmann 1994). In direct contrast to the effect of TGF-β on Th1 and Th2 cells, TGF-β has a positive effect on Th17 cell differentiation; TGF-β and IL-6 induce the Th17 differentiation program (Bettelli et al. 2006). How TGF-β regulates the differentiation of Tregs and Th17 cells with seemingly opposing functions, remains unresolved, but Foxp3 has been shown to interact with RORγt, a Th17 lineage specific transcription factor (Zhou et al. 2008). However, it seems that the presence of pro-inflammatory cytokines, indicative of infection, would determine whether TGF-β induces the differentiation of Th17 or induced Tregs. This results in a situation in which a reciprocal relationship between Treg induction and Th subset differentiation exists with the outcome of TCR stimulation being heavily dependent on the cytokine milieu, in which TGF-β plays a dominant role.

4.2 Treg Derived TGF-β

Despite the plethora of potential sources of TGF-β within the body, TGF-β produced by Tregs is suggested to be vital in maintaining peripheral tolerance. Mice in which only T cells fail to make TGF-β developed a chronic wasting colitis and had high levels of auto-antibody production (Li et al. 2007). In SCID mice, colitis induced by the transfer of $CD4^+CD45RB^{hi}$ cells can be prevented by the co-transfer of small numbers of Tregs; this Treg-mediated prevention is overcome by co-administration of anti-TGF-β (Powrie et al. 1996). So if Tregs produce TGF-β as a mechanism of immune suppression, an interesting question arises. Can Treg-derived TGF-β induce Foxp3 in naïve T cells and therefore expand the Treg pool? This is termed infectious tolerance (Qin et al. 1993) and has been shown to be dependent on LAP-TGF-β expressed by an activated Treg population (Andersson et al. 2008).

In addition, early studies on the differentiation of Th17 cells revealed that Treg-derived TGF-β could induce Th17 cells (Veldhoen et al. 2006a). Th17 differentiation was induced when naïve T cells were stimulated via the TCR in the presence of IL-6 produced from LPS-stimulated DC and Treg-derived TGF-β.

5 TGF-β and Aberrant Immune Responses

TGF-β can exert its influence on most cells of the immune system (Fig. 16.1). As such it is no surprise that aberrant immune responses occur in cases of TGF-β deregulation.

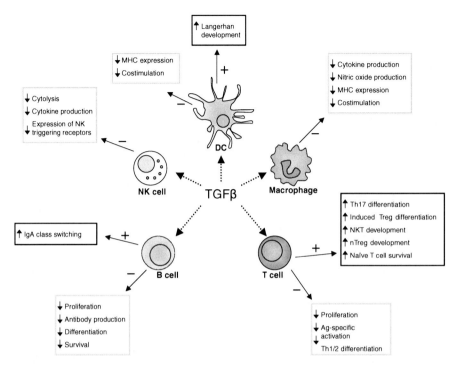

Fig. 16.1 TGF-β regulation of immune cells. Positive (*black boxes*) and negative (*gray boxes*) effects of TGF-β on populations of immune cells

5.1 Autoimmunity

Data from human patients and animal models of autoimmune disease have demonstrated a role for TGF-β in the regulation of autoimmune responses. TGF-β has been shown to be important in protecting against inflammation of the central nervous system (CNS); TGF-β protects against experimental autoimmune encephalomyelitis (EAE), a mouse model of Multiple Sclerosis (MS). Administration of TGF-β at initiation and during the course of passively induced EAE decreased disease severity, reduced relapse severity, and decreased T cell entry into the CNS (Racke et al. 1991). If TGF-β-signaling was blocked during EAE, disease incidence and severity were exacerbated (Johns and Sriram 1993). In contrast, in actively induced EAE TGF-β has been shown to be required for disease initiation, perhaps through the induction of Th17 cells (Veldhoen et al. 2006b). It is therefore a simplification to think that administration of TGF-β would consistently reduce inflammation and induce disease remission. The tangled web of TGF-β roles is further highlighted in the disease model of collagen-induced arthritis (CIA). Administration of TGF-β systemically before or during CIA protected against disease (Thorbecke et al. 1992); however, administration of TGF-β directly at the site of inflammation (the joint cavity) enhanced disease severity (Allen et al. 1990).

TGF-β has also been shown to be important in the induction and maintenance of oral tolerance; inactivation of TGF-β-signaling specifically in the intestine resulted in spontaneous colitis (Hahm et al. 2001), and T cells from the mucosa of patients with inflammatory bowel disease (IBD) demonstrated insensitivity to TGF-β signalling (Monteleone et al. 2001).

Collectively these data would caution the use of TGF-β as a treatment for autoimmune disease, but highlight the potential of manipulating the TGF-β-pathway in resolving autoimmunity. In line with this, recent data have demonstrated that administration of anti-CD3, a treatment shown to induce long-term remission from diabetes in mice and humans (Chatenoud and Bluestone 2007), promotes Treg development by increasing systemic levels of TGF-β (Perruche et al. 2008).

5.2 Cancer

An immune response would be mounted against tumors which express new antigens that may elicit tumor-specific immune response. However, tumor immunity is drastically limited. TGF-β contributes to the reduced anti-tumor response; malignant cells become resistant to TGF-β-mediated growth inhibition and TGF-β is secreted by tumor and non-tumor cells (Jakowlew 2006). In fact, TGF-β is associated with the growth of many types of tumor (Pasche 2001), and increased levels of TGF-β have been noted at the tumor and the site of tumor-Ag presentation. TGF-β hinders anti-tumor immunity through the direct deactivation of cells of the immune system. Moreover, tumor-induced TGF-β could also promote the induction of Tregs. Consequently, increased levels of TGF-β correlate with poor clinical outcome (Jakowlew 2006; Pasche 2001). Therefore TGF-β and its signaling intermediates are attractive molecular targets for cancer treatment strategies. Current therapeutics being tested in clinical setting include short peptide inhibitors of TGF-β (Gil-Guerrero et al. 2008), monoclonal antibodies blocking TGF-β, soluble TGFβRII and antisense oligonucleotides for TGF-β mRNA (Wrzesinski et al. 2007). However, it is important to remember the role of TGF-β in peripheral immune tolerance, and therefore acknowledge the risk associated with prolonged administration of drugs which target the TGF-β-pathway.

6 Concluding Remarks

Not simply an inhibitory cytokine, TGF-β exerts a variety of functions in the immune system. In the case of T cells, some of these functions would appear to directly contrast one and other, reinforcing the importance of TGF-β in mediating a balance within the immune system. Understanding the integration of these signals within a T cell remains a considerable hurdle. However, with the network of signals elucidated it may be possible to design strategies which specifically promote either Treg or Th17 cell expansion and thus develop tailored therapies for cancer, autoimmune diseases, and cases of chronic inflammation.

Acknowledgments We thank Drs. T. Maruyama and P. Zhang, MIS, NIDCR, NIH for critically reading the manuscript. This research was supported by the intramural Research program of the NIH, National Institute for Dental and Craniofacial Research.

References

Allen JB, Manthey CL, Hand AR, Ohura K, Ellingsworth L, Wahl SM (1990) Rapid onset synovial inflammation and hyperplasia induced by transforming growth factor beta. J Exp Med 171:231–247

Andersson J, Tran DQ, Pesu M, Davidson TS, Ramsey H, O'Shea JJ, Shevach EM (2008) CD4+ FoxP3+ regulatory T cells confer infectious tolerance in a TGF-beta-dependent manner. J Exp Med 205:1975–1981

Apostolou I, von Boehmer H (2004) In vivo instruction of suppressor commitment in naive T cells. J Exp Med 199:1401–1408

Bellone G, Aste-Amezaga M, Trinchieri G, Rodeck U (1995) Regulation of NK cell functions by TGF-beta 1. J Immunol 155:1066–1073

Bettelli E, Carrier Y, Gao W, Korn T, Strom TB, Oukka M, Weiner HL, Kuchroo VK (2006) Reciprocal developmental pathways for the generation of pathogenic effector TH17 and regulatory T cells. Nature 441:235–238

Bogdan C, Paik J, Vodovotz Y, Nathan C (1992) Contrasting mechanisms for suppression of macrophage cytokine release by transforming growth factor-beta and interleukin-10. J Biol Chem 267:23301–23308

Bommireddy R, Engle SJ, Ormsby I, Boivin GP, Babcock GF, Doetschman T (2004) Elimination of both CD4+ and CD8+ T cells but not B cells eliminates inflammation and prolongs the survival of TGF-beta1-deficient mice. Cell Immunol 232:96–104

Bommireddy R, Pathak LJ, Martin J, Ormsby I, Engle SJ, Boivin GP, Babcock GF, Eriksson AU, Singh RR, Doetschman T (2006) Self-antigen recognition by TGF-beta1-deficient T cells causes their activation and systemic inflammation. Lab Invest 86:1008–1019

Borkowski TA, Letterio JJ, Farr AG, Udey MC (1996) A role for endogenous transforming growth factor beta 1 in Langerhans cell biology: the skin of transforming growth factor beta 1 null mice is devoid of epidermal Langerhans cells. J Exp Med 184:2417–2422

Brabletz T, Pfeuffer I, Schorr E, Siebelt F, Wirth T, Serfling E (1993) Transforming growth factor beta and cyclosporin A inhibit the inducible activity of the interleukin-2 gene in T cells through a noncanonical octamer-binding site. Mol Cell Biol 13:1155–1162

Castriconi R, Cantoni C, Della Chiesa M, Vitale M, Marcenaro E, Conte R, Biassoni R, Bottino C, Moretta L, Moretta A (2003) Transforming growth factor beta 1 inhibits expression of NKp30 and NKG2D receptors: consequences for the NK-mediated killing of dendritic cells. Proc Natl Acad Sci USA 100:4120–4125

Cazac BB, Roes J (2000) TGF-beta receptor controls B cell responsiveness and induction of IgA in vivo. Immunity 13:443–451

Chatenoud L, Bluestone JA (2007) CD3-specific antibodies: a portal to the treatment of autoimmunity. Nat Rev Immunol 7:622–632

Chen W, Frank ME, Jin W, Wahl SM (2001a) TGF-beta released by apoptotic T cells contributes to an immunosuppressive milieu. Immunity 14:715–725

Chen W, Jin W, Tian H, Sicurello P, Frank M, Orenstein JM, Wahl SM (2001b) Requirement for transforming growth factor beta1 in controlling T cell apoptosis. J Exp Med 194:439–453

Chen W, Jin W, Hardegen N, Lei KJ, Li L, Marinos N, McGrady G, Wahl SM (2003) Conversion of peripheral CD4+CD25- naive T cells to CD4+CD25+ regulatory T cells by TGF-beta induction of transcription factor Foxp3. J Exp Med 198:1875–1886

Dennler S, Goumans MJ, ten Dijke P (2002) Transforming growth factor beta signal transduction. J Leukoc Biol 71:731–740

Derynck R, Zhang YE (2003) Smad-dependent and Smad-independent pathways in TGF-beta family signalling. Nature 425:577–584

Doisne JM, Bartholin L, Yan KP, Garcia CN, Duarte N, Le Luduec JB, Vincent D, Cyprian F, Horvat B, Martel S et al (2009) iNKT cell development is orchestrated by different branches of TGF-beta signaling. J Exp Med 206:1365–1378

Fadok VA, Bratton DL, Konowal A, Freed PW, Westcott JY, Henson PM (1998) Macrophages that have ingested apoptotic cells in vitro inhibit proinflammatory cytokine production through autocrine/paracrine mechanisms involving TGF-beta, PGE2, and PAF. J Clin Invest 101: 890–898

Fantini MC, Becker C, Monteleone G, Pallone F, Galle PR, Neurath MF (2004) Cutting edge: TGF-beta induces a regulatory phenotype in CD4+CD25- T cells through Foxp3 induction and down-regulation of Smad7. J Immunol 172:5149–5153

Faunce DE, Terajewicz A, Stein-Streilein J (2004) Cutting edge: in vitro-generated tolerogenic APC induce CD8+ T regulatory cells that can suppress ongoing experimental autoimmune encephalomyelitis. J Immunol 172:1991–1995

Fiorentino DF, Bond MW, Mosmann TR (1989) Two types of mouse T helper cell. IV. Th2 clones secrete a factor that inhibits cytokine production by Th1 clones. J Exp Med 170:2081–2095

Geissmann F, Revy P, Regnault A, Lepelletier Y, Dy M, Brousse N, Amigorena S, Hermine O, Durandy A (1999) TGF-beta 1 prevents the noncognate maturation of human dendritic Langerhans cells. J Immunol 162:4567–4575

Gil-Guerrero L, Dotor J, Huibregtse IL, Casares N, Lopez-Vazquez AB, Rudilla F, Riezu-Boj JI, Lopez-Sagaseta J, Hermida J, Van Deventer S et al (2008) In vitro and in vivo down-regulation of regulatory T cell activity with a peptide inhibitor of TGF-beta1. J Immunol 181:126–135

Hahm KB, Im YH, Parks TW, Park SH, Markowitz S, Jung HY, Green J, Kim SJ (2001) Loss of transforming growth factor beta signalling in the intestine contributes to tissue injury in inflammatory bowel disease. Gut 49:190–198

Jakowlew SB (2006) Transforming growth factor-beta in cancer and metastasis. Cancer Metastasis Rev 25:435–457

Johns LD, Sriram S (1993) Experimental allergic encephalomyelitis: neutralizing antibody to TGF beta 1 enhances the clinical severity of the disease. J Neuroimmunol 47:1 7

Kee BL, Rivera RR, Murre C (2001) Id3 inhibits B lymphocyte progenitor growth and survival in response to TGF-beta. Nat Immunol 2:242–247

Kehrl JH, Roberts AB, Wakefield LM, Jakowlew S, Sporn MB, Fauci AS (1986a) Transforming growth factor beta is an important immunomodulatory protein for human B lymphocytes. J Immunol 137:3855–3860

Kehrl JH, Wakefield LM, Roberts AB, Jakowlew S, Alvarez-Mon M, Derynck R, Sporn MB, Fauci AS (1986b) Production of transforming growth factor beta by human T lymphocytes and its potential role in the regulation of T cell growth. J Exp Med 163:1037–1050

Kretschmer K, Apostolou I, Hawiger D, Khazaie K, Nussenzweig MC, von Boehmer H (2005) Inducing and expanding regulatory T cell populations by foreign antigen. Nat Immunol 6:1219–1227

Kulkarni AB, Huh CG, Becker D, Geiser A, Lyght M, Flanders KC, Roberts AB, Sporn MB, Ward JM, Karlsson S (1993) Transforming growth factor beta 1 null mutation in mice causes excessive inflammatory response and early death. Proc Natl Acad Sci USA 90:770–774

Lee JC, Lee KM, Kim DW, Heo DS (2004) Elevated TGF-beta1 secretion and down-modulation of NKG2D underlies impaired NK cytotoxicity in cancer patients. J Immunol 172:7335–7340

Li MO, Sanjabi S, Flavell RA (2006) Transforming growth factor-beta controls development, homeostasis, and tolerance of T cells by regulatory T cell-dependent and -independent mechanisms. Immunity 25:455–471

Li MO, Wan YY, Flavell RA (2007) T cell-produced transforming growth factor-beta1 controls T cell tolerance and regulates Th1- and Th17-cell differentiation. Immunity 26:579–591

Liu Y, Zhang P, Li J, Kulkarni AB, Perruche S, Chen W (2008) A critical function for TGF-beta signaling in the development of natural CD4+CD25+Foxp3+ regulatory T cells. Nat Immunol 9:632–640

Marie JC, Liggitt D, Rudensky AY (2006) Cellular mechanisms of fatal early-onset autoimmunity in mice with the T cell-specific targeting of transforming growth factor-beta receptor. Immunity 25:441–454

McKarns SC, Schwartz RH, Kaminski NE (2004) Smad3 is essential for TGF-beta 1 to suppress IL-2 production and TCR-induced proliferation, but not IL-2-induced proliferation. J Immunol 172:4275–4284

Monteleone G, Kumberova A, Croft NM, McKenzie C, Steer HW, MacDonald TT (2001) Blocking Smad7 restores TGF-beta1 signaling in chronic inflammatory bowel disease. J Clin Invest 108:601–609

Morelli AE, Zahorchak AF, Larregina AT, Colvin BL, Logar AJ, Takayama T, Falo LD, Thomson AW (2001) Cytokine production by mouse myeloid dendritic cells in relation to differentiation and terminal maturation induced by lipopolysaccharide or CD40 ligation. Blood 98:1512–1523

Nandan D, Reiner NE (1997) TGF-beta attenuates the class II transactivator and reveals an accessory pathway of IFN-gamma action. J Immunol 158:1095–1101

Nelson BH, Martyak TP, Thompson LJ, Moon JJ, Wang T (2003) Uncoupling of promitogenic and antiapoptotic functions of IL-2 by Smad-dependent TGF-beta signaling. J Immunol 170:5563–5570

Pasche B (2001) Role of transforming growth factor beta in cancer. J Cell Physiol 186:153–168

Perruche S, Zhang P, Liu Y, Saas P, Bluestone JA, Chen W (2008) CD3-specific antibody-induced immune tolerance involves transforming growth factor-beta from phagocytes digesting apoptotic T cells. Nat Med 14:528–535

Powrie F, Carlino J, Leach MW, Mauze S, Coffman RL (1996) A critical role for transforming growth factor-beta but not interleukin 4 in the suppression of T helper type 1-mediated colitis by CD45RB(low) CD4+ T cells. J Exp Med 183:2669–2674

Qin S, Cobbold SP, Pope H, Elliott J, Kioussis D, Davies J, Waldmann H (1993) "Infectious" transplantation tolerance. Science 259:974–977

Racke MK, Dhib-Jalbut S, Cannella B, Albert PS, Raine CS, McFarlin DE (1991) Prevention and treatment of chronic relapsing experimental allergic encephalomyelitis by transforming growth factor-beta 1. J Immunol 146:3012–3017

Robinson RT, French MA, Kitzmiller TJ, Gorham JD (2006) Restriction of the CD4+ T-cell receptor repertoire prevents immune pathology in TGF-beta1 knockout mice. Lab Invest 86:815–828

Roes J, Choi BK, Cazac BB (2003) Redirection of B cell responsiveness by transforming growth factor beta receptor. Proc Natl Acad Sci USA 100:7241–7246

Rook AH, Kehrl JH, Wakefield LM, Roberts AB, Sporn MB, Burlington DB, Lane HC, Fauci AS (1986) Effects of transforming growth factor beta on the functions of natural killer cells: depressed cytolytic activity and blunting of interferon responsiveness. J Immunol 136:3916–3920

Sad S, Mosmann TR (1994) Single IL-2-secreting precursor CD4 T cell can develop into either Th1 or Th2 cytokine secretion phenotype. J Immunol 153:3514–3522

Shi Y, Massague J (2003) Mechanisms of TGF-beta signaling from cell membrane to the nucleus. Cell 113:685–700

Shull MM, Ormsby I, Kier AB, Pawlowski S, Diebold RJ, Yin M, Allen R, Sidman C, Proetzel G, Calvin D et al (1992) Targeted disruption of the mouse transforming growth factor-beta 1 gene results in multifocal inflammatory disease. Nature 359:693–699

Strobl H, Bello-Fernandez C, Riedl E, Pickl WF, Majdic O, Lyman SD, Knapp W (1997) flt3 Ligand in cooperation with transforming growth factor-beta1 potentiates in vitro development of Langerhans-type dendritic cells and allows single-cell dendritic cell cluster formation under serum-free conditions. Blood 90:1425–1434

Takeuchi M, Alard P, Streilein JW (1998) TGF-beta promotes immune deviation by altering accessory signals of antigen-presenting cells. J Immunol 160:1589–1597

Thorbecke GJ, Shah R, Leu CH, Kuruvilla AP, Hardison AM, Palladino MA (1992) Involvement of endogenous tumor necrosis factor alpha and transforming growth factor beta during induction of collagen type II arthritis in mice. Proc Natl Acad Sci USA 89:7375–7379

Tsunawaki S, Sporn M, Ding A, Nathan C (1988) Deactivation of macrophages by transforming growth factor-beta. Nature 334:260–262

Veldhoen M, Hocking RJ, Atkins CJ, Locksley RM, Stockinger B (2006a) TGF-beta in the context of an inflammatory cytokine milieu supports de novo differentiation of IL-17-producing T cells. Immunity 24:179–189

Veldhoen M, Hocking RJ, Flavell RA, Stockinger B (2006b) Signals mediated by transforming growth factor-beta initiate autoimmune encephalomyelitis, but chronic inflammation is needed to sustain disease. Nat Immunol 7:1151–1156

Vodovotz Y, Bogdan C, Paik J, Xie QW, Nathan C (1993) Mechanisms of suppression of macrophage nitric oxide release by transforming growth factor beta. J Exp Med 178:605–613

Wolfraim LA, Walz TM, James Z, Fernandez T, Letterio JJ (2004) p21Cip1 and p27Kip1 Act in synergy to alter the sensitivity of naive T cells to TGF-beta-mediated G1 arrest through modulation of IL-2 responsiveness. J Immunol 173:3093–3102

Wrzesinski SH, Wan YY, Flavell RA (2007) Transforming growth factor-beta and the immune response: implications for anticancer therapy. Clin Cancer Res 13:5262–5270

Yamagata T, Mathis D, Benoist C (2004) Self-reactivity in thymic double-positive cells commits cells to a CD8 alpha alpha lineage with characteristics of innate immune cells. Nat Immunol 5:597–605

Zhou L, Lopes JE, Chong MM, Ivanov II, Min R, Victora GD, Shen Y, Du J, Rubtsov YP, Rudensky AY et al (2008) TGF-beta-induced Foxp3 inhibits T(H)17 cell differentiation by antagonizing RORgammat function. Nature 453:236–240

Chapter 17
Indoleamine 2,3-Dioxygenase and Tumor-Induced Immune Suppression

David H. Munn

Abbreviations

DC   Dendritic cell
IDO   Indoleamine 2,3-dioxygenase
LN   Lymph node
1MT   1-Methyl-tryptophan
Tregs   Regulatory T cells

1 Introduction

Tumors express a variety of antigens to which the immune system should in theory be able to respond (Boon and van der Bruggen 1996), and tumor-bearing hosts possess T cells that are specific for a variety of tumor-associated antigens (Ercolini et al. 2005; Lurquin et al. 2005). Yet, despite this, hosts with an established tumor do not spontaneously reject their tumors. Instead, the immune system behaves as if it were tolerant (functionally unresponsive) to any antigen associated with the tumor.

This tolerance is not merely a passive failure to detect tumor antigens. Although in some cases the immune system does appear unaware of tumor antigens (Ochsenbein et al. 1999; Spiotto et al. 2002), in many cases the immune system is clearly aware of these antigens, but is somehow rendered unresponsive to them. This has been experimentally demonstrated with developing tumors in vivo

D.H. Munn (✉)
Cancer Immunotherapy Program, Room CN-4141, Augusta, GA 30912, USA
e-mail: dmunn@georgiahealth.edu

(Willimsky et al. 2008), and has been clearly shown in systems in which tumors were engineered to express a highly immunogenic foreign antigen: typically, in such cases the tumors are not rejected, but simply create de novo tolerance to the new antigen (Cuenca et al. 2003; Sotomayor et al. 2001; Yu et al. 2005). Even more dauntingly, once this acquired tolerance has been established, immunization with tumor-associated antigens may merely serve to intensify the antigen-specific suppression (Maksimow et al. 2006; Zhou et al. 2006). Taken together, these studies show that tumor-induced tolerance is an acquired state, reflecting active mechanisms of immunosuppression, and can represent a major impediment to clinical immunotherapy of cancer.

2 Characteristics of the IDO Enzyme

IDO is a monomeric enzyme that catalyzes the oxidative cleavage of the pyrrol (5-membered) ring of L-tryptophan. It is a ~42–45 kDa single-chain protein, with a heme prosthetic group forming part of the active site (Sugimoto et al. 2006). IDO uses molecular oxygen or oxygen radicals to convert L-tryptophan into kynurenine, which is then further metabolized by a series of enzymes along the kynurenine pathway (Stone and Darlington 2002). A similar reaction is catalyzed by the unrelated enzyme tryptophan oxygenase (TDO), which is constitutively expressed in the liver; however, TDO is not known to have an immunoregulatory function. IDO is inducible by interferons or other pro-inflammatory signals in cells of the immune system (macrophages and DCs), as well as keratinocytes, fibroblasts, endothelial cells, and other cells under certain conditions.

The molecular regulation of IDO is complex. There are two genes, termed IDO1 and IDO2, that share sequence homology but differ in their regulation and pattern of expression (Ball et al. 2009; Metz et al. 2007). Genetic polymorphisms exist in both human genes, and these polymorphisms affect IDO activity (Arefayene et al. 2009). IDO1 and IDO2 mRNAs show alternate splicing, and the IDO1 protein is post-translationally regulated by ubiquitin-mediated proteasomal degradation (Orabona et al. 2008) and protein nitration by iNOS (Fujigaki et al. 2006). It is likely that IDO2 is similarly regulated, but this is not yet known. Regulatory factors known to influence IDO expression and function include SOCS3, NF-κB, DAP12, and IRF8 (Orabona et al. 2006, 2008; Tas et al. 2007). Given this complexity, it is not surprising that IDO expression can differ widely between cell types, and even between different activation states of the same cell type. In the immune system, IDO is not usually expressed constitutively by cells at rest, but rather is inducible in certain specific cell types by certain stimuli (IFNγ, IFNα, and other signals). Thus, it is perhaps most accurate to say that specific cell types in the immune system are "IDO-competent," meaning that they are primed by their lineage differentiation and maturation status to up-regulate IDO in response to specific triggering signals.

3 IDO as an Endogenous Mechanism of Immune Tolerance

3.1 In Vivo Biologic Role of IDO in Mouse Models

IDO expression is an endogenous molecular mechanism contributing to immune regulation and tolerance in vivo (reviewed in refs. Mellor and Munn 2008; Munn and Mellor 2007). The effects of IDO are focused and selective, being required for specific kinds of acquired peripheral tolerance, but not required for constitutive tolerance to self antigens (as shown by the fact that IDO1-knockout mice or mice treated with IDO-inhibitor drugs do not develop spontaneous autoimmune disorders). However, in settings where IDO is important, its effects can be dramatic. IDO is expressed in the placenta, and pregnant mice treated with an IDO-inhibitor drug spontaneously reject fetuses that express foreign paternal alloantigens (Muller et al. 2005a; Munn et al. 1998). Similarly, blocking the endogenous host IDO pathway in mouse models of graft-versus-host disease (Jasperson et al. 2008), autoimmunity (Gurtner et al. 2003) or chronic infection (Grohmann et al. 2007; Romani et al. 2008) converts mild, survivable disease into rapidly lethal inflammation. In a variety of experimental models, it has been found that blocking IDO renders the host refractory to the creation of acquired peripheral tolerance: examples include mucosal tolerance (van der Marel et al. 2007), tolerance induced by CTLA4-Ig (Grohmann et al. 2002; Mellor et al. 2003), and tolerance induced by CD40 blockade (Guillonneau et al. 2007). Perhaps most dramatically, organ and tissue allografts that are engineered to overexpress IDO are accepted across full haplo-mismatched MHC barriers without any other immunosuppression (Guillonneau et al. 2007; Liu et al. 2006; Swanson et al. 2004).

The shared theme in each of these settings is that IDO contributes to an acquired state of unresponsiveness to a new set of antigens. Doubtless, IDO is only one contributing part of a multifactorial process of acquired tolerance. But the key finding is that IDO appears to be a *nonredundant* (not immediately dispensable) component in a number of systems, such that if IDO is suddenly inhibited, then tolerance is dramatically weakened or broken. This is of particular interest from the standpoint of tumor immunotherapy, because, as we will discuss below, IDO appears to contribute to tumor-induced tolerance.

3.2 Mechanism of Action of IDO

The molecular mechanism by which IDO regulates immune responses is still a subject of active research. Biochemically, IDO produces two effects: depletion of tryptophan and production of downstream kynurenine-pathway metabolites. Both of these effects appear to have immunoregulatory effects in vivo, and the two in combination may be synergistic. Several of the kynurenine metabolites produced by IDO are immunosuppressive (reviewed in ref. Belladonna et al. 2009), and it has been shown that local production of kynurenines by IDO is required for the control of certain forms of inflammation (Romani et al. 2008). The molecular mechanism of action of kynurenines has not been elucidated, but may involve a direct inhibitory effect on T cells and induction of apoptosis (Hayashi et al. 2007). In addition, IDO activity also depletes the local pool of tryptophan, both in the cell expressing IDO, and in neighboring cells (e.g., T cells to which an IDO-expressing cell is presenting antigen). This IDO-induced amino-acid withdrawal stress appears to activate the amino-acid sensitive GCN2 kinase pathway (Munn et al. 2005). The GCN2 pathway senses the level of uncharged transfer-RNA, and thus responds to any cellular deficiency in amino acids (Wek et al. 2006). In the immune system, GCN2 generates signals that affect both the cell that expresses IDO (Manlapat et al. 2007), and the neighboring T cell to which the IDO-expressing cell presents antigen (Munn et al. 2005; Sharma et al. 2007, 2009). The GCN2 pathway is also a mediator of the immunoregulatory effects of the enzyme arginase (Rodriguez et al. 2007), and thus may form part of a general system of amino-acid-based immune regulation (Cobbold et al. 2009). In general, immune cells appear particularly sensitive to regulation by GCN2 (Jalili et al. 2009; Sundrud et al. 2009). Thus, both tryptophan depletion and kynurenine-metabolite production contribute to the immunologic effects of IDO, and the combination of these pathways may be synergistic for immune regulation (Fallarino et al. 2006).

3.3 IDO and Tregs

In addition to the direct effects of IDO described above, IDO can also create potent collateral suppression via activation of the regulatory T cell (Treg) system. A number of groups have now shown that exposure of naive $CD4^+$ T cells to IDO during activation can bias their differentiation toward a $Foxp3^+$ Treg phenotype (Chen et al. 2008; Chung et al. 2009; Fallarino et al. 2006; Manches et al. 2008). In addition to this developmental effect on differentiation, we have shown that IDO can also directly activate the suppressive function of existing, mature Tregs (Sharma et al. 2007). This latter is not a gradual developmental change, but a rapid functional activation of pre-existing Tregs that allows them to become potently and constitutively suppressive (Sharma et al. 2007, 2009). IDO-activated Tregs are found in tumor-draining lymph nodes (LNs) in mice, where they may contribute to tumor-induced tolerance (Sharma et al. 2007). In addition, IDO appears to stabilize the suppressive phenotype of Tregs under conditions of inflammation, and prevent their spontaneous re-programming into pro-inflammatory Th17-like cells (Baban et al. 2009; Sharma et al. 2009).

3.4 IDO Expression by Human Cells

The mechanistic studies described above are based on mouse models. Fewer mechanistic studies exist in the human system, but it is well established that IDO can be expressed by a number of human cell types in vitro. The most extensively studied human cell type is monocyte-derived dendritic cells (DCs) (Beutelspacher et al. 2006b; Chung et al. 2009; Hwu et al. 2000; Munn et al. 2002, 2004b; Vacca et al. 2005; Wobser et al. 2007). In DC culture systems, there appears to be a number of variables that influence whether the cultured DCs will express IDO or not. Thus, certain cytokines and growth factors may induce IDO protein without functional enzymatic activity (Braun et al. 2005; Munn et al. 2002), while some culture conditions produce DCs that do not express IDO (Terness et al. 2005), or the DCs may express IDO but activity is not inhibited by the D isomer of 1MT (D-1MT) (Lob et al. 2008), or activity is inhibited by D-1MT but this does not result in enhanced T cell proliferation (Qian et al. 2009). However, numerous reports confirm that monocyte-derived DCs, as well as macrophages and other human cell types, are capable of expressing IDO under a variety of conditions (Beutelspacher et al. 2006a, b; Boasso et al. 2007; Braun et al. 2005; Brenk et al. 2009; Duluc et al. 2007; Hwu et al. 2000; Orabona et al. 2006; Rutella et al. 2006; Vacca et al. 2005; Wobser et al. 2007). IDO expression is able to inhibit proliferation of T cells in vitro (Beutelspacher et al. 2006b; Boasso et al. 2007; Duluc et al. 2007; Munn et al. 2002, 2004b). IDO can also promote the differentiation of Foxp3$^+$ Tregs from human CD4$^+$ T cells (Chen et al. 2008; Chung et al. 2009; Curti et al. 2007b; Manches et al. 2008). Depending on the experimental system, IDO expressed by human cells can be inhibited by D-1MT (Boasso et al. 2007; Curti et al. 2007b; Duluc et al. 2007; Hou et al. 2007; Munn et al. 2002, 2004b; Rutella et al. 2006); by L-1MT (Lob et al. 2008; Qian et al. 2009); or by the DL racemic mixture (Hwu et al. 2000; Vacca et al. 2005).

4 IDO and Tumors

4.1 IDO and Tolerance to Tumors

IDO can be expressed in tumor-draining (sentinel) lymph nodes of both humans (Lee et al. 2003, 2005; Munn et al. 2002; von Bergwelt-Baildon et al. 2006) and mice (Munn et al. 2004a). Tumor-draining LNs are immunologically important sites, because most studies suggest that resting T cells initially become aware of tumor antigens primarily through cross-presentation by host antigen-presenting cells (rather than by direct presentation by the tumor cells themselves) (Hildner et al. 2008; Huang et al. 1994; Sotomayor et al. 2001). Classically, this initial cross-presentation occurs in draining lymph nodes. Unfortunately, tumors frequently alter their draining LNs such that these become a potently immunosuppressive and tolerogenic milieu (Cochran et al. 2006; Mellor and Munn 2008). Mechanistic studies in mice suggest that IDO contributes to this local immune suppression in tumor-draining LNs.

In mice, the IDO-expressing cells in tumor-draining lymph nodes are phenotypically similar to plasmacytoid DCs, but with additional co-expression of the B cell-lineage marker CD19 (Munn et al. 2004a). Similar CD19$^+$ plasmacytoid DCs expressing IDO have been shown in other models of tolerance as well (Baban et al. 2005; Mellor et al. 2005). IDO$^+$ DCs from tumor-draining LNs actively suppress T cell responses in vitro, and induce antigen-specific T cell anergy when adoptively transferred into new hosts (Munn et al. 2004a, 2005). IDO$^+$ DCs also directly activate Tregs for potent suppression of bystander T cells, and IDO-activated Tregs can be isolated ex vivo from tumor-draining LNs (Sharma et al. 2007). Taken together, these studies suggest that IDO-expressing host DCs in tumor-draining LNs may help convert these LNs into sites of immunosuppression and tolerance induction rather than beneficial immune activation.

In humans, the specific cell type expressing IDO in tumor-draining LNs has not yet been definitively characterized. However, it is clear that these are frequently host cells (not metastatic tumor cells), and that they may display a "plasmacytoid" morphology (Lee et al. 2003). One recent study (Qian et al. 2009) has suggested that the IDO$^+$ cells infiltrating ovarian cancers may have a CD123$^+$ phenotype similar to the IDO-expressing monocyte-derived DCs described in vitro (Munn et al. 2002).

4.2 IDO Expression in Human Tumors

In 2003, Uyttenhove and colleagues reported that IDO was detectable by immunohistochemistry in a variety of human cancers (Uyttenhove et al. 2003). Since then, IDO has been described in biopsy material from patients with malignant melanoma (Brody et al. 2009; Polak et al. 2007), pancreatic cancer (Witkiewicz et al. 2008, 2009), ovarian cancer (Qian et al. 2009), acute myelogenous leukemia (Chamuleau et al. 2008; Corm et al. 2009; Curti et al. 2007b), colorectal cancer (Brandacher et al. 2006; Huang et al. 2002), prostate cancer (Feder-Mengus et al. 2008), endometrial cancer (Ino et al. 2006, 2008), and ovarian cancer (Okamoto et al. 2005). In several of these studies, the presence of IDO correlated with a worse clinical outcome (in some cases dramatically worse), and IDO was often independent of known adverse prognostic factors (Brandacher et al. 2006; Chamuleau et al. 2008; Corm et al. 2009; Ino et al. 2008; Munn et al. 2004a; Okamoto et al. 2005).

In the preceding studies, IDO was expressed by the tumor cells themselves. However, IDO has also been found in host cells associated with tumors. These host cells include the IDO$^+$ cells with a plasmacytoid DC morphology found in melanoma-draining LNs, as mentioned above (Lee et al. 2003; Munn et al. 2004a); IDO$^+$ macrophages isolated from human ovarian cancer (Duluc et al. 2007); and IDO$^+$ CD123$^+$ DCs from ovarian cancer (Qian et al. 2009). Thus, IDO can be expressed in both tumor cells and in cells of the host immune system. It is not yet known which is the more important site of IDO expression, but it seems likely that both may be important, depending on the biology of the particular tumor.

5 Chemo-Immunotherapy with IDO-Inhibitor Drugs

5.1 Immunologic Effects of Chemotherapy

One important development during the past several years is the realization that chemotherapy can potentially be synergistic with anti-tumor immunotherapy. This has profound practical implications for delivering immunotherapy in the clinic, since it means that patients may not need to be denied standard-of-care chemotherapy in order to receive immunotherapy; and, conversely, immunotherapy may be integrated at an earlier stage in the treatment sequence, when disease is less extensive and performance status is better.

The molecular mechanisms by which chemotherapy synergizes with immunotherapy are complex. Chemotherapy releases a wave of antigens from dying tumor cells (Lake and Robinson 2005), and, under the right conditions, this cell-death process may activate immune responses (Zitvogel et al. 2008). Chemotherapy may also at least partially deplete immunosuppressive Tregs (Zou 2006). Finally, chemotherapy induces transient lymphopenia followed by homeostatic recovery, which creates a cytokine-rich environment in which T cells are receptive to breaking tolerance (Williams et al. 2007). Although chemotherapy alone seldom triggers successful immune rejection of established tumors, chemotherapy may create a "window" in which tumor antigens are released, and the immune system is receptive to activation by immunotherapy.

5.2 1MT Plus Chemotherapy Can Break Tolerance to Tumors in Mouse Models

Preclinical studies in a variety of mouse tumor models demonstrate that 1-methyl-DL-tryptophan (1MT), an IDO inhibitor, displays synergy when combined with a number of chemotherapeutic drugs (Hou et al. 2007; Muller et al. 2005a) This was first demonstrated by Muller et al. using a model of autochthonous breast tumors in mice overexpressing the HER2/neu oncogene in mammary glands (Muller et al. 2005a). In this model (as in human tumors) each tumor is genetically different, arising through its own unique series of mutations, and thus develops its own strategy to evade immune surveillance. Despite this genetic diversity, tumors uniformly displayed growth delay or regressed in size when treated with 1MT plus any of several chemotherapy drugs (Muller et al. 2005a). Chemotherapy agents effective in this model included cyclophosphamide, doxorubicin, paclitaxel, and cisplatin. These findings have been confirmed and extended in a second report (Hou et al. 2007). The observed synergy was mediated by the host immune system, because the effect of 1MT was lost when tumors were grown in immunodeficient hosts, or when T cells were depleted (Hou et al. 2007; Muller et al. 2005b). Thus, adding 1MT to standard chemotherapy allows immune-mediated anti-tumor responses to occur which would otherwise be suppressed – in functional terms, tolerance to the tumor is transiently broken.

6 IDO-Inhibitor Drugs and Vaccines

Tumor-bearing hosts respond sub-optimally to anti-tumor vaccines. In many cases this appears to be due to the presence of Tregs that have been recruited or activated by the tumor (Quezada et al. 2008). We have recently shown that the IDO-inhibitor drug D-1MT is synergistic with anti-tumor immunization in a mouse model of established melanoma (Sharma et al. 2009). Encouragingly, blocking IDO allowed immunosuppressive Tregs to be converted ("re-programmed") into pro-inflammatory T-helper cells with a TH17-like phenotype, resulting in enhanced anti-tumor efficacy of the vaccine. Further studies will be required to optimize the combination of IDO-inhibitors and vaccination, but this could potentially be a clinically relevant combination.

7 IDO as a General Counter-regulatory Mechanism

The beneficial effect of blocking IDO at the time of vaccination raises a general point about IDO, which is that IDO is induced by a wide variety of inflammatory stimuli. We hypothesize that this is because IDO often functions as a counter-regulatory mechanism in the immune system, acting to limit dangerous or excessive inflammation (Mellor and Munn 2008). Support for this hypothesis comes from models in which IDO is absent or reduced, and inflammation becomes lethally dysregulated (Jasperson et al. 2008; Romani et al. 2008). Counter-regulation is important in the immune system because it protects the host from uncontrolled inflammation; but in the context of anti-tumor immunotherapy, counter-regulation has the potential to antagonize and suppress the desired pro-inflammatory effects of the immunotherapy.

Thus, for example, with regard to vaccine adjuvants, it is important to note that unmethylated CpG motifs – which are potent activators of vaccine responses, and are in clinical trials as vaccine adjuvants – are also potent inducers of IDO (Mellor et al. 2005). High-dose intravenous CpG can result in systemic immunosuppression and tolerance, due to systemic induction of IDO (Baban et al. 2009; Mellor et al. 2005). Similarly, type I and type II interferons (which are often induced by inflammation or vaccine adjuvants), and mycobacteria (which have strong adjuvant effects) are all inducers of IDO (Moreau et al. 2005). Even T cell stimulatory antibodies against CD137 (4-1BB) have been reported to unexpectedly induce IDO expression, and thereby cause collateral immunosuppression in certain settings (Kim et al. 2009). The implication of all these findings is that collateral IDO induction – with attendant immunosuppression – could potentially be an undesirable concomitant of a variety of existing immunotherapy strategies. Whether specific adjuvants or immunomodulators do, in fact, induce IDO will have to be empirically determined. But the corollary is that existing adjuvants, vaccines or immunostimulatory agents may potentially benefit from combination with an IDO-inhibitor drug, which could block the counter-regulatory effect of IDO and thereby enhance efficacy.

8 Preclinical and Clinical Studies of IDO-Inhibitor Drugs

8.1 1-Methyl-Tryptophan: D and L Isomers

Several biochemical inhibitors of IDO have been reported in the literature (reviewed in ref. Muller and Scherle 2006). Of these, the most extensively studied has been 1-methyl-tryptophan (1MT). 1MT exists in two stereoisomers, the D and L forms, with somewhat different biological properties. The L isomer has been found to be more potent at inhibiting the purified IDO enzyme in cell-free systems, and is also superior at inhibiting IDO expressed in cultured cell lines (Hou et al. 2007). However, the D isomer was somewhat more effective in reversing the inhibition of T cell proliferation created by IDO-expressing DCs, using both human monocyte-derived DCs and murine TDLN pDCs (Hou et al. 2007). In vivo, mouse studies directly comparing D with L isomer showed that the D isomer was more efficacious in chemo-immunotherapy regimens (Hou et al. 2007).

The molecular basis for the difference in biological properties of D and L 1MT has not yet been fully elucidated. There is evidence that the two isoforms of IDO (IDO1 and IDO2) may be differentially sensitive to the D vs. L isomers of 1MT (Metz et al. 2007). Thus, the relative potency of the D and L isomers may differ depending on which isoform of IDO is predominantly expressed by the target cell type (Lob et al. 2008). In addition, one or both stereoisomers of 1MT may affect the IDO pathway in a noncompetitive fashion (e.g., by affecting gene expression, enzyme regulation, cofactors, or other points upstream or downstream of the enzyme active site itself). Finally, since the desired effect of 1MT is successful immune activation, off-target toxicities of 1MT on T cells must be considered. In vitro, it appears that the D isomer of 1MT may have a somewhat lower off-target toxicity for activated T cells (Hou et al. 2007).

Overall, in a number of experimental systems, D-1MT appears to have good biological activity in mouse models and is also effective against human cells (Boasso et al. 2007; Chen et al. 2008; Curti et al. 2007a; Duluc et al. 2007; Munn et al. 2002; Rutella et al. 2006), at least when the target is IDO expressed by host DCs and macrophages. It is possible that IDO expressed by tumor cells themselves (rather than host immune cells) may behave differently (e.g., the tumor may express a different isoform of IDO, or different regulation of the enzyme), and in some cases tumor-associated IDO may not be susceptible to inhibition by D-1MT (Lob et al. 2009b). This caveat will need to be borne in mind if D-1MT does not show efficacy against tumors that express IDO (Lob et al. 2009a).

In preclinical pharmacology/toxicology testing, the D isomer of 1MT showed good oral bioavailability and a long half-life (suitable for once or twice-daily oral administration); no dose-limiting toxicity was observed in mice, rats or dogs (Jia et al. 2008).

8.2 Early-Phase Clinical Trials of D-1MT

The first human clinical trial of oral 1MT is ongoing, and interim results have been reported in a preliminary abstract (Soliman et al. 2009). No efficacy data is available from this Phase I dose-escalation study, but the drug appears well tolerated. Of interest, two patients who had received previous immunotherapy with other agents were reported to have developed Grade 2 hypophysitis while receiving 1MT. This perhaps represented a recall toxicity, because subsequent patients who had not received prior immunotherapy did not show toxicity. However, this study is currently ongoing and final outcome will provide valuable information.

9 Conclusions

Successful anti-tumor immunotherapy regimens will rely on a combination of multiple targeted strategies acting in synergy. Rationally designed regimens will require a mechanistic understanding of the specific immunologic barriers that need to be overcome in patients with established tumors. One key step will be overcoming the state of pre-existing functional tolerance toward tumor-associated antigens, in particular the suppression mediated by Tregs. IDO expression is a molecular mechanism that is positioned at the intersection of several key immunologic pathways, including the direct inhibition of effector T cells; the activation of suppressive Treg cells; and the control of Treg re-programming in the context of vaccine-induced inflammation. IDO can be expressed by the tumor itself, induced in host cells in the presence of tumor cells, or collaterally induced by vaccine adjuvants or other immunostimulatory interventions. Thus, blocking the IDO pathway may enhance immune-mediated responses against tumors – particularly when used in conjunction with conventional chemotherapeutic agents – and may also be beneficial in combination with other immunotherapy strategies, which may be restricted by collateral induction of IDO.

Conflict of interest statement: The author has intellectual property interests in the therapeutic use of IDO and IDO inhibitors, and receives consulting income and research support from NewLink Genetics, Inc.

References

Arefayene M, Philips S, Cao D, Mamidipalli S, Desta Z, Flockhart DA, Wilkes DS, Skaar TC (2009) Identification of genetic variants in the human indoleamine 2,3-dioxygenase (IDO1) gene, which have altered enzyme activity. Pharmacogenet Genomics 19:464–476

Baban B, Hansen A, Chandler P, Manlapat A, Bingaman A, Kahler D, Munn D, Mellor A(2005) A minor population of splenic dendritic cells expressing CD19 mediates IDO-dependent T cell suppression via type 1 interferon-signaling following B7 ligation. Int Immunol 17:909–919

Baban B, Chandler PR, Sharma MD, Pihkala J, Koni PA, Munn DH, Mellor AL (2009) IDO activates regulatory T cells and blocks their conversion into Th17-like T cells. J Immunol 183: 2475–2483

Ball HJ, Yuasa HJ, Austin CJ, Weiser S, Hunt NH (2009) Indoleamine 2,3-dioxygenase-2; a new enzyme in the kynurenine pathway. Int J Biochem Cell Biol 41:467–471

Belladonna ML, Orabona C, Grohmann U, Puccetti P (2009) TGF-beta and kynurenines as the key to infectious tolerance. Trends Mol Med 15:41–49

Beutelspacher SC, Pillai R, Watson MP, Tan PH, Tsang J, McClure MO, George AJ, Larkin DF (2006a) Function of indoleamine 2,3-dioxygenase in corneal allograft rejection and prolongation of allograft survival by over-expression. Eur J Immunol 36:690–700

Beutelspacher SC, Tan PH, McClure MO, Larkin DF, Lechler RI, George AJ (2006b) Expression of indoleamine 2,3-dioxygenase (IDO) by endothelial cells: implications for the control of alloresponses. Am J Transplant 6:1320–1330

Boasso A, Herbeuval JP, Hardy AW, Anderson SA, Dolan MJ, Fuchs D, Shearer GM (2007) HIV inhibits CD4+ T-cell proliferation by inducing indoleamine 2,3-dioxygenase in plasmacytoid dendritic cells. Blood 109:3351–3359

Boon T, van der Bruggen P (1996) Human tumor antigens recognized by T lymphocytes. J Exp Med 183:725–729

Brandacher G, Perathoner A, Ladurner R, Schneeberger S, Obrist P, Winkler C, Werner ER, Werner-Felmayer G, Weiss HG, Gobel G et al (2006) Prognostic value of indoleamine 2,3-dioxygenase expression in colorectal cancer: effect on tumor-infiltrating T cells. Clin Cancer Res 12:1144–1151

Braun D, Longman RS, Albert ML (2005) A two step induction of indoleamine 2,3 dioxygenase (IDO) activity during dendritic cell maturation. Blood 106:2375–2381

Brenk M, Scheler M, Koch S, Neumann J, Takikawa O, Hacker G, Bieber T, von Bubnoff D (2009) Tryptophan deprivation induces inhibitory receptors ILT3 and ILT4 on dendritic cells favoring the induction of human CD4+CD25+ Foxp3+ T regulatory cells. J Immunol 183: 145–154

Brody JR, Costantino CL, Berger AC, Sato T, Lisanti MP, Yeo CJ, Emmons RV, Witkiewicz AK (2009) Expression of indoleamine 2,3-dioxygenase in metastatic malignant melanoma recruits regulatory T cells to avoid immune detection and affects survival. Cell Cycle 8: 1930–1934

Chamuleau ME, van de Loosdrecht AA, Hess CJ, Janssen JJ, Zevenbergen A, Delwel R, Valk PJ, Lowenberg B, Ossenkoppele GJ (2008) High INDO (indoleamine 2,3-dioxygenase) mRNA level in blasts of acute myeloid leukemic patients predicts poor clinical outcome. Haematologica 93:1894–1898

Chen W, Liang X, Peterson AJ, Munn DH, Blazar BR (2008) The indoleamine 2,3-dioxygenase pathway is essential for human plasmacytoid dendritic cell-induced adaptive T regulatory cell generation. J Immunol 181:5396–5404

Chung DJ, Rossi M, Romano E, Ghith J, Yuan J, Munn DH, Young JW (2009) Indoleamine 2,3-dioxygenase-expressing mature human monocyte-derived dendritic cells expand potent autologous regulatory T cells. Blood 114:555–563

Cobbold SP, Adams E, Farquhar CA, Nolan KF, Howie D, Lui KO, Fairchild PJ, Mellor AL, Ron D, Waldmann H (2009) Infectious tolerance via the consumption of essential amino acids and mTOR signaling. Proc Natl Acad Sci USA 106:12055–12060

Cochran AJ, Huang RR, Lee J, Itakura E, Leong SP, Essner R (2006) Tumour-induced immune modulation of sentinel lymph nodes. Nat Rev Immunol 6:659–670

Corm S, Berthon C, Imbenotte M, Biggio V, Lhermitte M, Dupont C, Briche I, Quesnel B (2009) Indoleamine 2,3-dioxygenase activity of acute myeloid leukemia cells can be measured from patients' sera by HPLC and is inducible by IFN-gamma. Leuk Res 33:490–494

Cuenca A, Cheng F, Wang H, Brayer J, Horna P, Gu L, Bien H, Borrello IM, Levitsky HI, Sotomayor EM (2003) Extra-lymphatic solid tumor growth is not immunologically ignored and results in early induction of antigen-specific T-cell anergy: dominant role of cross-tolerance to tumor antigens. Cancer Res 63:9007–9015

Curti A, Aluigi M, Pandolfi S, Ferri E, Isidori A, Salvestrini V, Durelli I, Horenstein AL, Fiore F, Massaia M et al (2007a) Acute myeloid leukemia cells constitutively express the immunoregulatory enzyme indoleamine 2,3-dioxygenase. Leukemia 21:353–355

Curti A, Pandolfi S, Valzasina B, Aluigi M, Isidori A, Ferri E, Salvestrini V, Bonanno G, Rutella S, Durelli I et al (2007b) Modulation of tryptophan catabolism by human leukemic cells results in the conversion of CD25- into CD25+ T regulatory cells. Blood 109:2871–2877

Duluc D, Delneste Y, Tan F, Moles MP, Grimaud L, Lenoir J, Preisser L, Anegon I, Catala L, Ifrah N et al (2007) Tumor-associated leukemia inhibitory factor and IL-6 skew monocyte differentiation into tumor-associated-macrophage-like cells. Blood 110:4319–4330

Ercolini AM, Ladle BH, Manning EA, Pfannenstiel LW, Armstrong TD, Machiels JP, Bieler JG, Emens LA, Reilly RT, Jaffee EM (2005) Recruitment of latent pools of high-avidity CD8(+) T cells to the antitumor immune response. J Exp Med 201:1591–1602

Fallarino F, Grohmann U, You S, McGrath BC, Cavener DR, Vacca C, Orabona C, Bianchi R, Belladonna ML, Volpi C et al (2006) The combined effects of tryptophan starvation and tryptophan catabolites down-regulate T cell receptor zeta-chain and induce a regulatory phenotype in naive T cells. J Immunol 176:6752–6761

Feder-Mengus C, Wyler S, Hudolin T, Ruszat R, Bubendorf L, Chiarugi A, Pittelli M, Weber WP, Bachmann A, Gasser TC et al (2008) High expression of indoleamine 2,3-dioxygenase gene in prostate cancer. Eur J Cancer 44:2266–2275

Fujigaki H, Saito K, Lin F, Fujigaki S, Takahashi K, Martin BM, Chen CY, Masuda J, Kowalak J, Takikawa O et al (2006) Nitration and inactivation of IDO by peroxynitrite. J Immunol 176:372–379

Grohmann U, Orabona C, Fallarino F, Vacca C, Calcinaro F, Falorni A, Candeloro P, Belladonna ML, Bianchi R, Fioretti MC, Puccetti P (2002) CTLA-4-Ig regulates tryptophan catabolism in vivo. Nat Immunol 3:1097–1101

Grohmann U, Volpi C, Fallarino F, Bozza S, Bianchi R, Vacca C, Orabona C, Belladonna ML, Ayroldi E, Nocentini G et al (2007) Reverse signaling through GITR ligand enables dexamethasone to activate IDO in allergy. Nat Med 13:579–586

Guillonneau C, Hill M, Hubert FX, Chiffoleau E, Herve C, Li XL, Heslan M, Usal C, Tesson L, Menoret S et al (2007) CD40Ig treatment results in allograft acceptance mediated by CD8CD45RC T cells, IFN-gamma, and indoleamine 2,3-dioxygenase. J Clin Invest 117: 1096–1106

Gurtner GJ, Newberry RD, Schloemann SR, McDonald KG, Stenson WF (2003) Inhibition of indoleamine 2,3-dioxygenase augments trinitrobenzene sulfonic acid colitis in mice. Gastroenterology 125:1762–1773

Hayashi T, Mo JH, Gong X, Rossetto C, Jang A, Beck L, Elliott GI, Kufareva I, Abagyan R, Broide DH et al (2007) 3-Hydroxyanthranilic acid inhibits PDK1 activation and suppresses experimental asthma by inducing T cell apoptosis. Proc Natl Acad Sci USA 104:18619–18624

Hildner K, Edelson BT, Purtha WE, Diamond M, Matsushita H, Kohyama M, Calderon B, Schraml BU, Unanue ER, Diamond MS et al (2008) Batf3 deficiency reveals a critical role for CD8alpha+ dendritic cells in cytotoxic T cell immunity. Science 322:1097–1100

Hou DY, Muller AJ, Sharma MD, Duhadaway JB, Banerjee T, Johnson M, Mellor AL, Prendergast GC, Munn DH (2007) Inhibition of IDO in dendritic cells by stereoisomers of 1-methyl-tryptophan correlates with anti-tumor responses. Cancer Res 67:792–801

Huang AY, Golumbek P, Ahmadzadeh M, Jaffee E, Pardoll D, Levitsky H (1994) Role of bone marrow-derived cells in presenting MHC class I-restricted tumor antigens. Science 264: 961–965

Huang A, Fuchs D, Widner B, Glover C, Henderson DC, Allen-Mersh TG (2002) Serum tryptophan decrease correlates with immune activation and impaired quality of life in colorectal cancer. Br J Cancer 86:1691–1696

Hwu P, Du MX, Lapointe R, Do M, Taylor MW, Young HA (2000) Indoleamine 2,3-dioxygenase production by human dendritic cells results in the inhibition of T cell proliferation. J Immunol 164:3596–3599

Ino K, Yoshida N, Kajiyama H, Shibata K, Yamamoto E, Kidokoro K, Takahashi N, Terauchi M, Nawa A, Nomura S et al (2006) Indoleamine 2,3-dioxygenase is a novel prognostic indicator for endometrial cancer. Br J Cancer 95:1555–1561

Ino K, Yamamoto E, Shibata K, Kajiyama H, Yoshida N, Terauchi M, Nawa A, Nagasaka T, Takikawa O, Kikkawa F (2008) Inverse correlation between tumoral indoleamine 2,3-dioxygenase expression and tumor-infiltrating lymphocytes in endometrial cancer: its association with disease progression and survival. Clin Cancer Res 14:2310–2317

Jalili RB, Forouzandeh F, Moeenrezakhanlou A, Rayat GR, Rajotte RV, Uludag H, Ghahary A (2009) Mouse pancreatic islets are resistant to indoleamine 2,3 dioxygenase-induced general control nonderepressible-2 kinase stress pathway and maintain normal viability and function. Am J Pathol 174:196–205

Jasperson LK, Bucher C, Panoskaltsis-Mortari A, Taylor PA, Mellor AL, Munn DH, Blazar BR (2008) Indoleamine 2,3-dioxygenase is a critical regulator of acute GVHD lethality. Blood 111:3257–3265

Jia L, Schweikart K, Tomaszewski J, Page JG, Noker PE, Buhrow SA, Reid JM, Ames MM, Munn DH (2008) Toxicology and pharmacokinetics of 1-methyl-D-tryptophan: absence of toxicity due to saturating absorption. Food Chem Toxicol 46:203–211

Kim YH, Choi BK, Kang WJ, Kim KH, Kang SW, Mellor AL, Munn DH, Kwon BS (2009) IFN-{gamma}-indoleamine-2,3 dioxygenase acts as a major suppressive factor in 4–1BB-mediated immune suppression in vivo. J Leukoc Biol 85(5):817–825

Lake RA, Robinson BW (2005) Immunotherapy and chemotherapy – a practical partnership. Nat Rev Cancer 5:397–405

Lee JR, Dalton RR, Messina JL, Sharma MD, Smith DM, Burgess RE, Mazzella F, Antonia SJ, Mellor AL, Munn DH (2003) Pattern of recruitment of immunoregulatory antigen presenting cells in malignant melanoma. Lab Invest 83:1457–1466

Lee JH, Torisu-Itakara H, Cochran AJ, Kadison A, Huynh Y, Morton DL, Essner R (2005) Quantitative analysis of melanoma-induced cytokine-mediated immunosuppression in melanoma sentinel nodes. Clin Cancer Res 11:107–112

Liu H, Liu L, Fletcher BS, Visner GA (2006) Novel action of indoleamine 2,3-dioxygenase attenuating acute lung allograft injury. Am J Respir Crit Care Med 173:566–572

Lob S, Konigsrainer A, Schafer R, Rammensee HG, Opelz G, Terness P (2008) Levo- but not dextro-1-methyl tryptophan abrogates the IDO activity of human dendritic cells. Blood 111: 2152–2154

Lob S, Konigsrainer A, Rammensee HG, Opelz G, Terness P (2009a) Inhibitors of indoleamine-2,3-dioxygenase for cancer therapy: can we see the wood for the trees? Nat Rev Cancer 9: 445–452

Lob S, Konigsrainer A, Zieker D, Brucher BL, Rammensee HG, Opelz G, Terness P (2009b) IDO1 and IDO2 are expressed in human tumors: levo- but not dextro-1-methyl tryptophan inhibits tryptophan catabolism. Cancer Immunol Immunother 58:153–157

Lurquin C, Lethe B, De Plaen E, Corbiere V, Theate I, van Baren N, Coulie PG, Boon T (2005) Contrasting frequencies of antitumor and anti-vaccine T cells in metastases of a melanoma patient vaccinated with a MAGE tumor antigen. J Exp Med 201:249–257

Maksimow M, Miiluniemi M, Marttila-Ichihara F, Jalkanen S, Hanninen A (2006) Antigen targeting to endosomal pathway in dendritic cell vaccination activates regulatory T cells and attenuates tumor immunity. Blood 108:1298–1305

Manches O, Munn D, Fallahi A, Lifson J, Chaperot L, Plumas J, Bhardwaj N (2008) HIV-activated human plasmacytoid DCs induce Tregs through an indoleamine 2,3-dioxygenase-dependent mechanism. J Clin Invest 118:3431–3439

Manlapat AK, Kahler DJ, Chandler PR, Munn DH, Mellor AL (2007) Cell-autonomous control of interferon type I expression by indoleamine 2,3-dioxygenase in regulatory CD19(+) dendritic cells. Eur J Immunol 37:1064–1071

Mellor AL, Munn DH (2008) Creating immune privilege: active local suppression that benefits friends, but protects foes. Nat Rev Immunol 8:74–80

Mellor AL, Baban B, Chandler P, Marshall B, Jhaver K, Hansen A, Koni PA, Iwashima M, Munn DH (2003) Cutting edge: induced indoleamine 2,3 dioxygenase expression in dendritic cell subsets suppresses T cell clonal expansion. J Immunol 171:1652–1655

Mellor AL, Baban B, Chandler PR, Manlapat A, Kahler DJ, Munn DH (2005) Cutting edge: CpG oligonucleotides induce splenic CD19+ dendritic cells to acquire potent indoleamine 2,3-dioxygenase-dependent T cell regulatory functions via IFN type 1 signaling. J Immunol 175:5601–5605

Metz R, Duhadaway JB, Kamasani U, Laury-Kleintop L, Muller AJ, Prendergast GC (2007) Novel tryptophan catabolic enzyme IDO2 is the preferred biochemical target of the antitumor indoleamine 2,3-dioxygenase inhibitory compound D-1-methyl-tryptophan. Cancer Res 67: 7082–7087

Moreau M, Lestage J, Verrier D, Mormede C, Kelley KW, Dantzer R, Castanon N (2005) Bacille Calmette-Guerin inoculation induces chronic activation of peripheral and brain indoleamine 2,3-dioxygenase in mice. J Infect Dis 192:537–544

Muller AJ, Scherle PA (2006) Targeting the mechanisms of tumoral immune tolerance with small-molecule inhibitors. Nat Rev Cancer 6:613–625

Muller AJ, Duhadaway JB, Donover PS, Sutanto-Ward E, Prendergast GC (2005a) Inhibition of indoleamine 2,3-dioxygenase, an immunoregulatory target of the cancer suppression gene Bin1, potentiates cancer chemotherapy. Nat Med 11:312–319

Muller AJ, Malachowski WP, Prendergast GC (2005b) Indoleamine 2,3-dioxygenase in cancer: targeting pathological immune tolerance with small-molecule inhibitors. Expert Opin Ther Targets 9:831–849

Munn DH, Mellor AL (2007) Indoleamine 2,3-dioxygenase and tumor-induced tolerance. J Clin Invest 117:1147–1154

Munn DH, Zhou M, Attwood JT, Bondarev I, Conway SJ, Marshall B, Brown C, Mellor AL (1998) Prevention of allogeneic fetal rejection by tryptophan catabolism. Science 281:1191–1193

Munn DH, Sharma MD, Lee JR, Jhaver KG, Johnson TS, Keskin DB, Marshall B, Chandler P, Antonia SJ, Burgess R et al (2002) Potential regulatory function of human dendritic cells expressing indoleamine 2,3-dioxygenase. Science 297:1867–1870

Munn DH, Sharma MD, Hou D, Baban B, Lee JR, Antonia SJ, Messina JL, Chandler P, Koni PA, Mellor A (2004a) Expression of indoleamine 2,3-dioxygenase by plasmacytoid dendritic cells in tumor-draining lymph nodes. J Clin Invest 114:280–290

Munn DH, Sharma MD, Mellor AL (2004b) Ligation of B7-1/B7-2 by human CD4+ T cells triggers indoleamine 2,3-dioxygenase activity in dendritic cells. J Immunol 172:4100–4110

Munn DH, Sharma MD, Baban B, Harding HP, Zhang Y, Ron D, Mellor AL (2005) GCN2 kinase in T cells mediates proliferative arrest and anergy induction in response to indoleamine 2,3-dioxygenase. Immunity 22:633–642

Ochsenbein AF, Klenerman P, Karrer U, Ludewig B, Pericin M, Hengartner H, Zinkernagel RM (1999) Immune surveillance against a solid tumor fails because of immunological ignorance. Immunology 96:2233–2238

Okamoto A, Nikaido T, Ochiai K, Takakura S, Saito M, Aoki Y, Ishii N, Yanaihara N, Yamada K, Takikawa O et al (2005) Indoleamine 2,3-dioxygenase serves as a marker of poor prognosis in gene expression profiles of serous ovarian cancer cells. Clin Cancer Res 11:6030–6039

Orabona C, Puccetti P, Vacca C, Bicciato S, Luchini A, Fallarino F, Bianchi R, Velardi E, Perruccio K, Velardi A et al (2006) Toward the identification of a tolerogenic signature in IDO-competent dendritic cells. Blood 107:2846–2854

Orabona C, Pallotta MT, Volpi C, Fallarino F, Vacca C, Bianchi R, Belladonna ML, Fioretti MC, Grohmann U, Puccetti P (2008) SOCS3 drives proteasomal degradation of indoleamine 2,3-dioxygenase (IDO) and antagonizes IDO-dependent tolerogenesis. Proc Natl Acad Sci USA 105:20828–20833

Polak ME, Borthwick NJ, Gabriel FG, Johnson P, Higgins B, Hurren J, McCormick D, Jager MJ, Cree IA (2007) Mechanisms of local immunosuppression in cutaneous melanoma. Br J Cancer 96:1879–1887

Qian F, Villella J, Wallace PK, Mhawech-Fauceglia P, Tario JD Jr, Andrews C, Matsuzaki J, Valmori D, Ayyoub M, Frederick PJ et al (2009) Efficacy of levo-1-methyl tryptophan and dextro-1-methyl tryptophan in reversing indoleamine-2,3-dioxygenase-mediated arrest of T-cell proliferation in human epithelial ovarian cancer. Cancer Res 69(13):5498–504

Quezada SA, Peggs KS, Simpson TR, Shen Y, Littman DR, Allison JP (2008) Limited tumor infiltration by activated T effector cells restricts the therapeutic activity of regulatory T cell depletion against established melanoma. J Exp Med 205:2125–2138

Rodriguez PC, Quiceno DG, Ochoa AC (2007) L-arginine availability regulates T-lymphocyte cell-cycle progression. Blood 109:1568–1573

Romani L, Fallarino F, De Luca A, Montagnoli C, D'Angelo C, Zelante T, Vacca C, Bistoni F, Fioretti MC, Grohmann U et al (2008) Defective tryptophan catabolism underlies inflammation in mouse chronic granulomatous disease. Nature 451:211–215

Rutella S, Bonanno G, Procoli A, Mariotti A, de Ritis DG, Curti A, Danese S, Pessina G, Pandolfi S, Natoni F et al (2006) Hepatocyte growth factor favors monocyte differentiation into regulatory interleukin (IL)-10++IL-12low/neg accessory cells with dendritic-cell features. Blood 108:218–227

Sharma MD, Baban B, Chandler P, Hou DY, Singh N, Yagita H, Azuma M, Blazar BR, Mellor AL, Munn DH (2007) Plasmacytoid dendritic cells from mouse tumor-draining lymph nodes directly activate mature Tregs via indoleamine 2,3-dioxygenase. J Clin Invest 117:2570–2582

Sharma MD, Hou DY, Liu Y, Koni PA, Metz R, Chandler P, Mellor AL, He Y, Munn DH (2009) Indoleamine 2,3-dioxygenase controls conversion of Foxp3+ Tregs to TH17-like cells in tumor-draining lymph nodes. Blood 113:6102–6111

Soliman HH, Antonia SJ, Sullivan D, Vanahanian N, Link C (2009) Overcoming tumor antigen anergy in human malignancies using the novel indeolamine 2,3-dioxygenase (IDO) enzyme inhibitor, 1-methyl-D-tryptophan (1MT). J Clin Oncol 27:3004

Sotomayor EM, Borrello I, Rattis FM, Cuenca AG, Abrams J, Staveley-O'Carroll K, Levitsky HI (2001) Cross-presentation of tumor antigens by bone marrow-derived antigen-presenting cells is the dominant mechanism in the induction of T-cell tolerance during B-cell lymphoma progression. Blood 98:1070–1077

Spiotto MT, Yu P, Rowley DA, Nishimura MI, Meredith SC, Gajewski TF, Fu YX, Schreiber H (2002) Increasing tumor antigen expression overcomes "ignorance" to solid tumors via crosspresentation by bone marrow-derived stromal cells. Immunity 17:737–747

Stone TW, Darlington LG (2002) Endogenous kynurenines as targets for drug discovery and development. Nat Rev Drug Discov 1:609–620

Sugimoto H, Oda S, Otsuki T, Hino T, Yoshida T, Shiro Y (2006) Crystal structure of human indoleamine 2,3-dioxygenase: catalytic mechanism of O2 incorporation by a heme-containing dioxygenase. Proc Natl Acad Sci USA 103:2611–2616

Sundrud MS, Koralov SB, Feuerer M, Calado DP, Kozhaya AE, Rhule-Smith A, Lefebvre RE, Unutmaz D, Mazitschek R, Waldner H et al (2009) Halofuginone inhibits TH17 cell differentiation by activating the amino acid starvation response. Science 324:1334–1338

Swanson KA, Zheng Y, Heidler KM, Mizobuchi T, Wilkes DS (2004) CD11c+cells modulate pulmonary immune responses by production of indoleamine 2,3-dioxygenase. Am J Respir Cell Mol Biol 30:311–318

Tas SW, Vervoordeldonk MJ, Hajji N, Schuitemaker JH, van der Sluijs KF, May MJ, Ghosh S, Kapsenberg ML, Tak PP, de Jong EC (2007) Noncanonical NF-kappaB signaling in dendritic cells is required for indoleamine 2,3-dioxygenase (IDO) induction and immune regulation. Blood 110:1540–1549

Terness P, Chuang JJ, Bauer T, Jiga L, Opelz G (2005) Regulation of human auto- and alloreactive T cells by indoleamine 2,3-dioxygenase (IDO)-producing dendritic cells: too much ado about IDO? Blood 105:2480–2486

Uyttenhove C, Pilotte L, Theate I, Stroobant V, Colau D, Parmentier N, Boon T, Van Den Eynde BJ (2003) Evidence for a tumoral immune resistance mechanism based on tryptophan degradation by indoleamine 2,3-dioxygenase. Nat Med 9:1269–1274

Vacca C, Fallarino F, Perruccio K, Orabona C, Bianchi R, Gizzi S, Velardi A, Fioretti MC, Puccetti P, Grohmann U (2005) CD40 ligation prevents onset of tolerogenic properties in human dendritic cells treated with CTLA-4-Ig. Microbes Infect 7:1040–1048

van der Marel AP, Samsom JN, Greuter M, van Berkel LA, O'Toole T, Kraal G, Mebius RE (2007) Blockade of IDO inhibits nasal tolerance induction. J Immunol 179:894–900

von Bergwelt-Baildon MS, Popov A, Saric T, Chemnitz J, Classen S, Stoffel MS, Fiore F, Roth U, Beyer M, Debey S et al (2006) CD25 and indoleamine 2,3-dioxygenase are up-regulated by prostaglandin E2 and expressed by tumor-associated dendritic cells in vivo: additional mechanisms of T-cell inhibition. Blood 108:228–237

Wek RC, Jiang HY, Anthony TG (2006) Coping with stress: eIF2 kinases and translational control. Biochem Soc Trans 34:7–11

Williams KM, Hakim FT, Gress RE (2007) T cell immune reconstitution following lymphodepletion. Semin Immunol 19:318–330

Willimsky G, Czeh M, Loddenkemper C, Gellermann J, Schmidt K, Wust P, Stein H, Blankenstein T (2008) Immunogenicity of premalignant lesions is the primary cause of general cytotoxic T lymphocyte unresponsiveness. J Exp Med 205:1687–1700

Witkiewicz A, Williams TK, Cozzitorto J, Durkan B, Showalter SL, Yeo CJ, Brody JR (2008) Expression of indoleamine 2,3-dioxygenase in metastatic pancreatic ductal adenocarcinoma recruits regulatory T cells to avoid immune detection. J Am Coll Surg 206:849–854; discussion 854–846

Witkiewicz AK, Costantino CL, Metz R, Muller AJ, Prendergast GC, Yeo CJ, Brody JR (2009) Genotyping and expression analysis of IDO2 in human pancreatic cancer: a novel, active target. J Am Coll Surg 208:781–787; discussion 787–789

Wobser M, Voigt H, Houben R, Eggert AO, Freiwald M, Kaemmerer U, Kaempgen E, Schrama D, Becker JC (2007) Dendritic cell based antitumor vaccination: impact of functional indoleamine 2,3-dioxygenase expression. Cancer Immunol Immunother 56:1017–1024

Yu P, Lee Y, Liu W, Krausz T, Chong A, Schreiber H, Fu YX (2005) Intratumor depletion of CD4+ cells unmasks tumor immunogenicity leading to the rejection of late-stage tumors. J Exp Med 201:779–791

Zhou G, Drake CG, Levitsky HI (2006) Amplification of tumor-specific regulatory T cells following therapeutic cancer vaccines. Blood 107:628–636

Zitvogel L, Apetoh L, Ghiringhelli F, Kroemer G (2008) Immunological aspects of cancer chemotherapy. Nat Rev Immunol 8:59–73

Zou W (2006) Regulatory T cells, tumour immunity and immunotherapy. Nat Rev Immunol 6: 295–307

Chapter 18
Myeloid-Derived Suppressor Cells in Cancer: Mechanisms and Therapeutic Perspectives

Paulo C. Rodríguez and Augusto C. Ochoa

1 Introduction

Modern concepts in carcinogenesis including the viral etiology of certain malignancies, the presence of mutated onco-proteins, and the overexpression of certain normal antigens, lead support to the concept that antigen-specific immune responses can be generated against these targets to control tumor growth. However, three decades of clinical trials in cancer immunotherapy and recent research have made evident that tumor cells have sophisticated mechanisms to evade the immune response. Recent findings have characterized multiple molecular mechanisms triggered by the tumor microenvironment resulting in the impairment of T cell antitumor responses. The molecular and cellular bases underlying these mechanisms are a matter of extensive research, and may hold the key to being able to modulate the immune response for the therapeutic benefit of cancer patients. Even though most researchers agree that malignant cells trigger the events that ultimately lead to T cell dysfunction, the mediators of this process vary from regulatory T cells and suppressor macrophages to the more recently described

P.C. Rodríguez
Department of Microbiology, Immunology and Parasitology,
Louisiana State University Health Sciences Center, New Orleans, LA, USA

Stanley S. Scott Cancer Center, Louisiana State University Health Sciences Center,
New Orleans, LA, USA

A.C. Ochoa (✉)
Stanley S. Scott Cancer Center, Louisiana State University Health Sciences Center,
New Orleans, LA, USA

Department of Pediatrics, Louisiana State University Health Sciences Center,
New Orleans, LA, USA
e-mail: aochoa@lsuhsc.edu

myeloid-derived suppressor cells (MDSC). The latter subpopulation of immune cells has been of great interest because of their ability to regulate T cell responses by controlling the availability of the amino acid L-Arginine (L-Arg). The demonstration of this mechanism in tumor models, patients with cancer and various other chronic inflammatory diseases, and the potential for therapeutic intervention has created a major interest in MDSC. We will discuss some of the most recent concepts of how MDSC regulate T cell function in disease, and suggest possible therapeutic applications to inhibit their suppressive activity.

2 Alterations of the Immune Response in Cancer

A dysfunctional immune response in cancer patients manifested by the loss of delayed type hypersensitivity was demonstrated several decades ago (Miescher et al. 1986, 1988; Whiteside et al. 1988; Whiteside and Rabinowich 1998). Initial explanations included the development of "blocking antibodies," the production of suppressor factors by tumor cells, and the generation of suppressor macrophages (Hellstrom et al. 1971, 1983; Varesio et al. 1979). However, the significance of these findings on the progression of the disease was unknown. Although cancer patients generally do not develop the characteristic opportunistic infections seen in patients immunosuppressed by high doses of chemotherapy, they show impaired T cell responses against bacterial and/or chemical antigens (Miescher et al. 1986, 1988; Whiteside et al. 1988; Whiteside and Rabinowich 1998). Therefore, tumors significantly impair T cell responses. In fact, several animal tumor models and many clinical trials demonstrated that immunotherapy in mice or patients with advanced tumors failed to achieve a therapeutic response as a result of the loss of T cell responses (reviewed in ref. Gattinoni et al. 2006). In addition, several vaccine trials demonstrated the progression of tumors in spite of a robust T cell response (Stevenson 2005). The development of cellular and molecular models leading to T cell anergy provided important insights on how cancer (and chronic inflammatory diseases) could selectively cause T cell dysfunction (Rabinovich et al. 2007). This provided the basis for the discovery of new mechanisms including the role of the immunoregulatory B7 family of molecules (Dong et al. 1999; Klausner et al. 1990; Kryczek et al. 2006a, b), the development of regulatory T cells (McHugh et al. 2001; McHugh and Shevach 2002), and the generation of MDSC (Bronte and Zanovello 2005; Gabrilovich 2004; Pekarek et al. 1995; Seung et al. 1995). Young and colleagues demonstrated that suppressor macrophages blocked T cell responses by producing IL-10, TGF-β, and prostaglandin E_2 (PGE_2) (Young et al. 1987). Gabrilovich et al. (1996) demonstrated that VEGF produced by tumor cells arrested the differentiation of dendritic cells, resulting in immature myeloid cells that induce T cell dysfunction. These immature myeloid cells were found to be increased in patients with breast, head and neck, and lung cancer (Almand et al. 2000, 2001). More recently, Mellor and Munn demonstrated that an impaired T cell response can also occur as a result of the depletion of the essential amino acid tryptophan by plasmacytoid dendritic cells producing indoleamine 2,3-dioxygenase (IDO) (Mellor and Munn 2004; Munn et al. 2005).

3 Mechanisms of T cell Anergy in Cancer

In the 1990s, we and others showed that T cells from cancer patients and tumor-bearing mice had multiple, but discrete changes in the expression of signal transduction molecules, including a decreased expression of the T cell receptor ζ chain (CD3ζ), low expression of tyrosine kinases p56^{lck} and p59^{fyn}, and an inability to upregulate Jak-3 and to translocate NF-kB (p65), all of which resulted in diminished in vitro T cell response (Ghosh et al. 1994; Li et al. 1994; Mizoguchi et al. 1992). These alterations were accompanied by a decreased ability to mobilize Ca^{++} and diminished tyrosine phosphorylation (Mizoguchi et al. 1992), which provided a possible molecular explanation for T cell dysfunction in cancer. These initial findings in mice were confirmed in patients with renal cell carcinoma, melanoma, Hodgkin's disease, ovarian cancer, colon carcinoma, and cervical cancer among others (Finke et al. 1993; Kono et al. 1996a; Zea et al. 1995). Preliminary studies also showed that patients with renal cell carcinoma or head and neck tumors had a decreased survival time if expressing low levels of CD3ζ (Zea et al. 1995; Kuss et al. 1999). The absence of a mechanism to explain these changes and the apparent lack of specificity of these alterations created some initial controversy around these observations.

Otsuji et al. (1996) and Kono et al. (1996a, b) first demonstrated that the co-incubation of activated murine peritoneal macrophages with T cells induced the loss of CD3ζ chain. This phenomenon could be blocked by oxygen radical scavengers and was therefore thought to be mediated by H_2O_2 (Corsi et al. 1998). Similarly, Schmielau and Finn described an increased number of activated neutrophils in peripheral blood of pancreatic and breast cancer patients who had a diminished expression of CD3ζ chain (Schmielau and Finn 2001). Another mechanism suggested that the loss of CD3ζ chain was a consequence of Fas–FasL-induced T cell apoptosis (Rabinowich et al. 1998; Uzzo et al. 1999). In addition, Baniyash and colleagues proposed that chronic stimulation of T cells by specific antigens led to decreased expression of CD3ζ chain leading to induction of anergy (Bronstein-Sitton et al. 2003). However, none of these models fully reproduced the multiple alterations found in T cells of cancer patients.

Reports from other diseases also suggested that the loss of CD3ζ was not unique to cancer. Zea et al. (1998, 2006) described that patients with lepromatous leprosy or active pulmonary tuberculosis presented with similar alterations in T cells. In addition, mice with severe trauma were shown to have decreased CD3ζ expression and diminished T cell function (Makarenkova et al. 2006). Furthermore, trauma patients showed a rapid depletion of L-Arg levels in serum which was paralleled by the loss of T cell function. Animal trauma models also showed that replenishment of L-Arg reestablished normal T cell function and increased the number of CD4$^+$ cells (Kirk et al. 1992; Ochoa et al. 2000, 2001).

3.1 L-Arginine and Immune Response

The association between L-Arg and the immune system was initially suggested by experiments showing that the thymic involution and decrease in T cells seen in mice undergoing extensive surgery was prevented by the injection of L-Arg (Barbul et al. 1977). Albina and Mills (Albina et al. 1989) later demonstrated that L-Arg was fundamental for wound healing. In addition, a study in liver transplant and trauma patients showed that rapid depletion of plasma levels of L-Arg was accompanied by a markedly decreased T cell function (Kirk et al. 1992; Ochoa et al. 2000, 2001).

Our initial experiments demonstrated that culturing Jurkat T cells in tissue culture medium with L-Arg levels <50 µM resulted in the gradual loss of CD3ζ and caused a significant decrease in proliferation (Taheri et al. 2001). Experiments using primary T cells did not show any effects of L-Arg deprivation on resting T cells. However, T cells activated in an L-Arg free environment developed all the alterations previously described in tumor-bearing mice and cancer patients, i.e. decreased expression of CD3ζ, an inability to upregulate Jak-3 and decreased translocation of NF-kB-p65. T cells cultured without L-Arg also failed to proliferate and did not produce IFN-γ. However, these changes were selective since other functions, including the production of IL2 and the upregulation and expression of the IL-2 receptor chains (CD25, CD122, CD132), were similar to cells cultured in medium with L-Arg. These results suggested a potential role for L-Arg depletion as a mechanism for the inhibition of T cell function. However, it was unclear how L-Arg levels might be regulated in vivo.

In healthy adults, L-Arg is considered to be a nonessential amino acid. It is synthesized endogenously from citrulline produced by epithelial cells of the small intestine which is then metabolized by the proximal tubules of the kidney to produce L-Arg de novo (reviewed in ref. Brosnan and Brosnan 2004). Normal levels of L-Arg in serum range between 50 and 150 µM. However, L-Arg is also classified as a conditional essential amino acid in certain conditions such as trauma and cancer where changes in the systemic levels of L-Arg cause major alterations in the immune response (Nieves and Langkamp-Henken 2002). L-Arg is the substrate for four enzymes that exist as multiple isoforms: nitric oxide synthases (NOS1, NOS2, and NOS3), arginases (Arginase I and II), Arginine: glycine amidinotransferase (AGAT), and L-Arg decarboxylase (ADC). Dietary L-Arg is taken up by intestinal epithelial cells and traverses the plasma membrane via the y+system of cationic amino acid transporters (CAT) (Closs et al. 2004). Inside the cell L-Arg is metabolized by NOS enzymes to produce citrulline and nitric oxide, the latter of which plays an important role in cytotoxic mechanisms and vasodilatation (Amber et al. 1991; Hibbs et al. 1987). Alternatively, arginase I and arginase II metabolize L-Arg to L-ornithine and urea, the first being the precursor for the production of polyamines essential for cell proliferation and the second an important mechanism for detoxification of protein degradation (Morris 2002). ADC converts L-Arg to agmatine, which in turn is converted to putrescine and urea by agmatinase. ADC and AGAT appear to be less involved in immune reponse. Mammalian ADC is highly expressed in the brain (Iyo et al. 2006; Zhu et al. 2004), while AGAT is expressed in the brain and the heart (Cullen et al. 2006; Item et al. 2001).

Arginase I and NOS2 play important roles in immune response. The expression of arginase I and NOS2 in murine macrophages is differentially regulated by Th1 and Th2 cytokines (Hesse et al. 2001; Munder et al. 1999). Stimulation of murine macrophages with IFN-γ upregulates NOS2 exclusively, while IL-4, IL-10, and IL-13 (Munder et al. 1998; Rutschman et al. 2001) induce arginase I. The mitochondrial isoform of arginase II is not significantly modulated by cytokines (Rodriguez et al. 2003). The inhibition of arginase I leads to increased NOS2 expression and consequently promotes NO production (Chicoine et al. 2004). Conversely, upregulation of arginase I inhibits NOS activity and contributes to the pathophysiology of several disease processes, including vascular dysfunction and asthma (Zhang et al. 2004). The mechanisms of inhibition of NOS2 expression by arginase I appears to be mediated by L-Arg depletion which blocks the induction of NOS2 expression and subsequent NO production in macrophages (Lee et al. 2003). In addition, low levels of NOS induce nitrosylation of cysteine residues of arginase I, which increases the biological activity of arginase I and reduces L-Arg (Santhanam et al. 2007).

Activation of peritoneal macrophages with Th1 or Th2 cytokines also has different effects on the extracellular levels of L-Arg. Peritoneal macrophages stimulated with IL-4 plus IL-13 increase the expression of Arginase I and CAT-2B, which results in a rapid increase in the uptake of extracellular L-Arg with the consequent reduction of L-Arg in the microenvironment. In contrast, macrophages stimulated with IFN-γ preferentially express NOS2, do not increase CAT-2B, and do not deplete L-Arg from the microenvironment (Rodriguez et al. 2003). Recent data from arginase I and arginase II knockout mice confirm that only arginase I is able to deplete serum levels of L-Arg (Deignan et al. 2006; Iyer et al. 2002). Similarly, in vitro coculture experiments (using transwells) showed that only macrophages producing arginase I, but not macrophages expressing NOS2, caused prolonged loss of CD3ζ and inhibited T cell proliferation. The addition of arginase inhibitors N-Hydroxy-nor-L-Arg (Nor-NOHA) and N-Hydroxy-L-Arg (NOHA) or exogenous L-Arg reversed the CD3ζ loss and reestablished T cell proliferation (Rodriguez et al. 2003). These results were confirmed with macrophages from arginase I conditional knockout mice (P. Rodriguez, personal communication).

4 Molecular Effects of L-Arg Starvation on T Cells

Jurkat cells and primary T cells cultured in medium lacking L-Arg show decreased expression of CD3ζ and proliferation that was not associated with increased apoptosis (Taheri et al. 2001; Rodriguez et al. 2002, 2003; Zea et al. 2004). Replenishment of L-Arg at physiologic concentrations (50–150 µM) resulted in the rapid recovery of CD3ζ expression and T cell proliferation (Zea et al. 2004). The initial hypothesis suggested that low T cell proliferation was the result of decreased CD3ζ, however, this failed to explain how T cells cultured in the absence of L-Arg, and activated with PMA, (which bypasses the TCR), also failed to proliferate. In addition, T cells cultured in the absence of L-Arg had similar patterns of calcium flux and tyrosine phosphorylation as T cells cultured with L-Arg, and were able to upregulate the expression of activation markers CD25 and CD69, suggesting that signaling through the T cell receptor was intact during the early stages of culture without L-Arg (Zea et al. 2004).

Recent work by Rodriguez et al. showed instead that activated T cells cultured in the absence of L-Arg were arrested at the G_0–G_1 phase of the cell cycle, while cells cultured with L-Arg progressed into the S and G_2–M phases (Rodriguez et al. 2007). T cells cultured in the absence of L-Arg were unable to upregulate the expression of cyclin D3 and cyclin-dependent kinase 4 (cdk4), but not cdk6 (Rodriguez et al. 2007). Cyclin D3 and Cdk4 are closely associated with the D-type cyclins (Cyclins D1, D2 and D3) and regulate progression through early G_1 and later into the S phase of the cell cycle (Kato 1997; Sicinska et al. 2003). In fact, silencing of cyclin D3 in Jurkat cells induced a similar inhibition of proliferation as that seen with L-Arg starvation. It was unclear however why L-Arg starvation decreased the expression of cyclin D3 and cdk4 mRNA, but not cdk6. Results demonstrated that L-Arg starvation decreased cyclin D3 mRNA stability and diminished cyclin D3 translational rate. Therefore, the absence of L-Arg decreases expression of cyclin D3 and cdk4 through posttranscriptional and translational mechanisms (Rodriguez et al. 2007). Recent studies suggest that arginine depletion activates GCN2 kinase and the translation initiation factor eIF2α.

In eukaryotes, the accumulation of empty aminoacyl tRNAs caused by amino acid starvation activates GCN2 kinase which phosphorylates the translation initiation factor eIF2α. The phosphorylated form of eIF2α binds with high affinity to eIF2B blocking its ability to exchange GDP for GTP, which inhibits the binding of the eIF2 complex to Methionine aminoacyl tRNA, which in turn blocks the initiation of protein translation. However, it is unclear whether a similar event occurs in the T cells cultured in the absence of L-Arg.

We have defined some of the initial mediators of these events. The absence of L-Arg leads to the activation of GCN2 as shown by a significant increase in the phosphorylation of eIF2α. This was observed in activated T cells cultured in the absence of L-Arg, but not in cells cultured in the presence of L-Arg (Rodriguez et al. 2007). Indeed, it appears that GCN2 is a central mediator of the effects of low L-Arg on T cells since T cells from GCN2 KO mice do not show an arrest in cell cycle or a decreased proliferation when cultured in medium without L-Arg. (Rodriguez et al. 2007). These results support the role of GCN2 in T cells as the sensing protein in conditions of amino acid starvation.

How amino acid availability modulates mRNA stability is still unclear. In fact, some mRNA are more stable under conditions of L-Arg starvation. This was shown using the CAT-1 transporter where amino acid limitation increases its mRNA stability and translation, at a time when global protein synthesis decreases. The increased mRNA stability requires an 11 nucleotide AU-rich element within the distal 217 bases of the 3'-untranslated region (Yaman et al. 2002). In addition, amino acid starvation triggers increased translocation of the DNA binding protein HuR from the nucleus to the cytoplasm which increases CAT-1 mRNA stability (Yaman et al. 2002).

5 Arginase Expression in Tumors

Several tumors including some non-small lung carcinomas and breast carcinomas have been shown to express arginase (Chang et al. 2001; Suer et al. 1999; Singh et al. 2000). This has been thought to be a mechanism for the production of polyamines needed to sustain the rapid proliferation of tumor cells. Results from our laboratory suggest instead that arginase I is preferentially expressed in myeloid cells infiltrating tumors, which inhibits T cell function and represents a possible mechanism of tumor evasion (Rodriguez et al. 2004). Myeloid cells infiltrating murine 3LL lung carcinoma and expressing arginase I have the morphology and express the markers of mature macrophages. However, myeloid cells found in the spleen of tumor-bearing mice (including 3LL tumors) and expressing arginase I, appear to be immature myeloid cells and express granulocytic marker LY6G (Rodriguez et al. 2004). Even though there are variations in cell morphology and maturation markers between different tumor models and between murine and human tumors, these myeloid cells suppress T cell function. Recently, a panel of leading investigators in the field agreed to use the common term "MDSCs" (Gabrilovich et al. 2007). Two important subsets of MDSC have been reported based on their expression of CD11b, LY6G, and LY6C. Granulocytic MDSC have a CD11b$^+$ LY6G$^+$ LY6C^{low} phenotype, whereas monocytic MDSC are CD11b$^+$ LY6G$^-$ LY6C^{high} (Youn et al. 2008). Furthermore, we and others previously reported the existence of CD11b$^+$ LY6G$^-$ LY6C$^-$ MDSC in tumors, which have a similar phenotype to alternatively activated macrophages (Rodriguez et al. 2004; Dolcetti et al. 2010). Granulocytic and monocytic MDSC are present in the bone marrow of healthy mice, and accumulate in the spleen and tumors of tumor-bearing mice (Bronte et al. 2000; Kusmartsev et al. 2004; Sinha et al. 2005a). Depletion of MDSC using anti-Gr-1 antibodies induced an antitumor effect mediated by CD8$^+$ T cells (Pekarek et al. 1995; Seung et al. 1995; Holda et al. 1985).

Our data suggests that the primary mechanism by which MDSCs induce T cell tolerance is by depleting extracellular L-Arg through arginase I (Rodriguez et al. 2003, 2004, 2005). The addition of arginase I inhibitors Nor-NOHA or NOHA in vitro, or its injection into tumor-bearing mice prevents the loss of T cell function and results in an immune-mediated antitumor response which inhibits tumor growth in a dose dependent manner. The inhibition of tumor growth caused by Nor NOHA, does not happen in tumor-bearing *scid* mice, strongly suggesting that the antitumor effect caused by arginase inhibition is dependent on lymphocyte function (Rodriguez et al. 2004).These results were recently confirmed by data showing a significant inhibition of tumor growth in arginase I conditional knockout mice (P. Rodriguez personal communication).

MDSC may also cause T cell tolerance through cell–cell contact. This mechanism appears to require the co-expression of arginase I and NOS2 (Bronte and Zanovello

2005). The addition of NOS2 and arginase inhibitors to cocultures of MDSC and activated T cells completely reestablishes T cell function (Bronte et al. 2003). It is possible that this phenomenon is in part mediated by the production of peroxynitrites. Under limiting amounts of L-Arg, NOS2 produces peroxynitrites ($ONOO_2$), a highly reactive oxidizing agent that nitrates proteins and induces T cell apoptosis (Kusmartsev and Gabrilovich 2005). This appears to affect the conformational flexibility of the T cell antigen receptor (TCR) and its interaction with MHC by inducing nitration of TCR proteins in $CD8^+$ cells. Thus, MDSC directly disrupt the binding of specific peptides on MHC to $CD8^+$ T cells (Nagaraj et al. 2007). MDSC co-expression of arginase I and NOS2 primarily impair $CD8^+$ T cell function (Rodriguez et al. 2004; Sinha et al. 2005a; Kusmartsev and Gabrilovich 2005; Van Ginderachter et al. 2006) by blocking their ability to secrete IFN-γ when stimulated with specific antigens (Kusmartsev et al. 2004; Gabrilovich et al. 2001), and inducing apoptosis (Kusmartsev and Gabrilovich 2005). This suppression requires the production of IL-13 and IFN-γ (Sinha et al. 2005a, b; Gallina et al. 2006) and signaling through STAT1 transcription factor (Kusmartsev and Gabrilovich 2005). In addition, MDSCs have been shown to produce high levels of stem cell factor (SCF) when stimulated with IFN-γ and IL-10 (Huang et al. 2006). Blocking of stem cell factor signaling in MDSC significantly impairs their ability to generate regulatory T cells (Pan et al. 2008).

6 MDSC in Human Tumors

Human MDSC phenotypes vary significantly ranging from immature dendritic cells (Sica and Bronte 2007) to activated granulocytes. They have been reported to express a wide range of markers including CD11b, CD15, CD34, CD33, and CD13 (Zea et al. 2005). A retrospective study of patients with metastatic renal cell carcinoma (RCC) demonstrated a six- to ten-fold increase in arginase activity in the peripheral blood mononuclear cells (PBMC), compared to normal controls (Zea et al. 2005). Separation of the different subpopulations in the PBMC of these patients demonstrated that the cells containing high arginase activity were activated granulocytes which separated with the PBMC when centrifuged over ficoll-hypaque (Rodriguez et al. 2009). These patients also had a significantly diminished expression of CD3ζ chain in T and NK cells. There was an inverse statistical correlation between arginase activity and MDSC numbers with the expression of CD3ζ chain. T cell proliferation and IFN-γ production in vitro was reestablished after the depletion of MDSC. A similar subpopulation of activated granulocytes had previously been described in patients with pancreatic cancer, where they also demonstrated a correlation between the presence of activated granulocytes and alterations in T cells such as reduced CD3ζ expression and decreased cytokine production (Schmielau and Finn 2001). In fact, clinical trials with IL-2 in patients with renal cell carcinoma and melanoma have shown an association between a poor clinical response and an increased numbers of granulocytes in the periphery of these patients (Rodgers et al. 1994).

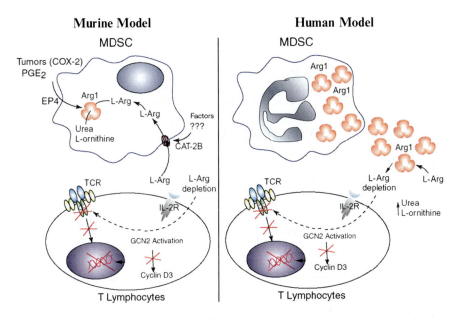

Fig. 18.1 MDSC from mice and humans differ in their mechanisms of arginine depletion. Murine MDSC rapidly incorporate L-Arg, while human MDSC release arginase I into the microenvironment (tumor and serum)

Although human MDSC also express high levels of arginase I, this does not appear to be upregulated by cytokines or other signals once these cells are in circulation. Furthermore human MDSC do not uptake L-Arg. Instead, arginase I stored in primary (Munder et al. 2005) or gelatinase granules (Jacobsen et al. 2007) is released to the microenvironment inducing a significant decrease in L-Arg levels, which impairs T cell function and CD3ζ chain expression (Zea et al. 2005; Kropf et al. 2007; Munder et al. 2006) (Fig. 18.1). In fact, the release of arginase I into the sera of renal cell carcinoma patients induced a decrease in plasma of L-Arg levels to <50 μM and an increase in ornithine levels demonstrating that arginase I not only had a metabolic effect (L-Arg depletion), but also a negative effect on T cell response (Zea et al. 2005). In fact, MDSC also appear to release arginase I in placenta as a mechanism for the development of tolerance in pregnancy (Kropf et al. 2007).

7 Regulation and Activation of MDSC in Cancer

Different cytokines participate in the recruitment of MDSC from the bone marrow, including VEGF and GM-CSF (Dolcetti et al. 2010). In fact, serum levels of VEGF directly correlated with numbers of MDSC in the blood and spleen (Ohm and Carbone 2001) and have been associated with poor prognosis in cancer patients. Tumor-derived VEGF has been previously associated with an arrest in DC maturation

(Gabrilovich et al. 1998; Oyama et al. 1998) through inhibition in NF-κβ signaling. Treatment of MDSC with all-*trans* retinoic acid appears to counter this inhibition and promotes MDSC differentiation into mature APC (Kusmartsev et al. 2003). Increased levels of GM-CSF have also been associated with MDSC-dependent suppression which was reversed by the use of neutralizing antibodies to GM-CSF (Bronte et al. 2000). Similar effects on MDSC have been suggested with other growth factors including Fms-like tyrosine kinase 3 (Flt3) ligand (Solheim et al. 2007), FSC (Pan et al. 2008), and S100A9 protein (Cheng et al. 2008).

We used the 3LL murine lung carcinoma model to further determine what factors might be inducing the production of arginase I in the MDSC infiltrating tumors. MDSC isolated from 3LL tumors and cultured with regular RPMI medium, loose arginase I expression within 24 h. However, if freshly isolated MDSC were cocultured in transwells with 3LL cells or with 3LL supernatants they maintained arginase I expression, suggesting that the induction of arginase I was caused by soluble factor (s) produced by tumor cells (Rodriguez et al. 2005). Cytokines such as IL-4, IL-13, TGF-β, and others were not detected in the supernatants of the 3LL single cell suspensions. Instead, we detected a very high expression of the inducible cyclooxygenase-2 (COX-2) and an increased production of prostanoids including PGE_2. The addition of COX-2 inhibitors or silencing of COX-2 in 3LL cells, completely blocked their ability to induce arginase I in MDSC (Rodriguez et al. 2005). The effect of PGE_2 on MDSC was dependent on the expression of the E-prostanoid receptor (EP4) on MDSC and was associated with an increased cAMP levels (Rodriguez et al. 2005). Consequently, treatment of tumor-bearing mice with COX-2 inhibitor SC-58125 decreased the expression of arginase I in MDSC infiltrating the tumor and induced immune-mediated antitumor effects (Rodriguez et al. 2005). Similar results have been reported in mice-bearing 4T1 breast carcinoma cells where the treatment with the COX-2 inhibitor SC-58236 reduced accumulation of MDSC in the spleen in an EP2-dependent manner (Sinha et al. 2007). In addition celecoxib, a selective COX-2 inhibitor was able to inhibit the induction of colon tumors in Swiss mice treated with 1,2-dimethylhydrazine diHCl-(1,2-DMH) (Talmadge et al. 2007). Other factors may also play a role in the induction of arginase in MDSC including hypoxia-inducible factor 1 (HIF-1) and HIF-2 (reviewed in ref. Semenza 2003), IL-4, IL-13, and IFN-γ (Gallina et al. 2006). In conclusion, although the mechanisms of induction of arginase I in MDSC have been partially identified in mice, the factors inducing the activation of MDSC in patients are still unclear. A recent publication by Rotondo et al. suggests a possible role for tumor-derived IL-8 on release of arginase from human MDSC (Rotondo et al. 2009).

7.1 *MDSC: Lessons from Other Diseases and Future Applications*

The advent of immunotherapy of cancer made apparent that in spite of powerful biological agents that could prime tumor-specific T cells, tumors had sophisticated mechanisms to escape the immune response, including MDSC. MDSC however are not unique to cancer. Trauma patients and patients with chronic infections including active pulmonary tuberculosis also have increased numbers of MDSC expressing arginase I that inhibit T cell function. This data suggests that MDSCs may represent a normal process triggered by tissue damage (danger signal) with the aim of protecting the integrity of the tissues and "healing" the initial injury. A demonstration of this mechanism was described in the late 1980s by Albina et al. (1989) studying the healing of surgical wounds. They described that the tissue surrounding a surgical wound was initially infiltrated by cells expressing iNOS, which most likely eliminate offending agents contaminating the wound. This is followed by cells expressing arginase I which would metabolize L-Arg to ornithine and proline which in turn would trigger the synthesis of collagen by fibroblasts, ultimately leading to healing of the surgical wound. The local depletion of L-Arg would also prevent T cells from infiltrating a healing tissue. In cancer or chronic infections, tissue damage would also trigger a similar response with the proliferation of fibroblasts producing collagen aimed at isolating and healing the damaged tissue (i.e., malignant growth). As a matter of fact, many tumors are surrounded by dense fibrous tissue that makes surgical excision difficult. The major difference between both disease processes (surgical wound vs. malignant tumor) is that surgical wounds heal thus, ending the role for arginase producing MDSC, while malignant tumors do not stop growing and destroying tissue (do not "heal") promoting instead a chronic inflammatory process mediated by MDSC. The continuous production of arginase I would ultimately lead to depletion of L-Arg from the microenvironment and the development of T cell anergy. Therefore, it is our hypothesis that tumors "hijack" a normal healing process making it instead a vicious cycle that results in the inhibition of a potentially protective T cell antitumor response. Although this is an oversimplified version of the complex mechanisms triggered in vivo, it provides a model with which to understand a complex event involved in the development of cancer and probably design new therapeutic approaches that may interrupt this dysfunctional response.

Much has been learned about the role of MDSC in the progression of tumors in the last 10 years. Multiple approaches have been taken to block MDSC suppression using all trans retinoic acid (Kusmartsev et al. 2003), inhibiting nitric oxide function with nitro-aspirin (De et al. 2005), inhibiting phosphodiesterase-5 (Serafini et al. 2006) and blocking arginase activity with specific arginase inhibitors such as Nor-NOHA (Rodriguez et al. 2004). It is likely that the appropriate combination of inhibitors blocking MDSC function and stimuli protecting T cells may overcome this powerful tumor-derived mechanism that impairs the promise of cancer immunotherapy.

Acknowledgments This work was supported by NIH/NCI Grants 5R01CA082689, 5R01CA107974 and 5P20RR021970,

References

Albina JE, Caldwell MD, Henry WL Jr, Mills CD (1989) Regulation of macrophage functions by L-arginine. J Exp Med 169:1021–1029
Almand B, Resser JR, Lindman B et al (2000) Clinical significance of defective dendritic cell differentiation in cancer. Clin Cancer Res 6:1755–1766

Almand B, Clark JI, Nikitina E et al (2001) Increased production of immature myeloid cells in cancer patients: a mechanism of immunosuppression in cancer. J Immunol 166:678–689

Amber IJ, Hibbs JB Jr, Parker CJ, Johnson BB, Taintor RR, Vavrin Z (1991) Activated macrophage conditioned medium: identification of the soluble factors inducing cytotoxicity and the L-arginine dependent effector mechanism. J Leukoc Biol 49:610–620

Barbul A, Rettura G, Levenson SM, Seifter E (1977) Arginine: a thymotropic and wound-healing promoting agent. Surg Forum 28:101–103

Bronstein-Sitton N, Cohen-Daniel L, Vaknin I et al (2003) Sustained exposure to bacterial antigen induces interferon-gamma-dependent T cell receptor zeta down-regulation and impaired T cell function. Nat Immunol 4:957–964

Bronte V, Zanovello P (2005) Regulation of immune responses by L-arginine metabolism. Nat Rev Immunol 5:641–654

Bronte V, Apolloni E, Cabrelle A et al (2000) Identification of a CD11b (+)/Gr-1 (+)/CD31 (+) myeloid progenitor capable of activating or suppressing CD8 (+) T cells. Blood 96:3838–3846

Bronte V, Serafini P, De Santo C et al (2003) IL-4-induced arginase 1 suppresses alloreactive T cells in tumor-bearing mice. J Immunol 170:270–278

Brosnan ME, Brosnan JT (2004) Renal arginine metabolism. J Nutr 134:2791S–2795S

Chang CI, Liao JC, Kuo L (2001) Macrophage arginase promotes tumor cell growth and suppresses nitric oxide-mediated tumor cytotoxicity. Cancer Res 61:1100–1106

Cheng P, Corzo CA, Luetteke N et al (2008) Inhibition of dendritic cell differentiation and accumulation of myeloid-derived suppressor cells in cancer is regulated by S100A9 protein. J Exp Med 205:2235–2249

Chicoine LG, Paffett ML, Young TL, Nelin LD (2004) Arginase inhibition increases nitric oxide production in bovine pulmonary arterial endothelial cells. Am J Physiol Lung Cell Mol Physiol 287:L60–L68

Closs EI, Simon A, Vekony N, Rotmann A (2004) Plasma membrane transporters for arginine. J Nutr 134:2752S–2759S

Corsi MM, Maes HH, Wasserman K, Fulgenzi A, Gaja G, Ferrero ME (1998) Protection by L-2-oxothiazolidine-4-carboxylic acid of hydrogen peroxide-induced CD3zeta and CD16zeta chain down-regulation in human peripheral blood lymphocytes and lymphokine-activated killer cells. Biochem Pharmacol 56:657–662

Cullen ME, Yuen AH, Felkin LE et al (2006) Myocardial expression of the arginine:glycine amidinotransferase gene is elevated in heart failure and normalized after recovery: potential implications for local creatine synthesis. Circulation 114:I16–I20

De SC, Serafini P, Marigo I et al (2005) Nitroaspirin corrects immune dysfunction in tumor-bearing hosts and promotes tumor eradication by cancer vaccination. Proc Natl Acad Sci U S A 102:4185–4190

Deignan JL, Livesay JC, Yoo PK et al (2006) Ornithine deficiency in the arginase double knockout mouse. Mol Genet Metab 89:87–96

Dolcetti L, Peranzoni E, Ugel S et al (2010) Hierarchy of immunosuppressive strength among myeloid-derived suppressor cell subsets is determined by GM-CSF. Eur J Immunol 40:22–35

Dong H, Zhu G, Tamada K, Chen L (1999) B7-H1, a third member of the B7 family, co-stimulates T-cell proliferation and interleukin-10 secretion. Nat Med 5:1365–1369

Finke JH, Zea AH, Stanley J et al (1993) Loss of T-cell receptor zeta chain and p56 lck in T-cells infiltrating human renal cell carcinoma. Cancer Res 53:5613–5616

Gabrilovich D (2004) Mechanisms and functional significance of tumour-induced dendritic-cell defects. Nat Rev Immunol 4:941–952

Gabrilovich D, Ishida T, Oyama T et al (1998) Vascular endothelial growth factor inhibits the development of dendritic cells and dramatically affects the differentiation of multiple hematopoietic lineages in vivo. Blood 92:4150–4166

Gabrilovich DI, Velders MP, Sotomayor EM, Kast WM (2001) Mechanism of immune dysfunction in cancer mediated by immature Gr-1+ myeloid cells. J Immunol 166:5398–5406

Gabrilovich DI, Bronte V, Chen SH et al (2007) The terminology issue for myeloid-derived suppressor cells. Cancer Res 67:425

Gallina G, Dolcetti L, Serafini P et al (2006) Tumors induce a subset of inflammatory monocytes with immunosuppressive activity on CD8+ T cells. J Clin Invest 116:2777–2790

Gattinoni L, Powell DJ Jr, Rosenberg SA, Restifo NP (2006) Adoptive immunotherapy for cancer: building on success. Nat Rev Immunol 6:383–393

Ghosh P, Sica A, Young HA et al (1994) Alterations in NF kappa B/Rel family proteins in splenic T-cells from tumor-bearing mice and reversal following therapy. Cancer Res 54:2969–2972

Hellstrom I, Sjogren HO, Warner G, Hellstrom KE (1971) Blocking of cell-mediated tumor immunity by sera from patients with growing neoplasms. Int J Cancer 7:226–237

Hellstrom KE, Hellstrom I, Nelson K (1983) Antigen-specific suppressor ("blocking") factors in tumor immunity. Biomembranes 11:365–388

Hesse M, Modolell M, La Flamme AC et al (2001) Differential regulation of nitric oxide synthase-2 and arginase-1 by type 1/type 2 cytokines in vivo: granulomatous pathology is shaped by the pattern of L-arginine metabolism. J Immunol 167:6533–6544

Hibbs JB Jr, Taintor RR, Vavrin Z (1987) Macrophage cytotoxicity: role for L-arginine deiminase and imino nitrogen oxidation to nitrite. Science 235:473–476

Holda JH, Maier T, Claman HN (1985) Murine graft-versus-host disease across minor barriers: immunosuppressive aspects of natural suppressor cells. Immunol Rev 88:87–105

Huang B, Pan PY, Li Q et al (2006) Gr-1+CD115+ immature myeloid suppressor cells mediate the development of tumor-induced T regulatory cells and T-cell anergy in tumor-bearing host. Cancer Res 66:1123–1131

Item CB, Stockler-Ipsiroglu S, Stromberger C et al (2001) Arginine:glycine amidinotransferase deficiency: the third inborn error of creatine metabolism in humans. Am J Hum Genet 69:1127–1133

Iyer RK, Yoo PK, Kern RM et al (2002) Mouse model for human arginase deficiency. Mol Cell Biol 22:4491–4498

Iyo AH, Zhu MY, Ordway GA, Regunathan S (2006) Expression of arginine decarboxylase in brain regions and neuronal cells. J Neurochem 96:1042–1050

Jacobsen LC, Theilgaard-Monch K, Christensen EI, Borregaard N (2007) Arginase 1 is expressed in myelocytes/metamyelocytes and localized in gelatinase granules of human neutrophils. Blood 109:3084–3087

Kato JY (1997) Control of G1 progression by D-type cyclins: key event for cell proliferation. Leukemia 11(Suppl 3):347–351

Kirk SJ, Regan MC, Wasserkrug HL, Sodeyama M, Barbul A (1992) Arginine enhances T-cell responses in athymic nude mice. JPEN J Parenter Enteral Nutr 16:429–432

Klausner RD, Lippincott-Schwartz J, Bonifacino JS (1990) The T cell antigen receptor: insights into organelle biology. Annu Rev Cell Biol 6:403–431

Kono K, Ressing ME, Brandt RM et al (1996a) Decreased expression of signal-transducing zeta chain in peripheral T cells and natural killer cells in patients with cervical cancer. Clin Cancer Res 2:1825–1828

Kono K, Salazar-Onfray F, Petersson M et al (1996b) Hydrogen peroxide secreted by tumor-derived macrophages down-modulates signal-transducing zeta molecules and inhibits tumor-specific T cell-and natural killer cell-mediated cytotoxicity. Eur J Immunol 26:1308–1313

Kropf P, Baud D, Marshall SE et al (2007) Arginase activity mediates reversible T cell hyporesponsiveness in human pregnancy. Eur J Immunol 37:935–945

Kryczek I, Wei S, Zou L et al (2006a) Cutting edge: induction of B7-H4 on APCs through IL-10: novel suppressive mode for regulatory T cells. J Immunol 177:40–44

Kryczek I, Zou L, Rodriguez P et al (2006b) B7-H4 expression identifies a novel suppressive macrophage population in human ovarian carcinoma. J Exp Med 203:871–881

Kusmartsev S, Gabrilovich DI (2005) STAT1 signaling regulates tumor-associated macrophage-mediated T cell deletion. J Immunol 174:4880–4891

Kusmartsev S, Cheng F, Yu B et al (2003) All-trans-retinoic acid eliminates immature myeloid cells from tumor-bearing mice and improves the effect of vaccination. Cancer Res 63:4441–4449

Kusmartsev S, Nefedova Y, Yoder D, Gabrilovich DI (2004) Antigen-specific inhibition of CD8+ T cell response by immature myeloid cells in cancer is mediated by reactive oxygen species. J Immunol 172:989–999

Kuss I, Saito T, Johnson JT, Whiteside TL (1999) Clinical significance of decreased zeta chain expression in peripheral blood lymphocytes of patients with head and neck cancer. Clin Cancer Res 5:329–334

Lee J, Ryu H, Ferrante RJ, Morris SM Jr, Ratan RR (2003) Translational control of inducible nitric oxide synthase expression by arginine can explain the arginine paradox. Proc Natl Acad Sci U S A 100:4843–4848

Li X, Liu J, Park JK et al (1994) T cells from renal cell carcinoma patients exhibit an abnormal pattern of kappa B-specific DNA-binding activity: a preliminary report. Cancer Res 54: 5424–5429

Makarenkova VP, Bansal V, Matta BM, Perez LA, Ochoa JB (2006) CD11b+/Gr-1+ myeloid suppressor cells cause T cell dysfunction after traumatic stress. J Immunol 176:2085–2094

McHugh RS, Shevach EM (2002) Cutting edge: depletion of CD4+CD25+ regulatory T cells is necessary, but not sufficient, for induction of organ-specific autoimmune disease. J Immunol 168:5979–5983

McHugh RS, Shevach EM, Margulies DH, Natarajan K (2001) A T cell receptor transgenic model of severe, spontaneous organ-specific autoimmunity. Eur J Immunol 31:2094–2103

Mellor AL, Munn DH (2004) IDO expression by dendritic cells: tolerance and tryptophan catabolism. Nat Rev Immunol 4:762–774

Miescher S, Whiteside TL, Carrel S, von FV (1986) Functional properties of tumor-infiltrating and blood lymphocytes in patients with solid tumors: effects of tumor cells and their supernatants on proliferative responses of lymphocytes. J Immunol 136:1899–1907

Miescher S, Stoeck M, Qiao L, Barras C, Barrelet L, von FV (1988) Preferential clonogenic deficit of CD8-positive T-lymphocytes infiltrating human solid tumors. Cancer Res 48:6992–6998

Mizoguchi H, O'Shea JJ, Longo DL, Loeffler CM, McVicar DW, Ochoa AC (1992) Alterations in signal transduction molecules in T lymphocytes from tumor-bearing mice. Science 258:1795–1798

Morris SM Jr (2002) Regulation of enzymes of the urea cycle and arginine metabolism. Annu Rev Nutr 22:87–105

Munder M, Eichmann K, Modolell M (1998) Alternative metabolic states in murine macrophages reflected by the nitric oxide synthase/arginase balance: competitive regulation by CD4+ T cells correlates with Th1/Th2 phenotype. J Immunol 160:5347–5354

Munder M, Eichmann K, Moran JM, Centeno F, Soler G, Modolell M (1999) Th1/Th2-regulated expression of arginase isoforms in murine macrophages and dendritic cells. J Immunol 163:3771–3777

Munder M, Mollinedo F, Calafat J et al (2005) Arginase I is constitutively expressed in human granulocytes and participates in fungicidal activity. Blood 105:2549–2556

Munder M, Schneider H, Luckner C et al (2006) Suppression of T-cell functions by human granulocyte arginase. Blood 108:1627–1634

Munn DH, Sharma MD, Baban B et al (2005) GCN2 kinase in T cells mediates proliferative arrest and anergy induction in response to indoleamine 2,3-dioxygenase. Immunity 22:633–642

Nagaraj S, Gupta K, Pisarev V et al (2007) Altered recognition of antigen is a mechanism of CD8+ T cell tolerance in cancer. Nat Med 13:828–835

Nieves C Jr, Langkamp-Henken B (2002) Arginine and immunity: a unique perspective. Biomed Pharmacother 56:471–482

Ochoa JB, Bernard AC, Mistry SK et al (2000) Trauma increases extrahepatic arginase activity. Surgery 127:419–426

Ochoa JB, Strange J, Kearney P, Gellin G, Endean E, Fitzpatrick E (2001) Effects of L-arginine on the proliferation of T lymphocyte subpopulations. JPEN J Parenter Enteral Nutr 25:23–29

Ohm JE, Carbone DP (2001) VEGF as a mediator of tumor-associated immunodeficiency. Immunol Res 23:263–272

Otsuji M, Kimura Y, Aoe T, Okamoto Y, Saito T (1996) Oxidative stress by tumor-derived macrophages suppresses the expression of CD3 zeta chain of T-cell receptor complex and antigen-specific T-cell responses. Proc Natl Acad Sci U S A 93:13119–13124

Oyama T, Ran S, Ishida T et al (1998) Vascular endothelial growth factor affects dendritic cell maturation through the inhibition of nuclear factor-kappa B activation in hemopoietic progenitor cells. J Immunol 160:1224–1232

Pan PY, Wang GX, Yin B et al (2008) Reversion of immune tolerance in advanced malignancy: modulation of myeloid derived suppressor cell development by blockade of SCF function. Blood 111:219–228

Pekarek LA, Starr BA, Toledano AY, Schreiber H (1995) Inhibition of tumor growth by elimination of granulocytes. J Exp Med 181:435–440

Rabinovich GA, Gabrilovich D, Sotomayor EM (2007) Immunosuppressive strategies that are mediated by tumor cells. Annu Rev Immunol 25:267–296

Rabinowich H, Reichert TE, Kashii Y, Gastman BR, Bell MC, Whiteside TL (1998) Lymphocyte apoptosis induced by Fas- ligand expressing ovarian carcinoma cells. Implications for altered expression of T cell receptor in tumor-associated lymphocytes. J Clin Invest 101:2579–2588

Rodgers S, Rees RC, Hancock BW (1994) Changes in the phenotypic characteristics of eosinophils from patients receiving recombinant human interleukin-2 (rhIL-2) therapy. Br J Haematol 86:746–753

Rodriguez PC, Zea AH, Culotta KS, Zabaleta J, Ochoa JB, Ochoa AC (2002) Regulation of T cell receptor CD3 zeta chain expression by L-arginine. J Biol Chem 277:21123–21129

Rodriguez PC, Zea AH, DeSalvo J et al (2003) L-arginine consumption by macrophages modulates the expression of CD3zeta chain in T lymphocytes. J Immunol 171:1232–1239

Rodriguez PC, Quiceno DG, Zabaleta J et al (2004) Arginase I production in the tumor microenvironment by mature myeloid cells inhibits T-cell receptor expression and antigen-specific T-cell responses. Cancer Res 64:5839–5849

Rodriguez PC, Hernandez CP, Quiceno D et al (2005) Arginase I in myeloid suppressor cells is induced by COX-2 in lung carcinoma. J Exp Med 202:931–939

Rodriguez PC, Quiceno DG, Ochoa AC (2007) L-arginine availability regulates T-lymphocyte cell-cycle progression. Blood 109:1568–1573

Rodriguez PC, Ernstoff MS, Hernandez C et al (2009) Arginase I-producing myeloid-derived suppressor cells in renal cell carcinoma are a subpopulation of activated granulocytes. Cancer Res 69:1553–1560

Rotondo R, Barisione G, Mastracci L et al (2009) IL-8 induces exocytosis of arginase 1 by neutrophil polymorphonuclears in nonsmall cell lung cancer. Int J Cancer 125:887–893

Rutschman R, Lang R, Hesse M, Ihle JN, Wynn TA, Murray PJ (2001) Cutting edge: Stat6-dependent substrate depletion regulates nitric oxide production. J Immunol 166:2173–2177

Santhanam L, Lim HK, Lim HK et al (2007) Inducible NO synthase dependent S-nitrosylation and activation of arginase1 contribute to age-related endothelial dysfunction. Circ Res 101:692–702

Schmielau J, Finn OJ (2001) Activated granulocytes and granulocyte-derived hydrogen peroxide are the underlying mechanism of suppression of T-cell function in advanced cancer patients. Cancer Res 61:4756–4760

Semenza GL (2003) Targeting HIF-1 for cancer therapy. Nat Rev Cancer 3:721–732

Serafini P, Meckel K, Kelso M et al (2006) Phosphodiesterase-5 inhibition augments endogenous antitumor immunity by reducing myeloid-derived suppressor cell function. J Exp Med 203:2691–2702

Seung LP, Rowley DA, Dubey P, Schreiber H (1995) Synergy between T-cell immunity and inhibition of paracrine stimulation causes tumor rejection. Proc Natl Acad Sci U S A 92:6254–6258

Sica A, Bronte V (2007) Altered macrophage differentiation and immune dysfunction in tumor development. J Clin Invest 117:1155–1166

Sicinska E, Aifantis I, Le CL et al (2003) Requirement for cyclin D3 in lymphocyte development and T cell leukemias. Cancer Cell 4:451–461

Singh R, Pervin S, Karimi A, Cederbaum S, Chaudhuri G (2000) Arginase activity in human breast cancer cell lines: N (omega)-hydroxy-L-arginine selectively inhibits cell proliferation and induces apoptosis in MDA-MB-468 cells. Cancer Res 60:3305–3312

Sinha P, Clements VK, Ostrand-Rosenberg S (2005a) Reduction of myeloid-derived suppressor cells and induction of M1 macrophages facilitate the rejection of established metastatic disease. J Immunol 174:636–645

Sinha P, Clements VK, Ostrand-Rosenberg S (2005b) Interleukin-13-regulated M2 macrophages in combination with myeloid suppressor cells block immune surveillance against metastasis. Cancer Res 65:11743–11751

Sinha P, Clements VK, Fulton AM, Ostrand-Rosenberg S (2007) Prostaglandin E2 promotes tumor progression by inducing myeloid-derived suppressor cells. Cancer Res 67:4507–4513

Solheim JC, Reber AJ, Ashour AE et al (2007) Spleen but not tumor infiltration by dendritic and T cells is increased by intravenous adenovirus-Flt3 ligand injection. Cancer Gene Ther 14:364–371

Stevenson FK (2005) Update on cancer vaccines. Curr Opin Oncol 17:573–577

Suer GS, Yoruk Y, Cakir E, Yorulmaz F, Gulen S (1999) Arginase and ornithine, as markers in human non-small cell lung carcinoma. Cancer Biochem Biophys 17:125–131

Taheri F, Ochoa JB, Faghiri Z et al (2001) L-Arginine regulates the expression of the T-cell receptor zeta chain (CD3zeta) in Jurkat cells. Clin Cancer Res 7:958S–965S

Talmadge JE, Hood KC, Zobel LC, Shafer LR, Coles M, Toth B (2007) Chemoprevention by cyclooxygenase-2 inhibition reduces immature myeloid suppressor cell expansion. Int Immunopharmacol 7:140–151

Uzzo RG, Rayman P, Kolenko V et al (1999) Mechanisms of apoptosis in T cells from patients with renal cell carcinoma. Clin Cancer Res 5:1219–1229

Van Ginderachter JA, Meerschaut S, Liu Y et al (2006) Peroxisome proliferator-activated receptor gamma (PPARgamma) ligands reverse CTL suppression by alternatively activated (M2) macrophages in cancer. Blood 108:525–535

Varesio L, Giovarelli M, Landolfo S, Forni G (1979) Suppression of proliferative response and lymphokine production during the progression of a spontaneous tumor. Cancer Res 39:4983–4988

Whiteside TL, Rabinowich H (1998) The role of Fas/FasL in immunosuppression induced by human tumors. Cancer Immunol Immunother 46:175–184

Whiteside TL, Miescher S, Moretta L, von FV (1988) Cloning and proliferating precursor frequencies of tumor-infiltrating lymphocytes from human solid tumors. Transplant Proc 20:342–343

Yaman I, Fernandez J, Sarkar B et al (2002) Nutritional control of mRNA stability is mediated by a conserved AU-rich element that binds the cytoplasmic shuttling protein HuR. J Biol Chem 277:41539–41546

Youn JI, Nagaraj S, Collazo M, Gabrilovich DI (2008) Subsets of myeloid-derived suppressor cells in tumor-bearing mice. J Immunol 181:5791–5802

Young MR, Newby M, Wepsic HT (1987) Hematopoiesis and suppressor bone marrow cells in mice bearing large metastatic Lewis lung carcinoma tumors. Cancer Res 47:100–105

Zarour H, De SC, Lehmann F et al (1996) The majority of autologous cytolytic T-lymphocyte clones derived from peripheral blood lymphocytes of a melanoma patient recognize an antigenic peptide derived from gene Pmel17/gp100. J Invest Dermatol 107:63–67

Zea AH, Curti BD, Longo DL et al (1995) Alterations in T cell receptor and signal transduction molecules in melanoma patients. Clin Cancer Res 1:1327–1335

Zea AH, Ochoa MT, Ghosh P et al (1998) Changes in expression of signal transduction proteins in T lymphocytes of patients with leprosy. Infect Immun 66:499–504

Zea AH, Rodriguez PC, Culotta KS et al (2004) l-Arginine modulates CD3zeta expression and T cell function in activated human T lymphocytes. Cell Immunol 232:21–31

Zea AH, Rodriguez PC, Atkins MB et al (2005) Arginase-producing myeloid suppressor cells in renal cell carcinoma patients: a mechanism of tumor evasion. Cancer Res 65:3044–3048

Zea AH, Culotta KS, Ali J et al (2006) Decreased expression of CD3zeta and nuclear transcription factor kappa B in patients with pulmonary tuberculosis: potential mechanisms and reversibility with treatment. J Infect Dis 194:1385–1393

Zhang C, Hein TW, Wang W et al (2004) Upregulation of vascular arginase in hypertension decreases nitric oxide-mediated dilation of coronary arterioles. Hypertension 44:935–943

Zhu MY, Iyo A, Piletz JE, Regunathan S (2004) Expression of human arginine decarboxylase, the biosynthetic enzyme for agmatine. Biochim Biophys Acta 1670:156–164

Chapter 19
Human Tumor Antigens Recognized by T Cells and Their Implications for Cancer Immunotherapy

Ryo Ueda, Tomonori Yaguchi, and Yutaka Kawakami

1 Introduction

Recent clinical trials of immunotherapies indicate that tumor reactive autologous T cells are able to regress even advanced, large tumors in melanoma patients. For example, the adoptive transfer of CD8+ cytotoxic T lymphocytes (CTL) specifically targeted for identified tumor antigens following lymphodepletive treatment, such as fludarabine/cyclophosphamide administration and total body irradiation, led to objective tumor responses in more than 70% of patients with melanoma (Dudley et al. 2008). Immunological analyses on these tumor tissues demonstrated that administered T cells may eliminate tumor cells through direct killing and cytokine secretion. Therefore, CD8+ CTLs that recognize MHC class I positive cancer cells are important for in vivo tumor rejection. In addition, CD4+ helper T (Th) cells may also play a role in the induction and maintenance of final effectors including CD8+ T cells and macrophages, the accumulation of CD8+ T cells in tumor tissues, as well as the direct recognition of MHC class II positive malignant cells including most hematological malignancies. Thus, the identification of human tumor antigens recognized by CD8+ and CD4+ T cells is important for the assessment/quantification of in vivo anti-tumor T cell responses and the development of effective immunotherapies. A variety of human tumor antigens recognized by T cells, and their T cell epitopes, have been identified recently using various isolation methods. These studies have led to the understanding of molecular mechanisms underlying human cancer cell recognition by T cells, and to the development of novel immunotherapies (Kawakami et al. 2004). In this chapter, recent progress in human tumor antigen identification and its implication for immunotherapy will be discussed.

R. Ueda • T. Yaguchi • Y. Kawakami (✉)
Division of Cellular Signaling, Institute for Advanced Medical Research, Keio University School of Medicine, 35 Shinanomachi Shinjuku-ku, Tokyo 160-8582, Japan
e-mail: yutakawa@sc.itc.keio.ac.jp

2 Methods for the Identification of Human Tumor Antigens Recognized by T Cells

Human melanoma antigens recognized by T cells were first isolated by expression DNA cloning using tumor reactive T cells, and T cell epitopes were identified by narrowing down the DNA sequences encoding the epitopes (van der Bruggen et al. 1991; Kawakami et al. 1994a). T cell epitope peptides could also be identified directly using mass spectrometry (Cox et al. 1994). However, it is difficult to generate tumor reactive T cells against various cancers other than melanoma. Thus, various strategies not requiring tumor reactive T cells from patients have been attempted. One technique called SEREX (serological analysis of recombinant cDNA expression libraries) involves cDNA expression cloning using serum IgG from cancer patients (Kiniwa et al. 2001). IgG Ab induction indicates that $CD4^+$ helper T cells specific for the target antigens are activated in these patients. In fact, these antigens can induce not only $CD4^+$ helper T cells, but also $CD8^+$ CTL in vitro from PBMC of cancer patients or healthy individuals (Jager et al. 2000) (Reverse immunology). Candidates for T cell antigens such as tissue-specific antigens, cancer-testis antigens, and overexpressed antigens, can also be systematically identified using various genetic analyses, including various cDNA subtraction methods comparing normal tissues and cancer cells, such as classical cDNA subtraction, representational differential analysis (RDA), and differential PCR display. Other methods may involve the comparison of cDNA profiles obtained by SAGE (serial analysis of gene expression), DNA microarray analysis, and EST databases (Brinkmann et al. 1999; Hayashi et al. 2007; Matsuzaki et al. 2005; Goto et al. 2006). Allogeneic antigens such as minor histocompatibility antigen (mHa) may be identified through single nucleotide polymorphism (SNP) searches. Using these techniques, we have identified a variety of human tumor antigens and made catalogs of tumor antigens for various human cancers, which led to the development of novel immunotherapies. The identification of T epitopes revealed the molecular mechanisms by which T cells recognize human cancer cells.

3 The Mechanisms for T Cell Recognition of Human Cancer Cells

The identification of human tumor antigens helped elucidate the events leading to T cell recognition of human cancer cells, including mechanisms for T cell epitope generation (Table 19.1). T cells against tumor-specific mutated peptides (e.g., point mutations, frameshift mutations, and translocations), tissue-specific proteins (e.g., cryptic epitope of self-proteins), overexpressed proteins, and proteins preferentially expressed in germline cells such as testis cells (cancer-testis antigens, cancer-germline antigens, typically expressed by DNA demethylation) were found to be elicited in cancer patients. The identification of T cell epitope peptides also revealed

Table 19.1 Examples of the representative human tumor antigens recognized by T cells

Group	Antigen	Cancer
Mutated peptides	β-Catenin/CDK4	Melanoma
	bcr-abl	CML, ALL
Tissue-specific proteins	gp100/MART-1/melanA	Melanoma
	PSA	Prostate cancer
	Proteinase3	Myelogenous leukemia
Cancer-Testis antigens	MAGE-A3/NY-ESO-1	Various cancers
Oncogenic proteins	WT1/Survivin/hTERT	Various cancers
Oncofetal antigens	CEA/AFP	Colon cancer, hepatoma
Viral proteins	EBV-EBNA	B cell lymphoma
	HPV16-E7	Cervical cancer
Mucin	MUC-1	Breast, ovarian, pancreas cancers
Idiotype	antibody	B cell lymphoma, myeloma
Allogeneic antigen (mHa)	HA1	Various leukemia/lymphoma
Cancer stem cell antigens	SOX2/SOX6	Breast cancer, myeloma, glioma

Table 19.2 Mechanisms for generating T cell epitopes on human cancer cells

Mechanism	Tumor antigens
1. Translation of functional genes	
a. Tissue-specific proteins	Melanosomal proteins (e.g., gp100)
Cryptic epitopes	MART-1, gp100, neo-PAP, CDC27
b. Cancer-testis antigens	MAGEs, NY-ESO-1, CRT2, SOX6
c. Overexpressed antigens	Her2, WT1, Survivin, hTERT
2. Genetic alterations	
a. Pin-point mutation	BRAF, p53, K-ras, MUM-1/2
Acquired MHC binding	β-Catenin, CDK4, MART-2, MUM-3
Extended peptide	Caspase-8
b. Frameshift mutations	$p14^{ARF}$, $p16^{INKa}$, TGFbRII
c. Translocation	bcr-abl, SYT-SSX
3. Translation of alternative ORFs	TRP-1, NY-ESO-1
4. Translation of introns	
a. Incomplete splicing	gp100, TRP-2, MUM-1
b. Cryptic promoter	GnT-V
5. Post-translational modification	
a. Deamidation	Tyrosinase
b. Cysteine oxidation	Tyrosinase
c. Protein splicing	FGF5, gp100
6. Differential processing by proteasomes	MART-1, gp100, MAGE-A1/A3

the causes of low immunogenic responses to tumor antigens, including low HLA binding and low cleavage activity in professional antigen presenting cells (APCs).

In addition, we and others revealed many surprising mechanisms for T cell recognition of human cancer cells (Table 19.2). T cell epitope peptides may be derived from introns (e.g., due to incomplete mRNA splicing or cryptic promoter activation), alternative open reading frames (ORFs), or peptides with post-translational modifications such as protein splicing, deamidation, and cysteine oxidation. Differential cleavage of T cell epiotopes, by constitutive proteasomes expressed in cancer cells and by immunoproteasomes expressed in professional APCs such as dendritic cells, leads to the differential expression of T cell epitopes between cancer cells and professional APCs. This observation has important implications for clinical applications of tumor antigens. For instance, minimal peptide should be utilized for the immunization of some antigens, instead of whole antigens which require processing within APCs.

4 Implications of the Identified Human Tumor Antigens for the Development of Immunotherapies

The identification of tumor antigens allows for immunizations that can be appropriately controlled for the maximal induction of anti-tumor immune responses by adjusting the amount of administered antigen, immunization methods, and the schedule of administration. In addition, we can modify antigens to increase immunogenicity of the intrinsically low immunogenic tumor antigens (Parkhurst et al. 1996; Rosenberg et al. 1998). We and others have discovered that the induction of immune responses to multiple endogenous tumor antigens may be important for in vivo tumor rejection. Methods which can efficiently induce antigen spreading to endogenous tumer antigen; such as the use of highly immunogenic antigens in combination with appropriate *in situ* tumor destruction to release endogenous tumor antigens in an immunoge manner (Toda et al. 2002; Udagawa et al. 2006), should be developed. One recent technological advancement involves the adoptive transfer of peripheral blood T cells that were retrovirally transduced with T cell receptor (TCR) genes specific for identified tumor antigens including MART-1, gp100, and NY-ESO-1 melanoma antigens (Morgan et al. 2006; Johnson et al. 2009). The adoptive immunotherapy with TCR-transduced T cells has resulted in melanoma regression, suggesting that similar immunotherapy may be developed for patients with other common cancers such as lung cancer, for which the generation of large amounts of anti-tumor T cells is difficult.

In addition to the potential use of tumor antigens as targets for immunotherapy, it is worth emphasizing that the identification of tumor antigens allowed us to assess immune responses in patients both quantitatively and qualitatively during immunotherapy using various methods including ELISPOT, HLA tetramer analysis, and DTH skin tests (Romero et al. 1998). In particular, HLA tetramer analysis allowed for quantitative and qualitative evaluation of the in vivo immune status of tumor-specific T cells by assessing their phenotype (naïve/memory/effector), expression of adhesion/co-stimulatory molecules, production of cytokines and cytotoxic molecules, and anergy status (Lee et al. 1999). Qualitative analysis of T cells in vivo helped us gain a better understanding of anti-tumor immune responses in patients and of tumor escape mechanisms such as tolerance induction, thus leading to improvements in immunotherapy. The identification of tumor antigens or their immune responses (e.g., tumor antigen-specific IgG in serum) may also be useful as diagnostic biomarkers. They may also be targets for molecular targeting therapies.

Criteria for ideal tumor antigens to develop effective immunotherapy may include (1) high expression in all tumor cells including cancer stem cells (CSC) (no relapse cure), (2) limited expression in normal cells as antigens presented on cell surface by MHCs (no autoimmunity problems), (3) common expression in many patients' cancers (treatment applicable for many patients), (4) high immunogenicity in cancer patients (efficient induction of anti-tumor immune responses), and (5) involvement in tumor cell proliferation and survival (less likely occurrence of antigen loss variants). Although antigens completely satisfying all of these criteria may not be available, the characteristics of representative human tumor antigens have been described using these criteria (Table 19.3).

4.1 Tumor-Specific Antigens Derived from Genetic Alterations in Tumor Cells

Autologous tumor-specific peptides derived from genetic alterations in cancer cells, which are involved in cancer development, are often isolated using T cells and IgG Ab from patients with good prognosis after treatment. For example, we isolated mutated peptides of β-catenin (Robbins et al. 1996) and Ski acyltransferase (MART-2) (Kawakami et al. 2001), using melanoma-reactive T cells derived from tumor infiltrating lymphocytes (TIL). The administration of these peptides along with high doses of IL-2 resulted in tumor regression. An amino acid change from serine to phenylalanine as a result of the β-catenin mutation disrupted a phosphorylation site, resulting in increased β-catenin levels through the prevention of subsequent degradation by proteasomes. Elevated β-catenin levels may be involved in the formation of malignant melanoma phenotypes (Rubinfeld et al. 1997). Mutations in MART-2, which adds palmitate to the N-terminus of the Hedgehog protein, appear to have caused the enzyme to lose GTP binding activity, although MART-2 association with tumorigenesis was not clear (Kawakami et al. 2001; Chamoun et al. 2001). These mutations led to the generation of tumor-specific peptides capable of binding to the patients' HLA. Then, these peptides induced anti-tumor T cell responses. This sequence of events appears to be one of the common mechanisms for the recognition of mutated peptides by autologous T cells, as the same mechanism was found in other tumor antigens such as CDK4 and MUM3 (Kawakami et al. 2005).

We have also isolated a tumor-specific frameshift CDX2 peptide as a colon cancer antigen from a HNPCC patient who had microsatellite instability (MSI) and colon cancer with abundant CD8[+] T cell infiltration, and a good prognosis after surgical resection (Ishikawa et al. 2003). This type of colon cancer has unique clinicopathological features, including T cell infiltration, particularly by CD8[+] T cells, and relatively good prognosis after treatment despite pathologically malignant undifferentiated type. These observations may indicate that T cell responses to

Table 19.3 Clinical implications of the representative tumor antigens recognized by T cells

Antigens	Expression in		Immunogenicity	Occurrence of antigen loss variants	Autoimmune reaction
	Normal tissues	Cancers			
Tumor-specific unique antigens	None	Relatively homogenous	Intermediate	Low when involved in tumor cell proliferation/survival	None
Tissue-specific antigens	Expressed at low densities on cell surfaces		Intermediate	Relatively high	Relatively high
Cancer-testis antigens	Limited to testis and placenta	Relatively heterogeneous	Intermediate	Low when involved in tumor cell proliferation/survival	Low
Allogeneic antigens	Expressed at high densities on cell surfaces		High	Depending on antigens	GVHD

These characteristics are different among the antigens even in the same category groups frameshift peptides may contribute to the maintenance of a tumor-free status after treatment. Tumor-specific mutated antigens have also been reported in other cancers, including mutated Caspase-8 with reduced apoptotic activity in head and neck cancer, and bcr-abl oncogenic fusion peptides via translocation in leukemia.

One problem in immunotherapy is the appearance of tumor antigen loss variants sometimes observed in immunotherapy against tissue-specific antigens such as MART-1 and gp100, which are not required for cancer cell survival and proliferation. We have previously shown, using lentiviral siRNA, that mutations in BRAF (V600E) frequently detected in superficial spreading melanoma (SSM) are responsible for the augmented proliferation and invasion of melanoma cells. We could also detect serum IgG for BRAF in some melanoma patients (Sumimoto et al. 2004). Recognition of the mutated peptides by CD8$^+$ CTL and CD4$^+$ helper T cells has been reported (Sharkey et al. 2004; Somasundaram et al. 2006). These tumor-specific antigens involved in the proliferation or survival of cancer cells are attractive targets for immunotherapy, because cancer cells are less likely to lose these antigens. In addition, possible early occurrence of BRAF mutation in melanoma development (presence of mutated BRAF in benign nevi) may also suggest that mutated BRAF are present in melanoma stem cells. Since it is difficult to identify these common mutated antigens, most of which are quite unique to each patient, it may be necessary to develop immunization methods that induce T cells to such endogenous mutated antigens without the need for antigen identification. For example, we have previously reported a technique involving the administration of intratumoral dendritic cells following cryoablative tumor treatment (Udagawa et al. 2006).

4.2 Tissue-Specific Antigens

T cells specific for self peptide antigens derived from tissue-specific antigens, including MART-1, gp100, tyrosinase, TRP1, and TRP2, are frequently detected in melanoma patients (Kawakami et al. 1994a, 1995). Various observations, including the antigens' low HLA binding and the presence of high avidity naïve T cells in healthy individuals, suggest that these peptides are relatively cryptic epitopes that are not presented at high densities on the cell surfaces of melanocytes and professional APCs in healthy individuals (Kawakami and Rosenberg 1996). However, these T cells may be easily induced in patients with memory T cells primed with increased antigens from melanoma cells by immune augmentation methods, e.g., IL-2 administration. One of the mechanisms for the cryptic nature of some epitopes and their low immunogenicity is relatively low HLA binding ability due to misplaced amino acids at critical anchor regions for HLA-peptide binding (typically the second and last portions of the peptides) (Kawakami et al. 1995, 1994b). We have succeeded in generating highly immunogenic peptides by substituting the appropriate amino acids (Parkhurst et al. 1996), and the generated, modified peptides induced anti-tumor immune responses more effectively than the native peptides in vivo (Rosenberg et al. 1998). In other cancers, similar tissue-specific antigens have been identified, including PSA in prostate cancer and Proteinase 3 in myelogenous leukemia. Although these shared antigens are useful for the treatment of many patients, relatively low immunogenicity, possible autoimmune reactions, and the occurrence of antigen loss variants may be problematic for effective immunotherapy.

4.3 Cancer-Testis Antigens

Self peptides derived from cancer-testis (CT) antigens are tumor-specific shared tumor antigens and attractive targets for immunotherapy, because their expression is observed in various cancers and limited to a few cell types in normal tissue, e.g., immunoprivileged testis cells with low HLA expression. Recently, MAGEA3 (Atanackovic et al. 2008) and NY-ESO-1 (Hunder et al. 2008) were extensively studied and some positive results were obtained in a number of clinical trials. Using various methods, including SEREX with testis cDNA library screening, genechip, and RDA analysis comparing testis cDNA profiles, we have identified various CT antigens such as CAGE (Iwata et al. 2005), KU-TES1 (Okada et al. 2006), BORIS, CRT2 (Hayashi et al. 2007), and SOX6 (Ueda et al. 2004), which are recognized by IgG and/or CD8$^+$ CTLs.

SOX6 is an attractive antigen because it may be expressed in glioma stem cells (Ueda et al. 2009). CSC have recently been actively investigated as targets for treatment because of their high tumor initiating ability with resistance to chemotherapy and radiotherapy, thus leading to cancer relapse. SOX6 expression is developmentally regulated and its high expression in the adult was restricted to the testis and glioma tissues (Ueda et al. 2004). SOX6 was expressed in glioma stem cell-like cell lines obtained by the sphere forming method and CD133$^+$ phenotyping, and the giloma stem cell-like cells were lysed by SOX6-specific CTLs (Ueda et al. 2009). Thus, SOX6 may be a useful antigen for the development of immunotherapy for the treatment of glioma.

4.4 Allogeneic Antigens

In some circumstances, including allogeneic stem cell transplantations and donor leukocyte infusions (DLI), allogeneic antigens such as minor histocompatibility antigens (mHa) and mismatched MHCs can be tumor antigens for immunotherapy. Donor-derived T cells specific for recipient allogeneic antigens administered to recipient patients could eliminate residual leukemia cells. Compared to the autologous tumor antigens discussed above, the allogeneic antigens are highly immunogenic and are expressed at high densities on cell surfaces, indicating their strong anti-tumor activity. However, to avoid life-threatening graft-versus-host disease (GVHD) caused by the allogeneic immune responses to the recipient's normal tissues, additional strategies are required. We have demonstrated the presence of cytotoxic CD4⁺ T cells specific for mismatch HLA-DQ and mHa, which are preferentially expressed in hematopoietic cells including leukemia cells (Matsushita et al. 2006). These CD4⁺ T cells may induce strong graft vs. leukemia (GVL) effects on the residual MHC class II positive leukemia cells without developing severe GVHD.

5 Concluding Remarks

The identification of human tumor antigens by T cells allowed us to not only develop novel cancer immunotherapies, but also evaluate anti-tumor T cell responses in patients and clarify the problems underlying each step that leads to in vivo immunological tumor rejection. Although simple tumor antigen immunizations along with adjuvants and cytokines showed only limited anti-tumor activity, comprehensive immunotherapy combining various immune-augmenting interventions and methods to correct the immunosuppressive environment in cancer patients may result in the improvement of current immunotherapies.

Acknowledgments A part of this work was supported by grants from the Ministry of Education, Science, and Culture, the Ministry of Health and Welfare, and Keio University.

References

Atanackovic D, Altorki NK, Cao Y, Ritter E, Ferrara CA, Ritter G et al (2008) Booster vaccination of cancer patients with MAGE-A3 protein reveals long-term immunological memory or tolerance depending on priming. Proc Natl Acad Sci USA 105:1650–1655

Brinkmann U, Vasmatzis G, Lee B, Pastan I (1999) Novel genes in the PAGE and GAGE family of tumor antigens found by homology walking in the dbEST database. Cancer Res 59: 1445–1448

Chamoun Z, Mann RK, Nellen D, von Kessler DP, Bellotto M, Beachy PA et al (2001) Skinny hedgehog, an acyltransferase required for palmitoylation and activity of the hedgehog signal. Science 293:2080–2084

Cox AL, Skipper J, Chen Y, Henderson RA, Darrow TL, Shabanowitz J et al (1994) Identification of a peptide recognized by five melanoma-specific human cytotoxic T cell lines. Science 264: 716–719

Dudley ME, Yang JC, Sherry R, Hughes MS, Royal R, Kammula U et al (2008) Adoptive cell therapy for patients with metastatic melanoma: evaluation of intensive myeloablative chemoradiation preparative regimens. J Clin Oncol 26:5233–5239

Goto Y, Matsuzaki Y, Kurihara S, Shimizu A, Okada T, Yamamoto K et al (2006) A new melanoma antigen fatty acid-binding protein 7, involved in proliferation and invasion, is a potential target for immunotherapy and molecular target therapy. Cancer Res 66:4443–4449

Hayashi E, Matsuzaki Y, Hasegawa G, Yaguchi T, Kurihara S, Fujita T et al (2007) Identification of a novel cancer-testis antigen CRT2 frequently expressed in various cancers using representational differential analysis. Clin Cancer Res 13:6267–6274

Hunder NN, Wallen H, Cao J, Hendricks DW, Reilly JZ, Rodmyre R et al (2008) Treatment of metastatic melanoma with autologous CD4+ T cells against NY-ESO-1. N Engl J Med 358: 2698–2703

Ishikawa T, Fujita T, Suzuki Y, Okabe S, Yuasa Y, Iwai T et al (2003) Tumor-specific immunological recognition of frameshift-mutated peptides in colon cancer with microsatellite instability. Cancer Res 63:5564–5572

Iwata T, Fujita T, Hirao N, Matsuzaki Y, Okada T, Mochimaru H et al (2005) Frequent immune responses to a cancer/testis antigen, CAGE, in patients with microsatellite instability-positive endometrial cancer. Clin Cancer Res 11:3949–3957

Jager E, Nagata Y, Gnjatic S, Wada H, Stockert E, Karbach J et al (2000) Monitoring CD8 T cell responses to NY-ESO-1: correlation of humoral and cellular immune responses. Proc Natl Acad Sci USA 97:4760–4765

Johnson LA, Morgan RA, Dudley ME, Cassard L, Yang JC, Hughes MS et al (2009) Gene therapy with human and mouse T-cell receptors mediates cancer regression and targets normal tissues expressing cognate antigen. Blood 114:535–546

Kawakami Y, Rosenberg SA (1996) T-cell recognition of self peptides as tumor rejection antigens. Immunol Res 15:179–190

Kawakami Y, Eliyahu S, Delgado CH, Robbins PF, Rivoltini L, Topalian SL et al (1994a) Cloning of the gene coding for a shared human melanoma antigen recognized by autologous T cells infiltrating into tumor. Proc Natl Acad Sci USA 91:3515–3519

Kawakami Y, Eliyahu S, Sakaguchi K, Robbins PF, Rivoltini L, Yannelli JR et al (1994b) Identification of the immunodominant peptides of the MART-1 human melanoma antigen recognized by the majority of HLA-A2-restricted tumor infiltrating lymphocytes. J Exp Med 180:347–352

Kawakami Y, Eliyahu S, Jennings C, Sakaguchi K, Kang X, Southwood S et al (1995) Recognition of multiple epitopes in the human melanoma antigen gp100 by tumor-infiltrating T lymphocytes associated with in vivo tumor regression. J Immunol 154:3961–3968

Kawakami Y, Wang X, Shofuda T, Sumimoto H, Tupesis J, Fitzgerald E et al (2001) Isolation of a new melanoma antigen, MART-2, containing a mutated epitope recognized by autologous tumor-infiltrating T lymphocytes. J Immunol 166:2871–2877

Kawakami Y, Fujita T, Matsuzaki Y, Sakurai T, Tsukamoto M, Toda M et al (2004) Identification of human tumor antigens and its implications for diagnosis and treatment of cancer. Cancer Sci 95:784–791

Kawakami Y, Sumimoto H, Fujita T, Matsuzaki Y (2005) Immunological detection of altered signaling molecules involved in melanoma development. Cancer Metastasis Rev 24:357–366

Kiniwa Y, Fujita T, Akada M, Ito K, Shofuda T, Suzuki Y et al (2001) Tumor antigens isolated from a patient with vitiligo and T-cell-infiltrated melanoma. Cancer Res 61:7900–7907

Lee PP, Yee C, Savage PA, Fong L, Brockstedt D, Weber JS et al (1999) Characterization of circulating T cells specific for tumor-associated antigens in melanoma patients. Nat Med 5:677–685

Matsushita M, Yamazaki R, Ikeda H, Mori T, Sumimoto H, Fujita T et al (2006) Possible involvement of allogeneic antigens recognised by donor-derived CD4 cytotoxic T cells in selective GVL effects after stem cell transplantation of patients with haematological malignancy. Br J Haematol 132:56–65

Matsuzaki Y, Hashimoto S, Fujita T, Suzuki T, Sakurai T, Matsushima K et al (2005) Systematic identification of human melanoma antigens using serial analysis of gene expression (SAGE). J Immunother 28:10–19

Morgan RA, Dudley ME, Wunderlich JR, Hughes MS, Yang JC, Sherry RM et al (2006) Cancer regression in patients after transfer of genetically engineered lymphocytes. Science 314:126–129

Okada T, Akada M, Fujita T, Iwata T, Goto Y, Kido K et al (2006) A novel cancer testis antigen that is frequently expressed in pancreatic, lung, and endometrial cancers. Clin Cancer Res 12:191–197

Parkhurst MR, Salgaller ML, Southwood S, Robbins PF, Sette A, Rosenberg SA et al (1996) Improved induction of melanoma-reactive CTL with peptides from the melanoma antigen gp100 modified at HLA-A*0201-binding residues. J Immunol 157:2539–2548

Robbins PF, El-Gamil M, Li YF, Kawakami Y, Loftus D, Appella E et al (1996) A mutated beta-catenin gene encodes a melanoma-specific antigen recognized by tumor infiltrating lymphocytes. J Exp Med 183:1185–1192

Romero P, Cerottini JC, Waanders GA (1998) Novel methods to monitor antigen-specific cytotoxic T-cell responses in cancer immunotherapy. Mol Med Today 4:305–312

Rosenberg SA, Yang JC, Schwartzentruber DJ, Hwu P, Marincola FM, Topalian SL et al (1998) Immunologic and therapeutic evaluation of a synthetic peptide vaccine for the treatment of patients with metastatic melanoma. Nat Med 4:321–327

Rubinfeld B, Robbins P, El-Gamil M, Albert I, Porfiri E, Polakis P (1997) Stabilization of beta-catenin by genetic defects in melanoma cell lines. Science 275:1790–1792

Sharkey MS, Lizee G, Gonzales MI, Patel S, Topalian SL (2004) CD4(+) T-cell recognition of mutated B-RAF in melanoma patients harboring the V599E mutation. Cancer Res 64:1595–1599

Somasundaram R, Swoboda R, Caputo L, Otvos L, Weber B, Volpe P et al (2006) Human leukocyte antigen-A2-restricted CTL responses to mutated BRAF peptides in melanoma patients. Cancer Res 66:3287–3293

Sumimoto H, Miyagishi M, Miyoshi H, Yamagata S, Shimizu A, Taira K et al (2004) Inhibition of growth and invasive ability of melanoma by inactivation of mutated BRAF with lentivirus-mediated RNA interference. Oncogene 23:6031–6039

Toda M, Iizuka Y, Kawase T, Uyemura K, Kawakami Y (2002) Immuno-viral therapy of brain tumors by combination of viral therapy with cancer vaccination using a replication-conditional HSV. Cancer Gene Ther 9:356–364

Udagawa M, Kudo-Saito C, Hasegawa G, Yano K, Yamamoto A, Yaguchi M et al (2006) Enhancement of immunologic tumor regression by intratumoral administration of dendritic cells in combination with cryoablative tumor pretreatment and Bacillus Calmette-Guerin cell wall skeleton stimulation. Clin Cancer Res 12:7465–7475

Ueda R, Iizuka Y, Yoshida K, Kawase T, Kawakami Y, Toda M (2004) Identification of a human glioma antigen, SOX6, recognized by patients' sera. Oncogene 23:1420–1427

Ueda R, Ohkusu-Tsukada K, Fusaki N, Soeda A, Kawase T, Kawakami Y et al (2009) Identification of HLA-A2- and A24-restricted T-cell epitopes derived from SOX6 expressed in glioma stem cells for immunotherapy. Int J Cancer 126(4):919–929

van der Bruggen P, Traversari C, Chomez P, Lurquin C, De Plaen E, Van den Eynde B et al (1991) A gene encoding an antigen recognized by cytolytic T lymphocytes on a human melanoma. Science 254:1643–1647

Chapter 20
Cancer/Testis Antigens: Potential Targets for Immunotherapy

Otavia L. Caballero and Yao-Tseng Chen

Abbreviations

5DC	5-aza-2-deoxycytidine
CT	Cancer/testis
CTL	Cytotoxic T lymphocyte
HDAC	Histone deacetylase
IHC	Immunohistochemical
NSCLC	Non-small cell lung cancer
qRT-PCR	Quantitative reverse transcription-polymerase chain reaction
SEREX	Serological analysis of recombinant cDNA expression libraries

The search for human tumor antigens as potential immunotherapeutic targets, either for antibody-based therapy or for cancer vaccines, has been a continuous task in the field of tumor immunology for several decades. One crucial criterion for selection is that the antigen must have either no or highly restricted expression in normal tissues, so that autoimmunity can be prevented. Over the decades, several categories of antigens were found to fulfill this requirement, including uniquely mutated antigens (e.g., p53), viral antigens (e.g., human papillomavirus antigens in cervical cancer) and differentiation antigens (e.g., CD20 in B cell lymphoma). More recently, a new category of antigen, namely the cancer/testis (CT) antigen, has emerged to be a unique group of antigen that could potentially be important antigen targets for antigen-specific cancer immunotherapy.

O.L. Caballero
Ludwig Institute for Cancer Research, New York Branch at Memorial
Sloan-Kettering Cancer Center, New York, NY, USA

Y.-T. Chen (✉)
Department of Pathology and Laboratory Medicine, Weill Cornell Medical College,
New York, NY, USA
e-mail: ytchen@med.cornell.edu

1 Identification of CT antigens

A major breakthrough in identifying tumor antigens recognized by host cytotoxic T lymphocytes (CTL) was the molecular cloning of MAGE-1 by van der Bruggen et al. (1991). Using a melanoma cell line MZ2-MEL and autologous CTL clones cytolytic to this tumor cell line, a mixed lymphocyte tumor culture system was established. Most melanoma cells were lysed by the CTL following incubation, but variant cell lines emerged that were resistant to the lysis by the specific co-culturing CTL clone, but not by other CTL clones. These immunoselected variants were believed to have lost the genes that encode tumor antigen targets of the specific CTL clones (i.e., antigen-loss variants), and the sensitivity to CTL killing would be reconstituted following transfection of the tumor antigen-encoding genes into the variant cell lines. Using a cosmid genomic DNA transfection-based technology followed by the rescue of transfected DNA species from the recipient cells, MAGE-1 (subsequently renamed as MAGE-A1, Melanoma antigen A1) was discovered and molecularly characterized, representing the first immunogenic tumor antigen shown to elicit autologous cytotoxic T lymphocyte responses in a cancer patient. Pursuing the same strategy by using additional CTL clones and antigen-loss variants from this same patient, Boon and his co-workers successfully identified MAGE-A3, another member of the MAGE-A family, as well as two additional families of antigens, namely BAGE and GAGE protein families (Boel et al. 1995; Van den Eynde et al. 1995; Gaugler et al. 1994).

Analysis of the mRNA expression found an intriguing feature that *MAGE-A*, *BAGE*, and *GAGE* genes were expressed in testis, but not in any other normal somatic tissues or cells, including melanocytes. In contrast, these genes were found to be expressed not only in melanoma, but also in a proportion of many different types of cancers, including breast cancer, lung cancer, ovarian cancer etc., indicating that expression of these tumor antigens was shared by multiple tumor types and not cell lineage-specific. This expression pattern, in conjunction with the lack of MHC class I antigen in testicular germ cells, imply that the protein products of these gene families are tumor-specific antigens from the cancer vaccine perspective, and these antigens were referred to as "shared tumor-specific antigens" by Boon et al. (1997). Shortly after the discovery of tumor antigens by this transfection-based assay, Pfreundschuh and co-workers developed a serological approach to molecularly clone immunogenic tumor antigens that had elicited high-titer IgG immune responses in autologous cancer patients. This methodology, termed SEREX (Serological analysis of Recombinant cDNA EXpression libraries), was based on immunoscreening of tumor cDNA expression libraries with sera from the autologous patients (Sahin et al. 1997). In their first experiments, Sahin et al. (1995) analyzed melanoma, renal cell carcinoma, astrocytoma, and Hodgkin lymphoma, and a large number of tumor antigens were isolated, including MAGE-A1 and tyrosinase, two antigens previously shown to be targets for CTL, indicating that protein antigens that elicit antibody responses in cancer patients are likely to have elicited simultaneous T cell responses. This prompted a large scale SEREX screening of various cancer types, spearheaded by the Ludwig Institute for Cancer Research (LICR), and the screening strategy was broadened to include screening of cDNA libraries derived from allogeneic tumors, tumor cell lines, and testis (Obata 1999; Chen et al. 1997; Lee et al. 2003; Chen et al. 1998; Jager et al. 2001; Obata et al. 2000; Scanlan et al. 1999). This effort and similar efforts by other researchers led to the identification of more than one thousand SEREX-defined antigens in several years (http://ludwig-sun5.unil.ch/CancerImmunomeDB/; http://www.cancerimmunity.org/SEREX/). Intriguing, several of these newly defined tumor antigens, e.g., SSX2, NY-ESO-1, SCP1 and CT7, although structurally unrelated to each other, were all found to be similar to the MAGE family in that they all had normal mRNA expression restricted to testis, with abnormal expression detected in various cancers, including melanoma, esophageal cancer, etc. Recognizing this characteristic expression pattern and their potential as cancer vaccine targets, the term cancer/testis (CT) antigen was coined by Old and Chen (1998) and Chen et al. (1997) to encompass this expanding category of tumor antigens, and CT antigens identified by SEREX to date included MAGE-A (Chen et al. 1998), SSX2 (Tureci et al. 1996), SSX4, NY-ESO-1 (Chen et al. 1997), SCP1 (Tureci et al. 1998), CT7 (Chen et al. 1998), NY-SAR-35 (Lee et al. 2003), OY-TES-1 (Ono et al. 2001), SLCO6A1 (Lee et al. 2004), PASD1 (Liggins et al. 2004), CAGE-1 (Park et al. 2003), KK-LC-1 (Fukuyama et al. 2006), etc.

The recognition of this restricted mRNA expression pattern also provided opportunities to identify new CT antigens, and multiple studies were launched to identify CT genes based on their preferential expression in testis and cancer. By representational difference analysis and comparing melanoma vs. normal skin, Gure et al. (2000) cloned a MAGE-A related CT gene, CT10, and anti-CT10 antibody was found in a melanoma patient, establishing its immunogenicity. Using a similar approach, Lucas et al. (1998) independently isolated the same gene and CT7, and these two genes were later named MAGE-C1 (CT7) and MAGE-C2 (CT10). A second gene of the NY-ESO-1 family, LAGE1 (Lethe et al. 1998), as well as other new CT genes, e.g., SAGE1 (Martelange et al. 2000), were similarly identified. More recently, massively parallel signature sequencing (MPSS) was utilized to compare in detail the mRNA expression profiles between testis, melanoma cell lines, and other somatic tissues (Chen et al. 2005a). This resulted in the identification of >20 CT or CT-like genes, including CT45, a gene subsequently shown to have a prominent expression in Hodgkin lymphoma (Heidebrecht et al. 2006). In addition to these experimental approaches, silico analysis was also employed as a tool to identify new CT antigen genes, e.g., by analyzing the EST (expressed sequence tags) databases for genes with cancer/testis-restricted expression. This approach, taken by several groups, resulted in the identification of BRDT (Scanlan et al. 2000), CT46 (Chen et al. 2005b), XAGE1 (Brinkmann et al. 1999) and PLAC1 (Silva et al. 2007).

To comprehensively analyze the mRNA expression data at a genomic level and identify all potentially CT genes, Hofmann et al. (2008) recently analyzed all available data using a combination of four platforms: MPSS, ESTs, CAGE, and RT-PCR. This thorough analysis resulted in the cataloguing of a total of 153 genes with mRNA expression in normal tissues restricted to, or at least preferentially in, testis, with evidence of tumor expression.

With this expansion of the CT genes, it became evident that a CT database would be highly desirable so that information related to this group of genes can be organized, as this would allow a systematic evaluation and comparison of these genes, thus facilitating the identification of CT antigens that are most promising targets for cancer immunotherapy. Such a CT database has recently been established by LICR (http://www.cta.lncc.br/) (Almeida et al. 2009), and 110 CT genes or gene families are included, reflecting all antigens that were published as CT antigens in the literature. The CT database also includes the results of standardized RT-PCR analysis of each CT antigen in a panel of 22 normal tissues and 32 cancer cell lines.

2 Genomic Organization of CT Antigen Genes

Among the first several CT antigens identified, most of them were found to be encoded by multigene families on chromosome X, particularly on the telomeric end between Xq24 to Xq28. These included MAGE-A, NY-ESO-1, CT7/MAGE-C1, CT10, and SAGE. In addition, SSX and GAGE were located at a more centromeric position of X chromosome, Xp11.2-11.4. This unusual clustering of CT genes on the X chromosome was noticed repeatedly as additional CT genes and gene families were identified, leading to the classification of CT genes into CT-X and non-X CT genes by Simpson et al. (2005) in their review. Of the 110 CT genes listed in the current CT database, 30 were CT-X genes, with Xq24-q28 bearing the highest density of these genes (Fig. 20.1). One characteristic of the CT-X genes is that they are often multicopy genes that resulted from recent gene duplications. These repeats are often palindromic, an example of which being CT45 gene family, for which six almost exact gene copies were identified in tandem on Xq26, with the DNA segment containing CT45.1, CT45.2, and CT45.3 being the inverted repeat of the segment containing CT45.4, CT45.5, and CT45.6. CT47 is an example of direct repeats, consisting of 13 genes duplicated in tandem, spanning a contig of 60 Kb. Combining all multicopy CT-X genes, it has been estimated that CT genes comprise ~10% of DNA sequence on the X chromosome (Ross et al. 2005). Similar findings have been reported in mouse in which 36 multicopy genes were defined on chromosome X, with between 2 and 28 gene copies (Mueller et al. 2008). When tested for their expression by RT-PCR, 33 of the 36 genes were found to be exclusively or preferentially expressed in testis, including the homologs of human CT genes, e.g., MAGE, NXF2, and SSX genes. Twenty-eight of these genes were analyzed for the stage of spermatogenesis during which they were expressed, and eight of them were found to be expressed in the self-renewing spermatogonia. On the other hand, the mRNA expression of the remaining 20 genes coincided with the appearance of postmeiotic germ cells, i.e., secondary spermatocytes and spermatids, suggesting that they are only expressed in the haploid germ cells (Mueller et al. 2008).

In contrast to the CT-X genes, most of the non-X CTs genes are single copy genes, and no additional chromosomal clustering is found. This drastic difference indicates

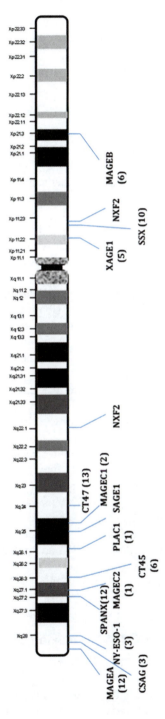

Fig. 20.1 Distribution of CT families on X-chromosome. The number of CT genes in each family is indicated in parenthesis

that CT-X and non-X CT genes are evolutionarily distinctive. Such differences are also reflected in their expression patterns and functional characteristics (see below), and CT-X antigens are currently considered to be more promising cancer vaccine targets.

3 Expression of CT Antigen mRNA in Normal Tissues

In addition to testicular expression, a subset of CT antigens has been found to be expressed in placenta. Examples include MAGEA3, MAGEA10, MAGEA8, XAGE2, and XAGE3. Conversely, placenta-specific genes, e.g., PLAC1, have been shown to be expressed in testis, but at a low abundance level (Silva et al. 2007). Besides placental expression, it has also become clear that many CT genes showed low-level mRNA expression in a limited number of somatic tissues, particularly if analyzed using a sensitive detection method such as quantitative RT-PCR. However, the mRNA expression levels of these genes in non-testicular tissues are usually at <1% of their expression level in testis. This low-level CT expression has never been confirmed at the protein level by immunohistochemical analysis with anti-CT antibodies, and whether such "leaky" RNA expression translates to a physiologically significant level of protein is debatable. Some of the genes originally described as CT genes have subsequently been shown to have a broader mRNA expression pattern than was initially recognized and these genes probably should not be grouped under CT antigen genes, and examples of this include JARID1B and SPA17. Recognizing this mRNA expression spectrum that ranged from testis-restricted to testis-predominant and testis-biased expression, Hofmann et al. (2008) classified the 153 CT genes that they analyzed into "testis-restricted" and "testis-selective" categories, with the latter being genes that are predominantly, but not exclusively expressed in testis. A third category, "testis/brain-selective," was also described in the study that encompassed a small number of genes that showed expression limited to testis and brain. When correlating to the chromosomal locations, it was found that of the 39 testis-restricted genes, 35 were CT-X genes and only four were non-CT-X genes. This disproportional enrichment of testis-restricted genes on the X chromosome, in conjunction to the fact that most immunogenic CT antigens identified to date, including MAGE-A, NY-ESO-1 and SSX, are all within this testis-restricted subgroup of CT-X genes, strongly imply that the CT-X genes are likely also the most interesting genes from the immunotherapeutic standpoint.

4 mRNA Expression of CT Antigens in Cancer

Aberrant activation and expression of mRNA transcripts in various human cancers in a lineage-independent fashion is the defining criterion of CT antigens. In addition, the following expression characteristics, pertinent to the consideration of CT antigens as immunotherapeutic targets, have been observed: (a) Different cancer types are significantly different in their frequency of CT mRNA expression; (b) For a given cancer type, tumors of higher histological grade and later clinical stage often show higher frequency of CT expression; and (c) CT antigens tend to be coordinated expressed, i.e., tumors that are positive for CT antigens often show simultaneous expression of more than one CT antigens.

Of the different types of cancers, melanoma, ovarian cancer, and lung cancer, particularly the squamous cell type, have been found to have the highest frequency of CT expression, sometimes referred to as "CT-rich" tumor types. In contrast, hematopoietic malignancies, including lymphomas and leukemia as well as renal, colon, and pancreatic cancers, have notably low frequency of CT antigen expression. Other common epithelial cancer types, e.g., breast cancer, bladder cancer, and prostate cancer, appear to be intermediate in their CT expression frequency. For instance, *MAGE-A1* mRNA has been detected in around 48% of metastatic melanoma (Brasseur et al. 1995), 25% of ovarian cancer (Yamada et al. 1995), but only in 12% of colon cancer (Li et al. 2005) and 3.5% of leukemia from various subtypes (Martinez et al. 2007). Similarly, *NY-ESO-1* mRNA expression has been observed in 52% of melanoma (Goydos et al. 2001), 27% of non-small cell lung carcinoma (Gure et al. 2005), 35% of bladder cancer (Sharma et al. 2003), but only in 10% of the colon cancer (Li et al. 2005), and none of the renal cell carcinoma and lymphoma tested (Chen et al. 1997). Exceptions to this observation do occur, most notably the high frequency expression of NY-ESO-1 in synovial sarcoma (Jungbluth et al. 2001), CT7/MAGE-C1 in multiple myeloma (Jungbluth et al. 2005) and CT45 in classical Hodgkin lymphoma (Heidebrecht et al. 2006). It is possible that these CT antigens might have specific biological roles in these specific tumor types, but such roles, if they do exist, remain to be elucidated.

For a given cancer type, higher frequency of CT expression is often correlated with worse outcome (Table 20.1). Higher grade and metastatic tumors have also been found to have more frequent CT expression than the primary tumors. For example, NY-ESO-1 has been found to be expressed in 40% of grade 3 tumors, 23% of grade 2 tumors, but none of the grade 1 tumors (Kurashige et al. 2001). Similarly, in lung adenocarcinoma, significant CT antigen mRNA expression is less common in the well-differentiated group, i.e., the bronchioloalveolar carcinoma (BAC) and BAC-predominant adenocarcinomas. MAGE-A1 expression has been found in 48% of metastatic melanoma, vs. 16% of primary melanoma (Brasseur et al. 1995).

Another expression characteristic that has been observed in multiple tumor types is the tendency for CT antigens to be coordinately expressed. In the analysis of expression of nine CT-X genes in lung cancer, Gure et al. (2005) found that expression of one CT antigen by a tumor greatly enhanced the likelihood that it would also simultaneously express a second CT antigen. On the other hand, a subset of tumors showed no expression of any of the CT antigens tested. This phenomenon of coordinated expression (or nonexpression) has been observed in tumor samples as well as cell lines, the most striking example being SK-MEL-37, which has been found to express almost all the CT antigens tested (Chen et al. 1998).

Table 20.1 Correlation of CT expression with clinicopathologic parameters and prognosis

Tumor type	Antigen	Association	Reference
Melanoma	MAGEA1, MAGEA2, MAGEA3, MAGEA4	Tumor thickness and metastasis	(Brasseur et al. 1995)
NSCLC	MAGEA1,MAGEA3, MAGEA4,MAGEA10, MAGEC1	Advanced tumor type, nodal and pathologic stages as well as pleural invasion	(Gure et al. 2005)
Pancreatic cancer	MAGEA3	Poor survival	(Kim et al. 2006)
Hepatocellular carcinoma	MAGEC1	Reduced overall survival	(Riener et al. 2009)
Colorectal	MAGEA4	Presence of vessel emboli	(Li et al. 2005)
Multiple Myeloma	MAGEA1,MAGEA3, MAGEA4, MAGEC1	Stage and risk status of disease	(Atanackovic et al. 2009; Condomines et al. 2006; Dhodapkar et al. 2003)
Multiple Myeloma	CT-45	Poor outcome	(Andrade and Vettore 2009)
Serous ovarian carcinomas	MAGEA4	Inverse correlation between expression and patient survival	(Yakirevich et al. 2003)
Gastrointestinal stromal tumors	MAGEA1,MAGEA3, MAGEA4, MAGEC1	Early recurrence	(Perez et al. 2008)
Cervical cancer	MAGEA, NY-ESO-1	tumor size and lymph node metastases and tumor grading	(Napoletano et al. 2008)
Vulvar cancer	MAGEA, NY-ESO-1	lymph node metastases and poor tumor differentiation	(Bellati et al. 2007)
Melanoma	NY-ESO-1	thicker primary lesions and a higher frequency of metastatic disease	(Velazquez et al. 2007)
Multiple Myeloma	SSX	Reduced survival	(Taylor et al. 2005)

5 Protein Expression of CT Antigens in Testis and in Cancer

For CT antigens to be potential immunotherapeutic targets, demonstration of protein expression in tumor is prerequisite. For that reason, polyclonal and monoclonal antibodies have been generated against many CT antigens by us and others, and immunohistochemical staining has been the main methodology that CT antigen protein expression in testis and in cancer have been evaluated.

At least three common patterns of CT protein expression have been observed in testis (a) predominant expression in spermatogonia – the self-renewing stem cell population of germ cell in adult testis, mostly as nuclear protein, (b) predominant expression in primary and/or secondary spermatocytes, again as nuclear antigens, (c) restricted expression to the mature sperm cells, mostly as cytoplasmic protein. Figure 20.2 shows examples of each one of these categories. Most of the CT-X antigens, including NY-ESO-1, MAGE-A, CT7/MAGE-C1, CT10/MAGE-C2, GAGE, CT47, SAGE1, NXF2 etc., belong to the first group, with strongest expression seen in the spermatogonia. Most of these are mainly nuclear antigens, but not infrequently also present in the cytoplasmic compartment. However, predominant cytoplasmic expression is rare, with CT47 being an example. In comparison to this group, some CT antigens are expressed mainly or exclusively in the spermatocyte stage. This group is comprised mostly of nuclear proteins and includes meiosis-related proteins, e.g., SCP1 and CT46/HORMAD1, as well as rare CT antigens in the CT-X group, e.g., CT45. The third group consists of genes that are only expressed in the more mature, postmeiotic sperm cells. COX6B2, a testis-specific isoform of the cytochrome c oxidase subunit VIb, is an example of this group. The only CT-X antigen analyzed so far that belongs to this group is the SPANX family, a family on Xq27 with at least five members.

Expression of CT proteins in tumor has only been analyzed for few CT antigens, i.e., NY-ESO-1, MAGE-A, GAGE, CT7/MAGE-C1, CT10/MAGE-C2, and most recently CT45 (Chen et al. 2009), examples of which are depicted in Fig. 20.3. From these analyses and our own recent data, the following characteristics have been observed: (a) Most CT genes evaluated have demonstrable protein expression in cancer, but with important exceptions; (b) CT protein expression correlates to the mRNA expression level, and tumors with higher CT mRNA levels, in general >1–10% of testicular mRNA expression level, usually have demonstrable protein expression; and (c) CT protein expression in tumor is often heterogeneous, and strong expression in a very small subset of tumor cells are not infrequently observed.

Almost all CT antigen-based cancer vaccine trials that have been performed to date use CT mRNA expression in tumor as the inclusion criterion for patient enrollment, under the assumption that CT mRNA expression would imply protein expression. Studies to correlate CT mRNA and protein levels have been performed for NY-ESO-1, CT45 and GAGE, and results all support this concept of transcriptional regulation, with protein expression detectable by immunohistochemistry in most cases that have CT mRNA level at >10% of the testicular expression.

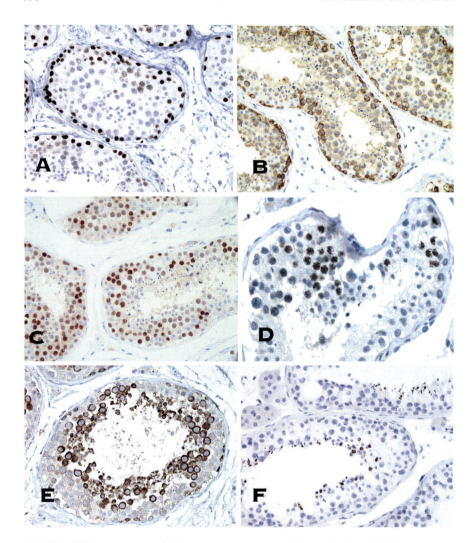

Fig. 20.2 Different patterns of CT antigen expression in adult testis. Many CT-X antigens are expressed as nuclear antigens in spermatogonia, including NXF2 (**a**), SAGE, and most MAGE-A antigens. An exception is CT47 (**b**), expressed as cytoplasmic antigens in spermatogonia. The third pattern is represented by CT45 (**c**), which shows strongest expression in the premeiotic spermatocytes as nuclear antigens. The fourth pattern is observed in meiosis-related CT antigens, which are expressed as nuclear antigens in cells undergoing meiosis, an example being CT46/HORMAD1 (**d**). THEG is the only antigen that show fifth pattern, being expressed as a cytoplasmic antigen in the postmeiotic spermatids as a cytoplasmic antigen (**e**). The last pattern, expression in the most mature sperm cells, is seen in SPANX (**f**), COX6B2 etc

Cases with 1–10% testicular level were borderline in their protein expression, and tumors with <1% testicular expression usually showed no detectable protein expression. In contrast to this mRNA-protein correlation, however, expression of some CT antigens may also be regulated posttranscriptionally, and the presence of CT mRNA

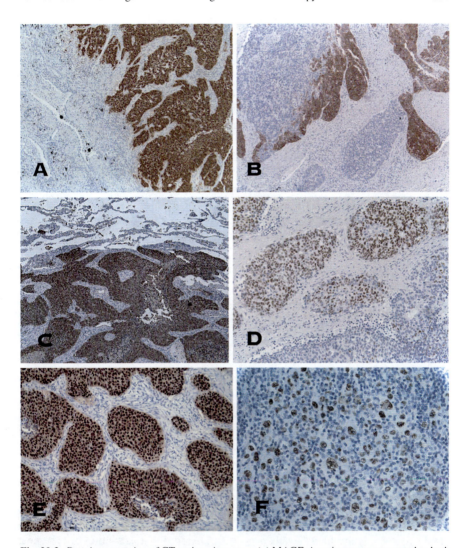

Fig. 20.3 Protein expression of CT antigen in cancer. (**a**) MAGE-A antigens are expressed as both nuclear and cytoplasmic proteins, showing diffuse expression in this lung cancer. (**b**) Similar nuclear and cytoplasmic expression is also seen in NY-ESO-1, which shows heterogeneous expression in this lung cancer. (**c**) Similar nuclear and cytoplasmic staining is observed for GAGE gene family, as well as other CT antigens, including CT7 (not shown). In comparison, pure nuclear staining is seen for CT10 (**d**) and CT45 (**e**). In Hodgkin lymphoma, CT45 often showed diffuse expression in the neoplastic Reed-Sternberg cells (**f**)

may not correlate with protein expression. For instance, despite the detection of substantial SCP1 and CT46 mRNA levels in some tumors and immunohistochemical detection of the protein expression in testicular spermatocytes, we have not been able to detect expression of these two proteins in mRNA-positive tumors (unpublished data). It is possible that these genes, given their specific functions in meiosis, are tightly controlled physiologically to prevent their aberrant expression, and this control might be exerted at both the transcriptional as well as at the translational levels, e.g., through translational suppression by microRNAs.

Two different spatial distribution patterns of CT protein expression have been observed in cancer. In some cases, CT antigens are diffusely and homogenously expressed in almost all tumor cells, suggesting that the gene activation is a clonal event, e.g., analogous to p53 overexpression as a result of mutated p53 gene. On the other hand, in many cases the CT expression are highly heterogeneous, ranging between patchy expression to cases in which a small cluster of tumor cells with strong expression is seen among a background of >99% of CT-negative tumor cells. This heterogeneous staining pattern suggests that the activation might be an epigenetic event in these cases, e.g., due to changes in DNA methylation. On the other hand, it has also been proposed that the CT-positive cells might represent the cancer stem cells in these cases (Gedye et al. 2009). From the immunotherapeutic standpoint, the heterogeneous staining pattern raises the concern of immunoselection of CT-negative cells clinically. However, the observation of "antigen-spreading" following killing of a subset of tumor cells would argue against this concern (Hunder et al. 2008), and if these CT-positive cells are indeed cancer stem cells, they would obviously be the crucial cells that should be targeted.

6 Regulation of CT Antigen Expression

One common future of CT antigen gene expression, particularly for the CT-X genes, is the induction by the DNA methyl-transferase 1 inhibitors, 5-aza-2-deoxycytidine (5DC), and/or by histone deacetylase (HDAC) inhibitors (De Smet et al. 1999). This has been shown for multiple CT genes, including *MAGE-A*, *NY-ESO-1*, and *SSX* (De Smet et al. 1999; Oi et al. 2009; Sigalotti et al. 2004). This finding, together with the inclination of global hypomethylation in cancer (Hoffmann and Schulz 2005), suggests CpG island hypomethylation at the promoter regions as the likely mechanism for transcriptional activation of CT genes in germ cells and in cancer. *SSX*, *MAGE*, and *LAGE1* promoter–reporter constructs were found to be active in all tumor cell lines regardless of the CT expression status of these cell lines (Lethe et al. 1998; De Smet et al. 1996), indicating that the essential transcriptional factors are universally present and that silencing mechanisms, e.g., CpG methylation, are in effect in CT-negative cell lines. One the other hand, however, 5DC failed to induce CT expression in primary fibroblasts as it readily does in most tumor cell lines (Weber et al. 1994), and addition of HDAC also does not lead to significant expression of the CT genes. Although it is possible that CpG islands in the promoter regions of these genes are so densely methylated in normal cells that 5DC and HDAC were ineffective, other mechanisms of transcriptional, and even posttranscriptional, control of gene expression might exist.

An interesting theory that has been proposed to explain the activation of CT antigens in cancer is that this activation may be the consequence of induction of a gametogenic program in cancer (Simpson et al. 2005; Old 2001). According to this hypothesis, the different CT expression profiles seen in cancer may correspond to the profiles of CT antigens normally expressed at various stages of gametogenesis or trophoblastic development, and the triggering event for this activation could be the switch-on of a master gene in germ cell development, e.g., by a mutational event. Supporting this hypothesis is the finding of CT antigens that are known to play specific roles in germ cell development, e.g., meiosis proteins SCP1 and HORMAD1/CT46, as well as normal trophoblastic protein PLAC1. In addition, the finding that BORIS, a germ cell specific protein and a CT antigen itself, can cause epigenetic reprogramming and might thus control the expression of other CT antigens (Vatolin et al. 2005), is also in line with the concept of a "master-switch" for CT activation in cancer.

7 Functions of CT Antigens

The biological role of CT-X in both germ line tissues and tumors remains poorly understood. Recent studies have provided some evidence that CT antigens may play a role in human tumorigenesis. In yeast, two-hybrid studies using cancer-related genes as bait have twice pulled out MAGE proteins: MAGE-A11 and MAGE-A4 (Bai et al. 2005; Nagao et al. 2003). MAGE-A11 was found to have a role in the regulation of androgen-receptor function by modulating its internal domain interactions and was found to have a dual amplifying effect on androgen signaling (Bai et al. 2005). MAGE-A4 was identified in a search for binding partners of the oncoprotein gankyrin (Nagao et al. 2003). Overexpression of MAGE-A4 in a human embryonic kidney cells (293 cells) was found to increase apoptosis while MAGE-A4 silencing using a small interfering RNA approach resulted in decreased caspase-3 activity in a squamous cell lung cancer and in 293/MAGE-A4 cells (Peikert et al. 2006). MAGE-A2 protein was shown to strongly downregulate p53 transactivation function and association between MAGEA expression levels and resistance to etoposide (ET) treatment was shown in short-term cell lines obtained from melanoma biopsies harboring wild-type-p53 (Monte et al. 2006). Multiple MAGE proteins including human MAGE-A3, MAGE-C2, and murine mage-b1 (mMage-b) proteins were shown to form complexes with Kap-1, a known corepressor of p53, and siRNA suppression of MAGE-A3, mMage-b, and MAGE-C2 genes induces apoptosis and causes increased p53 expression in vitro. Thus, MAGE gene expression may protect cells from programmed cell death and may actively contribute to the development of malignancies by promoting survival (Yang et al. 2007). In pituitary tumors, a reciprocal profile of FGFR2-IIIb and MAGE-A3 expression was identified (Zhu et al. 2008). Whereas, FGFR2-IIIb plays a growth-inhibitory tumor-suppressive role, MAGE-A3 is considered to have growth-promoting oncogenic functions. Downregulation of MAGE-A3 resulted in p53 transcriptional induction and p21 accumulation (Zhu et al. 2008). Similarly, MAGE-A3 was shown to be significantly upregulated in response to FN silencing in thyroid carcinoma cells (Liu et al. 2008). Forced expression of MAGE-A3 resulted in p21 downregulation, accelerated cell cycle progression, increased cell migration rate, and invasion in vitro and in vivo that recapitulated progression of thyroid cancer. Both *MAGE* and *GAGE* genes have been found to show significantly higher expression in paclitaxel- and doxorubicin-resistant cells lines than in the parental cell lines (Duan et al. 2003). The function of GAGE proteins also remains largely unknown, although anti-apoptotic properties of GAGE-7 have been reported (Cilensek et al. 2002). GAGE-7C was shown to render cells resistant to apoptosis mediated by IFN-γ or by Fas. In this study, the anti-apoptotic activity of GAGE was shown to reside downstream of caspase-8 activation and upstream of PARP cleavage in the Fas pathway. In addition, it was shown that GAGE renders cells resistant to Taxol and γ-irradiation. Its anti-apoptotic activity and the resistance to the clinically relevant agents may explain the reported correlation between GAGE expression and poor prognosis in some cancers.

We used the yeast two-hybrid system to identify putative novel MHD-interacting proteins (Cho et al. 2006). The MHD of MAGE-C1 was used as a bait to screen a human testis cDNA library. As a result of this investigation, we identified another member of the CT antigen family, CT-AG1B/NY-ESO-1 as a MAGE-C1 binding partner. This was the first report of a direct interaction between two CT antigens and may be pertinent in the light of the frequently coordinated expression of these proteins.

Overall, these findings indicate that CT-X antigens are functional integrators of diverse signals to modulate cancer progression and better insights in the function of these genes could hence be valuable for therapeutic considerations.

While few clues have emerged so far in relation to the function of the CT-X, most of the non-X CTs are conserved during evolution and have known roles in spermatogenesis and fertilization. OY-TES-1 (ACRBP) is similar to proacrosin binding protein sp32 precursor found in mouse, guinea pig, and pig. This protein is located in the sperm acrosome and is thought to function as a binding protein to proacrosin for packaging and condensation of the acrosin zymogen in the acrosomal matrix (Ono et al. 2001). Three proteins involved in germ cell meiosis were identified as CT antigens: SCP1, SYCE, and HORMAD1. SCP1 and SYCE are part of the synaptonemal complex lateral and central elements, respectively (Meuwissen et al. 1997; Hamer et al. 2006). ADAM2 (fertilin beta) and PRM2 were found to contribute to successful fertilization and also may have an important impact in development of preimplantation embryos (Depa-Martynow et al. 2007). Protamines are small sperm nuclear specific proteins that replace somatic histones and to chromatin remodeling during early spermiogenesis (Aoki et al. 2006). SEMG1 is the predominant protein in semen and it is involved in the formation of a gel matrix that encases ejaculated spermatozoa (Robert and Gagnon 1999). SEMG1 and/or its proteolytic fragments were also found be involved in regulating spermatozoon motility, capacitation and also to present antibacterial activity (Zhao et al. 2008).

8 Immunogenicity of CT Antigens

As potential cancer vaccine targets, the demonstration of immunogenicity in human host is considered crucial in the characterization of the CT antigens. Earlier CT antigens were cloned based on the spontaneous cytotoxic $CD8^+$ T cell response or antibody response that they have elicited in cancer patients, and several of them have subsequently been shown to elicit coordinated humoral and cell-mediated responses. The prototype examples include MAGE-A1, MAGE-A3, initially identified by cytotoxic T cell cloning, and NY-ESO-1 and SSX, initially identified by SEREX.

The T cell responses to CT antigens are typical investigated by the screening of overlapping peptide panels with peripheral blood $CD8^+$ T cells from either cancer patients or healthy donors, and similar studies were also extended to investigate $CD4^+$ T cell responses. Many HLA-restricted T cell epitopes have been identified this way, particularly for MAGE-A, NY-ESO-1, and SSX genes, forming the basis for peptide-based CT cancer vaccine trials and for the monitoring of postvaccination T cell responses (see below). These data on T cell epitopes have been compiled into the peptide database of T-cell defined tumor antigens (http://www.cancerimmunity.org/peptidedatabase/Tcellepitopes.htm). In contrast to this abundance of data on MAGE-A, NY-ESO-1, and SSX genes, studies to investigate T cell recognition of other CT antigens have been very limited (Fukuyama et al. 2006; Ait-Tahar et al. 2009; Xing et al. 2008; Frank et al. 2008), likely hindered by the technical complexity and cost of such studies.

In comparison, humoral immune responses have been investigated more broadly, usually by ELISA testing against recombinant CT proteins. NY-ESO-1 is the prototype example, and anti-NY-ESO-1 antibody has been detected in many cancer types, including lung cancer, ovarian cancer, breast cancer, bladder cancer, melanoma etc. The frequency of anti-NY-ESO-1 antibody response in patients with advanced NY-ESO-1 positive tumors has been estimated to be at the range of 25–50%, and the titer of the antibody appears to increase with progressive disease and decrease upon removal of the tumor or upon tumor regression (Jager et al. 1999). Investigation of anti-NY-ESO-1 T cell responses has demonstrated NY-ESO-1 specific $CD8^+$ T cells in the majority of patients with positive anti-NY-ESO-1 antibodies, whereas T cell response in the absence of a concurrent NY-ESO-1 antibody response is very rare. This high frequency of coordinated humoral and cell-mediated responses indicates that NY-ESO-1 the most immunogenic CT antigens known to date, making it one of the most attractive targets for cancer vaccines.

In addition to NY-ESO-1, coordinated antibody and T cell responses have also been observed for MAGE-A and SSX antigens. In contrast to NY-ESO-1, however, the frequency of antibody response appears to be much lower. For instance, MAGE-A genes are highly expressed in melanoma, and yet spontaneous MAGE-A1 and MAGE-A3 antibodies have only been found in <3% of these patients in our hands. However, after immunization with MAGE-A3 recombinant protein, many patients do develop MAGE-A3-specific antibodies, in most cases not accompanied by detectable $CD8^+$ T cell responses (Atanackovic et al. 2008).

Antibody responses to other CT antigens have been reported, some of them at very high frequencies, including SCP1 in 50% breast cancer patients (Mischo et al. 2006), cTAGE in 33% of cutaneous T cell lymphoma patients (Eichmuller et al. 2003), SSX2 in 18% of melanoma patients (Sahin et al. 1997) etc. However, since different assays with different sensitivity and specificity were used in various studies, it would be prudent to interpret these reports of exceptional high antibody frequency with caution, as much lower frequency of antibody response has also been reported.

9 Cancer Vaccine Trials Targeting CT Antigens

Restricted tissue expression and spontaneous immunogenicity in patients are crucial features for potential cancer vaccine targets, the best example being differentiation antigens, e.g., melanocyte antigens Melan-A and gp100, for the treatment of melanoma (Kawakami et al. 1998). For common epithelial cancers, however, such tumor antigen do not exist, and CT antigens thus provide the ideal antigenic target, with the caveat being that only a subset of patients will have tumors that express the CT antigen being targeted.

To evaluate CT antigens as therapeutic cancer vaccine targets, multiple clinical trials have been carried out against either MAGE-A3 or NY-ESO-1. For both antigens, the trials have tested peptide-based vaccines and recombinant protein vaccines. In one of the MAGE-A3 phase I/II trials, peptide-based vaccine was given to 25 stage III/IV melanoma patients, leading to regression of individual tumor nodules in seven patients, including three complete regressions. Similarly, disease stabilization and regression of isolated metastatic tumor nodules have been observed in the NY-ESO-1 peptide trials in some cases. One significant difference between MAGE-A3 and NY-ESO-1, however, was that postvaccination immune responses were more easily detectable following NY-ESO-1 vaccination, and peptide-specific CD8$^+$ T cell responses were detected in four of seven patients with no prior NY-ESO-1 immunity (Jager et al. 2006). In contrast, with one exception (Coulie et al. 2001), anti-MAGE-A3 CD8$^+$ T cell responses were essentially undetectable, even in patients with clinical response (Marchand et al. 1999).

While showing immunological and clinical responses in a subset of vaccine recipients, most peptide vaccines carry only one or few epitopes and cannot be expected to induce a broad spectrum CD8$^+$ and CD4$^+$ T immune responses. In contrast, protein antigens can be expected to elicit broader polyclonal CD8$^+$ and CD4$^+$ T responses against known and uncharacterized epitopes, with the additional advantage of being unrestricted by the HLA selection of the patients, thus suitable for a larger patient population.

For the first MAGE-A3 recombinant protein trial, a His-tag MAGE-A3 protein with protein D at N-terminus, produced by GlaxoSmithKline (gsk), was administered to stage III/IV melanoma patients, and clinical responses were seen in 5 of 26 patients, including one partial response and four mixed responses. This was followed by a phase II trial in 182 non-small cell lung cancer patients, for which an improvement of disease-free survival (hazard ratio=0.666, $p=0.12$) was observed at the interim analysis. Based on this promising result, a phase III trial that involves 2,270 lung cancer patients has been launched and is ongoing. Additional phase II melanoma trials on MAGE-A3 proteins have also been conducted to evaluate different immunological adjuvants (AS15 vs. AS02B), with clinical responses seen in 13 of 36 in the AS15 arm (3 complete responses, 1 partial response, 5 stable diseases, and 4 mixed responses), 9 of 36 in the AS02B arm (1 partial response, 5 stable diseases, and 3 mixed responses) (Lehmann et al. 2008).

For NY-ESO-1, the first recombinant protein trial was in 46 melanoma patients after complete excision of melanoma, using a His-tagged recombinant protein, either with or without ISCOMATRIX adjuvant (Davis et al. 2004). The results showed anti-NY-ESO-1 antibody responses in almost all patients receiving NY-ESO-1 with ISCOMATRIX, and integrated $CD4^+$ and $CD8^+$ T cell responses were also induced in a subset of patients, reacting to a broad range of NY-ESO-1 epitopes, most of them previously undefined. Clinically, it was found that 16 of 42 patients who completed the trial had tumor relapse within a 2-year interval, including 5 of 7 in the placebo group, 9 of 16 in the group of NY-ESO-1 protein alone, but only 2 of 19 in the group of NY-ESO-1 with ISCOMATRIX. This suggests that NY-ESO-1 vaccination might reduce the risk of recurrence in patients with fully resected melanoma. In comparison, a parallel study of the same vaccine on a group of 27 stage III/IV melanoma patients showed objective response in only one patient (in the form of stable disease), and T cell responses in these patients appeared to be inferior to those seen in the prior group of patients with minimal residual disease (Nicholaou et al. 2009). The reason for this inferior T cell response was attributed to immunosuppression by regulatory T cells, and the authors proposed that vaccine-based treatment might be more beneficial at the setting of early or minimal residual disease, when the tumor load and the extent of immunosuppression are both minimized.

In addition to the ISCOMATRIX adjuvants, other forms of NY-ESO-1 protein vaccine constructs are also being evaluated, including the fusion of NY-ESO-1 with cholesterol-bearing hydrophobized pullulan (CHP-NY-ESO-1) (Harada et al. 2008), or the use of other adjuvants, e.g., CpG, Montanide ISA-51, and/or imiquimod (Valmori et al. 2007; Odunsi et al. 2007). The possibility of producing NY-ESO-1 protein in vivo using DNA vaccine constructs has also been examined, either using naked plasmid DNA (Gnjatic et al. 2009), vaccinia/fowlpox viral constructs (Jager et al. 2006), or bacterial vectors such as *Salmonella typhimurium* (Nishikawa et al. 2006). Most of these phase I/II trials showed safety of the vaccine preparations, with variable capability of inducing anti-NY-ESO-1 specific immune responses. Whether the observed immune responses will correlate to beneficial clinical outcomes remains to be proven by larger schedule studies in defined patient populations.

Aside from its potential as antigen-specific cancer vaccines, NY-ESO-1 has also been found to be useful in adoptive immunotherapy. In the study of (Hunder et al. 2008), a $CD4^+$ T cell clone specifically targeting a HLA-DPB1*0401-restricted NY-ESO-1 epitope was isolated from a melanoma patient, expanded in vitro, and infused back to the patient in a single infusion. This adoptive transfer of clonal anti-NY-ESO-1 CD4⁺ T cells resulted in complete regression of pulmonary and nodal disease in this patient, who remains disease-free 2 years after treatment. In vitro testing showed that this patient has also generated previously undetected anti-MAGE-A3 and anti-Melan A T cell responses following the adoptive transfer, supporting the notion of "antigen-spreading."

Most recently, NY-ESO-1 has been found to be potentially useful if combined with nonspecific immunotherapeutic approaches such as CTLA-4 blockade (Yuan et al. 2008). In this study, 15 melanoma patients were treated with anti-CTLA4 monoclonal antibody (ipilimumab), and five of eight patients with evidence of clinical benefit were found to be NY-ESO-1 antibody positive, whereas none of seven clinical nonresponders had NY-ESO-1 antibody in serum. This finding suggests that anti-CTLA-4 therapy following induction of anti-NY-ESO-1 immune responses by vaccination could have a synergistic effect and this possibility should be further explored.

10 Concluding Remarks

Identification of appropriate target antigens is the first and most crucial step in the successful development of antigen-specific immunotherapy, and the discovery and characterization of CT antigens has provided the first group of target antigens that can be used in various common epithelial cancers. As none of the CT antigens appears to be cell surface antigens, they are currently considered cancer vaccine targets rather than targets for antibody-based therapy. However, recent studies have shown them to be potentially useful in adoptive T cell transfer approaches and in nonspecific immunotherapeutic approach that aims at CTLA-4 checkpoint blockade. This broadened role of CT antigens is exciting and will likely be fully explored in the coming years.

Acknowledgments The authors would like to thank Drs. Lloyd J. Old and Andy J. G. Simpson of the Ludwig Institute for Cancer Research for their unwavering support over the years.

References

Ait-Tahar K, Liggins AP, Collins GP et al (2009) Cytolytic T-cell response to the PASD1 cancer testis antigen in patients with diffuse large B-cell lymphoma. Br J Haematol 146(4):396–407

Almeida LG, Sakabe NJ (2009) deOliveira AR, et al. CTdatabase: a knowledge-base of high-throughput and curated data on cancer-testis antigens. Nucleic Acids Res 37:D816–D819

Andrade VC, Vettore AL (2009) Regis Silva MR, et al. Frequency and prognostic relevance of cancer testis antigen 45 expression in multiple myeloma. Exp Hematol 37:446–449

Aoki VW, Liu L, Jones KP et al (2006) Sperm protamine 1/protamine 2 ratios are related to in vitro fertilization pregnancy rates and predictive of fertilization ability. Fertil Steril 86:1408–1415

Atanackovic D, Altorki NK, Cao Y et al (2008) Booster vaccination of cancer patients with MAGE-A3 protein reveals long-term immunological memory or tolerance depending on priming. Proc Natl Acad Sci U S A 105:1650–1655

Atanackovic D, Luetkens T, Hildebrandt Y et al (2009) Longitudinal analysis and prognostic effect of cancer-testis antigen expression in multiple myeloma. Clin Cancer Res 15:1343–1352

Bai S, He B, Wilson EM (2005) Melanoma antigen gene protein MAGE-11 regulates androgen receptor function by modulating the interdomain interaction. Mol Cell Biol 25:1238–1257

Bellati F, Napoletano C, Tarquini E et al (2007) Cancer testis antigen expression in primary and recurrent vulvar cancer: association with prognostic factors. Eur J Cancer 43:2621–2627

Boel P, Wildmann C, Sensi ML et al (1995) BAGE: a new gene encoding an antigen recognized on human melanomas by cytolytic T lymphocytes. Immunity 2:167–175

Boon T, Coulie PG, Van den Eynde B (1997) Tumor antigens recognized by T cells. Immunol Today 18:267–268

Brasseur F, Rimoldi D, Lienard D et al (1995) Expression of MAGE genes in primary and metastatic cutaneous melanoma. Int J Cancer 63:375–380

Brinkmann U, Vasmatzis G, Lee B, Pastan I (1999) Novel genes in the PAGE and GAGE family of tumor antigens found by homology walking in the dbEST database. Cancer Res 59:1445–1448

Chen YT, Scanlan MJ, Sahin U et al (1997) A testicular antigen aberrantly expressed in human cancers detected by autologous antibody screening. Proc Natl Acad Sci U S A 94:1914–1918

Chen YT, Gure AO, Tsang S et al (1998) Identification of multiple cancer/testis antigens by allogeneic antibody screening of a melanoma cell line library. Proc Natl Acad Sci U S A 95:6919–6923

Chen YT, Scanlan MJ, Venditti CA et al (2005a) Identification of cancer/testis-antigen genes by massively parallel signature sequencing. Proc Natl Acad Sci U S A 102:7940–7945

Chen YT, Venditti CA, Theiler G et al (2005b) Identification of CT46/HORMAD1, an immunogenic cancer/testis antigen encoding a putative meiosis-related protein. Cancer Immun 5:9

Chen YT, Hsu M, Lee P et al (2009) Cancer/testis antigen CT45: analysis of mRNA and protein expression in human cancer. Int J Cancer 124:2893–2898

Cho HJ, Caballero OL, Gnjatic S et al (2006) Physical interaction of two cancer-testis antigens, MAGE-C1 (CT7) and NY-ESO-1 (CT6). Cancer Immun 6:12

Cilensek ZM, Yehiely F, Kular RK, Deiss LP (2002) A member of the GAGE family of tumor antigens is an anti-apoptotic gene that confers resistance to Fas/CD95/APO-1, Interferongamma, taxol and gamma-irradiation. Cancer Biol Ther 1:380–387

Condomines M, Quittet P, Lu ZY et al (2006) Functional regulatory T cells are collected in stem cell autografts by mobilization with high-dose cyclophosphamide and granulocyte colony-stimulating factor. J Immunol 176:6631–6639

Coulie PG, Karanikas V, Colau D et al (2001) A monoclonal cytolytic T-lymphocyte response observed in a melanoma patient vaccinated with a tumor-specific antigenic peptide encoded by gene MAGE-3. Proc Natl Acad Sci U S A 98:10290–10295

Davis ID, Chen W, Jackson H et al (2004) Recombinant NY-ESO-1 protein with ISCOMATRIX adjuvant induces broad integrated antibody and CD4(+) and CD8(+) T cell responses in humans. Proc Natl Acad Sci U S A 101:10697–10702

De Smet C, De Backer O, Faraoni I, Lurquin C, Brasseur F, Boon T (1996) The activation of human gene MAGE-1 in tumor cells is correlated with genome-wide demethylation. Proc Natl Acad Sci U S A 93:7149–7153

De Smet C, Lurquin C, Lethe B, Martelange V, Boon T (1999) DNA methylation is the primary silencing mechanism for a set of germ line- and tumor-specific genes with a CpG-rich promoter. Mol Cell Biol 19:7327–7335

Depa-Martynow M, Kempisty B, Lianeri M, Jagodzinski PP, Jedrzejczak P (2007) Association between fertilin beta, protamines 1 and 2 and spermatid-specific linker histone H1-like protein mRNA levels, fertilization ability of human spermatozoa, and quality of preimplantation embryos. Folia Histochem Cytobiol 45(Suppl 1):S79–S85

Dhodapkar MV, Osman K, Teruya-Feldstein J et al (2003) Expression of cancer/testis (CT) antigens MAGE-A1, MAGE-A3, MAGE-A4, CT-7, and NY-ESO-1 in malignant gammopathies is heterogeneous and correlates with site, stage and risk status of disease. Cancer Immun 3:9

Duan Z, Duan Y, Lamendola DE et al (2003) Overexpression of MAGE/GAGE genes in paclitaxel/doxorubicin-resistant human cancer cell lines. Clin Cancer Res 9:2778–2785

Eichmuller S, Usener D, Thiel D, Schadendorf D (2003) Tumor-specific antigens in cutaneous T-cell lymphoma: expression and sero-reactivity. Int J Cancer 104:482–487

Frank C, Hundemer M, Ho AD, Goldschmidt H, Witzens-Harig M (2008) Cellular immune responses against the cancer-testis antigen SPAN-XB in healthy donors and patients with multiple myeloma. Leuk Lymphoma 49:779–785

Fukuyama T, Hanagiri T, Takenoyama M et al (2006) Identification of a new cancer/germline gene, KK-LC-1, encoding an antigen recognized by autologous CTL induced on human lung adenocarcinoma. Cancer Res 66:4922–4928

Gaugler B, Van den Eynde B, van der Bruggen P et al (1994) Human gene MAGE-3 codes for an antigen recognized on a melanoma by autologous cytolytic T lymphocytes. J Exp Med 179:921–930

Gedye C, Quirk J, Browning J et al (2009) Cancer/testis antigens can be immunological targets in clonogenic CD133(+) melanoma cells. Cancer Immunol Immunother 58(10):1635–1646

Gnjatic S, Altorki NK, Tang DN et al (2009) NY-ESO-1 DNA vaccine induces T-cell responses that are suppressed by regulatory T cells. Clin Cancer Res 15:2130–2139

Goydos JS, Patel M, Shih W (2001) NY-ESO-1 and CTp11 expression may correlate with stage of progression in melanoma. J Surg Res 98:76–80

Gure AO, Stockert E, Arden KC et al (2000) CT10: a new cancer-testis (CT) antigen homologous to CT7 and the MAGE family, identified by representational-difference analysis. Int J Cancer 85:726–732

Gure AO, Chua R, Williamson B et al (2005) Cancer-testis genes are coordinately expressed and are markers of poor outcome in non-small cell lung cancer. Clin Cancer Res 11:8055–8062

Hamer G, Gell K, Kouznetsova A, Novak I, Benavente R, Hoog C (2006) Characterization of a novel meiosis-specific protein within the central element of the synaptonemal complex. J Cell Sci 119:4025–4032

Harada N, Hoshiai K, Takahashi Y et al (2008) Preclinical safety pharmacology study of a novel protein-based cancer vaccine CHP-NY-ESO-1. Kobe J Med Sci 54:E23–E34

Heidebrecht HJ, Claviez A, Kruse ML et al (2006) Characterization and expression of CT45 in Hodgkin's lymphoma. Clin Cancer Res 12:4804–4811

Hoffmann MJ, Schulz WA (2005) Causes and consequences of DNA hypomethylation in human cancer. Biochem Cell Biol 83:296–321

Hofmann O, Caballero OL, Stevenson BJ et al (2008) Genome-wide analysis of cancer/testis gene expression. Proc Natl Acad Sci U S A 105:20422–20427

Hunder NN, Wallen H, Cao J et al (2008) Treatment of metastatic melanoma with autologous CD4+ T cells against NY-ESO-1. N Engl J Med 358:2698–2703

Jager E, Stockert E, Zidianakis Z et al (1999) Humoral immune responses of cancer patients against "Cancer-Testis" antigen NY-ESO-1: correlation with clinical events. Int J Cancer 84:506–510

Jager D, Stockert E, Gure AO et al (2001) Identification of a tissue-specific putative transcription factor in breast tissue by serological screening of a breast cancer library. Cancer Res 61:2055–2061

Jager E, Karbach J, Gnjatic S et al (2006) Recombinant vaccinia/fowlpox NY-ESO-1 vaccines induce both humoral and cellular NY-ESO-1-specific immune responses in cancer patients. Proc Natl Acad Sci U S A 103:14453–14458

Jungbluth AA, Antonescu CR, Busam KJ et al (2001) Monophasic and biphasic synovial sarcomas abundantly express cancer/testis antigen NY-ESO-1 but not MAGE-A1 or CT7. Int J Cancer 94:252–256

Jungbluth AA, Ely S, DiLiberto M et al (2005) The cancer-testis antigens CT7 (MAGE-C1) and MAGE-A3/6 are commonly expressed in multiple myeloma and correlate with plasma-cell proliferation. Blood 106:167–174

Kawakami Y, Robbins PF, Wang RF, Parkhurst M, Kang X, Rosenberg SA (1998) The use of melanosomal proteins in the immunotherapy of melanoma. J Immunother 21:237–246

Kim J, Reber HA, Hines OJ et al (2006) The clinical significance of MAGEA3 expression in pancreatic cancer. Int J Cancer 118:2269–2275

Kurashige T, Noguchi Y, Saika T et al (2001) Ny-ESO-1 expression and immunogenicity associated with transitional cell carcinoma: correlation with tumor grade. Cancer Res 61:4671–4674

Lee SY, Obata Y, Yoshida M et al (2003) Immunomic analysis of human sarcoma. Proc Natl Acad Sci U S A 100:2651–2656

Lee SY, Williamson B, Caballero OL et al (2004) Identification of the gonad-specific anion transporter SLCO6A1 as a cancer/testis (CT) antigen expressed in human lung cancer. Cancer Immun 4:13

Lehmann F LJ, Gaulis S, Gruselle O, Brichard V. Clinical response to the MAGE-A3 immunotherapeutic in metastatic melanoma patients is associated with a specific gene profile present prior to treatment. XVIth Meeting in the cancer research institute international cancer immunotherapy symposium series and the 2008 meeting of the cancer vaccine consortium, New York City, 2008, S25.

Lethe B, Lucas S, Michaux L et al (1998) LAGE-1, a new gene with tumor specificity. Int J Cancer 76:903–908

Li M, Yuan YH, Han Y et al (2005) Expression profile of cancer-testis genes in 121 human colorectal cancer tissue and adjacent normal tissue. Clin Cancer Res 11:1809–1814

Liggins AP, Brown PJ, Asker K, Pulford K, Banham AH (2004) A novel diffuse large B-cell lymphoma-associated cancer testis antigen encoding a PAS domain protein. Br J Cancer 91:141–149

Liu W, Cheng S, Asa SL, Ezzat S (2008) The melanoma-associated antigen A3 mediates fibronectin-controlled cancer progression and metastasis. Cancer Res 68:8104–8112

Lucas S, De Smet C, Arden KC et al (1998) Identification of a new MAGE gene with tumor-specific expression by representational difference analysis. Cancer Res 58:743–752

Marchand M, van Baren N, Weynants P et al (1999) Tumor regressions observed in patients with metastatic melanoma treated with an antigenic peptide encoded by gene MAGE-3 and presented by HLA-A1. Int J Cancer 80:219–230

Martelange V, De Smet C, De Plaen E, Lurquin C, Boon T (2000) Identification on a human sarcoma of two new genes with tumor-specific expression. Cancer Res 60:3848–3855

Martinez A, Olarte I, Mergold MA et al (2007) mRNA expression of MAGE-A3 gene in leukemia cells. Leuk Res 31:33–37

Meuwissen RL, Meerts I, Hoovers JM, Leschot NJ, Heyting C (1997) Human synaptonemal complex protein 1 (SCP1): isolation and characterization of the cDNA and chromosomal localization of the gene. Genomics 39:377–384

Mischo A, Kubuschok B, Ertan K et al (2006) Prospective study on the expression of cancer testis genes and antibody responses in 100 consecutive patients with primary breast cancer. Int J Cancer 118:696–703

Monte M, Simonatto M, Peche LY et al (2006) MAGE-A tumor antigens target p53 transactivation function through histone deacetylase recruitment and confer resistance to chemotherapeutic agents. Proc Natl Acad Sci U S A 103:11160–11165

Mueller JL, Mahadevaiah SK, Park PJ, Warburton PE, Page DC, Turner JM (2008) The mouse X chromosome is enriched for multicopy testis genes showing postmeiotic expression. Nat Genet 40:794–799

Nagao T, Higashitsuji H, Nonoguchi K et al (2003) MAGE-A4 interacts with the liver oncoprotein gankyrin and suppresses its tumorigenic activity. J Biol Chem 278:10668–10674

Napoletano C, Bellati F, Tarquini E et al (2008) MAGE-A and NY-ESO-1 expression in cervical cancer: prognostic factors and effects of chemotherapy. Am J Obstet Gynecol 198:99e1–99e7

Nicholaou T, Ebert LM, Davis ID et al (2009) Regulatory T-cell-mediated attenuation of T-cell responses to the NY-ESO-1 ISCOMATRIX vaccine in patients with advanced malignant melanoma. Clin Cancer Res 15:2166–2173

Nishikawa H, Sato E, Briones G et al (2006) In vivo antigen delivery by a Salmonella typhimurium type III secretion system for therapeutic cancer vaccines. J Clin Invest 116:1946–1954

Obata Y, Takahashi T, Tamaki H et al (1999) Identification of Cancer Antigens in Breast Cancer by the SEREX Expression Cloning Method. Breast Cancer 6:305–311

Obata Y, Takahashi T, Sakamoto J et al (2000) SEREX analysis of gastric cancer antigens. Cancer Chemother Pharmacol 46(Suppl):S37–S42

Odunsi K, Qian F, Matsuzaki J et al (2007) Vaccination with an NY-ESO-1 peptide of HLA class I/II specificities induces integrated humoral and T cell responses in ovarian cancer. Proc Natl Acad Sci U S A 104:12837–12842

Oi S, Natsume A, Ito M et al (2009) Synergistic induction of NY-ESO-1 antigen expression by a novel histone deacetylase inhibitor, valproic acid, with 5-aza-2'-deoxycytidine in glioma cells. J Neurooncol 92:15–22

Old LJ (2001) Cancer/testis (CT) antigens - a new link between gametogenesis and cancer. Cancer Immun 1:1

Old LJ, Chen YT (1998) New paths in human cancer serology. J Exp Med 187:1163–1167

Ono T, Kurashige T, Harada N et al (2001) Identification of proacrosin binding protein sp32 precursor as a human cancer/testis antigen. Proc Natl Acad Sci U S A 98:3282–3287

Park S, Lim Y, Lee D et al (2003) Identification and characterization of a novel cancer/testis antigen gene CAGE-1. Biochim Biophys Acta 1625:173–182

Peikert T, Specks U, Farver C, Erzurum SC, Comhair SA (2006) Melanoma antigen A4 is expressed in non-small cell lung cancers and promotes apoptosis. Cancer Res 66:4693–4700

Perez D, Herrmann T, Jungbluth AA et al (2008) Cancer testis antigen expression in gastrointestinal stromal tumors: new markers for early recurrence. Int J Cancer 123:1551–1555

Riener MO, Wild PJ, Soll C et al (2009) Frequent expression of the novel cancer testis antigen MAGE-C2/CT-10 in hepatocellular carcinoma. Int J Cancer 124:352–357

Robert M, Gagnon C (1999) Semenogelin I: a coagulum forming, multifunctional seminal vesicle protein. Cell Mol Life Sci 55:944–960

Ross MT, Grafham DV, Coffey AJ et al (2005) The DNA sequence of the human X chromosome. Nature 434:325–337

Sahin U, Tureci O, Schmitt H et al (1995) Human neoplasms elicit multiple specific immune responses in the autologous host. Proc Natl Acad Sci U S A 92:11810–11813

Sahin U, Tureci O, Pfreundschuh M (1997) Serological identification of human tumor antigens. Curr Opin Immunol 9:709–716

Scanlan MJ, Gordan JD, Williamson B et al (1999) Antigens recognized by autologous antibody in patients with renal-cell carcinoma. Int J Cancer 83:456–464

Scanlan MJ, Altorki NK, Gure AO et al (2000) Expression of cancer-testis antigens in lung cancer: definition of bromodomain testis-specific gene (BRDT) as a new CT gene, CT9. Cancer Lett 150:155–164

Sharma P, Gnjatic S, Jungbluth AA et al (2003) Frequency of NY-ESO-1 and LAGE-1 expression in bladder cancer and evidence of a new NY-ESO-1 T-cell epitope in a patient with bladder cancer. Cancer Immun 3:19

Sigalotti L, Fratta E, Coral S et al (2004) Intratumor heterogeneity of cancer/testis antigens expression in human cutaneous melanoma is methylation-regulated and functionally reverted by 5-aza-2'-deoxycytidine. Cancer Res 64:9167–9171

Silva WA Jr, Gnjatic S, Ritter E et al (2007) PLAC1, a trophoblast-specific cell surface protein, is expressed in a range of human tumors and elicits spontaneous antibody responses. Cancer Immun 7:18

Simpson AJ, Caballero OL, Jungbluth A, Chen YT, Old LJ (2005) Cancer/testis antigens, gametogenesis and cancer. Nat Rev Cancer 5:615–625

Taylor BJ, Reiman T, Pittman JA et al (2005) SSX cancer testis antigens are expressed in most multiple myeloma patients: co-expression of SSX1, 2, 4, and 5 correlates with adverse prognosis and high frequencies of SSX-positive PCs. J Immunother 28:564–575

Tureci O, Sahin U, Schobert I et al (1996) The SSX-2 gene, which is involved in the t(X;18) translocation of synovial sarcomas, codes for the human tumor antigen HOM-MEL-40. Cancer Res 56:4766–4772

Tureci O, Sahin U, Zwick C, Koslowski M, Seitz G, Pfreundschuh M (1998) Identification of a meiosis-specific protein as a member of the class of cancer/testis antigens. Proc Natl Acad Sci U S A 95:5211–5216

Valmori D, Souleimanian NE, Tosello V et al (2007) Vaccination with NY-ESO-1 protein and CpG in Montanide induces integrated antibody/Th1 responses and CD8 T cells through cross-priming. Proc Natl Acad Sci U S A 104:8947–8952

Van den Eynde B, Peeters O, De Backer O, Gaugler B, Lucas S, Boon T (1995) A new family of genes coding for an antigen recognized by autologous cytolytic T lymphocytes on a human melanoma. J Exp Med 182:689–698

van der Bruggen P, Traversari C, Chomez P et al (1991) A gene encoding an antigen recognized by cytolytic T lymphocytes on a human melanoma. Science 254:1643–1647

Vatolin S, Abdullaev Z, Pack SD et al (2005) Conditional expression of the CTCF-paralogous transcriptional factor BORIS in normal cells results in demethylation and derepression of MAGE-A1 and reactivation of other cancer-testis genes. Cancer Res 65:7751–7762

Velazquez EF, Jungbluth AA, Yancovitz M et al (2007) Expression of the cancer/testis antigen NY-ESO-1 in primary and metastatic malignant melanoma (MM)–correlation with prognostic factors. Cancer Immun 7:11

Weber J, Salgaller M, Samid D et al (1994) Expression of the MAGE-1 tumor antigen is up-regulated by the demethylating agent 5-aza-2'-deoxycytidine. Cancer Res 54:1766–1771

Xing Q, Pang XW, Peng JR et al (2008) Identification of new cytotoxic T-lymphocyte epitopes from cancer testis antigen HCA587. Biochem Biophys Res Commun 372:331–335

Yakirevich E, Sabo E, Lavie O, Mazareb S, Spagnoli GC, Resnick MB (2003) Expression of the MAGE-A4 and NY-ESO-1 cancer-testis antigens in serous ovarian neoplasms. Clin Cancer Res 9:6453–6460

Yamada A, Kataoka A, Shichijo S et al (1995) Expression of MAGE-1, MAGE-2, MAGE-3/-6 and MAGE-4a/-4b genes in ovarian tumors. Int J Cancer 64:388–393

Yang B, O'Herrin SM, Wu J et al (2007) MAGE-A, mMage-b, and MAGE-C proteins form complexes with KAP1 and suppress p53-dependent apoptosis in MAGE-positive cell lines. Cancer Res 67:9954–9962

Yuan J, Gnjatic S, Li H et al (2008) CTLA-4 blockade enhances polyfunctional NY-ESO-1 specific T cell responses in metastatic melanoma patients with clinical benefit. Proc Natl Acad Sci U S A 105:20410–20415

Zhao H, Lee WH, Shen JH, Li H, Zhang Y (2008) Identification of novel semenogelin I-derived antimicrobial peptide from liquefied human seminal plasma. Peptides 29:505–511

Zhu X, Asa SL, Ezzat S (2008) Fibroblast growth factor 2 and estrogen control the balance of histone 3 modifications targeting MAGE-A3 in pituitary neoplasia. Clin Cancer Res 14:1984–1996

Chapter 21
Tumor Antigens and Immune Regulation in Cancer Immunotherapy

Rong-Fu Wang and Helen Y. Wang

1 Introduction

Host immune system plays an essential role in immunosurveillance and destruction of cancer cells in knockout mice which were deficient of important immune components (Shankaran et al. 2001). T-cell-mediated antitumor immunity has been demonstrated in murine tumor models by adoptive transfer experiments (Greenberg 1991); by contrast, depletion of T cells promotes tumor development in chemical-induced tumor models (Koebel et al. 2007). Similar strategies have been used to treat human cancer such as melanoma and renal carcinoma with various degrees of tumor regression as well as virus-induced tumors (Rosenberg 2001; Dudley et al. 2002). These animal experiments and clinical trials suggest the importance of T-cell-mediated antitumor immunity in controlling and destroying tumor cells. Using tumor-reactive T cells, we and other groups have identified immunogenic tumor antigens from many different types of cancer. These studies increase our understanding of antigen-specific tumor immunity and provide opportunity for the development of effective antigen-specific cancer therapy. However, clinical studies using molecularly defined tumor antigens have shown that antigen-specific T-cell responses are evident after vaccination, but overall immune responses are too weak and transient to eradicate tumor. To enhance antitumor immunity, it is necessary to induce both $CD4^+$ and $CD8^+$ T-cell responses against cancer cells in patients (Toes et al. 1999; Wang 2001). Recent studies indicate that these tumor antigens may induce $CD4^+$ regulator T (Treg) cells and IL-17-producing T (Th17) cells (Wang and Wang 2007; Miyahara et al. 2008). Indeed, tumor antigen-specific Treg cells as well as other Treg cells accumulate at tumor sites, inducing immune tolerance (Wang et al. 2004; Peng et al. 2007). Thus, immune suppression is one of the major

R.-F. Wang (✉) • H.Y. Wang
Department of Pathology and Immunology and Center for Cell and Gene Theraphy,
Baylor College of Medicine, Houston, TX 77030, USA
e-mail: rongfuw@bcm.edu

obstacles for the development of effective cancer vaccines. How to overcome such immune suppression is a fundamentally important research area in the field of cancer immunology. This chapter will summarize the current status of tumor antigen discovery, immune regulation, in particular immune suppression and inflammation in cancer, and future direction in cancer immunotherapy.

2 MHC Class I-Restricted Tumor Antigens and Mechanisms for Their Generation and Presentation

Because $CD8^+$ T cells can directly kill tumor cells, much attention has been paid to the role of $CD8^+$ T cells in the immunotherapy of cancer. Using tumor-reactive $CD8^+$ T cells derived from peripheral blood mononuclear cells (PBMCs) or TILs that exhibit antitumor activity, many MHC class I-restricted tumor antigens have been identified (Boon et al. 1994; Wang and Rosenberg 1999). These tumor antigens can be divided into several different classes based on the gene expression patterns of most antigens identified from melanoma (Table 21.1). The tissue-specific differentiation antigens, such as tyrosinase, MART-1, gp100, TRP-1/gp75, and TRP-2, are highly expressed in melanoma as well as normal melanocytes (Brichard et al. 1993; Kawakami et al. 1994; Wang et al. 1996a). The second class of tumor antigen is tumor-specific shared antigens such as MAGE-1 and NY-ESO-1. These tumor antigens are expressed in a wide variety of tumors such as breast cancer, prostate cancer, and lung cancer (Van der Bruggen et al. 1991; Jager et al. 1998; Wang et al. 1998a). The expression of these products is limited to cancer cells and normal testis. Thus, these tumor antigens are also called cancer-testis (CT) antigens. Tumor-specific unique or mutated antigens such as CDK4, β-catenin, and caspase 8 have also been described (Wolfel et al. 1995; Robbins et al. 1996; Mandruzzato et al. 1997).

Identification of tumor antigens and their corresponding T-cell epitopes has led to the discovery of several mechanisms by which MHC class I-restricted peptides are generated for T-cell recognition. T-cell epitopes can be generated at levels of transcription/splicing, translation or protein degradation or different mechanisms.

Transcriptional/splicing control: Several T-cell epitopes have been identified from aberrant mRNA or the intron of incompletely spliced mRNA. For example, a cryptic promoter present within one of the introns of the N-acetylglucosaminyltransferase V (GnT-V) gene appears to be responsible for the generation of an aberrant transcript, which translates a polypeptide with 74 amino acids (Guilloux et al. 1996). Similarly, gp100 and TRP-2 epitopes recognized by T cells have been identified from introns of an incomplete splicing form of the corresponding RNA (Robbins et al. 1997; Lupetti et al. 1998). These results indicate that cryptic promoters or aberrant splicing events can result in the translation of the intronic sequences of mRNA, thus generating T-cell epitopes for T-cell recognition (Table 21.2).

Translational control: T-cell epitopes may also be generated by the translation of an alternative open read frame of a gene. A T-cell epitope encoded by TRP-1/gp75

Table 21.1 Tumor antigens recognized by CD4+ and CD8+ T cells

Antigens	MHC class I restrictions	Peptide epitopes	References
Tissue-specific antigens			
gp100	A2	KTWGQYWQV	Bakker et al. (1994)
	A2	AMLGTHTMEV	Tsai et al. (1997)
	A2	MLGTHTMEV	Tsai et al. (1997)
	A2	SLADTNSLAV	Tsai et al. (1997)
	A2	ITDQVPFSV	Kawakami et al. (1995)
	A2	LLDGTATLRL	Kawakami et al. (1994)
	A2	YLEPGPVTA	Cox et al. (1994)
	A2	VLYRYGSFSV	Kawakami et al. (1995)
	A2	RLMKQDFSV	Kawakami et al. (1998)
	A2	RLPRIFCSC	Kawakami et al. (1998)
	A3	LIYRRRLMK	Kawakami et al. (1998)
	A3	ALNFPGSQK	Kawashima et al. (1998)
	A3	SLIYRRRLMK	Kawashima et al. (1998)
	A3	ALLAVGATK	Skipper et al. (1996)
	A24	VYFFLPDHL	Robbins et al. (1997)
	A*6801	HTMEVTVYHR	Sensi et al. (2002)
	B*3501	VPLDCVLYRY	Benlalam et al. (2003)
	Cw8	SNDGPTLI	Castelli et al. (1999)
MART-1/Melan-A	A2	AAGIGILTV	Coulie et al. (1994)
	A2	ILTVILGVL	Castelli et al. (1995)
	A2	EAAGIGILTV	Schneider et al. (1998)
	B45	AEEAAGIGIL	Schneider et al. (1998)
gp75/TRP-1	A31	MSLQRQFLR	Wang et al. (1996b)
TRP-2	A2	SVYDFFVWL	Parkhurst et al. (1998)
	A2	TLDSQVMSL	Noppen et al. (2000)
	A31	LLGPGRPYR	Wang et al. (1996a)
	A33	LLGPGRPYR	Wang et al. (1998b)
	A68	EVISCKLIKR	Lupetti et al. (1998)
	Cw8	ANDPIFVVL	Castelli et al. (1999)
Tyrosinase	A1	KCDICTDEY	Kittlesen et al. (1998)
	A1	SSDYVIPIGTY	Kawakami et al. (1998)
	A2	YMDGTMSQV	Wolfel et al. (1994)
	A2	MLLAVLYCL	Wolfel et al. (1994)
	A24	AFLPWHRLF	Kang et al. (1995)
	B44	SEIWRDIDF	Brichard et al. (1996)
	B*3501	TPRLPSSADVEF	Benlalam et al. (2003)
Tumor-specific shared antigens			
BAGE	Cw16	AARAVFLAL	Boel et al. (1995)
CAMEL	A2	MLMAQEALAFL	(Aarnoudse et al. (1999)

(continued)

Table 21.1 (continued)

Antigens	MHC class I restrictions	Peptide epitopes	References
MAGE-A1	A1	EADPTGHSY	Traversari et al. (1992)
	A3	SLFRAVITK	Chaux et al. (1999a)
	A24	NYKHCFPEI	Fujie et al. (1999)
	A28	EVYDGREHSA	Chaux et al. (1999a)
	B37	REPVTKAEML	Tanzarella et al. (1999)
	B53	DPARYEFLW	Chaux et al. (1999a)
	Cw2	SAFPTTINF	Chaux et al. (1999a)
	Cw3	SAYGEPRKL	Chaux et al. (1999a)
	Cw16	SAYGEPRKL	Van der Bruggen et al. (1994a)
MAGE-A2	A2	KMVELVHFL	Visseren et al. (1997)
	A2	YLQLVFGIEV	Visseren et al. (1997)
	A24	EYLQLVFGI	Tahara et al. (1999)
	B37	REPVTKAEML	Tanzarella et al. (1999)
MAGE-A3	A1	EADPIGHLY	Gaugler et al. (1994)
	A2	FLWGPRALV	Van der Bruggen et al. (1994b)
	A24	TFPDLESEF	Oiso et al. (1999)
	A24	IMPKAGLLI	Tanaka et al. (1997)
	B44	MEVDPIGHLY	Herman et al. (1996)
	B52	WQYFFPVIF	Russo et al. (2000)
	B37	REPVTKAEML	Tanzarella et al. (1999)
	B*3501	EVDPIGHLY	Benlalam et al. (2003)
MAGE-A4	A2	GVYDGREHTV	Duffour et al. (1999)
MAGE-A6	A34	MVKISGGPR	Zorn and Hercend (1999)
	B37	REPVTKAEML	Tanzarella et al. (1999)
	B*3501	EVDPIGHVY	Benlalam et al. (2003)
MAGE-A10	A2	GLYDGMEHL	Huang et al. (1999)
MAGE-A12	Cw7	VRIGHLYIL	Panelli et al. (2000)
NY-ESO-1	A2	SLLMWITQCFL	Jager et al. (1998)
	A2	SLLMWITQC	Jager et al. (1998)
	A2	QLSLLMWIT	Jager et al. (1998)
	A31	ASGPGGGAPR	Wang et al. (1998a)
	B*3501	MPFATPMEA	Benlalam et al. (2003)
SSX-2	A2	KASEKIFYV	Ayyoub et al. (2002)
Tumor-specific unique antigens			
β-Catenin	A24 S	YLDSGIHF	Robbins et al. (1996)
Caspase-8	B35	FPSDSWCYF	Mandruzzato et al. (1997)
DK-4	A2	ACDPHSGHFV	Wolfel et al. (1995)

gene is translated from gp75 mRNA by the use of an alternative reading frame (Wang et al. 1996b). An antigenic peptide recognized by TIL586 could not be found from peptides derived from the primary reading frame of gp75. Interestingly, one peptide MSLQRQFLR derived from ORF3 was capable of stimulating cytokine release from TIL586 (Wang et al. 1996b). This represented the first example that

Table 21.2 Molecular mechanisms for generating T-cell epitopes

Antigens	Restrictions	Peptide epitopes	Mechanisms	References
gp75/TRP-1	A31	MSLQRQFLR	Alternative ORFs	Wang et al. (1996b)
NY-ESO-1	A31	AAQERRVPR	Alternative ORFs	Wang et al. (1998a)
	A31	LAAQERRVPR	Alternative ORFs	Wang et al. (1998a)
CAMEL/LAGE	A2	MLMAQEALAFL	Alternative ORFs	Aarnoudse et al. (1999)
M-CSF	B35	LPAVVGLSPGEQEY	Alternative ORFs	Probst-Kepper et al. (2001)
BING-4	A2	MCQWGRLWQL	Alternative ORFs	Rosenberg et al. (2002)
GnT-V	A2	VLPDVFIRC	Intronic sequence	Guilloux et al. (1996)
AIM-2	A1	RSDSGQQARY	Intronic sequence	Harada et al. (2001)
TRP-2/INT2	A68	EVISCKLIKR	Intronic sequence	Lupetti et al. (1998)
TRP-2-6b	A2	ATTNILEHY	Alternatively splicing	Khong and Rosenberg (2002)
gp100	A24	VYFFLPDHL	Incompletely splicing	Robbins et al. (1997)
OGT	A2	SLYKFSPFPL	Frameshift	Ripberger et al. (2003)
TGFαRII	A2	RLSSCVPVA	Frameshift	Linnebacher et al. (2001)
TGFβRII	A24	RLSSCVPVA	Frameshift	Saeterdal et al. (2001)
FGF5	A3	NTYASPRFK	Protein splicing	Hanada et al. (2004)
gp100	A32	RTKQLYPEW	Protein splicing	Vigneron et al. (2004)
SP110	A3	SLPRGTSTPK	Protein splicing	Warren et al. (2006)

human cancer antigens can be generated from an alternative open reading frame. Similarly, we found that a T-cell epitope of tumor antigen NY-ESO-1 is generated from different open reading frames. Some TIL586 CTL clones recognized antigenic peptides derived from the primary ORF (180 amino acids) of NY-ESO-1, while other CTL clones did not recognize peptides from the NY-ESO-1 protein, but still recognized COS-7 cells transfected with the NY-ESO-1 cDNA (Wang et al. 1998a). Further experiments revealed that NY-ESO-1 mRNA can be translated into two gene products: a 180 amino acid protein translated from the primary ORF and a 58 amino acid polypeptide translated from ORF2. Although many CTL epitopes have been identified from the first gene product (180 amino acids), one T-cell epitope is identified from the second gene product (58 amino acids) encoded by ORF2 (Wang et al. 1998a). Similar to NY-ESO-1, LAGE-1, which shares 94% nucleotide and 87% amino acid homology to NY-ESO-1 (Lethe et al. 1998), also encodes T-cell epitope from the gene product translated from an alternative ORF2 of LAGE-1 (Aarnoudse et al. 1999; Rimoldi et al. 2000). Despite the fact that many examples of the use of alternative ORFs have been documented in the literature, the mechanisms of translational control of alternative open reading frame and biological significance of these gene products are still not clear.

Peptide splicing: Several examples have been reported for T-cell epitopes that are generated from different regions of the same protein by peptide splicing. For example, a T-cell epitope of FGF-5 recognized by T cells is generated by protein splicing. The FGF-5 polypeptide segment is excised and followed by ligation of the newly liberated carboxy-terminal and amino-terminal residues (Hanada et al. 2004). Similarly, a nonameric peptide that comprises two noncontiguous segments of melanocytic glycoprotein gp100 is generated by the excision of four amino acids and splicing of the fragments (Vigneron et al. 2004). In another study, the antigenic peptide comprises two noncontiguous SP110 peptide segments spliced together in reverse order. The antigenic peptide could be produced in vitro by the incubation of precursor peptides with highly purified 20S proteasomes (Warren et al. 2006). These studies suggest that amino acids in different regions of a protein can be spliced and ligated together to constitute a new T-cell epitope for T-cell recognition.

Proteolytic processing: It is well known that T-cell peptides are generated from the degradation of intracellular proteins by the 20S proteasome (Rock and Goldberg 1999). However, the composition of proteasome complex can be changed. Upon stimulation of cells with interferon gamma, three additional proteasome subunits (LMP2, LMP7, and MECL1) replace their constitutive homologs in newly formed proteasomes (Baumeister et al. 1998; Tanaka and Kasahara 1998). The incorporation of these inducible subunits in the so-called immunoproteasome changes the cleavage profiles of antigenic peptides (Tanaka and Kasahara 1998; Groettrup and Schmidtke 1999), thus leading to the generation of new epitopes, while some epitopes will be destroyed. Several such T-cell peptides have been identified and can be modulated by the immunoproteasome (Morel et al. 2000).

Taken together, these studies indicate that T-cell epitopes can be generated by many different mechanisms at different levels. It is increasingly clear that immune system samples or checks not only the conventional protein products but also alternative gene products, splicing peptides, and cryptic peptides as sources for T-cell epitopes.

3 Clinical Studies Using Molecularly Defined Tumor Antigens and Potential Problems

The majority of MHC class I-restricted tumor antigens identified to date are nonmutated self-proteins, which tend to elicit self-reactive T-cell responses and result in the potential development of autoimmune diseases (Boon et al. 1994; Wang and Rosenberg 1999). Clinical studies using these self-antigens as vaccines have showed some evidence for a therapeutic effect on tumor growth inhibition and regression (Jager et al. 1996; Rosenberg et al. 1998; Nestle et al. 1998), suggesting that immunization of patients with self-antigens can generate antitumor immunity, leading to tumor regression. However, the objective complete clinical responses were sporadic, even though CTL reactivity was clearly evident after one round of in vitro stimulation of PBMC from vaccinated patients (Rosenberg et al. 1998). Although DC-based immunotherapy represents a promising approach (Banchereau and Steinman 1998), clinical studies using mature DCs pulsed with tumor-associated self-antigens or peptides showed improved antitumor immunity, potent immune responses were only observed in a limited number of patients (Nestle et al. 1998; Bellone et al. 2000). These studies demonstrate the potential and feasibility of immunotherapy of cancer using molecularly identified tumor antigens, the overall immune responses, however, are still not sufficient to elicit therapeutic immunity against cancer (Rosenberg et al. 2004). Although there are many factors contributing to this failure, there are two major ones. The first one is that the current vaccine strategies focusing only on CD8$^+$ T cells can not generate long and long-lasting therapeutic immunity because optimal immunity requires both CD4$^+$ and CD8$^+$ T-cell responses. CD4$^+$ Th effector cells are critical for the subsequent expansion of memory CD8$^+$ T cells (Janssen et al. 2003), and are required for optimal antitumor immunity. The second major factor is the presence of immune suppression at tumor sites. One of the dominant immune suppressions is mediated by CD4$^+$ regulatory T (Treg) cells. The presence of CD4$^+$ Treg cells may significantly suppress immune responses, thus inducing immune tolerance at tumor sites.

4 Subsets of CD4$^+$ T Cells and Their Antigen Specificity

A growing body of evidence suggests that CD4$^+$ Th cells play a central role in initiating and maintaining immune responses against cancer (Wang 2001). Recent studies further demonstrate that CD4$^+$ T cells can be differentiated into different subsets of CD4$^+$ T cells – Th1, Th2, Th17, Tfth, and Treg. Treg cells significantly suppress immune responses, thus inducing immune tolerance at tumor sites, while Th17 cells have been linked to autoimmune diseases and cancer (Weaver et al. 2006; Langowski et al. 2006).

Th1 and Th2 cells: CD4$^+$ Th cells can be divided into Th1 and Th2 T cells based on their cytokine secretion profiles and transcriptional factors. CD4$^+$ Th1 cells secrete cytokines, such as IL-2 and IFN-γ, and express T-bet transcriptional factor. On the other hand, CD4$^+$ Th2 cells secrete IL-4, IL-5 and, IL-13, express a GATA-3 transcriptional factor and activate B cells to become antibody-secreting plasma cells (Weaver et al. 2006). Accumulating evidence indicates that Th1 immune response promotes or enhances antitumor immunity, while Th2-biased immune response inhibits antitumor immunity and promotes tumor growth.

Treg cells: CD4$^+$ Treg cells have been identified as a small (5–6%) subset in the total CD4$^+$ T-cell population. Expression of CD25 on T cells is used as a marker of Treg cells, but this expression is not necessarily associated with Treg cell function, in that it is also expressed by activated, nonregulatory effector lymphocytes. Foxp3 has been identified as a relatively specific marker of CD4$^+$ Treg cells (Wang et al. 2004; Hori et al. 2003). These Treg cells do not secrete IL-2 but express Foxp3 as a key regulator. Recent studies demonstrate an elevated proportion of CD4$^+$ CD25$^+$ Treg cells in the total CD4$^+$ T-cell population of several different human cancers, including lung, breast, and ovarian tumors (Woo et al. 2001).

Th17 cells: IL-17-producing T (Th17) cells are a distinct lineage of $CD4^+$ Th subsets, secreting a unique set of cytokines IL-17, IL-21, and IL-22 (Harrington et al. 2005). TGF-β, IL-6, and IL-23 are critical factors for Th17 cell differentiation (Veldhoen et al. 2006). The critical transcriptional factors for Th17 cells have been identified as RORγt and RORα (Ivanov et al. 2006). Because TGF-β is an important factor in the development and conversion of Treg cells, it may play a critical role in dictating the fate of $CD4^+$ T cells to become either Treg cells or Th17 cells. The transcriptional factor Foxp3 is upregulated in the presence of TGF-β, but inhibited by IL-6 through Stat3. In addition, IL-21 cooperates with TGF-β to promote the generation of Th17 cells and inhibit Treg cell differentiation (Korn et al. 2007). Interestingly, retinoic acid (RA) is capable of inhibiting the IL-6-driven induction of pro-inflammatory Th17 cells and promoting anti-inflammatory Treg differentiation (Mucida et al. 2007), while the ligands of aryl hydrocarbon receptor (AHR) enhance Th17 cell differentiation (Veldhoen et al. 2008). Infection of invading pathogens (bacteria and viruses) and danger signal stimulators, such as uric acid and ATP, can activate signaling pathways for the production of inflammatory cytokines, including IL-1 and IL-6 (Sutterwala et al. 2006). ATP has recently been shown to drive Th17 cell differentiation by activating DCs to secrete IL-6 and IL-23 (Atarashi et al. 2008). Despite the important role of Th17 cells in inflammation-mediated autoimmune diseases, their role in tumor development and progression is limited (Miyahara et al. 2008; Muranski et al. 2008).

5 Tumor Antigens Recognized by $CD4^+$ Th, Treg Cells or Both

Given the importance of $CD4^+$ T cells in antitumor immunity, it is critical to identify MHC class II-restricted tumor antigens capable of stimulating $CD4^+$ T cells. To facilitate the identification of MHC class II tumor antigens, we have developed genetic targeting expression (GTE) system (Wang and Rosenberg 1999; Wang et al. 1999a). The GTE system comprises two essential components: (1) generation of a highly transfectable HEK293IMDR cell line, and (2) the creation of an Ii fusion library from tumor cells such that the Ii fusion proteins are targeted to the endosomal/lysosomal compartment for efficient antigen processing and presentation for T-cell recognition (Wang and Rosenberg 1999; Wang et al. 1999a). Using this system, many tumor antigens have been identified, as described below.

Tumor antigens recognized by $CD4^+$ Th cells: Using tumor-reactive T cells, we screened an Ii-fusion expression library and identified a fusion gene product LDFP recognized by HLA-DR1-restricted $CD4^+$TIL. DNA sequencing analysis indicates that LDFP is generated by fusing a low-density-lipid receptor (LDLR) gene at the 5′ end to a GDP-L-Fucose:β-D-Galactoside 2-α-L-Fucosyltransferase (FUT) in an antisense orientation at the 3′ end (Wang et al. 1999a). Two overlapping minimal peptides (PVIWRRAPA and WRRAPAPGA) have been identified from the C-terminus of the fusion protein (Wang et al. 1999a). Using similar strategies, we have identified a mutated form of TPI identified by both biochemical and GTE approaches (Pieper et al. 1999; Wang et al. 1999b). This point mutation results in an amino acid substitution of Ile for Thr and thus creates an HLA-DR1-restricted peptide recognized by $CD4^+$ T cells. Using different tumor-reactive $CD4^+$ T cells, we also identified a mutated fibronectin (FN) as a tumor antigen recognized by HLA-DR2-restricted $CD4^+$ T cells. DNA sequencing analysis indicated that this gene contain a mutation, resulting in the substitution of lysine for glutamic acid and giving rise to a new T-cell epitope recognized by $CD4^+$ T cells (Wang et al. 2002). Analysis of cytokine profiles and suppressive activity of these T cells reveals that they are $CD4^+$ Th1 cells, secreting IFN-γ and IL-2, but no suppressive function.

Tumor antigens recognized by $CD4^+$ Treg cells: Despite the importance of $CD4^+$ Treg cells, their antigen specificity remains unknown for most natural Treg cells. Because elevated percentage of $CD4^+$ Treg cells are present in tumor tissues, tumor-infiltrating $CD4^+$ T cells provide an enriched source for establishing tumor-specific $CD4^+$ Treg cells. Indeed, we have recently generated many such tumor-/antigen-specific $CD4^+$ Treg cell clones from tumor-infiltrating lymphocytes (TILs) in surgically removed tumor samples. Using the same strategy for Th1 cells, we identified LAGE1 and ARTC1 as antigenic ligands for $CD4^+$ Treg cell clones established from the TIL102 and TIL164 lines, providing direct evidence that antigen-specific $CD4^+$ Treg cells are present at tumor sites and mediate antigen-specific and local immune suppression of antitumor immunity (Wang et al. 2004, 2005). Our previous study shows that the mutated CDC27 gives rise to a melanoma target antigen recognized by $CD4^+$ HLA-DR4-restricted T cells (Wang et al. 1999b). CDC27 is an important component of the anaphase-promoting complex involved in cell cycle regulation. Interestingly, the mutation itself does not constitute a T-cell epitope. Instead, T cells recognize a nonmutated peptide within CDC27 protein. Further analysis of T-cell property based on cytokine profiles and suppressive activity, found that like LAGE-specific T cells, they are antigen-specific Treg cells (unpublished data) (Table 21.3).

Tumor antigens recognized by Th1 and Treg cells: MHC class II-restricted epitopes can be identified by different approaches such as peptide stimulation in vitro or using HLA-DR transgenic (Tg) mice. We have recently used HLA-DR4-transgenic (Tg) mice to identify $CD4^+$ T-cell epitopes from candidate antigens (Touloukian et al. 2000; Zeng et al. 2000). HLA-DR-Tg mice might have advantages for identifying putative peptides, since they should have a high precursor frequency of antigen-specific T cells after immunization. Once candidate peptides are known, one can generate antigen-specific $CD4^+$ T cells from human PBMCs stimulated with synthetic candidate peptides. Therefore, the combined use of immunization of DR Tg mice with the intact protein antigens and stimulated with the peptides predicted by a computer-assisted algorithm may avoid the need to stimulate human PBMCs with a large number of peptides. Many antigen epitopes have been identified from known tumor antigens, including tyrosinase, MART-1, gp100, MAGE3, and NY-ESO-1 (Topalian et al. 1996; Touloukian et al. 2000; Zarour et al. 2000a, b; Manici et al. 1999; Chaux et al. 1999b; Schultz et al. 2000; Zeng et al. 2000; Kobayashi et al. 1998b). NY-ESO-1 is a potent immunogen recognized by both

Table 21.3 MHC class II-restricted melanoma antigens recognized by CD4+ T cells

Tumor antigens	HLA restrictions	Peptides	References
Mutated/fusion antigens			
TPI	HLA-DR1	GELIGILNAAKVPAD	Pieper et al. (1999); Wang et al. (1999b)
LDFP	HLA-DR1	PVIWRRAPA	Wang et al. (1999a)
	HLA-DR1	WRRAPAPGA	Wang et al. (1999a)
CDC27	HLA-DR4	FSWAMDLDPKGA	Wang et al. (1999b)
Fibronectin	HLA-DR2	PSVGQQMIFEKHGFRRTTPP	Wang et al. (2002)
Neo-PAP	HLA-DR7	RVIKNSIRLTL	Topalian et al. (2002)
ARTC1	HLA-DR1	YSVYFNLPADTIYTN	Wang et al. (2005)
Nonmutated antigens			
Tyrosinase	HLA-DR4	QNILLSNAPLGPQFP	Topalian et al. (1996)
	HLA-DR4	SYLQDSDPDSFQD	Topalian et al. (1996)
	HLA-DR15	FLLHHAFVDSIFEQWLQRHRP	Kobayashi et al. (1998a)
gp100	HLA-DR4	WNRQ**LYPEWTEAQ**RLD	Touloukian et al. (2000)
	HLA-DR7	GPT**LIGANASFS**IALN	Kobayashi et al. (2001a)
	HLA-DR7/DR53/DQW6	TGRA**MLGTHTMEV**TVYH	Lapointe et al. (2001); Kobayashi et al. (2001a)
	HLA-DR7	SLAV**VSTQLIMPGQE**	Kobayashi et al. (2001a)
MART-1	HLA-DR4	RNGYRALMDKSL HVGTQCALTRR	Zarour et al. (2000a)
MAGE-A1	HLA-DR13	LLKYRAREPVTKAE	Chaux et al. (1999a)
MAGE-A2	HAL-DR1	LLKYRAREPVTKAE	Chaux et al. (1999a)
MAGE-3	HLA-DR11	TSYVKVLHHMVKISG	Manici et al. (1999)
	HLA-DR13	AELVHFLLLKYRAR	Chaux et al. (1999b)
	HLA-DR13	FLLLKYRAREPVTKAE	Chaux et al. (1999b)
	HLA-DP4	TQHFVQENYLEY	Schultz et al. (2000)
	HLA-DR1,4,7,11	FFPVIFSKASSSLQL	Kobayashi et al. (2001b)
	HLA-DR1, 4, 11	RKVAELVHFLLLKYR	Consogno et al. (2003)
MAGE-A6	HLA-DR13	LLKYRAREPVTKAE	Chaux et al. (1999a)
LAGE1	HLA-DR13	RL**LQLHITMPF**SS	Wang et al. (2004)
CAMEL	HLA-DR11/12	PWKRSWSA	Slager et al. (2003)
NY-ESO-1	HLA-DR4	LPVPGV**LLKEFTVSG**NILTI	Zeng et al. (2000)
	HLA-DP4	**WITQCFLPV**FLAQPPSGQRR	Zeng et al. (2001)
hTRT	HLA-DR7	RPGLLGASVLGLDDI	Schroers et al. (2002)
Eph	HLA-DR11	DVTFNIACKKCG	Chiari et al. (2000)

antibody and T cells (Jager et al. 1998; Wang et al. 1998a; Chen et al. 1997). Of particular interest is that 10–13% of patients with advanced cancer developed a high titer of antibody (Zeng et al. 2000; Stockert et al. 1998). We identified a T-cell epitope presented by HLA-DP4, a predominant allele expressed in 40–70% of the population (Zeng et al. 2001). Identification of DP4-restricted T-cell peptides from MAGE-3 and NY-ESO-1 could be of great benefit for more than 50% of patients with cancer. All these studies suggest that unlike LAGE-1, NY-ESO-1 may preferentially activate CD4⁺ Th cells. However, a recent study shows that NY-ESO-1 can also induce Treg cells (Vence et al. 2007).

Besides tumor-derived antigens, our group and others have identified several T-cell epitopes from viral antigens recognized by CD4⁺ T cells. For example, several MHC class II peptides recognized by CD4⁺ T cells have been identified from EBNA1 as well as other viral antigens (Munz et al. 2000). T-cell peptides derived from EBV viral antigens are capable of stimulating CD4⁺ Th1 and Treg cells (Marshall et al. 2003; Voo et al. 2005). Interestingly, the same T-cell epitope from EBNA1 can stimulate both Th1 and Treg cells (Voo et al. 2005). Thus, it is likely that both tumor and viral antigens can activate effector and Treg cells, depending on particular epitope affinity and cytokine milieu.

6 Blocking Immune Suppression Mediated by Treg Cells

To block immune suppression mediated by Treg cells, we screened many cytokines and TLR ligands and found that Poly-G10 oligonucleotides can directly reverse their suppressive function in the absence of DCs. Using RNA interference technology, we identified the TLR8-MyD88 signaling pathway that is required for the reversal of Treg cell function by Poly-G oligonucleotides (Peng et al. 2005). Consistent with this observation, natural ligands for human TLR8, ssRNA40, and ssRNA33 derived from HIV viral sequences (Heil et al. 2004) could completely reverse the suppressive function of Treg cells as well. However, ligands for other human TLRs could not reverse the suppressive function of Treg cells, suggesting that TLR8 activation is specifically linked to regulation of Treg cell function. Instead, falgellin-mediated activation of TLR5 leads to enhanced proliferation and IL-2 secretion (Crellin et al. 2005). Since TLR8 is not functional in mice (Jurk et al. 2002), as expected, Poly-G oligonucleotides could not reverse the suppressive activity of murine Treg cells. However, other TLR ligands in mice may affect Treg cell function and growth. Recent studies show that murine TLR2-deficient mice reduce the number of CD4⁺ CD25⁺ Treg cells (Netea et al. 2004). Activation of TLR2 with its ligand (Pam3Cys) directly increases the proliferation of murine Treg cells and transiently reverses their suppressive function (Sutmuller et al. 2006). It has been reported that functional regulation of murine Treg cells is mainly achieved by TLR via DCs (Pasare and Medzhitov 2003), further studies are needed to determine whether control of Treg cell function by TLRs is directly acting on Treg and effector T cells or indirectly on DCs.

More importantly, we recently demonstrated that the suppressive function of CD8⁺ Treg cells and γδ-TCR Treg cells can also be reversed after Poly-G oligonucleotide treatment (Peng et al. 2007; Kiniwa et al. 2007), suggesting that these cells share a common TLR8 signaling-mediated mechanism with previously characterized CD4⁺ Treg cell subsets. Further dissection of the downstream pathways of TLR8-MyD88 using shRNA knockdown strategy suggests that TRAF6, p38, IKKα, and IKKβ are required to enable Treg cells to respond to Poly-G3 treatment, while

TAK1, JNK1, and ERK molecules are dispensable (Peng et al. 2007). Thus, it is possible that manipulation of the TLR8 signaling pathway through TLR-based ligands may allow one to block the suppressive function of Treg cells, thus improving the efficacy of cancer vaccines.

7 Future Directions

Development of potent therapeutic vaccines against cancer requires long-lasting antitumor immunity. However, overcoming immune suppression mediated by Treg and other immune cells such as myeloid-derived suppressor cells in the tumor microenvironment is one key factor determining whether we can induce potent antitumor immunity. Thus, the optimal strategy will be to block immune suppression, while stimulating maximal antigen-specific effector T-cell responses. To achieve these goals, we also need to block negative regulators of several key pathways such as NF-κB, type I interferon, and inflammasome at the molecular level to enhance the capacity of DCs to induce T-cell responses. More importantly, these novel concepts must be tested in the clinical setting for the development of effective therapeutic vaccines against cancer, and perhaps other diseases.

Acknowledgments We would like to thank many fellows working in the laboratory for their scientific contributions. This work is supported by grants from National Cancer Institute, NIH, American Cancer Society and Cancer Research Institute.

References

Aarnoudse CA, van den Doel PB, Heemskerk B, Schrier PI (1999) Interleukin-2-induced, melanoma-specific T cells recognize CAMEL, an unexpected translation product of LAGE-1. Int J Cancer 82(3):442–448

Atarashi K et al (2008) ATP drives lamina propria T(H)17 cell differentiation. Nature 455(7214): 808–812

Ayyoub M et al (2002) Proteasome-assisted identification of a SSX-2-derived epitope recognized by tumor-reactive CTL infiltrating metastatic melanoma. J Immunol 168(4):1717–1722

Bakker ABH et al (1994) Melanocyte lineage-specific antigen gp100 is recognized by melanocyte-derived tumor-infiltrating lymphocytes. J Exp Med 179:1005–1009

Banchereau J, Steinman RM (1998) Dendritic cells and the control of immunity. Nature 392(6673):245–252

Baumeister W, Walz J, Zuhl F, Seemuller E (1998) The proteasome: paradigm of a self-compartmentalizing protease. Cell 92(3):367–380

Bellone M et al (2000) Relevance of the tumor antigen in the validation of three vaccination strategies for melanoma. J Immunol 165(5):2651–2656

Benlalam H et al (2003) Identification of five new HLA-B*3501-restricted epitopes derived from common melanoma-associated antigens, spontaneously recognized by tumor-infiltrating lymphocytes. J Immunol 171(11):6283–6289

Bettelli E et al (2006) Reciprocal developmental pathways for the generation of pathogenic effector TH17 and regulatory T cells. Nature 441(7090):235–238

Bickham K et al (2001) EBNA1-specific CD4+ T cells in healthy carriers of Epstein-Barr virus are primarily Th1 in function. J Clin Invest 107(1):121–130

Boel P et al (1995) BAGE: a new gene encoding an antigen recognized on human melanomas by cytolytic T lymphocytes. Immunity 2:167–175

Boon T et al (1994) Tumor antigens recognized by T lymphocytes. Annu Rev Immunol 12: 337–365; Rosenberg SA (1999) A new era for cancer immunotherapy based on the genes that encode cancer antigens. Immunity 10(3):281–287

Brichard V et al (1993) The tyrosinase gene codes for an antigen recognized by autologous cytolytic T lymphocytes on HLA-A2 melanomas. J Exp Med 178:489–495

Brichard VG et al (1996) A tyrosinase nonpeptide presented by HLA-B44 is recognized on a human melanoma by autologous cytolytic T lymphocytes. Eur J Immunol 26:224–230

Castelli C et al (1995) Mass spectrometric identification of a naturally processed melanoma peptide recognized by CD8+ cytotoxic T lymphocytes. J Exp Med 181(1):363–368

Castelli C et al (1999) Novel HLA-Cw8-restricted T cell epitopes derived from tyrosinase-related protein-2 and gp100 melanoma antigens. J Immunol 162(3):1739–1748

Chaux P et al (1999a) Identification of five MAGE-A1 epitopes recognized by cytolytic T lymphocytes obtained by in vitro stimulation with dendritic cells transduced with MAGE-A1. J Immunol 163(5):2928–2936

Chaux P et al (1999b) Identification of MAGE-3 epitopes presented by HLA-DR molecules to CD4(+) T lymphocytes. J Exp Med 189(5):767–778

Chen YT et al (1997) A testicular antigen aberrantly expressed in human cancers detected by autologous antibody screening. Proc Natl Acad Sci USA 94:1914–1918

Chiari R et al (2000) Identification of a tumor-specific shared antigen derived from an Eph receptor and presented to CD4 T cells on HLA class II molecules. Cancer Res 60(17):4855–4863

Consogno G et al (2003) Identification of immunodominant regions among promiscuous HLA-DR-restricted CD4+ T-cell epitopes on the tumor antigen MAGE-3. Blood 101(3):1038–1044

Coulie PG et al (1994) A new gene coding for a differentiation antigen recognized by autologous cytolytic T lymphocytes on HLA-A2 melanomas. J Exp Med 180:35–42

Cox AL et al (1994) Identification of a peptide recognized by five melanoma-specific human cytotoxic T cell lines. Science 264:716–719

Crellin NK et al (2005) Human CD4+ T cells express TLR5 and its ligand flagellin enhances the suppressive capacity and expression of FOXP3 in CD4+CD25+ T regulatory cells. J Immunol 175(12):8051–8059

Curiel TJ et al (2004) Specific recruitment of regulatory T cells in ovarian carcinoma fosters immune privilege and predicts reduced survival. Nat Med 10(9):942–949

Dallal RM, Lotze MT (2000) The dendritic cell and human cancer vaccines. Curr Opin Immunol 12(5):583–588

Dudley ME et al (2002) Cancer regression and autoimmunity in patients after clonal repopulation with antitumor lymphocytes. Science 298(5594):850–854

Duffour MT et al (1999) A MAGE-A4 peptide presented by HLA-A2 is recognized by cytolytic T lymphocytes. Eur J Immunol 29(10):3329–3337

Fehervari Z, Sakaguchi S (2004) Control of Foxp3+ CD25+CD4+ regulatory cell activation and function by dendritic cells. Int Immunol 16(12):1769–1780

Fleischhauer K et al (1995) Characterization of natural peptide ligands for HLA-B*4402 and -B*4403: implications for peptide involvement in allorecognition of a single amino acid change in the HLA-B44 heavy chain. Tissue Antigens 44:311–317

Fontenot JD, Gavin MA, Rudensky AY (2003) Foxp3 programs the development and function of CD4(+)CD25(+) regulatory T cells. Nat Immunol 4:330–336

Fujie T et al (1999) A MAGE-1-encoded HLA-A24-binding synthetic peptide induces specific anti-tumor cytotoxic T lymphocytes. Int J Cancer 80(2):169–172

Gaugler B et al (1994) Human gene MAGE-3 codes for an antigen recognized on a melanoma by autologous cytolytic T lymphocytes. J Exp Med 179:921–930

Greenberg PD (1991) Adoptive T cell therapy of tumors: mechanisms operative in the recognition and elimination of tumor cells. Adv Immunol 49:281–355

Groettrup M, Schmidtke G (1999) Selective proteasome inhibitors: modulators of antigen presentation? Drug Discov Today 4(2):63–71

Guilloux Y et al (1996) A peptide recognized by human cytolytic T lymphocytes on HLA-A2 melanomas is encoded by an intron sequence of the N-acetylglucosaminyltransferase V gene. J Exp Med 183:1173–1183

Hanada K, Yewdell JW, Yang JC (2004) Immune recognition of a human renal cancer antigen through post-translational protein splicing. Nature 427(6971):252–256

Harada M et al (2001) Melanoma-reactive $CD8^+$ T cells recognize a novel tumor antigen expressed in a wide variety of tumor types. J Immunother 24(4):323–333

Harrington LE et al (2005) Interleukin 17-producing CD4+ effector T cells develop via a lineage distinct from the T helper type 1 and 2 lineages. Nat Immunol 6(11):1123–1132

Heidecker L et al (2000) Cytolytic T lymphocytes raised against a human bladder carcinoma recognize an antigen encoded by gene MAGE-A12. J Immunol 164(11):6041–6045

Heil F et al (2004) Species-specific recognition of single-stranded RNA via toll-like receptor 7 and 8. Science 303(5663):1526–1529

Herman J et al (1996) A peptide encoded by the human MAGE3 gene and presented by HLA-B44 induces cytolytic T lymphocytes that recognize tumor cells expressing MAGE3. Immunogenetics 43(6):377–383

Hori S, Nomura T, Sakaguchi S (2003) Control of regulatory T cell development by the transcription factor foxp3. Science 299(5609):1057–1061

Huang LQ et al (1999) Cytolytic T lymphocytes recognize an antigen encoded by MAGE-A10 on a human melanoma. J Immunol 162(11):6849–6854

Ivanov II et al (2006) The orphan nuclear receptor RORgammat directs the differentiation program of proinflammatory IL-17(+) T helper cells. Cell 126(6):1121–1133

Jager E et al (1996) Generation of cytotoxic T cell responses with synthetic melanoma-associated peptides in vivo: implication for tumor vaccines with melanoma-associated antigens. Int J Cancer 66:162–169

Jager E et al (1998) Simultaneous humoral and cellular immune response against cancer-testis antigen NY-ESO-1: definition of human histocompatibility leukocyte antigen (HLA)-A2-binding peptide epitopes. J Exp Med 187(2):265–270

Jager E et al (2000) Identification of NY-ESO-1 epitopes presented by human histocompatibility antigen (HLA)-DRB4*0101-0103 and recognized by CD4(+) T lymphocytes of patients with NY-ESO-1-expressing melanoma. J Exp Med 191(4):625–630

Janssen EM et al (2003) CD4(+) T cells are required for secondary expansion and memory in CD8(+) T lymphocytes. Nature 421(6925):852–856

Jurk M et al (2002) Human TLR7 or TLR8 independently confer responsiveness to the antiviral compound R-848. Nat Immunol 3(6):499

Kang XQ et al (1995) Identification of a tyrosinase epitope reocognized by HLA-A24 restricted tumor-infiltrating lymphocytes. J Immunol 155:1343–1348

Kawakami Y et al (1994) Identification of a human melanoma antigen recognized by tumor infiltrating lymphocytes associated with in vivo tumor rejection. Proc Natl Acad Sci USA 91:6458–6462

Kawakami Y et al (1994) Identification of the immunodominant peptides of the MART-1 human melanoma antigen recognized by the majority of HLA-A2 restricted tumor infiltrating lymphocytes. J Exp Med 180:347–352

Kawakami Y et al (1994) Cloning of the gene coding for a shared human melanoma antigen recognized by autologous T cells infiltrating into tumor. Proc Natl Acad Sci USA 91:3515–3519

Kawakami Y et al (1995) Recognition of multiple epitopes in the human melanoma antigen gp100 by tumor-infiltrating T lymphocytes associated with in vivo tumor regression. J Immunol 154:3961–3968

Kawakami Y et al (1998) Identification of new melanoma epitopes on melanosomal proteins recognized by tumor infiltrating T lymphocytes restricted by HLA-A1, -A2, and -A3 alleles. J Immunol 161(12):6985–6992

Kawashima I et al (1998) Identification of gp100-derived, melanoma-specific cytotoxic T- lymphocyte epitopes restricted by HLA-A3 supertype molecules by primary in vitro immunization with peptide-pulsed dendritic cells [In Process Citation]. Int J Cancer 78(4):518–524

Khattri R, Cox T, Yasayko SA, Ramsdell F (2003) An essential role for Scurfin in CD4(+)CD25(+) T regulatory cells. Nat Immunol 4:337–342

Khong HT, Rosenberg SA (2002) Pre-existing immunity to tyrosinase-related protein (TRP)-2, a new TRP- 2 isoform, and the NY-ESO-1 melanoma antigen in a patient with a dramatic response to immunotherapy. J Immunol 168(2):951–956

Kiniwa Y et al (2007) CD8$^+$ Foxp3$^+$ regulatory T cells mediate immunosuppression in prostate cancer. Clin Cancer Res 13:6947–6958

Kittlesen DJ et al (1998) Human melanoma patients recognize an HLA-A1-restricted CTL epitope from tyrosinase containing two cysteine residues: implications for tumor vaccine development. J Immunol 160(5):2099–2106

Kobayashi H et al (1998a) Tyrosinase epitope recognized by an HLA-DR-restricted T-cell line from a Vogt-Koyanagi-Harada disease patient. Immunogenetics 47(5):398–403

Kobayashi H et al (1998) CD4+ T cells from peripheral blood of a melanoma patient recognize peptides derived from nonmutated tyrosinase. Cancer Res 58(2):296–301

Kobayashi H, Lu J, Celis E (2001a) Identification of helper T-cell epitopes that encompass or lie proximal to cytotoxic T-cell epitopes in the gp100 melanoma tumor antigen. Cancer Res 61(20):7577–7584

Kobayashi H et al (2001b) Tumor-reactive T helper lymphocytes recognize a promiscuous MAGE-A3 epitope presented by various major histocompatibility complex class II alleles. Cancer Res 61(12):4773–4778

Koebel CM et al (2007) Adaptive immunity maintains occult cancer in an equilibrium state. Nature 450(7171):903–907

Korn T et al (2007) IL-21 initiates an alternative pathway to induce proinflammatory T(H)17 cells. Nature; Nurieva R et al (2007) Essential autocrine regulation by IL-21 in the generation of inflammatory T cells. Nature 448:484–487

Kubo T et al (2004) Regulatory T cell suppression and anergy are differentially regulated by proinflammatory cytokines produced by TLR-activated dendritic cells. J Immunol 173(12):7249–7258

Langowski JL et al (2006) IL-23 promotes tumour incidence and growth. Nature 442(7101):461–465

Lapointe R et al (2001) Retrovirally transduced human dendritic cells can generate T cells recognizing multiple MHC class I and class II epitopes from the melanoma antigen glycoprotein 100. J Immunol 167(8):4758–4764

Lau R et al (2001) Phase I trial of intravenous peptide-pulsed dendritic cells in patients with metastatic melanoma. J Immunother 24(1):66–78

Leen A et al (2001) Differential immunogenicity of Epstein-Barr virus latent-cycle proteins for human CD4(+) T-helper 1 responses. J Virol 75(18):8649–8659

Lethe B et al (1998) LAGE-1, a new gene with tumor specificity. Int J Cancer 76(6):903–908

Li K et al (1998) Tumour-specific MHC-class-II-restricted responses after in vitro sensitization to synthetic peptides corresponding to gp100 and Annexin II eluted from melanoma cells. Cancer Immunol Immunother 47(1):32–38

Linnebacher M et al (2001) Frameshift peptide-derived T-cell epitopes: a source of novel tumor-specific antigens. Int J Cancer 93(1):6–11

Liu H, Komai-Koma M, Xu D, Liew FY (2006) Toll-like receptor 2 signaling modulates the functions of CD4+CD25+ regulatory T cells. Proc Natl Acad Sci USA 103(18):7048–7053

Liyanage UK et al (2002) Prevalence of regulatory T cells is increased in peripheral blood and tumor microenvironment of patients with pancreas or breast adenocarcinoma. J Immunol 169(5):2756–2761

Lupetti R et al (1998) Translation of a retained intron in tyrosinase-related protein (TRP) 2 mRNA generates a new cytotoxic T lymphocyte (CTL)-defined and shared human melanoma antigen not expressed in normal cells of the melanocytic lineage. J Exp Med 188(6):1005–1016

Mandruzzato S et al (1997) A CASP-8 mutation recognized by cytolytic T lymphocytes on a human head and neck carcinoma. J Exp Med 186(5):785–793

Mangan PR et al (2006) Transforming growth factor-beta induces development of the T(H)17 lineage. Nature 441(7090):231–234

Manici S et al (1999) Melanoma cells present a MAGE-3 epitope to CD4(+) cytotoxic T cells in association with histocompatibility leukocyte antigen DR11. J Exp Med 189(5):871–876

Marchand M et al (1999) Tumor regressions observed in patients with metastatic melanoma treated with an antigenic peptide encoded by gene MAGE-3 and presented by HLA- A1. Int J Cancer 80(2):219–230

Mariathasan S et al (2006) Cryopyrin activates the inflammasome in response to toxins and ATP. Nature 440(7081):228–232

Marshall NA, Vickers MA, Barker RN (2003) Regulatory T cells secreting IL-10 dominate the immune response to EBV latent membrane protein 1. J Immunol 170(12):6183–6189

Martinon F et al (2006) Gout-associated uric acid crystals activate the NALP3 inflammasome. Nature 440(7081):237–241

Miyahara Y et al (2008) Generation and regulation of human CD4$^+$ IL-17-producing T cells in ovarian cancer. Proc Natl Acad Sci USA 105(40):15505–15510

Morel S et al (2000) Processing of some antigens by the standard proteasome but not by the immunoproteasome results in poor presentation by dendritic cells. Immunity 12(1):107–117

Mucida D et al (2007) Reciprocal TH17 and regulatory T cell differentiation mediated by retinoic acid. Science 317(5835):256–260

Munz C et al (2000) Human CD4(+) T lymphocytes consistently respond to the latent Epstein-Barr virus nuclear antigen EBNA1. J Exp Med 191(10):1649–1660

Muranski P et al (2008) Tumor-specific Th17-polarized cells eradicate large established melanoma. Blood 112(2):362–373

Nestle FO et al (1998) Vaccination of melanoma patients with peptide- or tumor lysate-pulsed dendritic cells. Nat Med 4(3):328–332

Netea MG et al (2004) Toll-like receptor 2 suppresses immunity against Candida albicans through induction of IL-10 and regulatory T cells. J Immunol 172(6):3712–3718

Noppen C et al (2000) Naturally processed and concealed HLA-A2.1-restricted epitopes from tumor-associated antigen tyrosinase-related protein-2. Int J Cancer 87(2):241–246

Oiso M et al (1999) A newly identified MAGE-3-derived epitope recognized by HLA-A24-restricted cytotoxic T lymphocytes. Int J Cancer 81(3):387–394

Paludan C, Munz C (2003) CD4+ T cell responses in the immune control against latent infection by Epstein-Barr virus. Curr Mol Med 3(4):341–347

Panelli MC et al (2000) A tumor-infiltrating lymphocyte from a melanoma metastasis with decreased expression of melanoma differentiation antigens recognizes MAGE-12. J Immunol 164(8):4382–4392

Park H et al (2005) A distinct lineage of CD4 T cells regulates tissue inflammation by producing interleukin 17. Nat Immunol 6(11):1133–1141

Parkhurst MR et al (1998) Identification of a shared HLA-A*0201-restricted T-cell epitope from the melanoma antigen tyrosinase-related protein 2 (TRP2). Cancer Res 58(21):4895–4901

Pasare C, Medzhitov R (2003) Toll pathway-dependent blockade of CD4+CD25+ T cell-mediated suppression by dendritic cells. Science 299(5609):1033–1036

Peng G et al (2005) Toll-like receptor 8 mediated-reversal of CD4$^+$ regulatory T cell function. Science 309:1380–1384

Peng G et al (2007) Tumor-infiltrating gamma-delta T cells suppress T and dendritic cell function via mechanisms controlled by a unique Toll-like receptor signaling pathway. Immunity 27:334–348

Pieper R et al (1999) Biochemical identification of a mutated human melanoma antigen recognized by CD4(+) T cells. J Exp Med 189(5):757–766

Probst-Kepper M et al (2001) An alternative open reading frame of the human macrophage colony – stimulating factor gene is independently translated and codes for an antigenic peptide of 14 amino acids recognized by tumor-infiltrating CD8 T lymphocytes. J Exp Med 193(10):1189–1198

Rimoldi D et al (2000) Efficient simultaneous presentation of NY-ESO-1/LAGE-1 primary and nonprimary open reading frame-derived CTL epitopes in melanoma. J Immunol 165(12): 7253–7261

Ripberger E et al (2003) Identification of an HLA-A0201-restricted CTL epitope generated by a tumor-specific frameshift mutation in a coding microsatellite of the OGT gene. J Clin Immunol 23(5):415–423

Robbins PF et al (1996) A mutated beta-catenin gene encodes a melanoma-specific antigen recognized by tumor infiltrating lymphocytes. J Exp Med 183:1185–1192

Robbins P et al (1997) The intronic region of an incompletely spliced gp100 gene transcript encodes an epitope recognized by melanoma-reactive tumor-infiltrating lymphocytes. J Immunol 159:303–308

Rock KL, Goldberg AL (1999) Degradation of cell proteins and the generation of MHC class I-presented peptides. Annu Rev Immunol 17:739–779

Rosenberg SA (2001) Progress in human tumour immunology and immunotherapy. Nature 411(6835):380–384

Rosenberg SA et al (1998) Immunologic and therapeutic evaluation of a synthetic tumor-associated peptide vaccine for the treatment of patients with metastatic melanoma. Nat Med 4:321–327

Rosenberg SA et al (2002) Identification of BING-4 cancer antigen translated from an alternative open reading frame of a gene in the extended MHC class II region using lymphocytes from a patient with a durable complete regression following immunotherapy. J Immunol 168(5):2402–2407

Rosenberg SA, Yang JC, Restifo NP (2004) Cancer immunotherapy: moving beyond current vaccines. Nat Med 10(9):909–915

Rosenberg SA et al (2008) Adoptive cell transfer: a clinical path to effective cancer immunotherapy. Nat Rev Cancer 8(4):299–308

Russo V et al (2000) Dendritic cells acquire the MAGE-3 human tumor antigen from apoptotic cells and induce a class I-restricted T cell response. Proc Natl Acad Sci USA 97(5):2185–2190

Saeterdal I et al (2001) A TGF betaRII frameshift-mutation-derived CTL epitope recognised by HLA-A2-restricted CD8$^+$ T cells. Cancer Immunol Immunother 50(9):469–476

Schneider J et al (1998) Overlapping peptides of melanocyte differentiation antigen Melan-A/MART-1 recognized by autologous cytolytic T lymphocytes in association with HLA-B45.1 and HLA-A2.1. Int J Cancer 75(3):451–458

Schreurs MW et al (2000) Dendritic cells break tolerance and induce protective immunity against a melanocyte differentiation antigen in an autologous melanoma model. Cancer Res 60(24):6995–7001

Schroers R et al (2002) Identification of HLA DR7-restricted epitopes from human telomerase reverse transcriptase recognized by CD4$^+$ T-helper cells. Cancer Res 62(9):2600–2605

Schultz ES et al (2000) A MAGE-A3 peptide presented by HLA-DP4 is recognized on tumor cells by CD4$^+$ cytolytic T lymphocytes. Cancer Res 60(22):6272–6275

Schultz ES et al (2002) The production of a new MAGE-3 peptide presented to cytolytic T lymphocytes by HLA-B40 requires the immunoproteasome. J Exp Med 195(4):391–399

Sensi M et al (2002) Identification of a novel gp100/pMel17 peptide presented by HLA-A*6801 and recognized on human melanoma by cytolytic T cell clones. Tissue Antigens 59(4):273–279

Shankaran V et al (2001) IFNgamma and lymphocytes prevent primary tumour development and shape tumour immunogenicity. Nature 410(6832):1107–1111

Shedlock DJ, Shen H (2003) Requirement for CD4 T cell help in generating functional CD8 T cell memory. Science 300(5617):337–339

Skipper JC et al (1996) Shared epitopes for HLA-A3-restricted melanoma-reactive human CTL include a naturally processed epitope from Pmel-17/gp100. J Immunol 157(11):5027–5033

Slager EH et al (2003) CD4$^+$ Th2 cell recognition of HLA-DR-restricted epitopes derived from CAMEL: a tumor antigen translated in an alternative open reading frame. J Immunol 170(3):1490–1497

Smyth MJ, Dunn GP, Schreiber RD (2006) Cancer immunosurveillance and immunoediting: the roles of immunity in suppressing tumor development and shaping tumor immunogenicity. Adv Immunol 90:1–50

Stockert E et al (1998) A survey of the humoral immune response of cancer patients to a panel of human tumor antigens. J Exp Med 187(8):1349–1354

Sun JC, Bevan MJ (2003) Defective CD8 T cell memory following acute infection without CD4 T cell help. Science 300(5617):339–342

Sutmuller RP et al (2006) Toll-like receptor 2 controls expansion and function of regulatory T cells. J Clin Invest 116(2):485–494

Sutterwala FS et al (2006) Critical role for NALP3/CIAS1/cryopyrin in innate and adaptive immunity through its regulation of caspase-1. Immunity 24(3):317–327

Tahara K et al (1999) Identification of a MAGE-2-encoded human leukocyte antigen-A24-binding synthetic peptide that induces specific antitumor cytotoxic T lymphocytes. Clin Cancer Res 5(8):2236–2241

Tanaka K, Kasahara M (1998) The MHC class I ligand-generating system: roles of immunoproteasomes and the interferon-gamma-inducible proteasome activator PA28. Immunol Rev 163:161–176

Tanaka F et al (1997) Induction of antitumor cytotoxic T lymphocytes with a MAGE-3-encoded synthetic peptide presented by human leukocytes antigen-A24. Cancer Res 57(20):4465–4468

Tanzarella S et al (1999) Identification of a promiscuous T-cell epitope encoded by multiple members of the MAGE family. Cancer Res 59(11):2668–2674

Thurner B et al (1999) Vaccination with mage-3A1 peptide-pulsed mature, monocyte-derived dendritic cells expands specific cytotoxic T cells and induces regression of some metastases in advanced stage IV melanoma. J Exp Med 190(11):1669–1678

Toes RE, Ossendorp F, Offringa R, Melief CJ (1999) CD4 T Cells and their role in antitumor immune responses. J Exp Med 189(5):753–756

Topalian SL et al (1996) Melanoma-specific CD4$^+$ T cells recognize nonmutated HLA-DR-restricted tyrosinase epitopes. J Exp Med 183:1965–1971

Topalian SL et al (2002) Revelation of a cryptic major histocompatibility complex class II-restricted tumor epitope in a novel RNA-processing enzyme. Cancer Res 62(19):5505–5509

Touloukian CE et al (2000) Identification of a MHC class II-restricted human gp100 epitope using DR4-IE transgenic mice. J Immunol 164(7):3535–3542

Traversari C et al (1992) A nonapeptide encoded by human gene MAGE-1 is recognized on HLA-A1 by cytolytic T lymphocytes directed against tumor antigen MZ2-E. J Exp Med 176:1453–1457

Tsai V et al (1997) Identification of subdominant CTL epitopes of the GP100 melanoma-associated tumor antigen by primary in vitro immunization with peptide-pulsed dendritic cells. J Immunol 158(4):1796–1802

Van der Bruggen P et al (1991) A gene encoding an antigen recognized by cytolytiv T lymphocytes on a hunan melanoma. Science 254:1643–1647

Van der Bruggen P et al (1994a) Autologous cytolytic T lymphocytes recognize a MAGE-1 nonapeptide on melanomas expressing Cw1601. Eur J Immunol 24:2134–2140

Van der Bruggen P et al (1994b) A peptide encoded by human gene MAGE-3 and presented by HLA-A2 induces cytolytic T lymphocytes that recognize tumor cells expressing MAGE-3. Eur J Immunol 24:3038–3043

Veldhoen M et al (2006) TGFbeta in the context of an inflammatory cytokine milieu supports de novo differentiation of IL-17-producing T cells. Immunity 24(2):179–189

Veldhoen M et al (2008) The aryl hydrocarbon receptor links TH17-cell-mediated autoimmunity to environmental toxins. Nature 453(7191):106–109

Vence L et al (2007) Circulating tumor antigen-specific regulatory T cells in patients with metastatic melanoma. Proc Natl Acad Sci USA 10:20884–20889

Vigneron N et al (2004) An antigenic peptide produced by peptide splicing in the proteasome. Science 304(5670):587–590

Visseren MJ et al (1997) Identification of HLA-A*0201-restricted CTL epitopes encoded by the tumor-specific MAGE-2 gene product. Int J Cancer 73(1):125–130

Voo KS et al (2002) Identification of HLA-DP3-restricted peptides from EBNA1 recognized by CD4(+) T cells. Cancer Res 62(24):7195–7199

Voo KS et al (2005) Functional characterization of EBV-encoded nuclear antigen 1-specific CD4⁺ helper and regulatory T cells elicited by in vitro peptide stimulation. Cancer Res 65(4): 1577–1586

Walker MR et al (2003) Induction of FoxP3 and acquisition of T regulatory activity by stimulated human CD4+CD25- T cells. J Clin Invest 112(9):1437–1443

Wang R-F et al (1995) Identification of a gene encoding a melanoma tumor antigen recognized by HLA-A31-restricted tumor-infiltrating lymphocytes. J Exp Med 181:799–804

Wang RF (2001) The role of MHC class II-restricted tumor antigens and CD4⁺ T cells in antitumor immunity. Trends Immunol 22:269–276

Wang RF, Rosenberg SA (1999) Human tumor antigens for cancer vaccine development. Immunol Rev 170:85–100

Wang HY, Wang RF (2007) Regulatory T cells and cancer. Curr Opin Immunol 19(2):217–223

Wang R-F et al (1996a) Identification of TRP-2 as a human tumor antigen recognized by cytotoxic T lymphocytes. J Exp Med 184:2207–2216

Wang RF et al (1996b) Utilization of an alternative open reading frame of a normal gene in generating a novel human cancer antigen. J Exp Med 183:1131–1140

Wang RF et al (1998a) A breast and melanoma-shared tumor antigen: T cell responses to antigenic peptides translated from different open reading frames. J Immunol 161:3596–3606

Wang RF et al (1998b) Recognition of an antigenic peptide derived from TRP-2 by cytotoxic T lymphocytes in the context of HLA-A31 and -A33. J Immunol 160:890–897

Wang RF, Wang X, Rosenberg SA (1999a) Identification of a novel MHC class II-restricted tumor antigen resulting from a chromosomal rearrangement recognized by CD4⁺ T cells. J Exp Med 189:1659–1667

Wang R-F et al (1999b) Cloning genes encoding MHC class II-restricted antigens: mutated CDC27 as a tumor antigen. Science 284:1351–1354

Wang HY et al (2002) Identification of a mutated fibronectin as a tumor antigen recognized by CD4⁺ T cells: its role in extracellular matrix formation and tumor metastasis. J Exp Med 195:1397–1406

Wang HY et al (2004) Tumor-specific human CD4⁺ regulatory T cells and their ligands: implication for immunotherapy. Immunity 20:107–118

Wang HY et al (2005) Recognition of a new ARTC1 peptide ligand uniquely expressed in tumor cells by antigen-specific CD4⁺ gegulatory T cells. J Immunol 174:2661–2670

Warren EH et al (2006) An antigen produced by splicing of noncontiguous peptides in the reverse order. Science 313(5792):1444–1447

Weaver CT et al (2006) Th17: an effector CD4 T cell lineage with regulatory T cell ties. Immunity 24(6):677–688

Wolfel T et al (1994) Two tyrosinase nonapeptides recognized on HLA-A2 melanomas by autologous cytolytic T lymphocytes. Eur J Immunol 24:759–764

Wolfel T et al (1995) A p16INK4a-insensitive CDK4 mutant targeted by cytolytic T lymphocytes in a human melanoma. Science 269:1281–1284

Woo EY et al (2001) Regulatory CD4(+)CD25(+) T cells in tumors from patients with early-stage non-small cell lung cancer and late-stage ovarian cancer. Cancer Res 61(12):4766–4772

Yang XO et al (2008) T helper 17 lineage differentiation is programmed by orphan nuclear receptors ROR alpha and ROR gamma. Immunity 28(1):29–39

Zarour HM et al (2000a) Melan-A/MART-1(51–73) represents an immunogenic HLA-DR4-restricted epitope recognized by melanoma-reactive CD4(+) T cells. Proc Natl Acad Sci USA 97(1):400–405

Zarour HM et al (2000) NY-ESO-1 encodes DRB1*0401-restricted epitopes recognized by melanoma-reactive CD4+ T cells. Cancer Res 60(17):4946–4952

Zeng G et al (2000) Identification of CD4⁺ T cell epitopes from NY-ESO-1 presented by HLA-DR molecules. J Immunol 165:1153–1159

Zeng G et al (2001) CD4+ T cell recognition of MHC class II-restricted epitopes from NY-ESO-1 presented by a prevalent HLA-DP4 allele: association with NY-ESO-1 antibody production. Proc Natl Acad Sci USA 98:3964–3969

Zhou L et al (2007) IL-6 programs T(H)-17 cell differentiation by promoting sequential engagement of the IL-21 and IL-23 pathways. Nat Immunol 8:967–974

Zorn E, Hercend T (1999) A MAGE-6-encoded peptide is recognized by expanded lymphocytes infiltrating a spontaneously regressing human primary melanoma lesion. Eur J Immunol 29(2):602–607

Chapter 22
Immunotherapy of Cancer

Michael Dougan and Glenn Dranoff

Immunotherapy is a central component of many cancer treatment regimens (Table 22.1) (Dougan and Dranoff 2009). Tumors can express microbial proteins, mutated proteins, and fusion proteins, as well as aberrantly expressed self proteins, all of which can be recognized by the immune system. Established therapies use a range of manipulations to activate antitumor immunity, including passive immunization with monoclonal antibodies, the introduction of adjuvants into the tumor microenvironment, and the systemic delivery of cytokines. Vaccination against and treatment for oncogenic microbial infections can act as tumor prophylaxis. Immune therapy is also an important component of bone marrow transplantations that are used to treat hematologic malignancies. Investigational immune therapies seek to build upon established treatments to generate more efficacious and less toxic cancer therapy. These novel strategies attempt to augment protective antitumor immunity and to disrupt the immune regulatory circuits critical for maintaining tumor tolerance (Dougan and Dranoff 2009).

1 Prophylactic Immune Therapy and Tumor Vaccines

A number of cancers are caused by microbial infections, either directly or through the induction of chronic inflammation (Lin and Karin 2007). As a result, therapies aimed at eradicating or preventing these infections act prophylactically against their associated tumors.

The hepatitis B virus (HBV) vaccine was the first vaccine to provide protection against an oncogenic infection. HBV infections of the liver can induce chronic

---

M. Dougan • G. Dranoff (✉)
Department of Medical Oncology and Cancer Vaccine Center, Dana-Farber Cancer Institute and Department of Medicine, Brigham and Women's Hospital and Harvard Medical School, Boston, MA 02115, USA
e-mail: glenn_dranoff@dfci.harvard.edu

Table 22.1 Clinically approved immunotherapy for cancer

Established therapies	Indication	References
Prophylactic therapy		
HBV vaccine	Hepatocellular carcinoma	Chang et al. (2000); Davis (2005)
HPV vaccine	Cervical cancer	Future, II Study Group (2007)
Antibiotics (*H. pylori*)	Gastric cancer, MALT lymphoma	Wong et al. (2004); Roggero et al. (1995)
NSAIDs (FAP, ulcerative colitis)	Colorectal cancer	Rostom et al. (2007); Steinbach et al. (2000); Turini and DuBois (2002); Velayos et al. (2005)
Adjuvants and cytokines		
BCG	Superficial bladder cancer	Bohle and Brandau (2003); Shelley et al. (2000); Herr et al. (1995); Sylvester et al. (2005)
Imiquimod	Basal cell carcinoma, VIN, actinic keratosis	van Seters et al. (2008)
IL-2	Melanoma, RCC	Atkins et al. (1999); Fyfe et al. (1995)
IFN-α	Melanoma, RCC	Kirkwood et al. (1996); Motzer et al. (2002)
TNF-α	Soft tissue sarcoma, melanoma	Lans et al. (2005)
Monoclonal antibodies		
Rituximab	NHL, CLL	Coiffier et al. (2002); Marcus and Hagenbeek (2007)
Ibritumomab tiuxetan	NHL	Witzig et al. (2002)
Tositumomab	NHL	Fisher et al. (2005)
Alemtuzumab	CLL	Keating et al. (2002)
Gentuzumab	AML	Bross et al. (2001)
Trastuzumab	Breast cancer	Hudis (2007)
Cetuximab	Colorectal cancer	Meyerhardt and Mayer (2005)
Panitumumab	Colorectal cancer	Van Cutsem et al. (2007)
Bevacizumab	Colorectal, lung	Bukowski et al. (2007); Kindler et al. (2005); Miller et al. (2005)
Bone marrow transplantation		
Allogeneic	Hematologic malignancies	Gale et al. (1994); Weiden et al. (1979); Wu and Ritz (2006)
DLI	Hematologic malignancies	Kolb et al. (1990)

AML acute myeloblastic leukemia; *BCG* bacilli Calmette-Guérin; *CLL* chronic lymphocytic leukemia; *DLI* donor lymphocyte infusion; *FAP* familial adenomatous polyposis; *HBV* hepatitis B virus; *HPV* human papilloma virus; *MALT* mucosal associated lymphoid tissue; *NHL* non Hodgkin's lymphoma; *NSAID* non steroidal anti-inflammatory drug; *RCC* renal cell carcinoma; *VIN* vulvar intraepithelial neoplasia hepatitis, which can, in turn, predispose people to hepatocellular carcinoma (Chang et al. 2000; Davis 2005). More recently, a vaccine against human papilloma virus (HPV) 16 and 18 has been developed specifically to prevent cervical cancer. Each year, cervical cancers cause more than 250,000 deaths worldwide, and HPV 16 and 18 are associated with 70% of these tumors, in addition to tumors of the vagina and vulva (Future II Study Group 2007; Garland et al. 2007; Parkin et al. 2005). Vaccination of girls against HPV prevents viral acquisition, leading to 98% efficacy against HPV 16 and 18 associated cervical intraepithelial neoplasia and cervical carcinoma (Future II Study Group 2007).

Like viruses, bacteria have also been associated with tumor development. The bacterium *Helicobacter pylori* is the principal cause of stomach cancer and is also an important cause of mucosal-associated lymphoid tissue (MALT) lymphomas (Parkin et al. 2005; Eslick 2006). *H. pylori* is treatable with antibiotics, and eradication of *H. pylori* prior to alterations in the gastric mucosa can decrease the risk of stomach cancer (Wong et al. 2004). Remarkably, MALT lymphomas are often treatable with antibiotics, and resistance to antibiotic therapy is associated with genomic alterations in the tumor cells (Liu et al. 2002; Roggero et al. 1995).

Even in the absence of a clear infection, chronic inflammation of the colon can substantially increase the risk of colorectal cancer, and several anti-inflammatory treatments are effective at reducing this risk (Dube et al. 2007; Higuchi et al. 2003; Rostom et al. 2007; Steinbach et al. 2000; Turini and DuBois 2002; Velayos et al. 2005). Treatment of patients with ulcerative colitis with the anti-inflammatory drug 5-aminosalicylic acid is associated with a 50% decrease in the odds of colorectal cancer development (Velayos et al. 2005). Similarly, anti-inflammatory cyclooxygenase-2 inhibitors are approved for reducing polyp formation in patients with familial adenomatous polyposis (Higuchi et al. 2003; Steinbach et al. 2000).

2 Immune Adjuvants and Cytokines

Although spontaneous immune responses to tumor antigens can occur, these reactions are typically unable to cause regression of established tumors; however, the introduction of immune adjuvants into the tumor microenvironment can boost these immune responses, leading to regression of some early stage tumors. The standard of care for superficial bladder cancer is surgical removal of the tumor followed by immune therapy with intra-vesicular bacilli Calmette-Guérin (BCG). In most patients, BCG provokes a local, self-limiting inflammatory reaction in the bladder wall, and the severity of this inflammation is correlated with clinical response (Bohle and Brandau 2003; Shelley et al. 2000). Several clinical trials have shown that, when combined with surgery, immune therapy with BCG is more effective than conventional chemotherapy, increasing progression-free survival over 10 years from 37 to 61.9% (Shelley et al. 2000; Herr et al. 1995; Sylvester et al. 2005).

Microbes can elicit immunity by activating pattern-recognition receptors, including Toll-like receptors (TLRs). Because of their substantial immune activating potential, purified TLR agonists are being evaluated as immune adjuvant therapy for cancer. The TLR7 agonist imiquimod, initially approved to treat dermal warts caused by HPV, has demonstrated efficacy against low-grade epithelial tumors and precancerous lesions (Geisse et al. 2004; Hadley et al. 2006). Imiquimod is approved for the treatment of basal cell carcinoma, as well as actinic keratosis, the precursor lesion of cutaneous squamous cell carcinoma (Geisse et al. 2004; Hadley et al. 2006). More recently, imiquimod has been evaluated as an alternative to surgical treatment for vulvar intraepithelial neoplasia as well as other tumors known to be associated with HPV infection (van Seters et al. 2008).

Like adjuvants, immune-modulating cytokines can activate antitumor immunity, though often with substantial systemic adverse effects. The cytokines IL-2 and interferon (IFN)-α have been used to treat advanced melanoma and renal cell carcinoma (RCC) where standard chemotherapy is generally ineffective, although response rates have been low (Atkins et al. 1999; Fyfe et al. 1995; Kirkwood et al. 1996; Motzer et al. 2002). IFN-α is most effective prior to distant metastasis (stage III disease); in this setting, IFN-α has a 16% overall response rate and a 5% complete response rate (Kirkwood et al. 1996). Effective IFN-α therapy is associated with an increased risk of autoimmunity, linking antitumor activity to the breaking of tolerance (Dunn et al. 2004, 2005; Gogas et al. 2006). Unlike IFN-α, IL-2 can induce responses in patients with metastatic melanoma, although the overall response rate (16%) and the complete response rate (6%) are similarly low (Atkins et al. 1999).

In contrast to systemic cytokine therapy used primarily for immune modulation, the direct cytotoxic effects of the cytokine tumor necrosis factor (TNF)-α have been used locally to treat soft tissue sarcomas of the limb and melanoma (Grunhagen et al. 2006; Lans et al. 2005). Isolated limb perfusion with TNF-α combined with the alkylating agent melphalan has a response rate of 70–85%, with a relatively high chance of limb preservation in patients who would typically require amputation (Grunhagen et al. 2006; Lans et al. 2005).

3 Monoclonal Antibodies

Tumor targeting monoclonal antibodies are among the most successful forms of cancer immunotherapy, partly because they can bypass limitations that impede endogenous immunity. Manufactured antibodies can target self-proteins to which the immune system is generally tolerant, and antibody specificity and affinity can be carefully selected. Biologically active antibody titers can also be achieved rapidly through direct infusion into the circulation. In general, monoclonal antibody therapies are less toxic than conventional chemotherapy, although significant adverse reactions can occur following binding to nonmalignant tissue (Byrd et al. 1999; Hurwitz et al. 2004; Robert et al. 2001; Slamon et al. 2001).

Nine monoclonal antibodies have been approved for cancer treatment; five of these bind membrane proteins expressed on hematologic tumors: CD52 in chronic lymphocytic leukemia (CLL) (alemtuzumab), CD33 in acute myelogenous leukemia (AML) (gentuzumab), and CD20 in non-Hodgkin's lymphoma (NHL) and CLL (rituximab, ibritumomab tiuxetan, and tositumomab) (Bross et al. 2001; Coiffier et al. 2002; Fisher et al. 2005; Keating et al. 2002; Witzig et al. 2002). Of these antibodies, rituximab is the most widely used and has now been added to cyclophosphamide, doxorubicin, vincristine, and prednisone as part of the standard treatment for NHL (Coiffier et al. 2002; Marcus and Hagenbeek 2007).

Four monoclonal antibodies have been approved for the treatment of solid tumors: trastuzumab, cetuximab, panitumumab, and bevacizumab (Cobleigh et al. 1999; Cohen et al. 2007a, b; Giusti et al. 2007; Hudis 2007; Jonker et al. 2007; Meyerhardt and Mayer 2005; Van Cutsem et al. 2007). Trastuzumab, cetuximab, and panitumumab target receptors of the epidermal growth factor (EGF) family, binding the EGF receptor itself (cetuximab and panitumumab) or HER2/neu (transtuzumab). Both EGFR-targeting antibodies have been approved for the treatment of metastatic colorectal cancer, and trastuzumab has been approved for the treatment of invasive, HER2/neu-positive breast cancer (Giusti et al. 2007; Hudis 2007; Jonker et al. 2007; Meyerhardt and Mayer 2005; Van Cutsem et al. 2007). Bevacizumab does not directly target malignant cells, binding to vascular endothelial growth factor (VEGF), a secreted angiogenic cytokine (Cohen et al. 2007a, b). Bevacizumab has shown some activity against several solid tumors, including tumors of the lung, colon, breast, kidney, and pancreas (Cohen et al. 2007a, b; Bukowski et al. 2007; Kindler et al. 2005; Miller et al. 2005).

Several monoclonal antibodies inhibit signaling downstream of their targets. Both cetuximab and pantitumumab inhibit EGFR signaling by blocking interactions with EGF and preventing conformational changes required for dimerization (Li et al. 2005; Sunada et al. 1986; Yang et al. 1999); similarly, rituximab and trastuzumab alter signaling downstream of their targets (Shan et al. 2000; Valabrega et al. 2007). Through VEGF binding, bevacizumab sterically inhibits VEGF-dependent angiogenesis (Kim et al. 1993). In addition to these direct effects, monoclonal antibodies may also facilitate the recruitment of immune effector cells to tumors. Ligation of fragment c receptors (FcRs) on innate immune cells can induce antibody-dependent cellular cytotoxicity, and clinical data now suggests a role for high affinity FcR polymorphisms in optimal responses to rituximab and trastuzumab (Cartron et al. 2002; Musolino et al. 2008). The link between FcR polymorphisms and clinical responses to these antibodies underscores the ability of innate immunity, when appropriately targeted, to have powerful antitumor effects. Given the capacity of immune cells to inhibit tumor growth, one of the principal goals of tumor immune therapy is to develop novel strategies for targeting immune cells to malignancies.

4 Bone Marrow Transplantation and Donor Leukocyte Infusion

Many hematologic malignancies are treated by bone marrow ablative therapy followed by bone marrow transplantation from a healthy donor. Despite a high response rate, tumor relapse following transplantation is still fairly common (Gale et al. 1994; Weiden et al. 1979). Intriguingly, for many tumors the risk of relapse is substantially higher for patients who receive a syngeneic transplant than for patients who receive allogeneic bone marrow, indicating a graft-versus-leukemia (GVL) effect in allogeneic transplantation (Gale et al. 1994; Wu and Ritz 2006). In acute lymphocytic leukemia (ALL), the risk of relapse is 36% with a syngeneic transplant, compared with 26% with an allogeneic transplant; in AML the difference in relapse rates is 52% compared with 16%; and in chronic myelocytic leukemia (CML) the difference is 40% compared with 7% (Gale et al. 1994). Allogeneic bone marrow recipients run the risk of developing graft-versus-host disease (GVHD), a potentially lethal disease caused by transplant-mediated immunity to recipient tissues. GVHD severity is inversely correlated with relapse risk, suggesting that similar immune mechanisms may be involved in GVHD and GVL (Weiden et al. 1979).

Perhaps the clearest evidence linking donor immunity to a reduction in relapse risk comes from the success of donor leukocyte infusion (DLI) (Kolb et al. 1990, 2004). In DLI, leukocytes are harvested from the peripheral blood of transplant donors and infused back into transplant recipients following relapse. This immune therapeutic approach has been remarkably successful in CML, leading to complete remission of relapsed disease in 70% of infused patients (Kolb et al. 2004). DLI is also effective in ALL, AML, and multiple myeloma, although complete remissions of relapsed disease are less common (15–29%) (Kolb et al. 2004). Because of its success, immune therapy with DLI is now a standard treatment for relapsed leukemia following bone marrow transplantation.

5 Investigational Approaches to Immune Therapy

By building upon advances in basic research, a range of novel strategies for eliciting protective antitumor immune responses are being developed. Although tumor-reactive cells are likely present in many therapeutic settings, regulatory pathways appear to prevent these cells from generating productive antitumor responses; circumventing these pathways is thus an important goal of many novel strategies for cancer immunotherapy. Even in the absence of regulation, the antigenic targets and frequency of tumor-reactive cells may be insufficient to inhibit tumor growth. As a result, several therapeutic strategies seek to increase the number of tumor-reactive cells through either vaccination or ex vivo expansion.

6 Immune-Modulating Antibodies

Many monoclonal antibodies with immune-modulating activity are under development for the treatment of cancer. Several of these antibodies antagonize negative regulatory circuits that are thought to be important in limiting antitumor responses; similarly, agonistic antibodies to T cell coreceptors are being developed to stimulate antitumor cytotoxicity.

6.1 Negative Regulatory Receptors

The most clinically advanced immune-modulating antibodies block cytotoxic T lymphocyte antigen (CTLA)-4, an important inhibitory receptor expressed on activated T cells and Tregs (Greenwald et al. 2005). In the absence of CTLA-4, mice develop a lethal multiorgan inflammatory disease, underscoring the central importance of CTLA-4 in immune homeostasis, and many studies have demonstrated enhanced antitumor activity following CTLA-4 blockade in animal models (Greenwald et al. 2005; van Elsas et al. 1999; Tivol et al. 1995; Waterhouse et al. 1995).

Two CTLA-4-blocking antibodies (ipilimumab and tremelimumab) have entered clinical testing predominantly in advanced melanoma (van Elsas et al. 1999; Korman et al. 2006; O'Day et al. 2007). A series of phase I and phase II trials have demonstrated clinical activity for both antibodies, with objective responses, including complete responses, in 5–15% of patients. On the basis of these trials, advanced registration trials for these antibodies are currently underway (O'Day et al. 2007). In addition to single-agent trials, some early trials have shown evidence for enhanced activity when anti-CTLA-4 therapy is combined with other immune-modulating therapy (O'Day et al. 2007).

CTLA-4 blockade has been associated with grade 3 and grade 4 autoimmune toxicities, establishing the importance of this negative regulatory pathway in maintaining normal immune homeostasis (van Elsas et al. 1999; Korman et al. 2006; O'Day et al. 2007). The most significant autoimmune reaction following CTLA-4 antibody administration has been colitis; however, other significant autoimmune reactions have been observed (van Elsas et al. 1999; Korman et al. 2006; O'Day et al. 2007).

The inhibitory receptor PD-1 is also under evaluation as a target for cancer immune therapy. PD-1 is expressed on a variety of immune effector cells, and one of its ligands, PD-L1, is often abundantly expressed on tumors, where expression is correlated with an unfavorable prognosis (Keir et al. 2008). Consistent with the importance of PD-1/PD-L1 in tumor development, blockade of PD-1 in animal models can improve antitumor immunity (Keir et al. 2008; Hirano et al. 2005).

A fully human PD-1-blocking monoclonal antibody has been developed that can enhance T cell responses in vitro (Wong et al. 2007). A phase I trial of the PD-1-blocking antibody CT-011 was recently completed in 17 patients with hematologic malignancies (Berger et al. 2008). In this population, PD-1 blockade was safe and associated with a complete response in one patient with NHL (Berger et al. 2008).

6.2 TNF Family Costimulatory Receptors

Agonistic antibodies that bind costimulatory receptors can directly enhance antitumor immunity. Several antibodies targeting TNF family costimulatory receptors are under development, including antibodies to glucocorticoid-induced tumor necrosis factor receptor (GITR), CD134 (OX40), CD137 (4-1BB), and CD40.

GITR, CD134, and CD137 are each costimulatory receptors expressed on T cells, and ligation of these receptors enhances antitumor immunity in animal models (Cohen et al. 2006; Lynch 2008; Piconese et al. 2008; Ramirez-Montagut et al. 2006; Sugamura et al. 2004). An anti-CD137 antibody (BMS-663513) is now in phase I and phase II testing for melanoma and NSCLC as well as other solid tumors, and clinical trials are planned for both GITR- and CD134-specific antibodies (Dougan and Dranoff 2009). CD40 is a critical receptor linking CD4$^+$ T cell, dendritic cell (DC), and B cell immunity, and activating antibodies against CD40 have shown efficacy in animal tumor models (French et al. 1999). In addition, a recent phase I trial of the anti-CD40 antibody CP-870893 showed encouraging results in patients with advanced melanoma (Vonderheide et al. 2007).

7 Novel Adjuvants

Imiquimod and BCG have proven useful in the treatment of a range of early stage tumors; however, neither adjuvant is suitable for systemic delivery. Consequently, current research has focused on identifying systemically active adjuvants that could be used to treat a wider range of tumors, including agonists of TLR9 and the NKT cell agonist α-galactosylceramide (α-galcer, KRN7000).

Agonists of TLR9, a receptor required for the recognition of microbial CpG DNA, can activate immune responses when delivered into the circulation (Iwasaki and Medzhitov 2004; Krieg 2006). Several TLR9 agonists are undergoing clinical testing in a range of tumors, including non-small cell lung carcinoma (NSCLC), basal cell carcinoma, metastatic melanoma, NHL, and cutaneous T cell lymphoma (Kim et al. 2004; Leonard et al. 2007; Manegold et al. 2005; Hofmann et al. 2008; Pashenkov et al. 2006). Currently, TLR9 agonist treatment has been associated with immune reactions and some evidence of antitumor activity, though complete responses have been rare (Kim et al. 2004; Leonard et al. 2007; Manegold et al. 2005; Hofmann et al. 2008; Pashenkov et al. 2006).

α-galcer, a lipid derived from marine sponges, was originally isolated more than a decade ago in a screen for biological molecules with anticancer activity (Kobayashi et al. 1995; Smyth et al. 2002). α-galcer is a specific agonist for NKT cells, a subset of T cells that recognize lipid antigens (Smyth et al. 2002). Administration of α-galcer can have potent antitumor effects in many murine cancer models, suggesting that NKT cells may play a broad role in antitumor immunity (Smyth et al. 2002). Several phase I clinical trials have investigated the potential for using α-galcer-mediated NKT cell activation as cancer therapy (Chang et al. 2005; Giaccone et al. 2002; Ishikawa et al. 2005; Motohashi et al. 2006; Nieda et al. 2004). Both direct infusion of α-galcer and infusion of α-galcer-loaded DCs have been used safely in patients, and produce signs of immune activation (Chang et al. 2005; Giaccone et al. 2002; Ishikawa et al. 2005; Nieda et al. 2004; Uchida et al. 2008). Autologous NKT cells have also been cultured ex vivo and then reintroduced into patients in an attempt to boost NKT cell numbers (Motohashi et al. 2006).

8 Antagonizing T Regulatory Cells

Regulatory T cells appear to play an important function in dampening antitumor immunity. Tregs infiltrate a wide range of tumors, and large Treg infiltrates are associated with poor prognosis in a variety of cancers (Bates et al. 2006; Curiel et al. 2004; Kobayashi et al. 2007; Wolf et al. 2005). In addition to inhibiting spontaneous immunity, Tregs may also pose a barrier to vaccination strategies, which can induce antigen-specific Tregs (Zhou et al. 2006). Given the potential role of Tregs in limiting antitumor immunity, methods for directly targeting these cells may be clinically useful.

The drug denileukin diftitox is a conjugate of Diphtheria toxin and IL-2 initially developed to treat T cell malignancies, yet this drug has shown some selective toxicity for Tregs (Dannull et al. 2005; Mahnke et al. 2007). Inclusion of denileukin diftitox in a vaccine setting may enhance the magnitude of stimulated antitumor responses (Dannull et al. 2005). Additional Treg-targeted therapies are also under investigation, including strategies to block Treg chemotaxis through CCL22 and CCR4, Treg function through IL-35, or Treg induction following the phagocytosis of apoptotic cells using a dominant negative form of milk fat globule EGF E8 (Collison et al. 2007; Iellem et al. 2001; Jinushi et al. 2007).

9 Adoptive T Cell Therapy

Adoptive T cell therapies generate productive antitumor immunity using the in vitro expansion of endogenous, cancer-reactive T cells, which are harvested from patients, manipulated, and then reintroduced. Adoptive T cell therapy has had promising early clinical results, showing an association with clinical responses in a substantial minority of patients with metastatic melanoma (Mackensen et al. 2006; Yee et al. 2000, 2002). $CD8^+$ cytotoxic T cells are the principal effectors in adoptive T cell therapy (June 2007; Klebanoff et al. 2005); however, $CD4^+$ T cells may also play an important role, given that transplantation of tumor-reactive $CD4^+$ T cells in metastatic melanoma has been associated with some efficacy (Hunder et al. 2008). T cells used in adoptive therapy can be harvested from the peripheral blood, resected lymph nodes, tumor biopsies, and malignant effusions. Peripheral blood is the most accessible site for obtaining T cells for transplant; however, tumor-infiltrating lymphocytes obtained from biopsies may contain the highest concentration of tumor-reactive cells (Dudley et al. 2003). Obtaining sufficient cells from tumor biopsies can be difficult, though this approach has been used successfully in patients with melanoma (Dudley et al. 2003).

Two alternative approaches seek to circumvent the low frequency of tumor reactive T cells in the peripheral blood by directly supplying tumor specificity to T cells. In the first approach, peripheral blood T cells are engineered to express tumor-reactive T cell receptors (TCRs); however, since TCR recognition of antigen is MHC allele specific, each engineered TCR can only be used in MHC matched patients (Morgan et al. 2006). Early tests of this approach have been conducted in metastatic melanoma (Morgan et al. 2006). The second approach bypasses MHC restriction by engineering T cells to express chimeric fusion proteins that link the antigen-binding domain of the B cell receptor with the signaling component of the TCR complex (Kershaw et al. 2006; Park et al. 2007; Lamers et al. 2006). These "T-bodies" can bind tumor antigens and activate T cells in an MHC independent fashion. Therapy with T-body-expressing T cells has been tested in RCC, ovarian carcinoma, and pediatric neuroblastoma. T-body-expressing cells are typically well tolerated; however, severe autoimmune hepatitis occurred in patients with RCC, likely resulting from expression of the target antigen in the biliary tract (Lamers et al. 2006). This adverse event indicates the reactive potential of T-body engineered T cells, but also underscores the importance of antigen selection.

Once harvested, T cells can be expanded through stimulation with activating antibodies or through exposure to tumor antigens (Mackensen et al. 2006; Yee et al. 2000, 2002). Thus far, adoptive T cell therapies have been limited by the replicative potential of cultured T cells. Several strategies to extend the lifespan of cultured T cells have been attempted including the introduction of telomerase or costimulatory receptors into cultured cells as well as the use of IL-15 as an additive to cultures (Hooijberg et al. 2000; Topp et al. 2003; June 2007). Engraftment of adoptively transferred T cells may also be enhanced in lymphodepleted hosts, and combining lymphodepleting chemotherapy with adoptive T cell transplantation appears to augment treatment efficacy (Dudley et al. 2002, 2005).

Combining adoptive T cell therapy with other immune-modulating strategies may augment treatment responses. Using an autologous tumor vaccine mixed with BCG in combination with adoptive T cell therapy has produced promising results in RCC, where treatment was associated with a 27% objective response rate in a recent phase II trial (Chang et al. 2003).

10 Tumor Antigens and Therapeutic Cancer Vaccines

Because of the investigational nature of current therapies, vaccination strategies for cancer have been limited to patients with advanced disease. Therapeutic vaccination represents a significant challenge, given that it must bypass established immune regulatory mechanisms that have already led to tumor tolerance. Many vaccination strategies for generating therapeutic antitumor immunity are being investigated; antigen-specific vaccines, DC vaccines, and cytokine-based, whole tumor cell vaccines are among the most promising and best studied of these strategies to date.

10.1 Antigen-Specific Vaccines

Several vaccination strategies based on a specific antigen are currently in clinical trials. These vaccines, which use recombinant proteins or antigenic peptides formulated with adjuvants, can elicit immune responses and have shown some efficacy in a variety of human tumors. The targets selected for these vaccines have been diverse, although many are cancer testes antigens. Cancer testes antigens are expressed by tumor cells as well as within the immune-privileged environment of the testes, making immune response against them relatively specific for tumor tissue.

Two cancer testes antigens, MAGE-A3 and NY-ESO-1, have been explored as targets in a series of clinical vaccine trials. MAGE-A3 is expressed by an array of tumors (Atanackovic et al. 2008; Brichard and Lejeune 2007), and MAGE-A3 targeting vaccines have led to potent antitumor immunity that can be associated with objective responses (Atanackovic et al. 2008). Phase I and II MAGE-A3 vaccine trials have been completed in melanoma and NSCLC, and a phase III trial in NSCLC is currently underway (Atanackovic et al. 2008; Brichard and Lejeune 2007). Similar to MAGE-A3, NY-ESO-1 is widely expressed in human cancers (Gnjatic et al. 2006; Valmori et al. 2007). Multiple clinical trials have examined NY-ESO-1-based vaccines in a diverse group of tumors, including melanoma, ovarian carcinoma, and NSCLC (Gnjatic et al. 2006; Valmori et al. 2007). These vaccines have elicited strong immune reactions, including coordinated antibody and cytotoxic T cell responses (Valmori et al. 2007). In addition to cancer testes antigens, tumors can express proteins with a narrow distribution in nonmalignant tissues; these tissue-restricted proteins have been targeted in melanoma, where melanocyte-specific proteins often continue to be expressed (Slingluff et al. 2006).

In addition to cancer testes antigens, antigens that are uniquely expressed on tumor cells have also been targeted by cancer vaccines. In particular, B cell lymphomas express specific, clonal rearrangements of the B cell receptor (idiotype) that can be targeted by antitumor vaccines, leading to specific immune responses against the tumor (Weng et al. 2004). Recent trials examining the efficacy of this approach have been promising, and suggest that anti-idiotype vaccines may be effective therapy for lymphomas in some settings.

10.2 Dendritic Cell Vaccines

The ability to culture DCs from human peripheral blood monocytes has led to interest in DC-based cancer vaccines (Schuler et al. 2003). Antigenic peptides or proteins can be readily loaded onto immature monocyte-derived DCs in culture, and these antigen-loaded DCs can then be used in an autologous transplant to activate antigen-specific T cells (Schuler et al. 2003).

DCs require activation before they can induce immune responses, and this activation can occur following a range of stimuli, including cytokines and microbial products (Napolitani et al. 2005; Sporri and Reis e Sousa 2005). Most trials generate mature DCs using a cytokine cocktail, although other approaches, including the use of microbial pattern-recognition receptor agonists and introduction of immature DCs into inflamed tissue, have also been considered (Mailliard et al. 2004; O'Neill et al. 2004; MartIn-Fontecha et al. 2003; Nair et al. 2003). Antigens can also be delivered directly to DCs in vivo through antibodies that bind surface receptors such as DEC205; this strategy for targeting DCs has proved successful in experimental models and is under development for use in patients (Jiang et al. 1995; Bonifaz et al. 2002; Mahnke et al. 2005). Antigen delivery to cultured DCs has been accomplished through direct loading of antigenic peptides or long overlapping peptide mixtures, exposure to whole recombinant protein, transfection with antigen-encoding mRNA, and fusion with tumor cells (Schuler et al. 2003; Rosenblatt et al. 2005; Vambutas et al. 2005; Van Tendeloo et al. 2001).

Many DC vaccination trials in cancer patients have been conducted using a range of protocols with some encouraging preliminary results (Andrews et al. 2008); however, to date phase III trials of DC vaccines, including a trial in metastatic melanoma, have yet to demonstrate clinical benefit (Andrews et al. 2008; Schadendorf et al. 2006). DC vaccination protocols are not yet optimized, though, and the creation of more effective vaccines continues to be an active area of investigation.

Recently a vaccination approach similar to DC vaccines has shown efficacy against recurrent, hormone-resistant prostate cancer (Small et al. 2006). This vaccine, called sipuleucel-T, uses autologous monocytes cultured in a fusion protein comprising GM-CSF and prostatic acid phosphatase to activate antitumor responses. Although a phase III trial of sipuleucel-T failed to meet its primary endpoint of delayed time to cancer progression, a post hoc analysis found that patients treated with sipuleucel-T showed increased survival (median survival = 25.9 months) compared to placebo (median survival 21.4 months) (Small et al. 2006). Similar results have been reported in a second trial that used survival as a primary endpoint, indicating that this approach may be clinically beneficial; both of these trials were the basis for the recent FDA approval of sipuleucel-T for the treatment of metastatic, hormone-resistant prostate cancer (Kantoff 2010).

10.3 Cytokine-Based Tumor Vaccines

The cytokines IL-2, IL-12, IFN-α, and GM-CSF have all been evaluated as cancer vaccine adjuvants; among these, GM-CSF has been the most widely studied (Berinstein 2007). GM-CSF has, thus far, been most potent when used to prime immune responses against irradiated whole tumor cells. GM-CSF primarily acts to recruit and mature DCs, enhancing tumor antigen presentation. In mouse models, prophylactic vaccines using GM-CSF-transfected tumor cells can engender protective immunity, while therapeutic use can delay tumor growth (Jinushi et al. 2008). Similarly, in cancer patients, injection of autologous, irradiated, whole tumor cells engineered to produce GM-CSF (GVAX) can induce coordinated adaptive immunity to a wide range of tumor antigens. In melanoma patients, these immune reactions have been associated with both partial and complete responses (Soiffer et al. 1998).

Autologous whole-cell vaccines have the advantage of providing multiple tumor antigens, yet large scale manufacturing of patient-specific vaccines also presents a significant challenge. To facilitate vaccine production, GM-CSF secreting allogeneic tumor vaccines have also been developed for clinical testing. These vaccines, which are derived from tumor cell lines, are under evaluation in pancreatic cancer, breast cancer, and hormone-resistant prostate cancer (Jaffee et al. 2001; Michael et al. 2005; Simons et al. 2006).

Although encouraging responses to GVAX have occurred in some patients, these vaccines may be most effective when used in combination with other immune-modulating therapies (Jinushi et al. 2008; Hodi et al. 2003, 2008). The anti-CTLA-4 monoclonal antibody ipilimumab has been tested in patients previously vaccinated using DCs or GVAX (Hodi et al. 2003, 2008). In these patients, ipilimumab is associated with enhanced antitumor immunity and objective responses in some patients (Hodi et al. 2003, 2008). Inflammatory reactions in nonmalignant tissues were associated with therapy, yet treatment did not provoke severe autoimmunity (Hodi et al. 2003, 2008). Intriguingly, tumor necrosis was associated with an increased ratio of tumor infiltrating $CD8^+$ T effectors to $FoxP3^+$ regulatory T cells (Fig. 22.1), suggesting that clinical responses to GVAX and CTLA-4 blockade follow from a loss of immune suppression in conjunction with enhanced cytotoxic immunity (Hodi et al. 2003, 2008). These preliminary results suggest that combination immune therapies may have significant clinical efficacy, although this potential remains to be tested in randomized clinical trials.

11 Conclusion

Single modality immune therapies have been successful in treating cancer in some settings, yet combination therapy may often be necessary in order to generate protective antitumor immunity (Dougan and Dranoff 2009). Combining strategies to expand and activate tumor-reactive cells with therapies designed to disable regulatory pathways may substantially improve cancer immunotherapy, though such combinations may also increase the risk of autoimmunity. Further research identifying the mechanisms of immune suppression that are most valuable to tumors and least necessary for the maintenance of tolerance should further expand the scope of effective immune therapies for cancer.

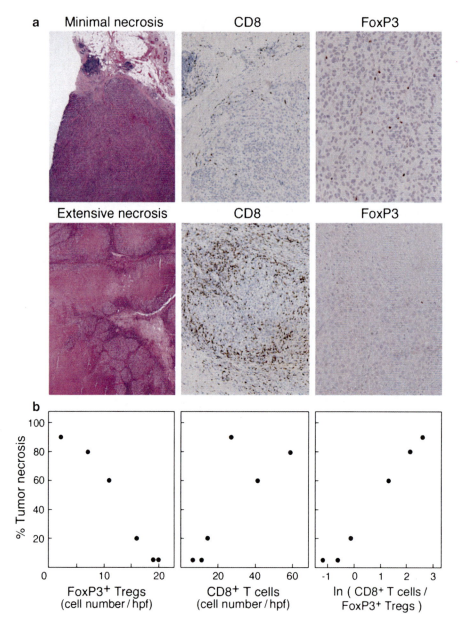

Fig. 22.1 The ratio of tumor-infiltrating CD8+ T cells to FoxP3+ Tregs after GVAX followed by ipilimumab infusion is tightly correlated with the extent of tumor necrosis. (**a**) *Upper row*: minimal necrosis of melanoma metastasis. *Lower row*: extensive necrosis of melanoma metastasis (magnification: H&E, ×4; CD8, ×20; FoxP3, ×40). (**b**) Numbers of tumor-infiltrating FoxP3+ Tregs and CD8+ T cells vs. tumor necrosis (reprinted from (Hodi et al. 2008))

References

Andrews DM, Maraskovsky E, Smyth MJ (2008) Cancer vaccines for established cancer: how to make them better? Immunol Rev 222:242–255

Atanackovic D, Altorki NK, Cao Y, Ritter E, Ferrara CA, Ritter G, Hoffman EW, Bokemeyer C, Old LJ, Gnjatic S (2008) Booster vaccination of cancer patients with MAGE-A3 protein reveals long-term immunological memory or tolerance depending on priming. Proc Natl Acad Sci USA 105:1650–1655

Atkins MB, Lotze MT, Dutcher JP, Fisher RI, Weiss G, Margolin K, Abrams J, Sznol M, Parkinson D, Hawkins M, Paradise C, Kunkel L, Rosenberg SA (1999) High-dose recombinant interleukin 2 therapy for patients with metastatic melanoma: analysis of 270 patients treated between 1985 and 1993. J Clin Oncol 17:2105–2116

Bates GJ, Fox SB, Han C, Leek RD, Garcia JF, Harris AL, Banham AH (2006) Quantification of regulatory T cells enables the identification of high-risk breast cancer patients and those at risk of late relapse. J Clin Oncol 24:5373–5380

Berger R, Rotem-Yehudar R, Slama G, Landes S, Kneller A, Leiba M, Koren-Michowitz M, Shimoni A, Nagler A (2008) Phase I safety and pharmacokinetic study of CT-011, a humanized antibody interacting with PD-1, in patients with advanced hematologic malignancies. Clin Cancer Res 14:3044–3051

Berinstein NL (2007) Enhancing cancer vaccines with immunomodulators. Vaccine 25(Suppl 2):B72–B88

Bohle A, Brandau S (2003) Immune mechanisms in bacillus Calmette-Guerin immunotherapy for superficial bladder cancer. J Urol 170:964–969

Bonifaz L, Bonnyay D, Mahnke K, Rivera M, Nussenzweig MC, Steinman RM (2002) Efficient targeting of protein antigen to the dendritic cell receptor DEC-205 in the steady state leads to antigen presentation on major histocompatibility complex class I products and peripheral CD8+ T cell tolerance. J Exp Med 196:1627–1638

Brichard VG, Lejeune D (2007) GSK's antigen-specific cancer immunotherapy programme: pilot results leading to Phase III clinical development. Vaccine 25(Suppl 2):B61–B71

Bross PF, Beitz J, Chen G, Chen XH, Duffy E, Kieffer L, Roy S, Sridhara R, Rahman A, Williams G, Pazdur R (2001) Approval summary: gemtuzumab ozogamicin in relapsed acute myeloid leukemia. Clin Cancer Res 7:1490–1496

Bukowski RM, Kabbinavar FF, Figlin RA, Flaherty K, Srinivas S, Vaishampayan U, Drabkin HA, Dutcher J, Ryba S, Xia Q, Scappaticci FA, McDermott D (2007) Randomized phase II study of erlotinib combined with bevacizumab compared with bevacizumab alone in metastatic renal cell cancer. J Clin Oncol 25:4536–4541

Byrd JC, Waselenko JK, Maneatis TJ, Murphy T, Ward FT, Monahan BP, Sipe MA, Donegan S, White CA (1999) Rituximab therapy in hematologic malignancy patients with circulating blood tumor cells: association with increased infusion-related side effects and rapid blood tumor clearance. J Clin Oncol 17:791–795

Cartron G, Dacheux L, Salles G, Solal-Celigny P, Bardos P, Colombat P, Watier H (2002) Therapeutic activity of humanized anti-CD20 monoclonal antibody and polymorphism in IgG Fc receptor FcgammaRIIIa gene. Blood 99:754–758

Chang MH, Shau WY, Chen CJ, Wu TC, Kong MS, Liang DC, Hsu HM, Chen HL, Hsu HY, Chen DS (2000) Hepatitis B vaccination and hepatocellular carcinoma rates in boys and girls. JAMA 284:3040–3042

Chang AE, Li Q, Jiang G, Sayre DM, Braun TM, Redman BG (2003) Phase II trial of autologous tumor vaccination, anti-CD3-activated vaccine-primed lymphocytes, and interleukin-2 in stage IV renal cell cancer. J Clin Oncol 21:884–890

Chang DH, Osman K, Connolly J, Kukreja A, Krasovsky J, Pack M, Hutchinson A, Geller M, Liu N, Annable R, Shay J, Kirchhoff K, Nishi N, Ando Y, Hayashi K, Hassoun H, Steinman RM, Dhodapkar MV (2005) Sustained expansion of NKT cells and antigen-specific T cells after injection of alpha-galactosyl-ceramide loaded mature dendritic cells in cancer patients. J Exp Med 201:1503–1517

Cobleigh MA, Vogel CL, Tripathy D, Robert NJ, Scholl S, Fehrenbacher L, Wolter JM, Paton V, Shak S, Lieberman G, Slamon DJ (1999) Multinational study of the efficacy and safety of humanized anti-HER2 monoclonal antibody in women who have HER2-overexpressing metastatic breast cancer that has progressed after chemotherapy for metastatic disease. J Clin Oncol 17:2639–2648

Cohen AD, Diab A, Perales MA, Wolchok JD, Rizzuto G, Merghoub T, Huggins D, Liu C, Turk MJ, Restifo NP, Sakaguchi S, Houghton AN (2006) Agonist anti-GITR antibody enhances vaccine-induced CD8(+) T-cell responses and tumor immunity. Cancer Res 66:4904–4912

Cohen MH, Gootenberg J, Keegan P, Pazdur R (2007a) FDA drug approval summary: bevacizumab (Avastin) plus Carboplatin and Paclitaxel as first-line treatment of advanced/metastatic recurrent nonsquamous non-small cell lung cancer. Oncologist 12:713–718

Cohen MH, Gootenberg J, Keegan P, Pazdur R (2007b) FDA drug approval summary: bevacizumab plus FOLFOX4 as second-line treatment of colorectal cancer. Oncologist 12:356–361

Coiffier B, Lepage E, Briere J, Herbrecht R, Tilly H, Bouabdallah R, Morel P, Van Den Neste E, Salles G, Gaulard P, Reyes F, Lederlin P, Gisselbrecht C (2002) CHOP chemotherapy plus rituximab compared with CHOP alone in elderly patients with diffuse large-B-cell lymphoma. N Engl J Med 346:235–242

Collison LW, Workman CJ, Kuo TT, Boyd K, Wang Y, Vignali KM, Cross R, Sehy D, Blumberg RS, Vignali DA (2007) The inhibitory cytokine IL-35 contributes to regulatory T-cell function. Nature 450:566–569

Curiel TJ, Coukos G, Zou L, Alvarez X, Cheng P, Mottram P, Evdemon-Hogan M, Conejo-Garcia JR, Zhang L, Burow M, Zhu Y, Wei S, Kryczek I, Daniel B, Gordon A, Myers L, Lackner A, Disis ML, Knutson KL, Chen L, Zou W (2004) Specific recruitment of regulatory T cells in ovarian carcinoma fosters immune privilege and predicts reduced survival. Nat Med 10:942–949

Dannull J, Su Z, Rizzieri D, Yang BK, Coleman D, Yancey D, Zhang A, Dahm P, Chao N, Gilboa E, Vieweg J (2005) Enhancement of vaccine-mediated antitumor immunity in cancer patients after depletion of regulatory T cells. J Clin Invest 115:3623–3633

Davis JP (2005) Experience with hepatitis A and B vaccines. Am J Med 118(Suppl 10A):7S–15S

Dougan M, Dranoff G (2009) Immune therapy for cancer. Annu Rev Immunol 27:83–117

Dube C, Rostom A, Lewin G, Tsertsvadze A, Barrowman N, Code C, Sampson M, Moher D (2007) The use of aspirin for primary prevention of colorectal cancer: a systematic review prepared for the U.S. Preventive Services Task Force. Ann Intern Med 146:365–375

Dudley ME, Wunderlich JR, Robbins PF, Yang JC, Hwu P, Schwartzentruber DJ, Topalian SL, Sherry R, Restifo NP, Hubicki AM, Robinson MR, Raffeld M, Duray P, Seipp CA, Rogers-Freezer L, Morton KE, Mavroukakis SA, White DE, Rosenberg SA (2002) Cancer regression and autoimmunity in patients after clonal repopulation with antitumor lymphocytes. Science 298:850–854

Dudley ME, Wunderlich JR, Shelton TE, Even J, Rosenberg SA (2003) Generation of tumor-infiltrating lymphocyte cultures for use in adoptive transfer therapy for melanoma patients. J Immunother 26:332–342

Dudley ME, Wunderlich JR, Yang JC, Sherry RM, Topalian SL, Restifo NP, Royal RE, Kammula U, White DE, Mavroukakis SA, Rogers LJ, Gracia GJ, Jones SA, Mangiameli DP, Pelletier MM, Gea-Banacloche J, Robinson MR, Berman DM, Filie AC, Abati A, Rosenberg SA (2005) Adoptive cell transfer therapy following non-myeloablative but lymphodepleting chemotherapy for the treatment of patients with refractory metastatic melanoma. J Clin Oncol 23:2346–2357

Dunn GP, Old LJ, Schreiber RD (2004) The three Es of cancer immunoediting. Annu Rev Immunol 22:329–360

Dunn GP, Bruce AT, Sheehan KC, Shankaran V, Uppaluri R, Bui JD, Diamond MS, Koebel CM, Arthur C, White JM, Schreiber RD (2005) A critical function for type I interferons in cancer immunoediting. Nat Immunol 6:722–729

Eslick GD (2006) *Helicobacter pylori* infection causes gastric cancer? A review of the epidemiological, meta-analytic, and experimental evidence. World J Gastroenterol 12:2991–2999

Fisher RI, Kaminski MS, Wahl RL, Knox SJ, Zelenetz AD, Vose JM, Leonard JP, Kroll S, Goldsmith SJ, Coleman M (2005) Tositumomab and iodine-131 tositumomab produces durable complete remissions in a subset of heavily pretreated patients with low-grade and transformed non-Hodgkin's lymphomas. J Clin Oncol 23:7565–7573

French RR, Chan HT, Tutt AL, Glennie MJ (1999) CD40 antibody evokes a cytotoxic T-cell response that eradicates lymphoma and bypasses T-cell help. Nat Med 5:548–553

Future, II Study Group (2007) Quadrivalent vaccine against human papillomavirus to prevent high-grade cervical lesions. N Engl J Med 356:1915–1927

Fyfe G, Fisher RI, Rosenberg SA, Sznol M, Parkinson DR, Louie AC (1995) Results of treatment of 255 patients with metastatic renal cell carcinoma who received high-dose recombinant interleukin-2 therapy. J Clin Oncol 13:688–696

Gale RP, Horowitz MM, Ash RC, Champlin RE, Goldman JM, Rimm AA, Ringden O, Stone JA, Bortin MM (1994) Identical-twin bone marrow transplants for leukemia. Ann Intern Med 120:646–652

Garland SM, Hernandez-Avila M, Wheeler CM, Perez G, Harper DM, Leodolter S, Tang GW, Ferris DG, Steben M, Bryan J, Taddeo FJ, Railkar R, Esser MT, Sings HL, Nelson M, Boslego J, Sattler C, Barr E, Koutsky LA (2007) Quadrivalent vaccine against human papillomavirus to prevent anogenital diseases. N Engl J Med 356:1928–1943

Geisse J, Caro I, Lindholm J, Golitz L, Stampone P, Owens M (2004) Imiquimod 5% cream for the treatment of superficial basal cell carcinoma: results from two phase III, randomized, vehicle-controlled studies. J Am Acad Dermatol 50:722–733

Giaccone G, Punt CJ, Ando Y, Ruijter R, Nishi N, Peters M, von Blomberg BM, Scheper RJ, van der Vliet HJ, van den Eertwegh AJ, Roelvink M, Beijnen J, Zwierzina H, Pinedo HM (2002) A phase I study of the natural killer T-cell ligand alpha-galactosylceramide (KRN7000) in patients with solid tumors. Clin Cancer Res 8:3702–3709

Giusti RM, Shastri KA, Cohen MH, Keegan P, Pazdur R (2007) FDA drug approval summary: panitumumab (Vectibix). Oncologist 12:577–583

Gnjatic S, Nishikawa H, Jungbluth AA, Gure AO, Ritter G, Jager E, Knuth A, Chen YT, Old LJ (2006) NY-ESO-1: review of an immunogenic tumor antigen. Adv Cancer Res 95:1–30

Gogas H, Ioannovich J, Dafni U, Stavropoulou-Giokas C, Frangia K, Tsoutsos D, Panagiotou P, Polyzos A, Papadopoulos O, Stratigos A, Markopoulos C, Bafaloukos D, Pectasides D, Fountzilas G, Kirkwood JM (2006) Prognostic significance of autoimmunity during treatment of melanoma with interferon. N Engl J Med 354:709–718

Greenwald RJ, Freeman GJ, Sharpe AH (2005) The B7 family revisited. Annu Rev Immunol 23:515–548

Grunhagen DJ, de Wilt JH, Graveland WJ, Verhoef C, van Geel AN, Eggermont AM (2006) Outcome and prognostic factor analysis of 217 consecutive isolated limb perfusions with tumor necrosis factor-alpha and melphalan for limb-threatening soft tissue sarcoma. Cancer 106:1776–1784

Hadley G, Derry S, Moore RA (2006) Imiquimod for actinic keratosis: systematic review and meta-analysis. J Invest Dermatol 126:1251–1255

Herr HW, Schwalb DM, Zhang ZF, Sogani PC, Fair WR, Whitmore WF Jr, Oettgen HF (1995) Intravesical bacillus Calmette-Guerin therapy prevents tumor progression and death from superficial bladder cancer: ten-year follow-up of a prospective randomized trial. J Clin Oncol 13:1404–1408

Higuchi T, Iwama T, Yoshinaga K, Toyooka M, Taketo MM, Sugihara K (2003) A randomized, double-blind, placebo-controlled trial of the effects of rofecoxib, a selective cyclooxygenase-2 inhibitor, on rectal polyps in familial adenomatous polyposis patients. Clin Cancer Res 9:4756–4760

Hirano F, Kaneko K, Tamura H, Dong H, Wang S, Ichikawa M, Rietz C, Flies DB, Lau JS, Zhu G, Tamada K, Chen L (2005) Blockade of B7-H1 and PD-1 by monoclonal antibodies potentiates cancer therapeutic immunity. Cancer Res 65:1089–1096

Hodi FS, Mihm MC, Soiffer RJ, Haluska FG, Butler M, Seiden MV, Davis T, Henry-Spires R, MacRae S, Willman A, Padera R, Jaklitsch MT, Shankar S, Chen TC, Korman A, Allison JP, Dranoff G (2003) Biologic activity of cytotoxic T lymphocyte-associated antigen 4 antibody

blockade in previously vaccinated metastatic melanoma and ovarian carcinoma patients. Proc Natl Acad Sci USA 100:4712–4717
Hodi FS, Butler M, Oble DA, Seiden MV, Haluska FG, Kruse A, Macrae S, Nelson M, Canning C, Lowy I, Korman A, Lautz D, Russell S, Jaklitsch MT, Ramaiya N, Chen TC, Neuberg D, Allison JP, Mihm MC, Dranoff G (2008) Immunologic and clinical effects of antibody blockade of cytotoxic T lymphocyte-associated antigen 4 in previously vaccinated cancer patients. Proc Natl Acad Sci USA 105:3005–3010
Hodi FS, O'Day SJ, McDermott DF, Weber RW, Sosman JA, Haanen JB, Gonzalez R, Robert C, Schadendorf D, Hassel JC, Akerley W, van den Eertwegh AJ, Lutzky J, Lorigan P, Vaubel JM, Linette GP, Hogg D, Ottensmeier CH, Lebbé C, Peschel C, Quirt I, Clark JI, Wolchok JD, Weber JS, Tian J, Yellin MJ, Nichol GM, Hoos A, Urba WJ (2010) Improved survival with ipilimumab in patients with metastatic melanoma. N Engl J Med 19;363(8):711–723
Hofmann MA, Kors C, Audring H, Walden P, Sterry W, Trefzer U (2008) Phase 1 evaluation of intralesionally injected TLR9-agonist PF-3512676 in patients with basal cell carcinoma or metastatic melanoma. J Immunother 31:520–527
Hooijberg E, Ruizendaal JJ, Snijders PJ, Kueter EW, Walboomers JM, Spits H (2000) Immortalization of human CD8+ T cell clones by ectopic expression of telomerase reverse transcriptase. J Immunol 165:4239–4245
Hudis CA (2007) Trastuzumab – mechanism of action and use in clinical practice. N Engl J Med 357:39–51
Hunder NN, Wallen H, Cao J, Hendricks DW, Reilly JZ, Rodmyre R, Jungbluth A, Gnjatic S, Thompson JA, Yee C (2008) Treatment of metastatic melanoma with autologous CD4+ T cells against NY-ESO-1. N Engl J Med 358:2698–2703
Hurwitz H, Fehrenbacher L, Novotny W, Cartwright T, Hainsworth J, Heim W, Berlin J, Baron A, Griffing S, Holmgren E, Ferrara N, Fyfe G, Rogers B, Ross R, Kabbinavar F (2004) Bevacizumab plus irinotecan, fluorouracil, and leucovorin for metastatic colorectal cancer. N Engl J Med 350:2335–2342
Iellem A, Mariani M, Lang R, Recalde H, Panina-Bordignon P, Sinigaglia F, D'Ambrosio D (2001) Unique chemotactic response profile and specific expression of chemokine receptors CCR4 and CCR8 by CD4(+)CD25(+) regulatory T cells. J Exp Med 194:847–853
Ishikawa A, Motohashi S, Ishikawa E, Fuchida H, Higashino K, Otsuji M, Iizasa T, Nakayama T, Taniguchi M, Fujisawa T (2005) A phase I study of alpha-galactosylceramide (KRN7000)-pulsed dendritic cells in patients with advanced and recurrent non-small cell lung cancer. Clin Cancer Res 11:1910–1917
Iwasaki A, Medzhitov R (2004) Toll-like receptor control of the adaptive immune responses. Nat Immunol 5:987–995
Jaffee EM, Hruban RH, Biedrzycki B, Laheru D, Schepers K, Sauter PR, Goemann M, Coleman J, Grochow L, Donehower RC, Lillemoe KD, O'Reilly S, Abrams RA, Pardoll DM, Cameron JL, Yeo CJ (2001) Novel allogeneic granulocyte-macrophage colony-stimulating factor-secreting tumor vaccine for pancreatic cancer: a phase I trial of safety and immune activation. J Clin Oncol 19:145–156
Jiang W, Swiggard WJ, Heufler C, Peng M, Mirza A, Steinman RM, Nussenzweig MC (1995) The receptor DEC-205 expressed by dendritic cells and thymic epithelial cells is involved in antigen processing. Nature 375:151–155
Jinushi M, Nakazaki Y, Dougan M, Carrasco DR, Mihm M, Dranoff G (2007) MFG-E8-mediated uptake of apoptotic cells by APCs links the pro- and antiinflammatory activities of GM-CSF. J Clin Invest 117:1902–1913
Jinushi M, Hodi FS, Dranoff G (2008) Enhancing the clinical activity of granulocyte-macrophage colony-stimulating factor-secreting tumor cell vaccines. Immunol Rev 222:287–298
Jonker DJ, O'Callaghan CJ, Karapetis CS, Zalcberg JR, Tu D, Au HJ, Berry SR, Krahn M, Price T, Simes RJ, Tebbutt NC, van Hazel G, Wierzbicki R, Langer C, Moore MJ (2007) Cetuximab for the treatment of colorectal cancer. N Engl J Med 357:2040–2048
June CH (2007) Principles of adoptive T cell cancer therapy. J Clin Invest 117:1204–1212

Kantoff PW, Higano CS, Shore ND, Berger ER, Small EJ, Penson DF, Redfern CH, Ferrari AC, Dreicer R, Sims RB, Xu Y, Frohlich MW, Schellhammer PF (2010). Sipuleucel-T immunotherapy for castration-resistant prostate cancer. N Engl J Med 363(5):411–422

Keating MJ, Flinn I, Jain V, Binet JL, Hillmen P, Byrd J, Albitar M, Brettman L, Santabarbara P, Wacker B, Rai KR (2002) Therapeutic role of alemtuzumab (Campath-1H) in patients who have failed fludarabine: results of a large international study. Blood 99:3554–3561

Keir ME, Butte MJ, Freeman GJ, Sharpe AH (2008) PD-1 and its ligands in tolerance and immunity. Annu Rev Immunol 26:677–704

Kershaw MH, Westwood JA, Parker LL, Wang G, Eshhar Z, Mavroukakis SA, White DE, Wunderlich JR, Canevari S, Rogers-Freezer L, Chen CC, Yang JC, Rosenberg SA, Hwu P (2006) A phase I study on adoptive immunotherapy using gene-modified T cells for ovarian cancer. Clin Cancer Res 12:6106–6115

Kim KJ, Li B, Winer J, Armanini M, Gillett N, Phillips HS, Ferrara N (1993) Inhibition of vascular endothelial growth factor-induced angiogenesis suppresses tumour growth in vivo. Nature 362:841–844

Kim Y, Girardi M, McAuley S, Schmalbach T (2004) Cutaneous T-cell lymphoma (CTCL) responses to a TLR9 agonist CPG immunomodulator (CPG 7909), a phase I study. J Clin Oncol 22:6600

Kindler HL, Friberg G, Singh DA, Locker G, Nattam S, Kozloff M, Taber DA, Karrison T, Dachman A, Stadler WM, Vokes EE (2005) Phase II trial of bevacizumab plus gemcitabine in patients with advanced pancreatic cancer. J Clin Oncol 23:8033–8040

Kirkwood JM, Strawderman MH, Ernstoff MS, Smith TJ, Borden EC, Blum RH (1996) Interferon alfa-2b adjuvant therapy of high-risk resected cutaneous melanoma: the Eastern Cooperative Oncology Group Trial EST 1684. J Clin Oncol 14:7–17

Klebanoff CA, Gattinoni L, Torabi-Parizi P, Kerstann K, Cardones AR, Finkelstein SE, Palmer DC, Antony PA, Hwang ST, Rosenberg SA, Waldmann TA, Restifo NP (2005) Central memory self/tumor-reactive CD8+ T cells confer superior antitumor immunity compared with effector memory T cells. Proc Natl Acad Sci USA 102:9571–9576

Kobayashi E, Motoki K, Uchida T, Fukushima H, Koezuka Y (1995) KRN7000, a novel immunomodulator, and its antitumor activities. Oncol Res 7:529–534

Kobayashi N, Hiraoka N, Yamagami W, Ojima H, Kanai Y, Kosuge T, Nakajima A, Hirohashi S (2007) FOXP3+ regulatory T cells affect the development and progression of hepatocarcinogenesis. Clin Cancer Res 13:902–911

Kolb HJ, Mittermuller J, Clemm C, Holler E, Ledderose G, Brehm G, Heim M, Wilmanns W (1990) Donor leukocyte transfusions for treatment of recurrent chronic myelogenous leukemia in marrow transplant patients. Blood 76:2462–2465

Kolb HJ, Schmid C, Barrett AJ, Schendel DJ (2004) Graft-versus-leukemia reactions in allogeneic chimeras. Blood 103:767–776

Korman AJ, Peggs KS, Allison JP (2006) Checkpoint blockade in cancer immunotherapy. Adv Immunol 90:297–339

Krieg AM (2006) Therapeutic potential of Toll-like receptor 9 activation. Nat Rev Drug Discov 5:471–484

Lamers CH, Sleijfer S, Vulto AG, Kruit WH, Kliffen M, Debets R, Gratama JW, Stoter G, Oosterwijk E (2006) Treatment of metastatic renal cell carcinoma with autologous T-lymphocytes genetically retargeted against carbonic anhydrase IX: first clinical experience. J Clin Oncol 24:e20–e22

Lans TE, Grunhagen DJ, de Wilt JH, van Geel AN, Eggermont AM (2005) Isolated limb perfusions with tumor necrosis factor and melphalan for locally recurrent soft tissue sarcoma in previously irradiated limbs. Ann Surg Oncol 12:406–411

Leonard JP, Link BK, Emmanouilides C, Gregory SA, Weisdorf D, Andrey J, Hainsworth J, Sparano JA, Tsai DE, Horning S, Krieg AM, Weiner GJ (2007) Phase I trial of toll-like receptor 9 agonist PF-3512676 with and following rituximab in patients with recurrent indolent and aggressive non Hodgkin's lymphoma. Clin Cancer Res 13:6168–6174

Li S, Schmitz KR, Jeffrey PD, Wiltzius JJ, Kussie P, Ferguson KM (2005) Structural basis for inhibition of the epidermal growth factor receptor by cetuximab. Cancer Cell 7:301–311

Lin WW, Karin M (2007) A cytokine-mediated link between innate immunity, inflammation, and cancer. J Clin Invest 117:1175–1183

Liu H, Ye H, Ruskone-Fourmestraux A, De Jong D, Pileri S, Thiede C, Lavergne A, Boot H, Caletti G, Wundisch T, Molina T, Taal BG, Elena S, Thomas T, Zinzani PL, Neubauer A, Stolte M, Hamoudi RA, Dogan A, Isaacson PG, Du MQ (2002) T(11;18) is a marker for all stage gastric MALT lymphomas that will not respond to *H. pylori* eradication. Gastroenterology 122:1286–1294

Lynch DH (2008) The promise of 4-1BB (CD137)-mediated immunomodulation and the immunotherapy of cancer. Immunol Rev 222:277–286

Mackensen A, Meidenbauer N, Vogl S, Laumer M, Berger J, Andreesen R (2006) Phase I study of adoptive T-cell therapy using antigen-specific CD8+ T cells for the treatment of patients with metastatic melanoma. J Clin Oncol 24:5060–5069

Mahnke K, Qian Y, Fondel S, Brueck J, Becker C, Enk AH (2005) Targeting of antigens to activated dendritic cells in vivo cures metastatic melanoma in mice. Cancer Res 65:7007–7012

Mahnke K, Schonfeld K, Fondel S, Ring S, Karakhanova S, Wiedemeyer K, Bedke T, Johnson TS, Storn V, Schallenberg S, Enk AH (2007) Depletion of CD4+ CD25+ human regulatory T cells in vivo: kinetics of Treg depletion and alterations in immune functions in vivo and in vitro. Int J Cancer 120:2723–2733

Mailliard RB, Wankowicz-Kalinska A, Cai Q, Wesa A, Hilkens CM, Kapsenberg ML, Kirkwood JM, Storkus WJ, Kalinski P (2004) Alpha-type-1 polarized dendritic cells: a novel immunization tool with optimized CTL-inducing activity. Cancer Res 64:5934–5937

Manegold C, Leichman G, Gravenor D, Woytowitz D, Mezger J, Albert G, Schmalbach T, Al-Adhami M (2005) Addition of CpG 7909 to taxane/platinum regimen for first-line treatment of unresectable NSCLC improves objective response in phase II clinical trial [abstract]. Eur J Cancer 3:326

Marcus R, Hagenbeek A (2007) The therapeutic use of rituximab in non-Hodgkin's lymphoma. Eur J Haematol Suppl (67):5–14

MartIn-Fontecha A, Sebastiani S, Hopken UE, Uguccioni M, Lipp M, Lanzavecchia A, Sallusto F (2003) Regulation of dendritic cell migration to the draining lymph node: impact on T lymphocyte traffic and priming. J Exp Med 198:615–621

Meyerhardt JA, Mayer RJ (2005) Systemic therapy for colorectal cancer. N Engl J Med 352:476–487

Michael A, Ball G, Quatan N, Wushishi F, Russell N, Whelan J, Chakraborty P, Leader D, Whelan M, Pandha H (2005) Delayed disease progression after allogeneic cell vaccination in hormone-resistant prostate cancer and correlation with immunologic variables. Clin Cancer Res 11:4469–4478

Miller KD, Chap LI, Holmes FA, Cobleigh MA, Marcom PK, Fehrenbacher L, Dickler M, Overmoyer BA, Reimann JD, Sing AP, Langmuir V, Rugo HS (2005) Randomized phase III trial of capecitabine compared with bevacizumab plus capecitabine in patients with previously treated metastatic breast cancer. J Clin Oncol 23:792–799

Morgan RA, Dudley ME, Wunderlich JR, Hughes MS, Yang JC, Sherry RM, Royal RE, Topalian SL, Kammula US, Restifo NP, Zheng Z, Nahvi A, de Vries CR, Rogers-Freezer LJ, Mavroukakis SA, Rosenberg SA (2006) Cancer regression in patients after transfer of genetically engineered lymphocytes. Science 314:126–129

Motohashi S, Ishikawa A, Ishikawa E, Otsuji M, Iizasa T, Hanaoka H, Shimizu N, Horiguchi S, Okamoto Y, Fujii S, Taniguchi M, Fujisawa T, Nakayama T (2006) A phase I study of in vitro expanded natural killer T cells in patients with advanced and recurrent non-small cell lung cancer. Clin Cancer Res 12:6079–6086

Motzer RJ, Bacik J, Murphy BA, Russo P, Mazumdar M (2002) Interferon-alfa as a comparative treatment for clinical trials of new therapies against advanced renal cell carcinoma. J Clin Oncol 20:289–296

Musolino A, Naldi N, Bortesi B, Pezzuolo D, Capelletti M, Missale G, Laccabue D, Zerbini A, Camisa R, Bisagni G, Neri TM, Ardizzoni A (2008) Immunoglobulin G fragment C receptor polymorphisms and clinical efficacy of trastuzumab-based therapy in patients with HER-2/neu-positive metastatic breast cancer. J Clin Oncol 26:1789–1796

Nair S, McLaughlin C, Weizer A, Su Z, Boczkowski D, Dannull J, Vieweg J, Gilboa E (2003) Injection of immature dendritic cells into adjuvant-treated skin obviates the need for ex vivo maturation. J Immunol 171:6275–6282

Napolitani G, Rinaldi A, Bertoni F, Sallusto F, Lanzavecchia A (2005) Selected Toll-like receptor agonist combinations synergistically trigger a T helper type 1-polarizing program in dendritic cells. Nat Immunol 6:769–776

Nieda M, Okai M, Tazbirkova A, Lin H, Yamaura A, Ide K, Abraham R, Juji T, Macfarlane DJ, Nicol AJ (2004) Therapeutic activation of Valpha24+ Vbeta11+ NKT cells in human subjects results in highly coordinated secondary activation of acquired and innate immunity. Blood 103:383–389

O'Day SJ, Hamid O, Urba WJ (2007) Targeting cytotoxic T-lymphocyte antigen-4 (CTLA-4): a novel strategy for the treatment of melanoma and other malignancies. Cancer 110:2614–2627

O'Neill DW, Adams S, Bhardwaj N (2004) Manipulating dendritic cell biology for the active immunotherapy of cancer. Blood 104:2235–2246

Park JR, Digiusto DL, Slovak M, Wright C, Naranjo A, Wagner J, Meechoovet HB, Bautista C, Chang WC, Ostberg JR, Jensen MC (2007) Adoptive transfer of chimeric antigen receptor re-directed cytolytic T lymphocyte clones in patients with neuroblastoma. Mol Ther 15:825–833

Parkin DM, Bray F, Ferlay J, Pisani P (2005) Global cancer statistics, 2002. CA Cancer J Clin 55:74–108

Pashenkov M, Goess G, Wagner C, Hormann M, Jandl T, Moser A, Britten CM, Smolle J, Koller S, Mauch C, Tantcheva-Poor I, Grabbe S, Loquai C, Esser S, Franckson T, Schneeberger A, Haarmann C, Krieg AM, Stingl G, Wagner SN (2006) Phase II trial of a toll-like receptor 9-activating oligonucleotide in patients with metastatic melanoma. J Clin Oncol 24:5716–5724

Piconese S, Valzasina B, Colombo MP (2008) OX40 triggering blocks suppression by regulatory T cells and facilitates tumor rejection. J Exp Med 205:825–839

Ramirez-Montagut T, Chow A, Hirschhorn-Cymerman D, Terwey TH, Kochman AA, Lu S, Miles RC, Sakaguchi S, Houghton AN, van den Brink MR (2006) Glucocorticoid-induced TNF receptor family related gene activation overcomes tolerance/ignorance to melanoma differentiation antigens and enhances antitumor immunity. J Immunol 176:6434–6442

Robert F, Ezekiel MP, Spencer SA, Meredith RF, Bonner JA, Khazaeli MB, Saleh MN, Carey D, LoBuglio AF, Wheeler RH, Cooper MR, Waksal HW (2001) Phase I study of anti-epidermal growth factor receptor antibody cetuximab in combination with radiation therapy in patients with advanced head and neck cancer. J Clin Oncol 19:3234–3243

Robert C, Thomas L, Bondarenko I, O'Day S, M D JW, Garbe C, Lebbe C, Baurain JF, Testori A, Grob JJ, Davidson N, Richards J, Maio M, Hauschild A, Miller WH Jr, Gascon P, Lotem M, Harmankaya K, Ibrahim R, Francis S, Chen TT, Humphrey R, Hoos A, Wolchok JD (2011) Ipilimumab plus dacarbazine for previously untreated metastatic melanoma. N Engl J Med 30;364(26):2517–2526

Roggero E, Zucca E, Pinotti G, Pascarella A, Capella C, Savio A, Pedrinis E, Paterlini A, Venco A, Cavalli F (1995) Eradication of *Helicobacter pylori* infection in primary low-grade gastric lymphoma of mucosa-associated lymphoid tissue. Ann Intern Med 122:767–769

Rosenblatt J, Kufe D, Avigan D (2005) Dendritic cell fusion vaccines for cancer immunotherapy. Expert Opin Biol Ther 5:703–715

Rostom A, Dube C, Lewin G, Tsertsvadze A, Barrowman N, Code C, Sampson M, Moher D (2007) Nonsteroidal anti-inflammatory drugs and cyclooxygenase-2 inhibitors for primary prevention of colorectal cancer: a systematic review prepared for the U.S. Preventive Services Task Force. Ann Intern Med 146:376–389

Schadendorf D, Ugurel S, Schuler-Thurner B, Nestle FO, Enk A, Brocker EB, Grabbe S, Rittgen W, Edler L, Sucker A, Zimpfer-Rechner C, Berger T, Kamarashev J, Burg G, Jonuleit H, Tuttenberg A, Becker JC, Keikavoussi P, Kampgen E, Schuler G (2006) Dacarbazine (DTIC) versus vaccination with autologous peptide-pulsed dendritic cells (DC) in first-line treatment of patients with metastatic melanoma: a randomized phase III trial of the DC study group of the DeCOG. Ann Oncol 17:563–570

Schwartzentruber DJ, Lawson DH, Richards JM, Conry RM, Miller DM, Treisman J, Gailani F, Riley L, Conlon K, Pockaj B, Kendra KL, White RL, Gonzalez R, Kuzel TM, Curti B, Leming PD, Whitman ED, Balkissoon J, Reintgen DS, Kaufman H, Marincola FM, Merino MJ, Rosenberg SA, Choyke P, Vena D, Hwu P (2011) gp100 peptide vaccine and interleukin-2 in patients with advanced melanoma. N Engl J Med 2;364(22):2119–2227

Schuler G, Schuler-Thurner B, Steinman RM (2003) The use of dendritic cells in cancer immunotherapy. Curr Opin Immunol 15:138–147

Schuster SJ, Neelapu SS, Gause BL, Janik JE, Muggia FM, Gockerman JP, Winter JN, Flowers CR, Nikcevich DA, Sotomayor EM, McGaughey DS, Jaffe ES, Chong EA, Reynolds CW, Berry DA, Santos CF, Popa MA, McCord AM, Kwak LW (2011) Vaccination with patient-specific tumor-derived antigen in first remission improves disease-free survival in follicular lymphoma. J Clin Oncol 10;29(20):2787–2794

Shan D, Ledbetter JA, Press OW (2000) Signaling events involved in anti-CD20-induced apoptosis of malignant human B cells. Cancer Immunol Immunother 48:673–683

Shelley MD, Court JB, Kynaston H, Wilt TJ, Fish RG, Mason M (2000) Intravesical Bacillus Calmette-Guerin in Ta and T1 bladder cancer. Cochrane Database Syst Rev CD001986

Simons JW, Carducci MA, Mikhak B, Lim M, Biedrzycki B, Borellini F, Clift SM, Hege KM, Ando DG, Piantadosi S, Mulligan R, Nelson WG (2006) Phase I/II trial of an allogeneic cellular immunotherapy in hormone-naive prostate cancer. Clin Cancer Res 12:3394–3401

Slamon DJ, Leyland-Jones B, Shak S, Fuchs H, Paton V, Bajamonde A, Fleming T, Eiermann W, Wolter J, Pegram M, Baselga J, Norton L (2001) Use of chemotherapy plus a monoclonal antibody against HER2 for metastatic breast cancer that overexpresses HER2. N Engl J Med 344:783–792

Slingluff CL Jr, Chianese-Bullock KA, Bullock TN, Grosh WW, Mullins DW, Nichols L, Olson W, Petroni G, Smolkin M, Engelhard VH (2006) Immunity to melanoma antigens: from self-tolerance to immunotherapy. Adv Immunol 90:243–295

Small EJ, Schellhammer PF, Higano CS, Redfern CH, Nemunaitis JJ, Valone FH, Verjee SS, Jones LA, Hershberg RM (2006) Placebo-controlled phase III trial of immunologic therapy with sipuleucel-T (APC8015) in patients with metastatic, asymptomatic hormone refractory prostate cancer. J Clin Oncol 24:3089–3094

Smyth MJ, Crowe NY, Hayakawa Y, Takeda K, Yagita H, Godfrey DI (2002) NKT cells – conductors of tumor immunity? Curr Opin Immunol 14:165–171

Soiffer R, Lynch T, Mihm M, Jung K, Rhuda C, Schmollinger JC, Hodi FS, Liebster L, Lam P, Mentzer S, Singer S, Tanabe KK, Cosimi AB, Duda R, Sober A, Bhan A, Daley J, Neuberg D, Parry G, Rokovich J, Richards L, Drayer J, Berns A, Clift S, Cohen LK, Mulligan RC, Dranoff G (1998) Vaccination with irradiated autologous melanoma cells engineered to secrete human granulocyte-macrophage colony-stimulating factor generates potent antitumor immunity in patients with metastatic melanoma. Proc Natl Acad Sci USA 95:13141–13146

Sporri R, Reis e Sousa C (2005) Inflammatory mediators are insufficient for full dendritic cell activation and promote expansion of CD4+ T cell populations lacking helper function. Nat Immunol 6:163–170

Steinbach G, Lynch PM, Phillips RK, Wallace MH, Hawk E, Gordon GB, Wakabayashi N, Saunders B, Shen Y, Fujimura T, Su LK, Levin B (2000) The effect of celecoxib, a cyclooxygenase-2 inhibitor, in familial adenomatous polyposis. N Engl J Med 342:1946–1952

Sugamura K, Ishii N, Weinberg AD (2004) Therapeutic targeting of the effector T-cell co-stimulatory molecule OX40. Nat Rev Immunol 4:420–431

Sunada H, Magun BE, Mendelsohn J, MacLeod CL (1986) Monoclonal antibody against epidermal growth factor receptor is internalized without stimulating receptor phosphorylation. Proc Natl Acad Sci USA 83:3825–3829

Sylvester RJ, van der Meijden AP, Witjes JA, Kurth K (2005) Bacillus calmette-guerin versus chemotherapy for the intravesical treatment of patients with carcinoma in situ of the bladder: a meta-analysis of the published results of randomized clinical trials. J Urol 174:86–91; discussion 91–82

Tivol EA, Borriello F, Schweitzer AN, Lynch WP, Bluestone JA, Sharpe AH (1995) Loss of CTLA-4 leads to massive lymphoproliferation and fatal multiorgan tissue destruction, revealing a critical negative regulatory role of CTLA-4. Immunity 3:541–547

Topp MS, Riddell SR, Akatsuka Y, Jensen MC, Blattman JN, Greenberg PD (2003) Restoration of CD28 expression in CD28- CD8+ memory effector T cells reconstitutes antigen-induced IL-2 production. J Exp Med 198:947–955

Turini ME, DuBois RN (2002) Cyclooxygenase-2: a therapeutic target. Annu Rev Med 53:35–57

Uchida T, Horiguchi S, Tanaka Y, Yamamoto H, Kunii N, Motohashi S, Taniguchi M, Nakayama T, Okamoto Y (2008) Phase I study of alpha-galactosylceramide-pulsed antigen presenting cells administration to the nasal submucosa in unresectable or recurrent head and neck cancer. Cancer Immunol Immunother 57:337–345

Valabrega G, Montemurro F, Aglietta M (2007) Trastuzumab: mechanism of action, resistance and future perspectives in HER2-overexpressing breast cancer. Ann Oncol 18:977–984

Valmori D, Souleimanian NE, Tosello V, Bhardwaj N, Adams S, O'Neill D, Pavlick A, Escalon JB, Cruz CM, Angiulli A, Angiulli F, Mears G, Vogel SM, Pan L, Jungbluth AA, Hoffmann EW, Venhaus R, Ritter G, Old LJ, Ayyoub M (2007) Vaccination with NY-ESO-1 protein and CpG in Montanide induces integrated antibody/Th1 responses and CD8 T cells through cross-priming. Proc Natl Acad Sci USA 104:8947–8952

Vambutas A, DeVoti J, Nouri M, Drijfhout JW, Lipford GB, Bonagura VR, van der Burg SH, Melief CJ (2005) Therapeutic vaccination with papillomavirus E6 and E7 long peptides results in the control of both established virus-induced lesions and latently infected sites in a pre-clinical cottontail rabbit papillomavirus model. Vaccine 23:5271–5280

Van Cutsem E, Peeters M, Siena S, Humblet Y, Hendlisz A, Neyns B, Canon JL, Van Laethem JL, Maurel J, Richardson G, Wolf M, Amado RG (2007) Open-label phase III trial of panitumumab plus best supportive care compared with best supportive care alone in patients with chemotherapy-refractory metastatic colorectal cancer. J Clin Oncol 25:1658–1664

van Elsas A, Hurwitz AA, Allison JP (1999) Combination immunotherapy of B16 melanoma using anti-cytotoxic T lymphocyte-associated antigen 4 (CTLA-4) and granulocyte/macrophage colony-stimulating factor (GM-CSF)-producing vaccines induces rejection of subcutaneous and metastatic tumors accompanied by autoimmune depigmentation. J Exp Med 190:355–366

van Seters M, van Beurden M, ten Kate FJ, Beckmann I, Ewing PC, Eijkemans MJ, Kagie MJ, Meijer CJ, Aaronson NK, Kleinjan A, Heijmans-Antonissen C, Zijlstra FJ, Burger MP, Helmerhorst TJ (2008) Treatment of vulvar intraepithelial neoplasia with topical imiquimod. N Engl J Med 358:1465–1473

Van Tendeloo VF, Ponsaerts P, Lardon F, Nijs G, Lenjou M, Van Broeckhoven C, Van Bockstaele DR, Berneman ZN (2001) Highly efficient gene delivery by mRNA electroporation in human hematopoietic cells: superiority to lipofection and passive pulsing of mRNA and to electroporation of plasmid cDNA for tumor antigen loading of dendritic cells. Blood 98:49–56

Velayos FS, Terdiman JP, Walsh JM (2005) Effect of 5-aminosalicylate use on colorectal cancer and dysplasia risk: a systematic review and metaanalysis of observational studies. Am J Gastroenterol 100:1345–1353

Vonderheide RH, Flaherty KT, Khalil M, Stumacher MS, Bajor DL, Hutnick NA, Sullivan P, Mahany JJ, Gallagher M, Kramer A, Green SJ, O'Dwyer PJ, Running KL, Huhn RD, Antonia SJ (2007) Clinical activity and immune modulation in cancer patients treated with CP-870,893, a novel CD40 agonist monoclonal antibody. J Clin Oncol 25:876–883

Waterhouse P, Penninger JM, Timms E, Wakeham A, Shahinian A, Lee KP, Thompson CB, Griesser H, Mak TW (1995) Lymphoproliferative disorders with early lethality in mice deficient in Ctla-4. Science 270:985–988

Weiden PL, Flournoy N, Thomas ED, Prentice R, Fefer A, Buckner CD, Storb R (1979) Antileukemic effect of graft-versus-host disease in human recipients of allogeneic-marrow grafts. N Engl J Med 300:1068–1073

Weng WK, Czerwinski D, Timmerman J, Hsu FJ, Levy R (2004) Clinical outcome of lymphoma patients after idiotype vaccination is correlated with humoral immune response and immunoglobulin G Fc receptor genotype. J Clin Oncol 22:4717–4724

Witzig TE, Gordon LI, Cabanillas F, Czuczman MS, Emmanouilides C, Joyce R, Pohlman BL, Bartlett NL, Wiseman GA, Padre N, Grillo-Lopez AJ, Multani P, White CA (2002) Randomized controlled trial of yttrium-90-labeled ibritumomab tiuxetan radioimmunotherapy versus rituximab immunotherapy for patients with relapsed or refractory low-grade, follicular, or transformed B-cell non-Hodgkin's lymphoma. J Clin Oncol 20:2453–2463

Wolf D, Wolf AM, Rumpold H, Fiegl H, Zeimet AG, Muller-Holzner E, Deibl M, Gastl G, Gunsilius E, Marth C (2005) The expression of the regulatory T cell-specific forkhead box transcription factor FoxP3 is associated with poor prognosis in ovarian cancer. Clin Cancer Res 11:8326–8331

Wong BC, Lam SK, Wong WM, Chen JS, Zheng TT, Feng RE, Lai KC, Hu WH, Yuen ST, Leung SY, Fong DY, Ho J, Ching CK (2004) *Helicobacter pylori* eradication to prevent gastric cancer in a high-risk region of China: a randomized controlled trial. JAMA 291:187–194

Wong RM, Scotland RR, Lau RL, Wang C, Korman AJ, Kast WM, Weber JS (2007) Programmed death-1 blockade enhances expansion and functional capacity of human melanoma antigen-specific CTLs. Int Immunol 19:1223–1234

Wu CJ, Ritz J (2006) Induction of tumor immunity following allogeneic stem cell transplantation. Adv Immunol 90:133–173

Yang XD, Jia XC, Corvalan JR, Wang P, Davis CG, Jakobovits A (1999) Eradication of established tumors by a fully human monoclonal antibody to the epidermal growth factor receptor without concomitant chemotherapy. Cancer Res 59:1236–1243

Yee C, Thompson JA, Roche P, Byrd DR, Lee PP, Piepkorn M, Kenyon K, Davis MM, Riddell SR, Greenberg PD (2000) Melanocyte destruction after antigen-specific immunotherapy of melanoma: direct evidence of t cell-mediated vitiligo. J Exp Med 192:1637–1644

Younes A, Bartlett NL, Leonard JP, Kennedy DA, Lynch CM, Sievers EL, Forero-Torres A (2010) Brentuximab vedotin (SGN-35) for relapsed CD30-positive lymphomas. N Engl J Med 4;363(19):1812–1821

Yee C, Thompson JA, Byrd D, Riddell SR, Roche P, Celis E, Greenberg PD (2002) Adoptive T cell therapy using antigen-specific CD8+ T cell clones for the treatment of patients with metastatic melanoma: in vivo persistence, migration, and antitumor effect of transferred T cells. Proc Natl Acad Sci USA 99:16168–16173

Zhou G, Drake CG, Levitsky HI (2006) Amplification of tumor-specific regulatory T cells following therapeutic cancer vaccines. Blood 107:628–636

Chapter 23
Current Progress in Adoptive T-Cell Therapy of Lymphoma

Kenneth P. Micklethwaite, Helen E. Heslop, and Malcolm K. Brenner

1 Introduction

The lymphomas are a diverse group of malignancies arising from the lymphoreticular system. Individual subtypes have unique pathological features, clinical courses, and response to traditional chemotherapy agents.

Although many entities such as Hodgkin's Disease (HD) and Burkitt's lymphoma have an excellent response to standard therapy, and the development of tumor antigen-specific monoclonal antibodies has improved outcome for others, a significant proportion of lymphoma patients develop relapsed, resistant or progressive disease. The successful cure of lymphoma patients using allogeneic hemopoietic stem cell transplantation (HSCT) with unmanipulated donor lymphocyte infusions (DLI) (Mandigers et al. 2003; Bishop et al. 2008) and more recently, reduced intensity conditioning (Khouri et al. 2008), points to the potential for an immunologically mediated response to eradicate otherwise incurable lymphoma. The limited availability of HSCT donors and the toxicity of the procedure (with consequent unaltered overall survival of lymphoma patients irrespective of whether they are transplanted or not) means that the transplant option is suboptimal, and has prompted investigators to examine means of providing a more targeted antitumor immune response through the adoptive transfer of ex vivo generated lymphoma-specific T-cells.

Basing their initial approach on the causal association of many lymphomas with Epstein–Barr virus (EBV) and their subsequent viral antigen expression, groups have successfully treated many EBV-positive lymphomas with virus-specific cytotoxic T-lymphocytes (CTLs) (Heslop et al. 2010; Bollard et al. 2007; Wynn et al. 2005). The success and lack of toxicity of this approach has prompted

---

K.P. Micklethwaite • H.E. Heslop • M.K. Brenner (✉)
Center for Cell and Gene Therapy, Baylor College of Medicine, The Methodist Hospital and Texas Children's Hospital, Houston, TX USA
e-mail: mbrenner@bcm.edu

efforts to overcome the remaining challenges and broaden the availability of immunotherapy to all lymphoma patients, including subjects with EBV-negative disease.

2 Immunotherapy of EBV-Related Lymphoma

EBV is a ubiquitous gamma herpes virus which may present acutely with an infectious mononucleosis syndrome or be asymptomatic. Upon resolution of acute infection, EBV establishes latency in B-lymphocytes. The latent state is maintained by the expression of a limited number of viral antigens including Epstein–Barr nuclear antigens (EBNA); Epstein–Barr encoded RNAs (EBERs), and latent membrane protein (LMP) antigens. Four patterns of latent antigen expression exist, corresponding to different phases of the viral life cycle: Type 0 with no antigen expression; Type 1 with EBNA1 alone; Type 2 with EBNA1 and LMP1 and LMP2; Type 3 with EBNA1-6 and LMP1 and LMP2. Types 0–2 may be present in healthy seropositive individuals whereas Type 3 expression is associated with the immunocompromised state (Heslop 2009). There is a well-established causal relationship between EBV and a number of lymphomas including HD, Burkitt's lymphoma, and immunodeficiency or immunosuppression-related non-Hodgkin's lymphoma (NHL). Each of these malignancies is associated with a specific latency type (Fig. 23.1).

Active viral replication during acute and latent infection is controlled by a large number of EBV-specific CD4+ and CD8+ T-lymphocytes circulating in the peripheral blood. These T-cells can be isolated and expanded ex vivo by stimulating them with B lymphoblastoid cell lines (LCLs) which are B-cells transformed with a laboratory strain of EBV. LCLs have a Type 3 pattern of antigen expression and elicit a CTL response directed to immunodominant antigens such as EBNA3A with much less response to subdominant antigens such as EBNA1, LMP1, and LMP2 (Roskrow et al. 1998; Rooney et al. 2002; Bollard et al. 2004; Merlo et al. 2008; Pallesen et al. 1993).

Both autologous and allogeneic EBV CTLs generated by stimulation with EBV LCLs have been successfully utilized to treat EBV-related lymphomas, particularly posttransplant lymphoproliferative disease (PTLD) (Heslop et al. 2010; Haque et al. 2001, 2002, 2007; Sherritt et al. 2003; Savoldo et al. 2006).

3 Posttransplant Lymphoproliferative Disease (PTLD)

PTLD refers to the presence of uncontrolled proliferation of B-lymphocytes following HSCT or solid organ transplant (SOT) (Heslop 2009). The majority of PTLDs are due to proliferation of EBV-infected B-lymphocytes (Paya et al. 1999;

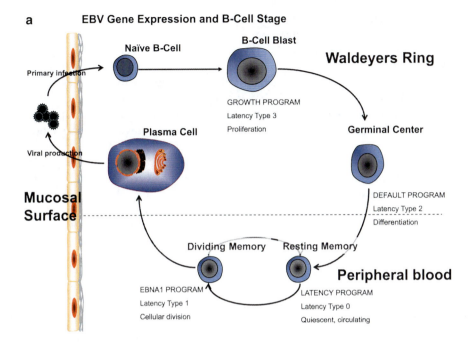

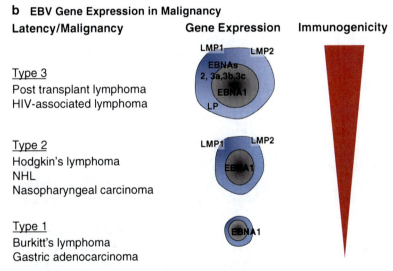

Fig. 23.1 (a) EBV gene expression and B-cell stage. Viral gene expression programs and their association with type of latent antigen expression and infected B-cell maturation stage. Type 0 = no viral gene expression, Type 1 = EBNA1, Type 2 = EBNA1, LMP1 and LMP2, Type 3 = EBNA1-6, LMP1 and LMP2. Adapted from Thorley-Lawson 2004 and 2008 (Thorley-Lawson and Gross 2004; Thorley-Lawson et al. 2008). (b) EBV gene expression in malignancy. Immunogenicity of viral antigens and their expression patterns in different EBV-associated malignancies. Adapted from Heslop (2009) and Merlo et al. (2008)

Opelz and Dohler 2004; Curtis et al. 1999), and the histological spectrum ranges from polyclonal B-cell proliferation to aggressive NHL (Tsao and Hsi 2007). Proliferation occurs because of low circulating T-cell numbers coupled with the immunosuppressive drugs used in HSCT and SOT. Hence the incidence of PTLD increases with the intensity and length of time of immunosuppression. Following HSCT, PTLD is mostly of donor origin and usually occurs within the first 6 months, corresponding with the time of most profound lymphopenia (Curtis et al. 1999; Tsao and Hsi 2007). Following SOT, however, PTLD arises mostly in recipient B-cells and occurs after the first year posttransplant (Opelz and Dohler 2004; Tsao and Hsi 2007). Therapy aims to restore the balance between proliferating EBV-infected B-lymphocytes and EBV-specific T-cells. Standard means of achieving this balance have included decreasing immunosuppression, or administration of cytotoxic chemotherapy or the CD20-specific monoclonal antibody rituximab. Even with these measures, PTLD has an overall mortality of up to 50% (Opelz and Dohler 2004).

Initial attempts to bolster EBV-specific immunity after HSCT included infusion of unmanipulated DLI which produced remission in 5/5 patients (Papadopoulos et al. 1994). Unfortunately this approach was also associated with morbidity and mortality from graft-versus host disease (GVHD) (Heslop et al. 1994; O'Reilly et al. 2007) due to alloreactive T-cells in the DLI. To circumvent this limitation, allogeneic EBV-specific CTLs, generated by stimulating peripheral blood mononuclear cells (PBMC) with LCLs, were given to ten HSCT recipients, three of whom had active EBV-PTLD at that time (Rooney et al. 1995). None of the recipients developed acute GVHD. All three recipients with PTLD had reduction of EBV DNA levels to normal and resolution of their disorder. The CTLs were genetically marked and could be detected for 10 weeks or more postinfusion.

A similar strategy has been used in SOT, but since the transformed B-cells are of recipient origin, CTLs were generated from the patients' own T-cells (Emanuel et al. 1997; Haque et al. 1998; Khanna et al. 1999). Although generating such CTLs from these patients requires longer culture periods due to the immunosuppression they receive, CTL production is nonetheless feasible and these effector cells have antitumor activity in vivo (Emanuel et al. 1997; Haque et al. 1998; Khanna et al. 1999) Multiple subsequent studies have demonstrated the safety of EBV-specific CTLs for the treatment of PTLD occurring after both HSCT and SOT (Heslop 2009; Merlo et al. 2008; O'Reilly et al. 2007) (Tables 23.1–23.4).

The efficacy of CTLs for EBV-PTLD can be explained by the fact that PTLD tumors have arisen in the context of a defective immune system and so largely lack the immune evasion strategies required by any equivalently immunogenic tumors that arise in the immunocompetent host. In addition, proliferating B-lymphocytes in PTLD have the same Type 3 pattern of EBV antigen expression as LCLs and are therefore both highly immunogenic and specifically targeted by CTLs expanded through LCL stimulation. Nonetheless, the success of this approach has stimulated interest in utilizing EBV CTL for therapy of other EBV-related lymphomas.

Table 23.1 Immunotherapy of established PTLD post-HSCT

Patient#	Indication for CTLs	CTL origin	Response	Adverse events	Reference
13	Elevated PB EBV DNA Fever Lymphadenopathy (nine patients) Pulmonary infiltrates (three patients) CNS lesions (two patients)	MUD	Complete remission (11 patients) Normalization of EBV DNA Gene marked CTL persistence to 5.5 years Gene marked CTLs infiltrating tumor biopsy Two died of progressive disease (one with virus mutation with deletion of HLA-restricted epitopes of EBNA3A)	Localized lymph node swelling (two patients) with airway obstruction (one patient) Pleural effusion (one patient) Transient elevated transaminases (one patient) Exacerbation of GVHD (one patient)	Rooney et al. (1995, 1998a); Gottschalk et al. (2001); Wagner et al. (2004); Pakakasama et al. (2004); Heslop et al. (2010)
1	Advanced PTLD Elevated PB EBV DNA Fever, lymphadenopathy Colonic mass	MMRD	Died of progressive disease 2.5 weeks after CTLs	Nil infusion related	Imashuku et al. (1997)
6	Resistance to rituximab Rising PB EBV DNA Fever Overt PTLD (five patients) Emergence of CD20-CD19+ phenotype	Haplotype-MMRD	Complete remission	Nil infusion related	Comoli et al. (2007, 2008)
3	PTLD unresponsive to conventional therapy	Third party	Two with complete remission, one died prior to the assessment of unrelated cause	Nil infusion related	Haque et al. (2002, 2007)

PTLD posttransplant lymphoproliferative disease; *PB* peripheral blood; *MUD* matched unrelated donor; *MMRD* mismatched related donor; *third party* closely matched allogeneic donor different to stem cell donor; *CNS* central nervous system, GVHD = graft versus host disease

Table 23.2 Immunoprophylaxis of PTLD post-HSCT

Patient#	Indication for CTLs	CTL origin	Response	Adverse events	Reference
101	High risk of PTLD: TCD MUD or MMRD, immune deficiencies, past EBV lymphoma	MUD MMRD	No PTLD post-CTLs Gene marked CTL persistence to 9 years	Nil infusion related	Rooney et al. (1995; 1998b); Heslop et al. (1996, 2010)
6	High risk of PTLD: TCD (five patients), MMUD EBV DNA level greater than 1,000 (five patients)	MMUD	No PTLD post-CTLs (five patients) Decreased EBV DNA (four patients) One patient received CTLs lacking EBV-specific killing died of disseminated EBV NHL	Nil infusion related	Gustafsson et al. (2000)

PTLD posttransplant lymphoproliferative disorder; *TCD* T-cell depleted; *MUD* matched unrelated donor; *MMRD* mismatched unrelated donor; *NHL* non-Hodgkin's lymphoma

Table 23.3 Immunotherapy of established PTLD post-SOT

Patient# (TP type)	Indication for CTLs	CTL origin	Response	Adverse events	Reference
1 (lung)	Multiple lymphoma deposits in liver and GIT Lung nodules	Autologous	Remission of GIT lymphoma followed by relapse in the lung 10 weeks after CTLs Reduction in lung nodules after repeat CTL infusion	Died of hemorrhage from necrotic nodule involving pulmonary vessel	Khanna et al. (1999)
1 (heart)	Multiple cutaneous PTLD deposits	Autologous	Complete remission of PTLD associated with increased EBV-CTLs in the peripheral blood	Nil infusion related	Sherritt et al. (2003)
2	Elevated EBV-DNA Ocular and liver PTLD	Autologous	Resolution of liver PTLD 50% Reduction in ocular PTLD then stable greater than 1 year	Nil infusion related	Savoldo et al. (2006)
2 (1 kidney, 1 liver)	PTLD unresponsive to conventional therapy	1 MRD 1 MMRD	Complete remission	Nil infusion related	Sun et al. (2002)
38 (2 heart, 12 liver, 6 liver + bowel, 15 kidney, 2 lung, 1 heart + lung)	PTLD unresponsive to conventional therapy	Third party	2 died of unrelated causes prior to assessment 15 complete remissions 3 partial remissions 18 no response Outcome better with higher degree of HLA matching	Nil infusion related	Haque et al. (2001, 2002, 2007)
3 (1 kidney, 1 heart, 1 heart + lung)	PTLD unresponsive to conventional therapy	Third party	2 complete remissions 1 died of complications of lung PTLD 11 days post CTLs- autopsy confirmed CTL homing to tumor	Nil infusion related	Gandhi et al. (2007)

PTLD posttransplant lymphoproliferative disease; *MUD* matched unrelated donor; *MMRD* mismatched related donor; *third party* closely matched allogeneic donor different to stem cell donor

Table 23.4 Immunoprophylaxis of PTLD post-SOT

Patient# (TP type)	Indication for CTLs	CTL origin	Response	Adverse events	Reference
3 (2 liver, 1 kidney)	Prophylaxis	Autologous	No PTLD post-CTLs Increased levels of EBV-CTLs in peripheral blood	Nil infusion related	Haque et al. (1998)
7 (5 heart, 1 liver, 1 kidney)	EBV-DNA level greater than 1,000 on two sequential occasions	Autologous	No PTLD post-CTLs Decreased viral load in 5 No reduction in viral load in 2	Nil infusion related	Comoli et al. (2002)
5 (kidney)	Secondary prophylaxis after standard therapy for PTLD	Autologous	No PTLD post-CTLs	Nil infusion related	Comoli et al. (2005)
10 (7 liver, 3 heart)	High risk of PTLD: persistent EBV-DNA Previous PTLD EBV seroconversion early posttransplant	Autologous	No PTLD post-CTLs Increased levels of EBV-CTLs in peripheral blood for 2 months postinfusion No consistent decrease in EBV-DNA	Nil infusion related	Savoldo et al. (2006)

PTLD posttransplant lymphoproliferative disorder

4 Hodgkin's Lymphoma

Up to 40% of patients with HD have Reed-Sternberg (RS) cells that are positive for EBV antigens (Huls et al. 2003); these RS cells, however, express the less immunogenic Type 2 latency pattern (Fig. 23.1b). Early trials of infusion of autologous EBV-specific CTLs in HD demonstrated increased virus-specific activity, decreased EBV viral load, persistence of infused cells, and some complete tumor responses (Roskrow et al. 1998; Rooney et al. 2002; Bollard et al. 2004). However, EBV-CTLs were less successful in eliminating tumor than in PTLD with only 2 out of 14 subjects achieving a durable complete remission (Table 23.5). This limited response is due to the fact that, unlike PTLD, HD arises in the context of an intact immune system and the tumor employs a variety of immunosuppressive and immune evasion strategies which impede the ability of infused CTLs to lyse tumor cells. In addition, the CTL response to LCLs is skewed toward immunodominant antigens such as EBNA3 which are absent on the tumor cells, rather than to the immunologically "weak" antigens, such as EBNA1 or LMP1 and LMP2 that are actually expressed by the malignant cells of HD. To address this problem of misdirected antigenic specificity, newer techniques to generate CTLs use vectors or plasmids to overexpress subdominant antigens such as LMP1 and LMP2 (Bollard et al. 2006, 2007; Rooney et al. 2002) in antigen presenting cells and thereby stimulate a more tumor-specific CTL population. Three patients with active EBV + HD and five in remission with high risk of relapse were given autologous CTLs generated using this technique, with a durable remission being present in two of the three with active disease and five of the five at high risk of relapse (Bollard et al. 2007). LMP-specific CTLs may also be produced by the introduction of an artificial T-cell receptor (TCR) specific for an HLA-restricted antigen epitope present in the viral protein (Orentas et al. 2001; Jurgens et al. 2006). This approach has yet to be validated clinically.

In an effort to increase the response rate still further, efforts are focusing on developing countermeasures to tumor immune evasion strategies, for example by making the T-cells resistant to the TGF-beta many of these lymphomas produce, (Bollard et al. 2002) and to broadening the range of lymphomas that can be targeted by expressing transgenic chimeric antigen receptors (CARs) directed against antigens such as CD30 (Savoldo et al. 2007) that are also present on EBV-negative lymphomas.

5 Other EBV-Related Lymphomas

EBV-specific CTLs have been given to a small number of patients with the T-cell lymphomas that may develop in individuals with congenital immunodeficiencies. These include chronic active EBV (CAEBV) and NKT-cell lymphoma (Kuzushima et al. 1996; Hagihara et al. 2003; Savoldo et al. 2002; Cho et al. 2006) Durable complete remission was observed in a patient with severe CAEBV treated with LMP-2-specific CTLs (Bollard et al. 2007) and prolonged improvement in symptoms and

Table 23.5 Immunotherapy of HD

Patient#	Indication for CTLs	CTL origin	Response	Adverse events	Reference
13	Therapy for multiply relapsed EBV+HD (nine patients) Adjuvant therapy after autologous HSCT (five patients)	Autologous LCL stimulated	CTLs persisted up to 12 months and homed to tumor sites B symptoms improved (three of four patients) 11 patients with measurable disease 2 complete remission 1 partial response 5 stable disease 3 no response Three patients with no measurable disease remained in remission 24–38 months followup	Transient swelling and pain in cervical lymph nodes (one patient)	Roskrow et al. (1998); Rooney et al. (2002); Bollard et al. (2004)
1	Multiply relapsed EBV+HD	Autologous then allogeneic post-HSCT	Autologous CTLs persisted 12 months postinfusion Relapse 6 months post autologous CTLs In remission 5 years post allogeneic MUD-CTLs	Flu like symptoms	Bollard et al. (2006)
8	Measurable relapsed EBV+HD (three patients) High risk EBV+HD in remission (previous relapsed, immuno-suppression related)	Autologous CTLs stimulated with LMP2+ APC	Increased LMP2-specific CTLs in peripheral blood Three patients with measurable disease 2 Complete remissions 1 no response Five patients with no measurable disease remained in remission 6–24 months followup	Nil infusion related	Bollard et al. (2007)

6	Chemotherapy refractory EBV + HD	Allogeneic partially matched unrelated donor	EBV CTLs alone (three patients) 1 complete remission with 2.5 years followup 2 partial responses EBV CTLs after fludarabine (three patients) 2 partial responses 1 stable disease	Nil infusion related	Sun et al. (2002); Lucas et al. (2004)

HD Hodgkin's disease; *HSCT* hemopoietic stem cell transplantation; *LMP* lymphoblastoid cell line; *MUD* matched unrelated donor signs was documented in five patients with mild to moderate CAEBV (Savoldo et al. 2002). The more limited overall response of these lymphoproliferations may in part be a reflection of their low immunogenicity associated with their Type 2 latency pattern of antigen expression and their lack of co-stimulatory molecules. Treatment of EBV-positive B-cell lymphomas in patients with hereditary and acquired immunodeficiency has also had variable success (Wynn et al. 2005; Hong et al. 2001; Sun et al. 2002) although at least one patient with EBV+CNS lymphoma had a dramatic and sustained response following repeated infusions of partially matched EBV CTLs (Wynn et al. 2005).

The mixed results of treating lymphomas other than PTLD and HD with EBV-CTLs demonstrate the potential of the approach, but also stress the need for an improved understanding of tumor biology and the development of techniques that will enhance CTL activity in the face of multiple tumor immune evasion strategies (see Sect. 8.2 below).

6 EBV-Negative Lymphomas

Although the above studies show the utility of immunotherapy of EBV-positive lymphomas, the majority of lymphomas are EBV negative. Two possible solutions to the problem of immunotherapy of EBV-negative lymphomas are currently being explored: The first is the generation of tumor-specific T-cells by stimulation with whole tumor cells or antigen presenting cells expressing tumor-associated antigens such as SSX, MAGE, and bcl-2 (Chaperot et al. 1999; Chambost et al. 2000; Andersen et al. 2005); while the second is the genetic modification of T-cells to express antigen receptors directed against lymphoma antigens.

6.1 Expansion of Lymphoma-Specific T-Cells with Whole Tumor Cells

Several murine models of adoptive immunotherapy demonstrate that T-cells can effectively target EBV-negative lymphomas, but many of these bear little relevance to the feasibility or functionality of lymphoma-specific CTLs in humans (Leshem et al. 1999; Chamoto et al. 2004; Edinger et al. 2003). While groups have shown it is possible to generate lymphoma-specific T-cells through stimulation with whole tumor cells (Chaperot et al. 1999), the lack of appropriate co-stimulatory molecules on tumor cells produces suboptimal tumor-specific T-cell expansion. This can be overcome by the upregulation of co-stimulatory molecule expression on lymphoma cells by stimulation with CD40 ligand (Schmitter et al. 1999; Hoogendoorn et al. 2004, 2005; Mohty et al. 2002) or by the genetic modification of the tumor cells to express co-stimulatory molecules. No clinical trials of T-cells stimulated with whole lymphoma cells have been reported, but the potential efficacy of this technique has been demonstrated in melanoma, in which the infusion of ex vivo expanded tumor infiltrating lymphocytes has led to regression of advanced tumors (Rosenberg et al. 1986; Dudley et al. 2002, 2005).

6.2 Nonviral Tumor Antigens

Cancer testis antigens (CTAs) such as MAGE-A4 and SSX are expressed by many solid tumors and by RS cells up to 50% of Hodgkin's Lymphomas (Chambost et al. 2000; Colleoni et al. 2002). CTA-specific CTLs can be detected in the peripheral blood of cancer patients, and can be expanded in vitro with tumor-specific cytotoxicity (Groeper et al. 2007). The relatively limited expression of these CTAs to tumor and germ cells makes them favourable candidates for immunotherapy of EBV-negative lymphoma. Of note, the expression of CTAs is increased on HL side population stem cells which are relatively chemoresistant (Shafer et al. 2008) and targeting these may be particularly beneficial to patients with persistent or relapsed disease, but the utility of CTA-specific CTLs awaits assessment in clinical trials.

The immunoglobulin idiotype or light chain isotype expressed by lymphoma cells is another possible target antigen (Harig et al. 2001; Armstrong et al. 2004) since these are restricted to the tumor cells themselves or to approximately half of normal mature B-lymphocytes respectively.

7 Transgenic Receptor Expression

Although it is possible to generate lymphoma-specific T-cells using whole tumor cells and CTAs, routine application is hampered by the time and labor required to expand the low frequency of often low affinity tumor antigen-specific T-cells in peripheral blood. This has led investigators to explore the option of genetically engineering tumor antigen-specific T-cells through the forced expression of transgenic TCRs or CARs.

7.1 Transgenic T-Cell Receptors

TCRs from CTL clones specific for epitopes of EBV or tumor-associated antigens have been isolated and cloned into retroviral vectors (Orentas et al. 2001). CTLs expressing these artificial TCRs are able to lyse target cells expressing the appropriate antigen and MHC molecules in an HLA restricted manner (Jurgens et al. 2006). This technique has been employed successfully in patients with metastatic melanoma (Morgan et al. 2006; Circosta et al. 2009). TCRs have also been cloned for minor histocompatibility antigens present on leukemia and lymphomas (Heemskerk et al. 2008) that are the targets of graft vs. leukemia activity, but these have not yet been tested clinically. The HLA restriction of conventional TCRs limits application to patients with HLA types for which antigenic epitopes have been identified and to which individual transgenic TCRs can be made.

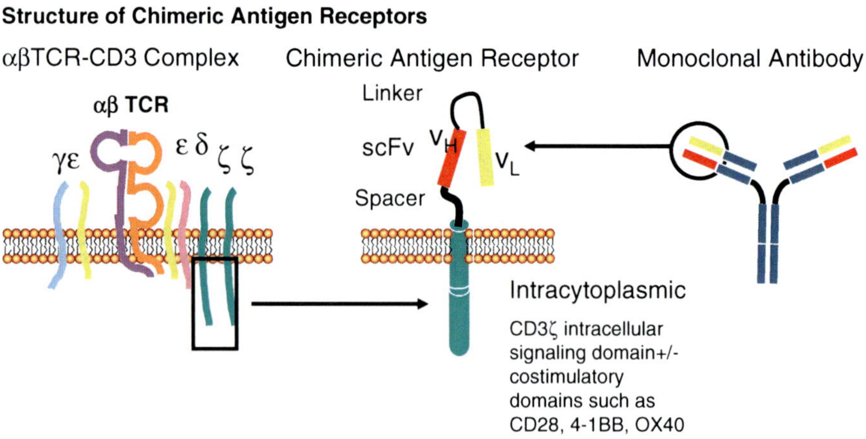

Structure of Chimeric Antigen Receptors

Fig. 23.2 Structure of chimeric antigen receptors. scFv = single chain variable fragment consisting of the variable regions of the heavy (V_H) and light (V_L) chains of a monoclonal antibody specific for the target antigen. αβ TCR = alpha and beta chains of the T-cell receptor. γ, ε, δ, ζ = gamma, epsilon, delta, and zeta chains of CD3. Adapted from Rossig et al. (2005) and Riddell (2007)

7.2 Artificial Chimeric Antigen Receptors

CARs afford an MHC-unrestricted alternative, and so are more universally applicable. First generation CARs consist of the single chain variable fragment (scFv) of an antibody specific for tumor antigen linked to the transmembrane and intracellular signaling domain of either CD3-zeta or FcR-gamma (Fig. 23.2) (Eshhar et al. 1993; Kuwana et al. 1987; Gross et al. 1989). This produces HLA unrestricted activation of the modified T-cells upon encounter with tumor antigen, leading to lysis of tumor cells in vitro (Hwu et al. 1993) and eradication of tumor in mice models (Brentjens et al. 2003). Lymphoma antigen-specific CARs have been produced for use in both B-cell NHL (CD20, CD19, CD22, immunoglobulin idiotype or light chain isotype specific) (Vera et al. 2006; Jensen et al. 1998; Cooper et al. 2003; James et al. 2008) and HD (CD30 specific) (Hombach et al. 1998). First generation CARs provide incomplete activation of T-cells with limited expansion and persistence in vivo (Mitsuyasu et al. 2000; Walker et al. 2000; Till et al. 2008), since normal T-cell activation is dependent on receipt of two classes of signal: one through the engagement of the TCR with antigen presented in the context of MHC, and a second through engagement of co-stimulatory molecules such as CD28, OX40, and CD40L (Sharpe 2009). Tumors often do not express appropriate ligands for co-stimulatory molecules and engagement of first generation CARs in the absence of co-stimulation leads to anergy and failure of in vivo expansion.

To address the above deficiency, second generation CARs incorporate the intracellular domains of one or more of these co-stimulatory molecules. This enhances T-cell proliferation and survival in vitro (Krause et al. 1998; Finney et al. 1998) and tumor killing and T-cell persistence in vivo (Kowolik et al. 2006; Milone et al. 2009). Other ways of enhancing CAR-T-cell persistence include CAR expression in CTLs specific for latent viruses such as EBV (Savoldo et al. 2007). CTL numbers are maintained through stimulation of their native TCRs by latent viral antigens and by concomitant co-stimulation provided by viral antigen presenting cells (Pule et al. 2008).

Many in vitro and in vivo murine studies have demonstrated the potential efficacy of CARs in eradicating lymphoma (Savoldo et al. 2007; Brentjens et al. 2003; Vera et al. 2006; Jensen et al. 1998; Cooper et al. 2003, 2006; James et al. 2008; Hombach et al. 1998; Cheadle et al. 2005; Rossig et al. 2005; Serrano et al. 2006; Wang et al. 2007; Cheadle et al. 2009; Huang et al. 2008). Most of these studies have focused on CD19 and CD20 as target antigens, both of which are stably expressed on the majority of B-cell malignancies. Moreover, targeting the CD20 antigen has been validated clinically, since the monoclonal antibody rituximab is now the standard of care for B-cell lymphomas.

CD19 has several potential advantages over CD20 as a target antigen, since it is expressed in acute lymphoblastic leukemia in addition to NHL and thus has a potentially broader application; it should also not be blocked by prior administration of CD20-specific monoclonal antibodies, allowing its use in combination therapy. Both of these antigens have the significant drawback of being present on normal B-cells and so treatment may be associated with prolonged B-lymphopenia. Targeting immunoglobulin light chains, the expression of which is clonally restricted to either lambda or kappa in lymphomas, may avoid this problem, since it will spare normal lymphocytes with the alternate light chain (Vera et al. 2006).

Multiple current clinical trials are examining the safety and efficacy of CAR expressing T-cells given to patients with B-cell malignancies (Table 23.6). Thus far, the results of one trial of CD20-specific CAR expressing T-cells for indolent lymphoma and mantle cell lymphoma are available (Till et al. 2008). Seven patients received a total of 19 infusions. CAR-T-cells were detectable for only 3 weeks post infusion. This increased to 5–9 weeks when exogenous IL-2 was added. Two patients continued in a previous complete response and one patient achieved a partial response. This demonstrates the safety of CARs expressing T-cells but does not bode well for effectiveness of these first generation CARs that lack co-stimulatory molecules and cannot sustain T-cell persistence.

Many of the trials in Table 23.6 incorporate co-stimulatory molecule endodomains in their CARs. A recent study in 6 patients with low-grade non-Hodgkin's lymphoma treated with CD19-specific CAR-T-cells directly compared first and second generation CARs administered to the same recipient (Savoldo, Ramos et al. 2011). This showed that the incorporation of the CD28 co-stimulatory endodomain enhanced T-cell expansion and persistence. Early reports from another trial using CARs incorporating the 4-1BB costimulatory endodomain, demonstrate massive in vivo proliferation corresponding to clinically significant reduction in size of malignant lymph nodes and clearance of leukemic deposits in the bone marrow of patients with multiply relapsed chronic lymphocytic leukemia (Kalos, Levine et al. 2011; Porter, Levine et al. 2011). These CART19 cells could be detected in the peripheral

Table 23.6 Current clinical trials of CAR expressing CTLs for B-cell malignancies registered with the U.S. government

Clinical trials identifier	Protocol title	Sponsor	Status
NCT00621452	A pilot study to evaluate the safety and feasibility of cellular immunotherapy using genetically modified autologous CD20-specific T cells for patients with relapsed or refractory mantle cell and indolent B-cell lymphomas	Fred Hutchinson Cancer Research Center	Recruiting
NCT00924326	Phase I/II study of B-cell malignancies using T cells expressing an anti-CD19 chimeric receptor: assessment of the impact of lymphocyte depletion prior to T cell transfer	National Cancer Institute	Recruiting
NCT00881920	Phase I study of adoptive transfer of autologous T lymphocytes engrafted with a chimeric antigen receptor targeting the kappa light chain of immunoglobulin expressed in patients with chronic lymphocytic leukemia or B-cell lymphoma	Baylor College of Medicine	Recruiting
NCT00709033	Phase I study of the administration of peripheral activated T-cells or EBV-specific CTLs expressing CD19 chimeric receptors for advanced B-cell non-Hodgkin's lymphoma and chronic lymphocytic leukemia (ATECRAB)	Baylor College of Medicine	Recruiting
NCT00968760	CD19-specific T cell infusion in patients with B-lineage lymphoid malignancies after autologous hematopoietic stem cell transplantation	M.D. Anderson Cancer Center	Not yet recruiting
NCT00608270	Phase I study of CD19 chimeric receptor expressing T lymphocytes in B-cell non Hodgkin's lymphoma and chronic lymphocytic leukemia [CRETI-NH]	Baylor College of Medicine	Recruiting
NCT00840853	Phase I/II study of the administration of multi-virus-specific cytotoxic T lymphocytes (CTLs) expressing CD19 chimeric receptors for prophylaxis of therapy of relapse of acute lymphoblastic leukemia post hemopoietic stem cell transplantation	Baylor College of Medicine	Recruiting
NCT00891215	Pilot study of redirected autologous T cells engineered to contain anti-CD19 attached to TCRζ and 4-1BB signaling domains in patients with chemotherapy resistant or refractory CD19+ leukemia and lymphoma	University of Pennsylvania	Recruiting

Source: http://www.clinicaltrials.gov

blood and bone marrow by flow cytometry for at least 6 months post infusion. It remains to be seen whether the enhanced activity these co-stimulatory signals produce will be adequate to provide durable antitumor activity or if further modifications allowing the T-cells to circumvent tumor escape mechanisms will be required.

8 Future Directions in Lymphoma Immunotherapy

The ultimate goal of tumor immunotherapy is to provide a safe and effective treatment for malignancy for as great a number of people as possible. In keeping with these goals work has focused on enhancing T-cell efficacy and simplifying production.

8.1 Enhancing T-Cell Efficacy and Safety

To be effective antitumor agents, adoptively transferred T-cells must be able to expand and persist in vivo, home to the tumor site, recognize appropriate tumor antigens while ignoring normal host antigens, and avoid the suppressive effects of the tumor microenvironment. It is now known that the in vitro manipulations used to generate antigen-specific CTLs can lead to their exhaustion and impaired longevity. Infused CTLs derived from the central memory compartment appear to have a greater potential for survival (Berger et al. 2008) and protocols with short culture time, and which selectively expand these in vitro may have greater success in vivo. In addition, the use of exogenous growth factors such as IL-2 and IL-15 may be needed initially to support engraftment and expansion of transferred CTLs (Emanuel et al. 1997; Brentjens et al. 2003; Till et al. 2008). Migration of T-cells and CTLs from the intravascular space to lymph nodes is a multistep process involving multiple chemotactic and adhesion molecules with CCR7 and CD62L being of central importance (Sackstein 2005). The ability of central memory derived CTLs to revert to a central memory phenotype once infused may also have an impact on expression of these adhesion molecules and allow egress to the tissues where lymphoma resides (Berger et al. 2008). Liver toxicity in recent studies using gene-modified T-cells directed against the carcino-embryonic (CEA) tumor antigen in patients with metastatic renal cell carcinoma highlights the necessity of choosing target antigens wisely (Lamers et al. 2006). Ideally these antigens should be unique to the tumor (such as the BCR-ABL product in CML) or have a limited expression in nonessential organs. Although CTAs and targets such as immunoglobulin light chain have been identified, further work is needed to define immunogenic tumor restricted targets. Other approaches to reducing the potential for damage to normal tissue include the use of suicide genes such as thymidine kinase or pharmacologically inducible Fas, or caspase 9, which can be activated by the administration of an appropriate pro-drug (Straathof et al. 2005; Riddell et al. 1996; Bonini et al. 1997; Quintarelli et al. 2007; Thomis et al. 2001; Berger et al. 2004).

8.2 Development of Countermeasures to Tumor Immune Evasion

Tumors arising in immunocompetent individuals must develop strategies to evade destruction by the hosts' immune system. Lymphoma cells use a variety of mechanisms including reduction in MHC and co-stimulatory molecule expression, upregulation of FasL, secretion of immunosuppressive cytokines such as TGF-beta and recruitment of T-regulatory cells. While the use of MHC independent CARs may overcome the lack of MHC expression, the other factors may prevent T-cells from destroying the tumor. Several approaches have been devised as counter measures. For example, the inhibitory effects of TGF-beta can be prevented by transducing T-cells with a dominant negative TGF-beta receptor making the T-cells resistant to the cytokine's immunosuppressive effects (Bollard et al. 2002). Alternatively T-regulatory cells at the tumor site (many of which also produce TGFβ), can be reduced by the use of immunodepleting strategies prior to CTL infusion such as fludarabine, cyclophosphamide, or leukapheresis (Awwad and North 1988), a strategy effective in immunotherapy of melanoma (Morgan et al. 2006) that may also be beneficial in lymphomas. In addition, cellular immunotherapy may be incorporated into standard chemotherapy regimens, or with monoclonal antibodies and other therapeutics that sensitize tumors to T-cell killing. CTAs, for example, are upregulated by demethylating agents such as 5-aza-2-deoxycytidine (Shichijo et al. 1996; De Smet et al. 1999) and histone de-acetylase inhibitors such as valproic acid and Suberoylanilide hydroxamic acid (O'Connor et al. 2006). These drugs also have cytotoxic and pro-apoptotic properties and their use in conjunction with standard therapy followed by the administration of CTA-specific CTLs may enhance long-term disease control with minimal increase in therapy-related toxicity (Gattei et al. 2005).

9 Towards Routine Application (from Boutique to Wholesale)

The routine incorporation of cellular therapies requires the rapid production of a standardized product in high volumes which can be given to multiple recipients. The safety of third party donor, partially HLA matched virus-specific CTLs is being established (Haque et al. 2001, 2007; Sun et al. 2002; Lucas et al. 2004; Gandhi et al. 2007) for an increasing number of indications. Combined with recently developed bioreactors which reduce manipulation and cost involved in tumor-specific T-cell production, there is great potential for broadening T-cell therapy for more widespread use. This will allow larger, more informative studies of efficacy to be performed and establish the approach as a standard therapeutic option rather than just for a select few.

References

Andersen MH, Svane IM, Kvistborg P et al (2005) Immunogenicity of Bcl-2 in patients with cancer. Blood 105:728–734

Armstrong AC, Dermime S, Mulryan K, Stern PL, Bhattacharyya T, Hawkins RE (2004) Adoptive transfer of anti-idiotypic T cells cure mice of disseminated B cell lymphoma. J Immunother 27:227–231

Awwad M, North RJ (1988) Cyclophosphamide (Cy)-facilitated adoptive immunotherapy of a Cy-resistant tumour. Evidence that Cy permits the expression of adoptive T-cell mediated immunity by removing suppressor T cells rather than by reducing tumour burden. Immunology 65:87–92

Berger C, Blau CA, Huang ML et al (2004) Pharmacologically regulated Fas-mediated death of adoptively transferred T cells in a nonhuman primate model. Blood 103:1261–1269

Berger C, Jensen MC, Lansdorp PM, Gough M, Elliott C, Riddell SR (2008) Adoptive transfer of effector CD8± T cells derived from central memory cells establishes persistent T cell memory in primates. J Clin Invest 118:294–305

Bishop MR, Dean RM, Steinberg SM et al (2008) Clinical evidence of a graft-versus-lymphoma effect against relapsed diffuse large B-cell lymphoma after allogeneic hematopoietic stem-cell transplantation. Ann Oncol 19:1935–1940

Bollard CM, Rossig C, Calonge MJ et al (2002) Adapting a transforming growth factor beta-related tumor protection strategy to enhance antitumor immunity. Blood 99:3179–3187

Bollard CM, Aguilar L, Straathof KC et al (2004) Cytotoxic T lymphocyte therapy for Epstein-Barr virus± Hodgkin's disease. J Exp Med 200:1623–1633

Bollard CM, Gottschalk S, Huls MH et al (2006) In vivo expansion of LMP 1- and 2-specific T-cells in a patient who received donor-derived EBV-specific T-cells after allogeneic stem cell transplantation. Leuk Lymphoma 47:837–842

Bollard CM, Gottschalk S, Leen AM et al (2007) Complete responses of relapsed lymphoma following genetic modification of tumor-antigen presenting cells and T-lymphocyte transfer. Blood 110:2838–2845

Bonini C, Ferrari G, Verzeletti S et al (1997) HSV-TK gene transfer into donor lymphocytes for control of allogeneic graft-versus-leukemia. Science 276:1719–1724

Brentjens RJ, Latouche JB, Santos E et al (2003) Eradication of systemic B-cell tumors by genetically targeted human T lymphocytes co-stimulated by CD80 and interleukin-15. Nat Med 9:279–286

Chambost H, Van Baren N, Brasseur F et al (2000) Expression of gene MAGE-A4 in Reed-Sternberg cells. Blood 95:3530–3533

Chamoto K, Tsuji T, Funamoto H et al (2004) Potentiation of tumor eradication by adoptive immunotherapy with T-cell receptor gene-transduced T-helper type 1 cells. Cancer Res 64:386–390

Chaperot L, Delfau-Larue MH, Jacob MC et al (1999) Differentiation of antitumor-specific cytotoxic T lymphocytes from autologous tumor infiltrating lymphocytes in non-Hodgkin's lymphomas. Exp Hematol 27:1185–1193

Cheadle EJ, Gilham DE, Thistlethwaite FC, Radford JA, Hawkins RE (2005) Killing of non-Hodgkin lymphoma cells by autologous CD19 engineered T cells. Br J Haematol 129:322–332

Cheadle EJ, Hawkins RE, Batha H, Rothwell DG, Ashton G, Gilham DE (2009) Eradication of established B-cell lymphoma by CD19-specific murine T cells is dependent on host lymphopenic environment and can be mediated by CD4± and CD8± T cells. J Immunother 32:207–218

Cho HI, Hong YS, Lee MA et al (2006) Adoptive transfer of Epstein-Barr virus-specific cytotoxic T-lymphocytes for the treatment of angiocentric lymphomas. Int J Hematol 83:66–73

Circosta P, Granziero L, Follenzi A et al (2009) T cell receptor (TCR) gene transfer with lentiviral vectors allows efficient redirection of tumor specificity in naive and memory T cells without prior stimulation of endogenous TCR. Hum Gene Ther 20(12):1576–1588

Colleoni GW, Capodieci P, Tickoo S, Cossman J, Filippa DA, Ladanyi M (2002) Expression of SSX genes in the neoplastic cells of Hodgkin's lymphoma. Hum Pathol 33:496–502

Comoli P, Labirio M, Basso S et al (2002) Infusion of autologous Epstein-Barr virus (EBV)-specific cytotoxic T cells for prevention of EBV-related lymphoproliferative disorder in solid organ transplant recipients with evidence of active virus replication. Blood 99:2592–2598

Comoli P, Maccario R, Locatelli F et al (2005) Treatment of EBV-related post-renal transplant lymphoproliferative disease with a tailored regimen including EBV-specific T cells. Am J Transplant 5:1415–1422

Comoli P, Basso S, Zecca M et al (2007) Preemptive therapy of EBV-related lymphoproliferative disease after pediatric haploidentical stem cell transplantation. Am J Transplant 7:1648–1655

Comoli P, Basso S, Labirio M, Baldanti F, Maccario R, Locatelli F (2008) T cell therapy of Epstein-Barr virus and adenovirus infections after hemopoietic stem cell transplant. Blood Cells Mol Dis 40:68–70

Cooper LJ, Topp MS, Serrano LM et al (2003) T-cell clones can be rendered specific for CD19: toward the selective augmentation of the graft-versus-B-lineage leukemia effect. Blood 101:1637–1644

Cooper LJ, Ausubel L, Gutierrez M et al (2006) Manufacturing of gene-modified cytotoxic T lymphocytes for autologous cellular therapy for lymphoma. Cytotherapy 8:105–117

Curtis RE, Travis LB, Rowlings PA et al (1999) Risk of lymphoproliferative disorders after bone marrow transplantation: a multi-institutional study. Blood 94:2208–2216

De Smet C, Lurquin C, Lethe B, Martelange V, Boon T (1999) DNA methylation is the primary silencing mechanism for a set of germ line- and tumor-specific genes with a CpG-rich promoter. Mol Cell Biol 19:7327–7335

Dudley ME, Wunderlich JR, Robbins PF et al (2002) Cancer regression and autoimmunity in patients after clonal repopulation with antitumor lymphocytes. Science 298:850–854

Dudley ME, Wunderlich JR, Yang JC et al (2005) Adoptive cell transfer therapy following nonmyeloablative but lymphodepleting chemotherapy for the treatment of patients with refractory metastatic melanoma. J Clin Oncol 23:2346–2357

Edinger M, Cao YA, Verneris MR, Bachmann MH, Contag CH, Negrin RS (2003) Revealing lymphoma growth and the efficacy of immune cell therapies using in vivo bioluminescence imaging. Blood 101:640–648

Emanuel DJ, Lucas KG, Mallory GB Jr et al (1997) Treatment of posttransplant lymphoproliferative disease in the central nervous system of a lung transplant recipient using allogeneic leukocytes. Transplantation 63:1691–1694

Eshhar Z, Waks T, Gross G, Schindler DG (1993) Specific activation and targeting of cytotoxic lymphocytes through chimeric single chains consisting of antibody-binding domains and the gamma or zeta subunits of the immunoglobulin and T-cell receptors. Proc Natl Acad Sci USA 90:720–724

Finney HM, Lawson AD, Bebbington CR, Weir AN (1998) Chimeric receptors providing both primary and costimulatory signaling in T cells from a single gene product. J Immunol 161:2791–2797

Gandhi MK, Wilkie GM, Dua U et al (2007) Immunity, homing and efficacy of allogeneic adoptive immunotherapy for posttransplant lymphoproliferative disorders. Am J Transplant 7:1293–1299

Gattei V, Fonsatti E, Sigalotti L et al (2005) Epigenetic immunomodulation of hematopoietic malignancies. Semin Oncol 32:503–510

Gottschalk S, Ng CY, Perez M et al (2001) An Epstein-Barr virus deletion mutant associated with fatal lymphoproliferative disease unresponsive to therapy with virus-specific CTLs. Blood 97:835–843

Groeper C, Gambazzi F, Zajac P et al (2007) Cancer/testis antigen expression and specific cytotoxic T lymphocyte responses in non small cell lung cancer. Int J Cancer 120:337–343

Gross G, Waks T, Eshhar Z (1989) Expression of immunoglobulin-T-cell receptor chimeric molecules as functional receptors with antibody-type specificity. Proc Natl Acad Sci USA 86:10024–10028

Gustafsson A, Levitsky V, Zou JZ et al (2000) Epstein-Barr virus (EBV) load in bone marrow transplant recipients at risk to develop posttransplant lymphoproliferative disease: prophylactic infusion of EBV-specific cytotoxic T cells. Blood 95:807–814

Hagihara M, Tsuchiya T, Hyodo O et al (2003) Clinical effects of infusing anti-Epstein-Barr virus (EBV)-specific cytotoxic T-lymphocytes into patients with severe chronic active EBV infection. Int J Hematol 78:62–68

Haque T, Amlot PL, Helling N et al (1998) Reconstitution of EBV-specific T cell immunity in solid organ transplant recipients. J Immunol 160:6204–6209

Haque T, Taylor C, Wilkie GM et al (2001) Complete regression of posttransplant lymphoproliferative disease using partially HLA-matched Epstein Barr virus-specific cytotoxic T cells. Transplantation 72:1399–1402

Haque T, Wilkie GM, Taylor C et al (2002) Treatment of Epstein-Barr-virus-positive post-transplantation lymphoproliferative disease with partly HLA-matched allogeneic cytotoxic T cells. Lancet 360:436–442

Haque T, Wilkie GM, Jones MM et al (2007) Allogeneic cytotoxic T-cell therapy for EBV-positive posttransplantation lymphoproliferative disease: results of a phase 2 multicenter clinical trial. Blood 110:1123–1131

Harig S, Witzens M, Krackhardt AM et al (2001) Induction of cytotoxic T-cell responses against immunoglobulin V region-derived peptides modified at human leukocyte antigen-A2 binding residues. Blood 98:2999–3005

Heemskerk MH, Griffioen M, Falkenburg JH (2008) T-cell receptor gene transfer for treatment of leukemia. Cytotherapy 10:108–115

Heslop HE (2009) How I treat EBV lymphoproliferation. Blood 114:4002–4008

Heslop HE, Brenner MK, Rooney CM (1994) Donor T cells to treat EBV-associated lymphoma. N Engl J Med 331:679–680

Heslop HE, Ng CY, Li C et al (1996) Long-term restoration of immunity against Epstein-Barr virus infection by adoptive transfer of gene-modified virus-specific T lymphocytes. Nat Med 2:551–555

Heslop HE, Slobod KS, Pule MA et al (2010) Long term outcome of EBV specific T-cell infusions to prevent or treat EBV-related lymphoproliferative disease in transplant recipients. Blood 115(5):925–935

Hombach A, Heuser C, Sircar R et al (1998) An anti-CD30 chimeric receptor that mediates CD3-zeta-independent T-cell activation against Hodgkin's lymphoma cells in the presence of soluble CD30. Cancer Res 58:1116–1119

Hong R, Shen V, Rooney C et al (2001) Correction of DiGeorge anomaly with EBV-induced lymphoma by transplantation of organ-cultured thymus and Epstein-Barr-specific cytotoxic T lymphocytes. Clin Immunol 98:54–61

Hoogendoorn M, Wolbers JO, Smit WM et al (2004) Generation of B-cell chronic lymphocytic leukemia (B-CLL)-reactive T-cell lines and clones from HLA class I-matched donors using modified B-CLL cells as stimulators: implications for adoptive immunotherapy. Leukemia 18:1278–1287

Hoogendoorn M, Olde Wolbers J, Smit WM et al (2005) Primary allogeneic T-cell responses against mantle cell lymphoma antigen-presenting cells for adoptive immunotherapy after stem cell transplantation. Clin Cancer Res 11:5310–5318

Huang X, Guo H, Kang J et al (2008) Sleeping Beauty transposon-mediated engineering of human primary T cells for therapy of CD19± lymphoid malignancies. Mol Ther 16:580–589

Huls MH, Rooney CM, Heslop HE (2003) Adoptive T-cell therapy for Epstein-Barr virus-positive Hodgkin's disease. Acta Haematol 110:149–153

Hwu P, Shafer GE, Treisman J et al (1993) Lysis of ovarian cancer cells by human lymphocytes redirected with a chimeric gene composed of an antibody variable region and the Fc receptor gamma chain. J Exp Med 178:361–366

Imashuku S, Goto T, Matsumura T et al (1997) Unsuccessful CTL transfusion in a case of post-BMT Epstein-Barr virus-associated lymphoproliferative disorder (EBV-LPD). Bone Marrow Transplant 20:337–340

James SE, Greenberg PD, Jensen MC et al (2008) Antigen sensitivity of CD22-specific chimeric TCR is modulated by target epitope distance from the cell membrane. J Immunol 180:7028–7038

Jensen M, Tan G, Forman S, Wu AM, Raubitschek A (1998) CD20 is a molecular target for scFvFc:zeta receptor redirected T cells: implications for cellular immunotherapy of CD20± malignancy. Biol Blood Marrow Transplant 4:75–83

Jurgens LA, Khanna R, Weber J, Orentas RJ (2006) Transduction of primary lymphocytes with Epstein-Barr virus (EBV) latent membrane protein-specific T-cell receptor induces lysis of virus-infected cells: a novel strategy for the treatment of Hodgkin's disease and nasopharyngeal carcinoma. J Clin Immunol 26:22–32

Kalos M, Levine BL et al (2011) T cells with chimeric antigen receptors have potent antitumor effects and can establish memory in patients with advanced leukemia. Sci Transl Med 3(95): 95ra73

Khanna R, Bell S, Sherritt M et al (1999) Activation and adoptive transfer of Epstein-Barr virus-specific cytotoxic T cells in solid organ transplant patients with posttransplant lymphoproliferative disease. Proc Natl Acad Sci USA 96:10391–10396

Khouri IF, McLaughlin P, Saliba RM et al (2008) Eight-year experience with allogeneic stem cell transplantation for relapsed follicular lymphoma after nonmyeloablative conditioning with fludarabine, cyclophosphamide, and rituximab. Blood 111:5530–5536

Kowolik CM, Topp MS, Gonzalez S et al (2006) CD28 costimulation provided through a CD19-specific chimeric antigen receptor enhances in vivo persistence and antitumor efficacy of adoptively transferred T cells. Cancer Res 66:10995–11004

Krause A, Guo HF, Latouche JB, Tan C, Cheung NK, Sadelain M (1998) Antigen-dependent CD28 signaling selectively enhances survival and proliferation in genetically modified activated human primary T lymphocytes. J Exp Med 188:619–626

Kuwana Y, Asakura Y, Utsunomiya N et al (1987) Expression of chimeric receptor composed of immunoglobulin-derived V regions and T-cell receptor-derived C regions. Biochem Biophys Res Commun 149:960–968

Kuzushima K, Yamamoto M, Kimura H et al (1996) Establishment of anti-Epstein-Barr virus (EBV) cellular immunity by adoptive transfer of virus-specific cytotoxic T lymphocytes from an HLA-matched sibling to a patient with severe chronic active EBV infection. Clin Exp Immunol 103:192–198

Lamers CH, Sleijfer S, Vulto AG et al (2006) Treatment of metastatic renal cell carcinoma with autologous T-lymphocytes genetically retargeted against carbonic anhydrase IX: first clinical experience. J Clin Oncol 24:e20–e22

Leshem B, Dorfman Y, Kedar E (1999) Induction of preferential cytotoxicity against allogeneic mouse lymphoma cells: in vitro and in vivo studies. Cancer Immunol Immunother 48: 179–188

Lucas KG, Salzman D, Garcia A, Sun Q (2004) Adoptive immunotherapy with allogeneic Epstein-Barr virus (EBV)-specific cytotoxic T-lymphocytes for recurrent, EBV-positive Hodgkin disease. Cancer 100:1892–1901

Mandigers CM, Verdonck LF, Meijerink JP, Dekker AW, Schattenberg AV, Raemaekers JM (2003) Graft-versus-lymphoma effect of donor lymphocyte infusion in indolent lymphomas relapsed after allogeneic stem cell transplantation. Bone Marrow Transplant 32:1159–1163

Merlo A, Turrini R, Dolcetti R, Zanovello P, Amadori A, Rosato A (2008) Adoptive cell therapy against EBV-related malignancies: a survey of clinical results. Expert Opin Biol Ther 8:1265–1294

Milone MC, Fish JD, Carpenito C et al (2009) Chimeric receptors containing CD137 signal transduction domains mediate enhanced survival of T cells and increased antileukemic efficacy in vivo. Mol Ther 17:1453–1464

Mitsuyasu RT, Anton PA, Deeks SG et al (2000) Prolonged survival and tissue trafficking following adoptive transfer of CD4zeta gene-modified autologous CD4(±) and CD8(±) T cells in human immunodeficiency virus-infected subjects. Blood 96:785–793

Mohty M, Isnardon D, Charbonnier A et al (2002) Generation of potent T(h)1 responses from patients with lymphoid malignancies after differentiation of B lymphocytes into dendritic-like cells. Int Immunol 14:741–750

Morgan RA, Dudley ME, Wunderlich JR et al (2006) Cancer regression in patients after transfer of genetically engineered lymphocytes. Science 314:126–129

O'Connor OA, Heaney ML, Schwartz L et al (2006) Clinical experience with intravenous and oral formulations of the novel histone deacetylase inhibitor suberoylanilide hydroxamic acid in patients with advanced hematologic malignancies. J Clin Oncol 24:166–173

O'Reilly RJ, Doubrovina E, Trivedi D, Hasan A, Kollen W, Koehne G (2007) Adoptive transfer of antigen-specific T-cells of donor type for immunotherapy of viral infections following allogeneic hematopoietic cell transplants. Immunol Res 38:237–250

Opelz G, Dohler B (2004) Lymphomas after solid organ transplantation: a collaborative transplant study report. Am J Transplant 4:222–230

Orentas RJ, Roskopf SJ, Nolan GP, Nishimura MI (2001) Retroviral transduction of a T cell receptor specific for an Epstein-Barr virus-encoded peptide. Clin Immunol 98:220–228

Pakakasama S, Eames GM, Morriss MC et al (2004) Treatment of Epstein-Barr virus lymphoproliferative disease after hematopoietic stem-cell transplantation with hydroxyurea and cytotoxic T-cell lymphocytes. Transplantation 78:755–757

Pallesen G, Hamilton-Dutoit SJ, Zhou X (1993) The association of Epstein-Barr virus (EBV) with T cell lymphoproliferations and Hodgkin's disease: two new developments in the EBV field. Adv Cancer Res 62:179–239

Papadopoulos EB, Ladanyi M, Emanuel D et al (1994) Infusions of donor leukocytes to treat Epstein-Barr virus-associated lymphoproliferative disorders after allogeneic bone marrow transplantation. N Engl J Med 330:1185–1191

Paya CV, Fung JJ, Nalesnik MA et al (1999) Epstein-Barr virus-induced posttransplant lymphoproliferative disorders. ASTS/ASTP EBV-PTLD Task Force and the Mayo Clinic Organized International Consensus Development Meeting. Transplantation 68:1517–1525

Porter DL, Levine BL et al (2011) Chimeric antigen receptor-modified T cells in chronic lymphoid leukemia. N Engl J Med 365(8):725–733

Pule MA, Savoldo B, Myers GD et al (2008) Virus-specific T cells engineered to coexpress tumor-specific receptors: persistence and antitumor activity in individuals with neuroblastoma. Nat Med 14:1264–1270

Quintarelli C, Vera JF, Savoldo B et al (2007) Co-expression of cytokine and suicide genes to enhance the activity and safety of tumor-specific cytotoxic T lymphocytes. Blood 110:2793–2802

Riddell SR (2007) Engineering antitumor immunity by T-cell adoptive immunotherapy. Hematology Am Soc Hematol Educ Program 250–256

Riddell SR, Elliott M, Lewinsohn DA et al (1996) T-cell mediated rejection of gene-modified HIV-specific cytotoxic T lymphocytes in HIV-infected patients. Nat Med 2:216–223

Rooney CM, Smith CA, Ng CY et al (1995) Use of gene-modified virus-specific T lymphocytes to control Epstein-Barr-virus-related lymphoproliferation. Lancet 345:9–13

Rooney CM, Smith CA, Ng CY et al (1998a) Infusion of cytotoxic T cells for the prevention and treatment of Epstein-Barr virus-induced lymphoma in allogeneic transplant recipients. Blood 92:1549–1555

Rooney CM, Heslop HE, Brenner MK (1998b) EBV specific CTL: a model for immune therapy. Vox Sang 74(Suppl 2):497–498

Rooney CM, Bollard C, Huls MH et al (2002) Immunotherapy for Hodgkin's disease. Ann Hematol 81(Suppl 2):S39–S42

Rosenberg SA, Spiess P, Lafreniere R (1986) A new approach to the adoptive immunotherapy of cancer with tumor-infiltrating lymphocytes. Science 233:1318–1321

Roskrow MA, Suzuki N, Gan Y et al (1998) Epstein-Barr virus (EBV)-specific cytotoxic T lymphocytes for the treatment of patients with EBV-positive relapsed Hodgkin's disease. Blood 91:2925–2934

Rossig C, Pscherer S, Landmeier S, Altvater B, Jurgens H, Vormoor J (2005) Adoptive cellular immunotherapy with CD19-specific T cells. Klin Padiatr 217:351–356

Sackstein R (2005) The lymphocyte homing receptors: gatekeepers of the multistep paradigm. Curr Opin Hematol 12:444–450

Savoldo B, Huls MH, Liu Z et al (2002) Autologous Epstein-Barr virus (EBV)-specific cytotoxic T cells for the treatment of persistent active EBV infection. Blood 100:4059–4066

Savoldo B, Goss JA, Hammer MM et al (2006) Treatment of solid organ transplant recipients with autologous Epstein Barr virus-specific cytotoxic T lymphocytes (CTLs). Blood 108:2942–2949

Savoldo B, Rooney CM, Di Stasi A et al (2007) Epstein Barr virus specific cytotoxic T lymphocytes expressing the anti-CD30zeta artificial chimeric T-cell receptor for immunotherapy of Hodgkin disease. Blood 110:2620–2630

Savoldo B, Ramos CA, et al (2011) CD28 costimulation improves expansion and persistence of chimeric antigen receptor-modified T cells in lymphoma patients. J Clin Invest 121(5): 1822–1826

Schmitter D, Bolliger U, Hallek M, Pichert G (1999) Involvement of the CD27-CD70 co-stimulatory pathway in allogeneic T-cell response to follicular lymphoma cells. Br J Haematol 106:64–70

Serrano LM, Pfeiffer T, Olivares S et al (2006) Differentiation of naive cord-blood T cells into CD19-specific cytolytic effectors for posttransplantation adoptive immunotherapy. Blood 107:2643–2652

Shafer JA, Leen AM, Cruz CR et al (2008) The "side-population" of human lymphoma cells have increased chemo-resistance, stem-cell like properties and are potential targets for immunotherapy. ASH Annu Meet Abstr 112:2620

Sharpe AH (2009) Mechanisms of costimulation. Immunol Rev 229:5–11

Sherritt MA, Bharadwaj M, Burrows JM et al (2003) Reconstitution of the latent T-lymphocyte response to Epstein-Barr virus is coincident with long-term recovery from posttransplant lymphoma after adoptive immunotherapy. Transplantation 75:1556–1560

Shichijo S, Yamada A, Sagawa K et al (1996) Induction of MAGE genes in lymphoid cells by the demethylating agent 5-aza-2'-deoxycytidine. Jpn J Cancer Res 87:751–756

Straathof KC, Pule MA, Yotnda P et al (2005) An inducible caspase 9 safety switch for T-cell therapy. Blood 105:4247–4254

Sun Q, Burton R, Reddy V, Lucas KG (2002) Safety of allogeneic Epstein-Barr virus (EBV)-specific cytotoxic T lymphocytes for patients with refractory EBV-related lymphoma. Br J Haematol 118:799–808

Thomis DC, Marktel S, Bonini C et al (2001) A Fas-based suicide switch in human T cells for the treatment of graft-versus-host disease. Blood 97:1249–1257

Thorley-Lawson DA, Gross A (2004) Persistence of the Epstein-Barr virus and the origins of associated lymphomas. N Engl J Med 350:1328–1337

Thorley-Lawson DA, Duca KA, Shapiro M (2008) Epstein-Barr virus: a paradigm for persistent infection – for real and in virtual reality. Trends Immunol 29:195–201

Till BG, Jensen MC, Wang J et al (2008) Adoptive immunotherapy for indolent non-Hodgkin lymphoma and mantle cell lymphoma using genetically modified autologous CD20-specific T cells. Blood 112:2261–2271

Tsao L, Hsi ED (2007) The clinicopathologic spectrum of posttransplantation lymphoproliferative disorders. Arch Pathol Lab Med 131:1209–1218

Vera J, Savoldo B, Vigouroux S et al (2006) T lymphocytes redirected against the kappa light chain of human immunoglobulin efficiently kill mature B lymphocyte-derived malignant cells. Blood 108:3890–3897

Wagner HJ, Cheng YC, Huls MH et al (2004) Prompt versus preemptive intervention for EBV lymphoproliferative disease. Blood 103:3979–3981

Walker RE, Bechtel CM, Natarajan V et al (2000) Long-term in vivo survival of receptor-modified syngeneic T cells in patients with human immunodeficiency virus infection. Blood 96:467–474

Wang J, Jensen M, Lin Y et al (2007) Optimizing adoptive polyclonal T cell immunotherapy of lymphomas, using a chimeric T cell receptor possessing CD28 and CD137 costimulatory domains. Hum Gene Ther 18:712–725

Wynn RF, Arkwright PD, Haque T et al (2005) Treatment of Epstein-Barr-virus-associated primary CNS B cell lymphoma with allogeneic T-cell immunotherapy and stem-cell transplantation. Lancet Oncol 6:344–346

Chapter 24
Adoptive Immunotherapy of Melanoma

Seth M. Pollack and Cassian Yee

1 Introduction

Adoptive immunotherapy involves the ex vivo manipulation and expansion of lymphocytes to treat cancer. These lymphocytes, or effector cells, are "adoptively" transferred into the recipient and may be infused alone or as part of a regimen that includes chemotherapy, radiation therapy, exogenous cytokines and/or other biologic agents (e.g., antibodies) designed to enhance their survival and killing potential in vivo.

One of the earliest forms of adoptive therapy involved infusions of donor lymphocytes. Donor lymphocyte infusions (DLI) can be used to treat recipient patients relapsing from leukemia after an allogeneic bone marrow transplant by eliminating residual *host* tumor through the alloreactive response mediated by *donor* T cells. In the autologous setting, some of the most dramatic and effective uses of adoptive cellular therapy have been seen in the treatment of virus-associated malignancies, most notably, EBV, as treatment for posttransplant lymphoproliferative disease (PTLD) and EBV-associated malignancies such as Hodgkin's disease and nasopharyngeal cancer. Eventually, the identification of potential tumor rejection antigens in melanoma and other solid tumors along with the development of methods to efficiently expand autologous lymphocytes ex vivo led to the use of adoptive cellular therapy as a feasible modality for the treatment of patients.

Although adoptive cellular therapy can be applied to the treatment of many nonviral-associated solid tumor malignances, the clinical experience has largely focused on melanoma. Melanoma is amenable to both specific and nonspecific immunomodulations (i.e., IFN-α, high-dose IL-2), and potential tumor rejection melanoma-associated antigens have been identified. These antigens are immunogenic and are

S.M. Pollack • C. Yee (✉)
Fred Hutchinson Cancer Research Center, University of Washington,
825 Eastlake Avenue East, G3630, Seattle, WA 98109-1023, USA
e-mail: cyee@fhcrc.org

represented by two broad classes of tumor-associated antigens: differentiation antigens linked to normal tissue development (in this case, melanocytes) and cancer-testis antigens whose expression is limited to germinal tissues and shared among many other solid tumors. For these reasons, melanoma represents a prototypic target cancer for adoptive immunotherapy and this chapter will focus on the use of adoptive T cell therapy of melanoma as a model for other malignancies.

In spite of recent successes, the most fundamental issues remain to be defined in T cell therapy. These include the cell phenotype, antigen specificity, timing and dose of infusion, factors associated with in vitro manipulation and expansion, role of genetic modification, modulation of the host environment, combinational modalities and the clinical setting most amenable to T cell therapy. Many of these questions are being addressed in murine models and in larger mammals such as nonhuman primates, thus facilitating translation into the patient setting as clinical grade reagents become available. For the purposes of instruction, these many factors influencing the efficacy of adoptive T cell therapy will be considered in this chapter as either "intrinsic" or "extrinsic" in nature. *Intrinsic factors* are those properties inherent to the effector cell itself – for example, the cell phenotype (CD4 or CD8), its differentiation state (effector memory vs. central memory), and properties arising from genetic modification. *Extrinsic factors* are those factors external to the cell, related to the in vivo environment receiving the transferred cells. Strategies to modulate that milieu use preinfusion conditioning regimens, exogenous cytokine administration, immune checkpoint inhibitors and the use of combined modality therapy.

Within this framework, an overview of adoptive therapy focused primarily on the treatment of patients with metastatic melanoma as well as fundamental issues related to the most relevant clinical studies and key scientific work underlying the field will be presented.

2 Intrinsic Factors

Those properties inherent to the effector cell and which can be manipulated or selected in vitro include 1) antigen specificity; 2) cell phenotype; and 3) differentiation state.

A nonexclusive distinction is made between "endogenous" effector T cells, i.e., those isolated or enriched from the naturally-arising population of lymphocytes collected from the patient and "genetically modified" effector T cells which have been altered to redirect antigen specificity, enhance safety or augment efficacy (see Fig. 24.1).

The use of endogenous effectors in adoptive therapy was first implemented using lymphokine-activated killer (LAK) and tumor-infiltrating lympocytes (TIL); this was followed by the development of methods to isolate and expand endogenous *antigen-specific* T cells, which was the direct result of studies identifying Class I and II-restricted tumor-associated epitopes. Subsequently, advances in genetic

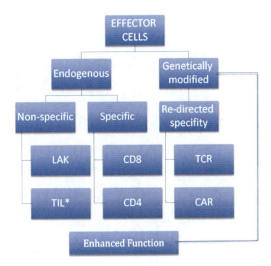

Fig. 24.1 Effector cells for adoptive therapy. Intrinsic factors associated with adoptive therapy are considered to be cell-specific *properties inherent to the effector cell*. These can be arbitrarily divided as those generated from an "Endogenous" source or those which are "Genetically Modified" to redirect specificity. A distinction is made between *endogenous* effectors that are treated in a nonspecific fashion in vitro (lymphokine-activated killer (LAK), tumor-infiltrating lympocytes (TIL)) and those that are expanded in an antigen-specific manner (CD8 or CD4⁺ T cells). Antigen specificity may also be endowed to an unselected population of peripheral blood lymphocytes by *redirected specificity*, i.e., genetically engineering them to express the tumor-cognate T cell receptor (TCR) or chimeric antigen receptor (CAR) (*Nonspecific vs. Specific categories are "empirical" definitions, for example, TIL effectors are generated in a nonspecific fashion, although antigen-specific T cells may exist among the population of expanded TIL)

modification and strategies to modulate T cell differentiation were applied to manipulate intrinsic factors associated with T cell therapy.

2.1 Effector Cells: Endogenous and Nonspecific (See Fig. 24.2)

2.1.1 Lymphokine-Activated Killer Cells

LAK Cells represent one of the earliest clinical uses of autologous lymphocytes for the treatment of patients with melanoma. Peripheral blood lymphocytes activated with IL-2 impart selective cytotoxicity against tumor cells in vitro. Much of the pioneering work on these cells performed at the NCI by the Surgery branch revealed that these cells were capable of lysing cell lines from multiple tumor types but not normal tissues (Lotze et al. 1981). Animal studies demonstrated efficacy of these cells in murine models of pulmonary and hepatic metastasis (Mule et al. 1984;

Endogenous Non-Specific

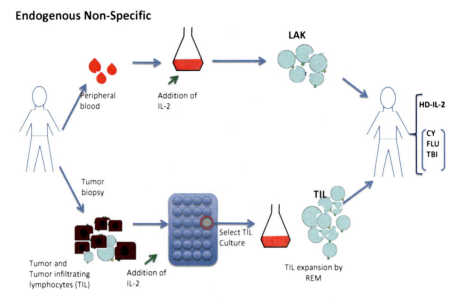

Fig. 24.2 Strategies for generating effector cells for adoptive therapy. The in vitro generation of lymphokine-activated killer, LAK cells (*top pathway*) or tumor-infiltrating lymphocytes, TIL (*bottom pathway*). LAK cells are generated by exposure of peripheral blood lymphocytes to high-dose IL-2 in vitro; after several weeks, an expanded LAK population can be harvested for infusion. TIL are generated from a starting population of mixed tumor cells and infiltrating lymphocytes from a fresh tumor biopsy. Following exposure to high-dose IL-2, tumor-reactive, expanding colonies are selected and expanded using anti-CD3 antibody, IL-2 and irradiated feeder cells to several billion ("Rapid Expansion Method," REM). Patients receiving LAK or TIL therapy are also treated with a 4–5 days regimen of high-dose IL-2 to sustain in vivo survival of transferred effectors. For TIL therapy, patients may be treated with a preinfusion conditioning regimen comprised of cyclophosphamide and fludarabine without or with total body irradiation (TBI), to induce lymphodepletion

Lafreniere and Rosenberg 1985) and concluded that the combination of LAK and IL-2 was synergistic in reducing the number of pulmonary metastases in a sarcoma mouse model, compared with either reagents given alone. Phase I studies found no toxicity other than transient fever and chills (Rosenberg 1984). However, objective clinical responses were not seen until LAK cells were combined with high-dose IL-2 (Rosenberg et al. 1985) but this was accompanied by serious toxicities associated with IL-2-induced vascular leak.

Initial reports suggested improved outcomes when LAK infusion was combined with high-dose IL-2 (Rosenberg et al. 1987), particularly in melanoma (Dillman et al. 1991), leading to a prospective trial (Rosenberg et al. 1993) randomizing patients with metastatic cancer (largely melanoma and renal cell carcinoma (RCC)) to high-dose IL-2 vs. high-dose IL-2, lymphocytopheresis, and LAK administration. A total of 181 patients were included in the study; 97 of the patients had RCC and 54 had melanoma. Ten CRs were seen in combined therapy compared with four seen in patients receiving IL-2 only. A total of 24 objective (CR plus PR) responses were seen with the combined therapy compared with 16 in the IL-2 only patients but this did not achieve statistical significance. A trend was also seen toward improved overall survival among the melanoma group for patients treated with both IL-2 and LAK cells compared to IL-2 alone but this was not statistically significant.

When TILs were found to have greater potency against tumors in murine models, (see below; Spiess et al. 1987; Rosenberg et al. 1986) attention shifted towards TIL-based adoptive immunotherapy trials. However, some groups have continued to investigate the use of LAK therapy for example as an adjunct to dendritic cell vaccination (Hirooka et al. 2009) or in combination with conventional therapies such as chemotherapy and surgery (Kobari et al. 2000; Weng et al. 2008) as well as its use as single-agent therapy, when administered intracranially following surgery for patients with glioblastoma (Dillman et al. 2004).

2.1.2 Tumor-Infiltrating Lymphocytes

TILs is the term applied to lymphocytes that can be cultured ex vivo from tumor fragments (Yron et al. 1980). Early studies involved enzymatic digestion of tumor fragments to create single cell suspensions which when cultured with IL-2 (6,000 U/mL) led to the outgrowth of potential tumor-reactive lymphocytes. TILs demonstrated cytolytic activity against tumor cell lines (Muul et al. 1987) in murine tumor models (Eberlein et al. 1982). In the mouse sarcoma model, antitumor activity of these cells was observed to be 50–100 times more potent than LAK cells (when considering the number of cells required to invoke tumor regression). In a colon adenocarcinoma model (MC-38), administration of either TIL or IL-2 alone had no statistically significant impact on the survival. However, when treated with a combination of LAK, TIL and IL-2, long-term regression was observed; a finding that was not reproduced with LAK cells.

Phenotypically, TIL cells are comprised of a mix of IL-2-responding effectors: CD8, CD4, NK, and NKT cells (Topalian et al. 1987; Yuen and Norris 2001; Schleypen et al. 2006; Malone et al. 2001) and can be expanded to achieve cell doses of up to 100 billion (Malone et al. 2001). TIL cells are cultured in high doses of IL-2 and their in vivo survival is dependent on co-administered high-dose IL-2 following adoptive transfer.

The first 20 patients with metastatic melanoma treated with TILs (along with high-dose IL-2) were described in a landmark 1987 *New England Journal of Medicine* article. Half of all patients in this study experienced an objective response including one complete response (Rosenberg et al. 1988). A follow-up report published in the Journal of the National Cancer Institute included the original patients among a total of 86 metastatic melanoma patients treated with 145 courses of TILs followed by high-dose IL-2. Despite a heavily pretreated population, 34% of patients achieved an objective response (CR or PR). Five patients had complete responses, all of which lasted at least 20 months (Rosenberg et al. 1994).

These results compared favorably to objective response rates from the NCI studies of high-dose IL-2 alone or with LAK and IL-2 (Rosenberg et al. 1989). Studies labeling transferred cells with Indium-111 demonstrated that unlike LAK cells, TILs trafficked to tumor sites (Fisher et al. 1989; Griffith et al. 1989). Clinical responses were more likely to be observed in patients whose TIL cultures grew more rapidly (Zhou et al. 2005; Rosenberg et al. 1994). In a follow-up analysis of these patients, a number of the patients had progressed, and ultimately 9 of 41 (22%) had what appeared to be sustained objective responses following TIL followed by high-dose IL-2 and in some cases with low-dose cyclophosphamide conditioning (Schwartzentruber et al. 1994). These results mirrored findings seen in the studies of LAK in which a number of patients who initially had objective responses subsequently progressed (Rosenberg et al. 1987).

In 2003, the Rosenberg group updated their method for generated TILs (Dudley et al. 2003). Multiple TIL cultures were evaluated for antitumor activity against at least two melanoma cell lines and those cultures with the best antitumor activity were selected. These tumor-reactive TIL cultures were then expanded using an adaptation of the "Rapid Expansion Method" (REM) protocol, previously developed by Riddell and Greenberg for expanding T cell clones, involving the use of a TCR trigger (anti-CD3 antibody), feeder cells, and lymphokine support (IL-2) (Crossland et al. 1991). The cultures grew in as little as 5 weeks and typically between 6 and 8 weeks.

Subsequent studies sought to optimize the potency of TILs by conditioning patients with increasing levels of lymphodepletion (Dudley et al. 2005, 2008) prior to cell infusion. These results are further discussed in Sect. 3.1.

Therapy with TIL has also been used as adjuvant therapy in patients with stage III melanoma (Khammari et al. 2007). Following lymph node excision, patients were randomly assigned to receive either TIL plus interleukin-2 (IL-2) for 2 months, or IL-2 alone. Eighty-eight patients were enrolled in the study. Although no significant difference in relapse-free interval or overall survival was observed, a significant difference was observed in the subset of patients with involvement of only one involved lymph node.

2.2 Effector Cells: Endogenous, Antigen-Specific (See Fig. 24.3)

In contrast to effector cells of undefined specificity generated under nonphysiologic conditions using very high doses of IL-2, antigen-specific T cells are elicited in vitro under more physiologic conditions involving cyclical antigen stimulation followed by exposure to low-dose IL-2 to expand T cells of defined specificity. Hence, one prerequisite in the development of antigen-specific effector cells for adoptive therapy is the identification of tumor-associated antigens recognized by endogenous T cells.

Endogenous Antigen-Specific

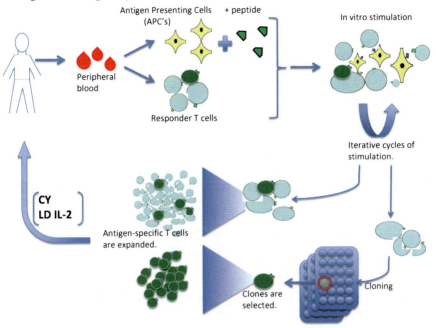

Fig. 24.3 The in vitro generation of antigen-specific T cells. Peripheral blood mononuclear cells collected from patients (by leukapheresis or serial phlebotomy), are used as a source of antigen-presenting cells (APCs) or responder T cells. After pulsing APCs with the tumor-associated epitope peptide, autologous T cells are cocultivated in vitro together with lymphokine cocktail (low-dose IL-2, IL-7) and restimulated for two to three cycles to enrich for the population of tumor antigen-specific T cells. The enriched T cell cultures may be expanded at this point for infusion (*upper path*) or cloned as single cells, selected for high affinity recognition of tumor antigen and expanded (*lower path*). T cell clones are typically expanded using the REM method (see above) to several billion in 2–4 weeks. Patients receive low-dose IL-2 for 1–2 weeks following adoptive transfer; this dose is sufficient to maintain in vivo persistence of T cells generated in this fashion. Long-term persistence may be achieved through the use lymphodepletion conditioning (e.g., cyclophosphamide) preinfusion

2.2.1 Identification of Target Antigens for Adoptive T Cell Therapy

Investigators had long sought to characterize specific tumor-associated antigens that would be considered "immunogenic," that is, capable of inducing an immune response, and therefore, potential tumor-rejection targets for immunotherapy. Early work performed by Thierry Boon and colleagues at the Ludwig Institute for Cancer Research in Brussels to elucidate tumor-associated antigens expressed by an immunogenic murine mastocytoma, P815, led to the discovery of four distinct antigens (A, B, C, and D) recognized by syngeneic cytotoxic T lymphocytes

(CTLs). Two of these antigens were found to be located on a single gene known as P1A. The identification of this gene as unmutated and expressed in normal tissues unveiled a novel paradigm in tumor immunology – that potential tumor rejection antigens may be represented by normal self proteins yet capable of provoking antigen-specific T cells that mediate tumor rejection; P1A elicited a dominant T cell response in >50% of P815 mice (Van den Eynde et al. 1991; Brandle et al. 1998) and in those mice where the tumor underwent partial regression only to regrow, these recrudescent tumors were found to have lost the P1A antigen (Uyttenhove et al. 1983).

Following on the heels of this discovery, the Boon group identified the first human tumor-associated T cell-defined antigen, MAGE-1 (Melanoma Antigen-1, subsequently renamed MAGE-A1) by screening target cells transfected with the cDNA library of a tumor line using autologous tumor reactive antigen-specific CTL. MAGE-A1 belongs to a class of "cancer-testis" antigens, a term first proposed by Lloyd Old to describe the family of tumor-associated antigens whose expression is restricted to germline tissues, placental trophoblasts, and a broad range of cancers. To date, there are more than 70 CT gene families, many of which are being developed as T cell targets for vaccine and adoptive cellular therapy (Simpson et al. 2005).

Subsequently, the first T cell-defined differentiation antigen in melanoma (MelanA or MART-1) was identified followed quickly by several other antigens associated with melanocyte differentiation with shared expression among melanoma cells (van der Bruggen et al. 1991).

Initially, Class I-restricted epitopes triggering $CD8^+$ T cells were identified because of the ease with which antigen specificity could be screened using chromium release assays; however, when Class II-restricted epitopes for several CT antigens and differentiation antigens were sequenced, it became possible to generate $CD4^+$ T cell responses in vitro (Hunder et al. 2008) as well as in vivo following vaccination (Topalian et al. 1996).

Other potential targets such as p53 and Her2 are expressed by some normal tissues but may be over expressed in tumor. "Universal antigens," described as those more uniformly expressed by tumors such as telomerase (hTERT) and survivin are associated with a tumorigenic advantage and targeting such antigens may circumvent the potential for outgrowth of antigen-loss variants (Vonderheide et al. 1999; Reker et al. 2004). Certain viral antigens from viruses such as EBV may also be potential targets in cancers associated with viral infection (Van den Eynde and van der Bruggen 1997).

2.2.2 Clinical Trials of Adoptive Therapy Using Antigen-Specific $CD8^+$ Cells

The identification of tumor-associated antigens, and immunogenic peptides representing Class I (and subsequently, Class II) restricted epitopes responsible for $CD8^+$ and $CD4^+$ T cell recognition, respectively, led to the development of methods to isolate and enrich for antigen-specific T cells ex vivo. For the most part, peptide epitopes presented by the more prevalent HLA alleles in the Caucasian population (who are most at risk for melanoma) such as HLA-A2 and -A24, have been identified for the melanocytes differentiation antigens and most cancer-testis antigens. The most straightforward approach requires autologous antigen-presenting cells, for example, dendritic cells, to be pulsed with the relevant MHC-restricted peptide and used to stimulate autologous responder T cells in vitro. This is taken through iterative cycles of restimulation until the population of peptide-specific, tumor-reactive T cells is expanded to sufficient numbers for adoptive transfer or for cloning and further expansion prior to adoptive transfer. By extrapolation from murine models, cell doses in the range of 5–50 billion have been used. This dose range is arbitrary and the requisite number is not known, but more likely dependent on other factors such as target avidity, replicative potential, and extrinsic factors. The use of peptides to generate a T cell response is the most easily translatable approach since clinical grade peptides are readily available. However, in cases where the MHC-restricting allele is not known, epitope peptides presented by any of the MHC alleles expressed by the patient have not been identified, or a more global response to the target antigen is desired, autologous antigen-presenting cells may be genetically engineered to present the target antigen of interest for in vitro stimulation. This may be achieved by transfecting antigen-presenting cells, such as dendritic cells, with RNA encoding the entire antigen (Liao et al. 2004), by lentiviral or retroviral transduction of target antigens (Specht et al. 1997), or cross-presentation of soluble antigen–antibody complexes (Groh et al. 2005). To date, however, the majority of clinical trials using antigen-specific T cells have used peptides corresponding to known antigenic epitopes.

The generation of antigen-specific T cells can be relatively facile, for example, in the case of MART-1/MelanA-specific T cells where the endogenous frequency is surprisingly high (0.2–1%); in other cases, where a self protein is more ubiquitously expressed in normal tissues (e.g., WT-1), and the extant T cell population is rare and of low avidity, it can be difficult or simply not feasible to isolate high avidity tumor-reactive T cells. Altman et al. in the Davis Lab generated multimers of soluble peptide-MHC complexes, initially as a means of enumerating by flow cytometry antigen-specific T cells through its cognate TCR (Altman et al. 1996); subsequently the use of peptide-MHC multimers was developed as a powerful means of sorting for rare and potentially highly avid antigen-specific T cells (Yee et al. 1999). In another embodiment, conjugation of the multimers to immunomagnetic particles would also allow for antigen-specific T cell enrichment (Bodinier et al. 2000). Initially designed as a tetramer complexed through avidin-biotin, peptide-MHC multimers can also take the form of pentamers and dimers with at least equal effectiveness in isolating antigen-specific T cells (Schneck et al. 2001) ; more recently, Class II multimers have been developed for isolating antigen-specific CD4$^+$ T cells (Gebe and Kwok 2007).

Mitchell et al. used insect cells transduced with HLA-A2, CD80, and CD54 pulsed with tyrosinase epitope peptide to generate cultures of tyrosinase-specific CTL for adoptive therapy of patients with refractory metastatic melanoma. Up to 5×10^8 T cells were administered (of which, 10–30% were tyrosinase-specific) without IL-2. Although Indium-labeled T cells could be seen in the liver and spleen and some lesions 48–72 h after infusion, infused cells were undetectable in the peripheral blood. Of ten patients treated, one experienced a partial response (Mitchell et al. 2002).

Mackensen et al. treated 11 patients with multiple infusions of MelanA specific T cells generated using peptide-pulsed DCs (and comprising on average, 38% of the infused cell product). The study demonstrated T cell trafficking to tumor sites (Meidenbauer et al. 2003) in vivo persistence for at least 24 h and up to 14 days post infusion, and significant clinical response: three patients had objective responses including one durable complete response (Mackensen et al. 2006).

Yee et al. generated antigen-specific CD8$^+$ T cell clones at doses up to 3.3×10^9 cells/m^2 that were administered together without and with low-dose IL-2 for 14 days (250,000 U/m^2 s.c. twice daily) for treatment of patients with progressive metastatic melanoma. Addition of IL-2 led to an extension of in vivo persistence from <7 to 17 days and was accompanied by disease stabilization, minor or mixed responses in eight of ten patients for up to 21 months with one long-term survivor, >7 years (Yee et al. 2002).

Khammari et al. recently published a trial in metastatic melanoma using MelanA specific CD8$^+$ CTL clones that were infused following 4 days of DTIC conditioning and a postinfusion course of IL-2 (9 mU (D1-4 and D8-12) and IFN-α (9 mU $\times$ 3$\times$/ week $\times$ 1 month)). T cells persisted for >30 days in 9 of 14 patients and clinical responses (PR and CR) were observed in 6 (43%) (Khammari et al. 2009).

In summary, these studies demonstrate that adoptive therapy with antigen-specific CD8$^+$ T cells leads to non-serious toxicities associated with cytokine release and depigmentation, can lead to the appearance of antigen-loss tumor variants following antigen-specific adoptive therapy, and the finding that in vivo persistence and measurable, durable antitumor responses are feasible when combined with conditioning (DTIC) and/or low-dose IL-2/IFN-α (Mackensen et al. 2006; Yee et al. 2002; Khammari et al. 2009).

2.2.3 Clinical Trials of Adoptive Therapy Using Antigen-Specific CD4$^+$ Cells

CD4$^+$ T cells play a critical role in the antitumor response by providing a helper function, increasing CD8$^+$ T cells potency and mediating a direct and indirect cytotoxic antitumor response (Hung et al. 1998; Giuntoli et al. 2002; Khanolkar et al. 2004; Wang and Livingstone 2003). Indeed, CD4$^+$ T cells are necessary for persistence of antigen-specific CD8 (Pardoll and Topalian 1998; Marzo et al. 2000) cells in vivo as well as infiltration of those cells into tumor (Greenberg 1991; Kalams and Walker 1998).

In some models, CD4$^+$ T cells have been shown to be more effective than CD8$^+$ T cells in eradicating tumor (Perez-Diez et al. 2007). Correlative studies in a number of vaccine trials have also underscored the pivotal role of CD4$^+$ T cell mediated (Mandic et al. 2005; Zhang et al. 2005) activity in cancer. For adoptive therapy, initial observations made in a murine leukemia model demonstrated that syngeneic CD4+ T cells alone were capable of inducing a complete response (Greenberg et al. 1985) in the absence of CD8+ T or NK cells, even against Class II-negative tumor (Greenberg et al. 1985; Plautz et al. 2000; Frey and Cestari 1997).

To more clearly define the requirements for effective CD4+ T cell therapy, a transgenic mouse model expressing the TCR for murine homolog of human TRP-1 was recently developed. Mice bearing large established B16 melanomas were cleared of disease after adoptive transfer of TRP-1-specific CD4+ T cells, in vivo immunization, and IL-2, an effect which was potentiated when using CD4+ T cells polarized to a Th17 phenotype in vitro (Muranski et al. 2008).

The discovery that several tumor-associated antigens capable of eliciting human CD8+ T cell responses were also immunogenic for CD4+ T cell responses and the identification of a number of Class II-restricted epitopes (e.g., tyrosinase, NY-ESO-1, MAGE-1) (Topalian et al. 1996), this led very quickly to vaccine studies designed to induce helper CD4+ T cell responses in patients with metastatic melanoma. In the case of NY-ESO-1, epitopes have been identified which are presented by commonly expressed Class II alleles (e.g., DP4) are capable of promiscuously binding multiple Class II alleles, and whose T cell immunogenicity is associated with an in vivo serologic response (Mandic et al. 2005; Zeng et al. 2001). The identification of these tumor-associated Class II-restricted epitopes also provided the opportunity to generate antigen-specific CD4+ T cells in vitro for adoptive therapy.

A first-in-human clinical trial using antigen-specific CD4+ T cells was completed recently. The Class II-restricted epitopes of NY-ESO-1 or tyrosinase were used to generate Th1-type CD4+ T cell clones to treat patients with refractory metastatic melanoma. At doses of up to 10^{10} cells/m^2, T cell frequencies up to 3% were observed for as long as 2 months after infusion. Four patients experienced a partial response or disease stabilization and one patient underwent complete durable response of >3 years. In some patients, induction of endogenous responses to non-targeted antigens was also observed (i.e., "antigen spreading") and may have contributed to a more complete response and the absence of antigen-loss tumor variants (Hunder et al. 2008).

2.2.4 T Cell Differentiation and In Vivo Persistence

The observation has been made in clinical trials and murine studies that persistence of adoptively transferred T cells correlates with antitumor activity (Klebanoff et al. 2006). When naïve T cells encounter antigen and undergo differentiation, the majority of T cells eventually progress to an effector memory (EM) subset with enhanced killing function (increase in granzyme and perforin expression) accompanied by a diminution of proliferative and trafficking properties. A smaller fraction of T cells develop into to a central memory (CM) pool, endowed with high replicative potential (CD28^{hi}, CD27^{hi}), expression of specialized chemokines receptors (CD62L, CCR7), and a latency to cytotoxicity (Murali-Krishna et al. 1999; Wherry and

Ahmed 2004); however, when rechallenged with antigen, these central memory T cells can rapidly proliferate and develop effector function (Barber et al. 2003).

Using T cells from transgenic mice expressing the TCR for the melanoma rejection antigen, p-mel (murine gp100 homolog), it was demonstrated that less differentiated effector cells, in particular, central memory CTL were more effective than CTL that had progressed to a more differentiated effector memory state, in eradicating (Gattinoni et al. 2005) established tumors from mice (Klebanoff et al. 2005). It was soon discovered that it was possible to generate antigen-specific T cells with central memory properties by in vitro exposure to IL-21 or pharmacologic modulators of the Wnt-β catenin pathway and that these CTL were more potent in eradicating established tumors than their more differentiated counterparts (Li and Yee 2008; Li et al. 2005). Finally, in nonhuman primates, it was recently demonstrated that effector CTLs derived from the CD8$^+$ *central memory* compartment recovered CD62L, CD27, and CCR7 expression in vivo following adoptive transfer, the ability to home to lymph nodes and bone marrow, and effect more potent antiviral immunity than CTL derived from the *effector memory* compartment (Berger et al. 2008).

Taken together, these data suggest that strategies to generate, maintain, or expand a population of T cells with high replicative potential would be instructive for the development of more effective adoptive cellular therapy trials.

2.3 Effector Cells: Genetically Modified (See Fig. 24.4)

The isolation of tumor-reactive T cells which exist at low frequency among the endogenous T cell repertoire can be a time- and resource-intensive process and most T cells that can be isolated recognizing tumor-associated normal self proteins can be of relatively low avidity. Redirecting the specificity of T cells by genetically modifying them to express the cognate TCR (Sect. 2.3.1) or antibody variable chains (Sect. 2.3.2) allows for greater flexibility in the antigens that can be targeted, and more rapid production of antigen-specific effector cells.

Genetic modification of T cells for adoptive therapy also provides the opportunity to enhance T cell function by endowing them with properties that *augment persistence* through costimulation or *confer resistance* to immunosuppressive or regulatory controls limiting T cell survival (Sect. 2.3.3).

2.3.1 Redirecting Specificity by Transfer of TCR

Once a T cell clone of desired specificity has been isolated, its TCR α and β chains can be sequenced and cloned into viral vectors to transfer antigen specificity. Patients with tumor expressing the shared target antigen and restricting allele can be treated using T cells transfected with these "universal" vectors obviating the requirement for extensive cell culture (Cooper et al. 2000; Stanislawski et al. 2001).

Genetically Modified

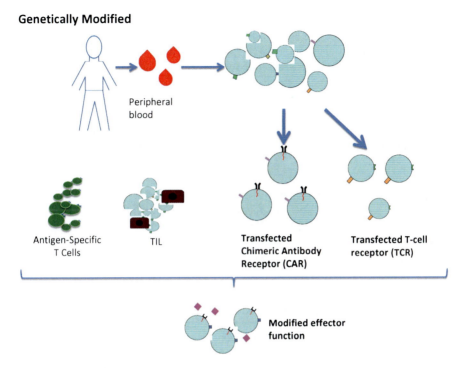

Fig. 24.4 The use of genetically modified T cells. Peripheral blood lymphocytes may be genetically modified to express a chimeric antigen receptor (extracellular antibody to surface tumor antigen fused to intracellular T cell signaling components) or T cell receptor (sequenced from a TCR recognizing an MHC-restricted tumor antigen-derived T cell epitope). Genetic modification to confer redirected specificity in this manner is a rapid means of achieving a population of antigen-specific effector cells for adoptive transfer. Effector cells genetically modified with redirected specificity or those endogenous effector cells (TIL or antigen-specific T cells) generated in vitro, can be modified with enhanced survival or antitumor function

Although the cloned TCR may be derived from a Class I-Restricted CD8[+] T cell, cognate antigen recognition can also be transferred to CD4[+] T cells, which retain properties of CD4 activation (i.e., IL-2 production) (Weber et al. 2005). The gene sequence of the cognate TCR responsible for peptide-MHC recognition can also be mutagenized to enhance avidity and molecular tools to rapidly screen for highly avid TCRs have been developed (Holler et al. 2000; Kessels et al. 2001).

Challenges to the development of TCR gene therapy include mispairing of the transduced α and β chains to endogenous α and β chains, resulting in nonfunctional TCRs or, in some cases, the possibility of generating TCRs reactive to autoantigens leading to unexpected autoimmune toxicities. The expression level of the desired TCR is also often much lower than that of endogenously expressed TCRs, and strategies to enhance expression in resting T cells using lentiviral vectors by optimizing vector promoters as well as codon sequences are being evaluated.

The first human study of TCR gene therapy using first generation TCR vectors demonstrated that specificity to the MART-1 antigen can be transferred to CD8⁺ and CD4⁺ T cells and that, these transduced T cells can persist for up to a month following adoptive transfer when infused in combination with nonablative conditioning and high-dose IL-2, Clinical responses were observed in 2 of 15 patients accompanied by the development of vitiligo (Morgan et al. 2003).

2.3.2 Redirecting Specificity Using Chimeric Antigen Receptors

The second strategy transduces the variable fragment (scFvs) from an antibody recognizing a tumor antigen coupled with an intracellular domain delivering a T cell activation signal (CD3ζ). These chimeric antigen receptors (also known as CARs) allow the targeting of surface proteins, generally with much higher affinity than TCRs (in the nanomolar vs. micromolar range) and mediate effector functions of a TCR (i.e., IFN-γ production or cytolysis) (Eshhar et al. 1993). The original CARs signaled solely through CD3, enabled only limited T cell proliferation following antigen exposure (Gong et al. 1999) and only modest clinical effects to date (Till et al. 2008). The development of second generation CAR coupled to the intracellular domain of costimulatory molecules such as CD28 and 41BB (Finney et al. 2004; Wang et al. 2007), have led to more potent in vitro effects and await clinical studies.

There are clear advantages to the use of CARs over transduced TCRs, including the capacity to target in a non-MHC-restricted fashion a broader pool of antigen targets and enhanced target affinity. However, as a fusion product, CARs are targets themselves for the endogenous immune response and in some clinical trials, host antibodies against the CAR gene product have been detected (Kershaw et al. 2006; Park et al. 2007; Lamers et al. 2006).

2.3.3 Genetic Modification: Enhanced Function

T cells can be modified to express autocrine growth factors including IL-2 or IL-15 to sustain survival following adoptive transfer. However, cytokine expression not coordinately regulated with antigen stimulation might result in T cell dysfunction or apoptosis and may induce cytokine-mediated toxicity. Signaling through the costimulatory molecule CD28 concurrent with T cell recognition of antigen would synchronize endogenous production of IL-2 with TCR signals (Topp et al. 2003). Reexpression of CD28 in human effector CD8⁺ T cells, via a retroviral vector, results in regulated IL-2 production. Unfortunately, tumors rarely express CD80 or CD86, the ligands for CD28, rendering this approach ineffective in a majority of cases. One solution to this problem would be to attach intracellular signaling domains from CD28 to the signaling TCR ζ domains of CARs, which can then provide both TCR and costimulation signals (Sadelain et al. 2003).

Alternatively, chimeric cytokine receptors (CCRs) may coordinate antigen stimulation with cytokine signaling. One such CCR employs the extracellular domain of the GM-CSF receptor fused to the intracellular signaling domains of the IL-2 receptor, so that GM-CSF, which is normally produced following TCR engagement in effector CD8⁺ T cells, can deliver, through the CCR, IL-2 prosurvival signals and enhance T cell proliferation in tumor-bearing mice (Cheng et al. 2002).

Other examples of using genetic modifications to increase effector function include the transduction of chemokine receptor CXCR2 to enable trafficking of T cells to tumor sites and strategies to increase in vivo survival and persistence by introducing proteins involved in apoptotic signaling pathways (Chiang et al. 2000; de Witte et al. 2008).

3 Extrinsic Factors

Manipulation of the host environment is critical to successful adoptive therapy. This was first demonstrated in several animal models where preinfusion conditioning with chemotherapy or radiation was required for full effector function and antitumor efficacy. Lymphodepletion, at least to some degree, appears to be critical to the success of adoptive T cell therapy by decreasing the impact of Tregs and other regulatory controls, removing a cytokine sink (Muranski et al. 2006) and creating a more favorable environment by upregulating homeostatic cytokines IL-15 and IL-7. Measures to achieve this include the use of nonspecific approaches to induce lymphodepletion such as chemotherapy or radiation therapy, and the use of more specific reagents that eliminate regulatory T cells (e.g., anti-CD25) (Mahnke et al. 2007; Dannull et al. 2005) or that interrupt autoregulatory or immune checkpoints (e.g., anti-CTLA4) (Peggs et al. 2006).

3.1 Lymphodepleting Conditioning

Some of the first observations demonstrating that manipulation of the host environment was essential for effective adoptive cellular therapy were made in mice implanted with the P815 mastocytoma tumors and treated with tumor-sensitized lymphocytes; complete tumor regression was observed only in mice that had been thymectomized prior to adoptive transfer (Berendt et al. 1978; Mills et al. 1981). For both adoptively transferred tumor-specific CD4 or CD8⁺ T cells, administration of cyclophosphamide prior to T cell infusion was critical for tumor eradication and cure of mice bearing FBL tumors. In other settings, where adoptively transferred LAK cells or TIL were used, sublethal irradiation (Mule et al. 1985) or cyclophosphamide conditioning (Rosenberg et al. 1986) were required. North demonstrated in a seminal study that suppressor cells played a role in mice bearing the cyclophosphamide-resistant lymphopma (L5178Y). Complete tumor regression was observed only when the combination of cyclophosphamide and tumor-sensitized T cells was administered (Awwad and North 1988). Furthermore, infusion of cyclophosphamide-sensitive CD4⁺ T cells from tumor-bearing hosts could inhibit this response providing the first evidence for the existence of regulatory cells. It would be more than 15 years before Sakaguchi et al. (1995) were able to phenotype and isolate the regulatory T cells responsible for tumor immune suppression.

3.1.1 Cyclophosphamide and Fludarabine

Among chemotherapy agents found to exhibit immunopotentiating properties, cyclophosphamide has been the most extensively studied (Machiels et al. 2001). Since the original observation almost 40 years ago that cyclophosphamide could augment immune responses (Maguire and Ettore 1967), this effect has been evaluated in animals and clinical studies at doses ranging from 40 to >6,000 mg/m^2 (Lutsiak et al. 2005; Vierboom et al. 1997; Greenberg et al. 1981; Proietti et al. 1998; Schiavoni et al. 2000). In murine models, some studies report cytoxan immunopotentiation only at high (175 mg/kg or >6 g/m^2) but not low doses (12.5 mg/kg or 40 mg/m^2) claiming only a "bystander" effect, while others demonstrate benefit at low doses (30 mg/kg) attributable to decreases in Treg numbers and/or function (Lutsiak et al. 2005; Ghiringhelli et al. 2004). In adoptive therapy studies, transferred memory T cells from tumor-sensitized mice are capable of eradicating disseminated cancer and providing long-term protection, but only when the mice were pretreated with cyclophosphamide; cyclophosphamide alone in these mice failed to protect (Greenberg 1991; Greenberg et al. 1981; Proietti et al. 1998; North 1982; Awwad and North 1989; Vierboom et al. 2000). This was observed for both prophylactic and challenge tumor models (i.e., mice with "large" tumor burdens). The immune-enhancing effects were believed to be dose-dependent and attributed to cyclophosphamide mediated elimination of "suppressor" or "regulatory" T cells (Ghiringhelli et al. 2004), a "bystander" effect leading to induction of homeostatic cytokines that support the growth of transferred T cells (Proietti et al. 1998), or immunologic "skewing" to a more favorable Th1 profile (Machiels et al. 2001), with upregulation of Type I interferon and augmentation in number of memory T cells in vivo (Schiavoni et al. 2000). Given an incomplete understanding of cyclophosphamide metabolism in murine models and the variable beneficial and adverse effects even among different mouse strains, translating these studies to clinical studies is not straightforward.

As early as the mid 1980s, Berd and Mastrangelo first demonstrated cyclophosphamide potentiation of DTH responses to a vaccine in patients with metastatic cancer at doses of 1,000 mg/m^2 (Berd et al. 1982) and later reported that a lower dose (300 mg/m^2) was also adequate, the latter being the result of a reduction in suppressor function based on in vitro functional studies (Berd and Mastrangelo 1987; Bast et al. 1983; Berd et al. 1984). It was suggested that lower doses of CY (200–400 mg/m^2) can selectively deplete suppressor activity (CD8) while higher doses may have a "bystander" homeostatic effect (Proietti et al. 1998; Bast et al. 1983), although at the time, regulatory T cell phenotypes had not been defined. Recently, Ghiringhelli et al. (2007) demonstrate Treg depletion as an important mechanism of action of cyclophosphamide and for vaccines, low-dose metronomic dosing (50 mg) would be sufficient to deplete regulatory T cells while preserving vaccine-elicited responses in vivo.

The Surgery Branch of the NCI was one of the first groups to combine a high-dose lymphodepletion regimen with *adoptive cellular therapy*. Patients received up to 60 mg/kg of cyclophosphamide in addition to fludarabine, which led to sustained functional and absolute lymphopenia. Tumor-infiltrating lymphocytes enriched in vitro with high-dose IL-2 were expanded, infused and supported in vivo by administering a course of high-dose IL-2 to patients. Serious life-threatening toxicities attributed to cytokine-induced vascular leak syndrome were observed, including respiratory failure and hypotension, while replacement of the immune repertoire with adoptively transferred oligoclonal T cells led to immune compromise and in some cases, opportunistic infections and lymphoproliferative disease. Among the 35 patients, more than 50% (18 patients) had experienced objective responses including 3 CRs, at least one of which was durable for over 2 years. Patients had clones persisting weeks and in some cases even months after TIL infusion (Dudley et al. 2002, 2008).

Whether the combination of both cyclophosphamide *and* fludarabine is required has not been comprehensively defined. Fludarabine when given as a single 5-day course is generally safe and has the capacity to cause profound lymphodepletion (Cheson 1995). One advantage of using fludarabine in immunotherapy trials is that fludarabine, unlike some modalities, has virtually no effect on most solid tumor malignancies including melanoma – making it easier to attribute clinical response to immunotherapy. In one study using fludarabine as the sole conditioning regimen, elevation of homeostatic cytokines was observed coincident with lymphopenia and led to extended persistence of transferred T cell clones (Wallen et al. 2009). Its clinical effect however was modest and may have been mitigated by a disproportionately greater fraction of regulatory T cells compared to effector T cells when recovering from lymphodepletion.

3.1.2 Radiation

In preclinical studies, adding radiation prior to T cell infusion resulted in greater antitumor efficacy (Wrzesinski et al. 2007a; Gattinoni et al. 2005). Radiation, by upregulating expression of local adhesion molecules and augmenting antigen presentation, can facilitate tumor infiltration and enhance immunogenicity (Lugade et al. 2005, 2008; Garnett et al. 2004).

In clinical studies, the NCI group incorporated total body irradiation (TBI) into the existing non-myeloablative regimen of cyclophosphamide and fludarabine. At doses of 2 Gy, no stem cell support was required; however, response rates did not improve over the non-TBI containing regimen. At a dose of 12 Gy, this chemoradiation regimen was myeloablative requiring co-administration of CD34+ hematopoietic stem cells. Among this select group of patients with metastatic melanoma, a historically significant response rate of >70% was observed (Dudley et al. 2008). These results, while highly promising, should be considered in the context of patients with accessible tumor, from whom TIL could be isolated and who meet restricted eligibility criteria on the basis of their ability to tolerate potentially life-threatening toxicities associated with high-dose IL-2 and in some cases ablative conditioning and stem cell transplantation. The durability of these responses and reproducibility of such a dramatically improved response rate remain to be evaluated in multi-institution-based, Phase II and III trials.

3.2 Future Prospects for Adoptive Cellular Therapy

In the last 20 years, the use of adoptive cellular therapy has progressed from animal models to anecdotal clinical results and presently to an emerging modality for the effective and durable treatment of late-stage solid tumors. During this time, advances in the understanding of antigen recognition by human T cells, identification of tumor target antigens, and the development of methods to expand the population of tumor-reactive T cells have led to successes in its clinical application. It has become apparent that immunomodulation of the host, in this case conditioning lymphodepletion, can significantly augment the in vivo persistence and antitumor efficacy of adoptively transferred T cell effectors. Nevertheless, the lack of uniform efficacy and the limited durability of the majority of responses have led researchers in this field to consider additional strategies to enhance persistence and overcome tumor immune resistance mechanisms.

Studies involving the use of a transgenic TCR model targeting the murine melanoma antigen, p-mel (murine homolog of human gp100), demonstrated that eradication of established tumor required the combination of adoptively transferred antigen-specific T cells, high-dose IL-2 *and* postinfusion vaccination (Overwijk et al. 2003). The use of vaccination has been described in clinical trials but only as a means to increase the frequency of an otherwise weak or rare tumor antigen-specific response (i.e., to increase T cell frequency in vivo prior to PBMC harvest) in order to increase the likelihood of generating a tumor-reactive effector population in vitro (Dudley et al. 2002). More recently, recombinant vaccines are being used in combination with high-dose IL-2, to expand and/or restimulate an adoptively transferred T cell population in vivo, thus recapitulating the murine model.

Strategies to circumvent tumor resistance mechanisms have been addressed in preclinical studies. Regulatory $CD25^{hi}$ T cells which impair the efficacy of an antigen-specific T cell response, may be partially depleted by cyclophosphamide conditioning, but can be more selectively depleted preinfusion using CD25 specific reagents such as Ontak, a fusion product of IL-2 linked to diphtheria toxin and Daclizumab (anti-CD25 Antibody).

Tumor-derived inhibitory products, such as TGF-β (known to be elevated in most human tumors) (Wrzesinski et al. 2007b) can be neutralized by genetically modifying T cells to express a dominant negative receptor for TGF-β (Foster et al. 2008) or through the co-administration of anti-TGF-β antibody (Terabe et al. 2009). For other products such as indoleamine 2, 3-dioxygenase (IDO), a metabolic inhibitor of T cell function (Munn and Mellor 2007), an antagonist analog of the IDO substrate can be used to mitigate immune resistance (Qian et al. 2009). Finally, antibodies that interrupt immune checkpoints in T cell proliferation – for example the CTLA4-B7 and PD1-PDL1 pathways, which normally apply a "brake" to overexuberant T cell proliferation, can be exploited to augment effector T cell expansion in vivo (Peggs et al. 2006; Hodi et al. 2008; Yuan et al. 2008; Fourcade et al. 2009; Wang et al. 2009; Zhang et al. 2009).

These examples illustrate that, having established reliable methods to generate effector cells for adoptive therapy, the availability of more and more clinically approved immunomodulatory reagents that address tumor-associated mechanisms of immune evasion, will lead to combination strategies capable of achieving consistent and durable clinical responses and position adoptive cellular therapy as a feasible therapeutic modality.

References

Altman JD, Moss PA, Goulder PJ, Barouch DH, McHeyzer-Williams MG, Bell JI, McMichael AJ, Davis MM (1996) Phenotypic analysis of antigen-specific T lymphocytes. Science 274:94–96

Awwad M, North RJ (1988) Cyclophosphamide (Cy)-facilitated adoptive immunotherapy of a Cy-resistant tumour. Evidence that Cy permits the expression of adoptive T-cell mediated immunity by removing suppressor T cells rather than by reducing tumour burden. Immunology 65:87–92

Awwad M, North RJ (1989) Cyclophosphamide-induced immunologically mediated regression of a cyclophosphamide-resistant murine tumor: a consequence of eliminating precursor L3T4+ suppressor T-cells. Cancer Res 49:1649–1654

Barber DL, Wherry EJ, Ahmed R (2003) Cutting edge: rapid in vivo killing by memory CD8 T cells. J Immunol 171:27–31

Bast RC Jr, Reinherz EL, Maver C, Lavin P, Schlossman SF (1983) Contrasting effects of cyclophosphamide and prednisolone on the phenotype of human peripheral blood leukocytes. Clin Immunol Immunopathol 28:101–114

Berd D, Mastrangelo MJ (1987) Effect of low dose cyclophosphamide on the immune system of cancer patients: reduction of T-suppressor function without depletion of the CD8+ subset. Cancer Res 47:3317–3321

Berd D, Mastrangelo MJ, Engstrom PF, Paul A, Maguire H (1982) Augmentation of the human immune response by cyclophosphamide. Cancer Res 42:4862–4866

Berd D, Maguire HC Jr, Mastrangelo MJ (1984) Potentiation of human cell-mediated and humoral immunity by low-dose cyclophosphamide. Cancer Res 44:5439–5443

Berendt MJ, North RJ, Kirstein DP (1978) The immunological basis of endotoxin-induced tumor regression. Requirement for a pre-existing state of concomitant anti-tumor immunity. J Exp Med 148:1560–1569

Berger C, Jensen MC, Lansdorp PM, Gough M, Elliott C, Riddell SR (2008) Adoptive transfer of effector CD8+ T cells derived from central memory cells establishes persistent T cell memory in primates. J Clin Invest 118:294–305

Bodinier M, Peyrat MA, Tournay C, Davodeau F, Romagne F, Bonneville M, Lang F (2000) Efficient detection and immunomagnetic sorting of specific T cells using multimers of MHC class I and peptide with reduced CD8 binding. Nat Med 6:707–710

Brandle D, Bilsborough J, Rulicke T, Uyttenhove C, Boon T, Van den Eynde BJ (1998) The shared tumor-specific antigen encoded by mouse gene P1A is a target not only for cytolytic T lymphocytes but also for tumor rejection. Eur J Immunol 28:4010–4019

Cheng LE, Ohlen C, Nelson BH, Greenberg PD (2002) Enhanced signaling through the IL-2 receptor in CD8+ T cells regulated by antigen recognition results in preferential proliferation and expansion of responding CD8+ T cells rather than promotion of cell death. Proc Natl Acad Sci U S A 99:3001–3006

Cheson BD (1995) Infectious and immunosuppressive complications of purine analog therapy. J Clin Oncol 13:2431–2448

Chiang YJ, Kole HK, Brown K, Naramura M, Fukuhara S, Hu RJ, Jang IK, Gutkind JS, Shevach E, Gu H (2000) Cbl-b regulates the CD28 dependence of T-cell activation. Nature 403:216–220

Cooper LJ, Kalos M, Lewinsohn DA, Riddell SR, Greenberg PD (2000) Transfer of specificity for human immunodeficiency virus type 1 into primary human T lymphocytes by introduction of T-cell receptor genes. J Virol 74:8207–8212

Crossland KD, Lee VK, Chen W, Riddell SR, Greenberg PD, Cheever MA (1991) T cells from tumor-immune mice nonspecifically expanded in vitro with anti-CD3 plus IL-2 retain specific function in vitro and can eradicate disseminated leukemia in vivo. J Immunol 146: 4414–4420

Dannull J, Su Z, Rizzieri D, Yang BK, Coleman D, Yancey D, Zhang A, Dahm P, Chao N, Gilboa E, Vieweg J (2005) Enhancement of vaccine-mediated antitumor immunity in cancer patients after depletion of regulatory T cells. J Clin Invest 115:3623–3633

de Witte MA, Jorritsma A, Swart E, Straathof KC, de Punder K, Haanen JB, Rooney CM, Schumacher TN (2008) An inducible caspase 9 safety switch can halt cell therapy-induced autoimmune disease. J Immunol 180:6365–6373

Dillman RO, Oldham RK, Tauer KW, Orr DW, Barth NM, Blumenschein G, Arnold J, Birch R, West WH (1991) Continuous interleukin-2 and lymphokine-activated killer cells for advanced cancer: a National Biotherapy Study Group trial. J Clin Oncol 9:1233–1240

Dillman RO, Duma CM, Schiltz PM, DePriest C, Ellis RA, Okamoto K, Beutel LD, De Leon C, Chico S (2004) Intracavitary placement of autologous lymphokine-activated killer (LAK) cells after resection of recurrent glioblastoma. J Immunother 27:398–404

Dudley ME, Wunderlich JR, Yang JC, Hwu P, Schwartzentruber DJ, Topalian SL, Sherry RM, Marincola FM, Leitman SF, Seipp CA, Rogers-Freezer L, Morton KE, Nahvi A, Mavroukakis SA, White DE, Rosenberg SA (2002) A phase I study of nonmyeloablative chemotherapy and adoptive transfer of autologous tumor antigen-specific T lymphocytes in patients with metastatic melanoma. J Immunother 25:243–251

Dudley ME, Wunderlich JR, Shelton TE, Even J, Rosenberg SA (2003) Generation of tumor-infiltrating lymphocyte cultures for use in adoptive transfer therapy for melanoma patients. J Immunother 26:332–342

Dudley ME, Wunderlich JR, Yang JC, Sherry RM, Topalian SL, Restifo NP, Royal RE, Kammula U, White DE, Mavroukakis SA, Rogers LJ, Gracia GJ, Jones SA, Mangiameli DP, Pelletier MM, Gea-Banacloche J, Robinson MR, Berman DM, Filie AC, Abati A, Rosenberg SA (2005) Adoptive cell transfer therapy following non-myeloablative but lymphodepleting chemotherapy for the treatment of patients with refractory metastatic melanoma. J Clin Oncol 23:2346–2357

Dudley ME, Yang JC, Sherry R, Hughes MS, Royal R, Kammula U, Robbins PF, Huang J, Citrin DE, Leitman SF, Wunderlich J, Restifo NP, Thomasian A, Downey SG, Smith FO, Klapper J, Morton K, Laurencot C, White DE, Rosenberg SA (2008) Adoptive cell therapy for patients with metastatic melanoma: evaluation of intensive myeloablative chemoradiation preparative regimens. J Clin Oncol 26:5233–5239

Eberlein TJ, Rosenstein M, Rosenberg SA (1982) Regression of a disseminated syngeneic solid tumor by systemic transfer of lymphoid cells expanded in interleukin 2. J Exp Med 156:385–397

Eshhar Z, Waks T, Gross G, Schindler DG (1993) Specific activation and targeting of cytotoxic lymphocytes through chimeric single chains consisting of antibody-binding domains and the gamma or zeta subunits of the immunoglobulin and T-cell receptors. Proc Natl Acad Sci U S A 90:720–724

Finney HM, Akbar AN, Lawson AD (2004) Activation of resting human primary T cells with chimeric receptors: costimulation from CD28, inducible costimulator, CD134, and CD137 in series with signals from the TCR zeta chain. J Immunol 172:104–113

Fisher B, Packard BS, Read EJ, Carrasquillo JA, Carter CS, Topalian SL, Yang JC, Yolles P, Larson SM, Rosenberg SA (1989) Tumor localization of adoptively transferred indium-111 labeled tumor infiltrating lymphocytes in patients with metastatic melanoma. J Clin Oncol 7:250–261

Foster AE, Dotti G, Lu A, Khalil M, Brenner MK, Heslop HE, Rooney CM, Bollard CM (2008) Antitumor activity of EBV-specific T lymphocytes transduced with a dominant negative TGF-beta receptor. J Immunother 31:500–505

Fourcade J, Kudela P, Sun Z, Shen H, Land SR, Lenzner D, Guillaume P, Luescher IF, Sander C, Ferrone S, Kirkwood JM, Zarour HM (2009) PD-1 is a regulator of NY-ESO-1-specific CD8+ T cell expansion in melanoma patients. J Immunol 182:5240–5249

Frey AB, Cestari S (1997) Killing of rat adenocarcinoma 13762 in situ by adoptive transfer of CD4+ anti-tumor T cells requires tumor expression of cell surface MHC class II molecules. Cell Immunol 178:79–90

Garnett CT, Palena C, Chakraborty M, Tsang KY, Schlom J, Hodge JW (2004) Sublethal irradiation of human tumor cells modulates phenotype resulting in enhanced killing by cytotoxic T lymphocytes. Cancer Res 64:7985–7994

Gattinoni L, Klebanoff CA, Palmer DC, Wrzesinski C, Kerstann K, Yu Z, Finkelstein SE, Theoret MR, Rosenberg SA, Restifo NP (2005) Acquisition of full effector function in vitro paradoxically impairs the in vivo antitumor efficacy of adoptively transferred CD8+ T cells. J Clin Invest 115:1616–1626

Gebe JA, Kwok WW (2007) Tracking antigen specific CD4+ T-cells with soluble MHC molecules. Methods Mol Med 136:39–50

Ghiringhelli F, Larmonier N, Schmitt E, Parcellier A, Cathelin D, Garrido C, Chauffert B, Solary E, Bonnotte B, Martin F (2004) CD4+CD25+ regulatory T cells suppress tumor immunity but are sensitive to cyclophosphamide which allows immunotherapy of established tumors to be curative. Eur J Immunol 34:336–344

Ghiringhelli F, Menard C, Puig PE, Ladoire S, Roux S, Martin F, Solary E, Le Cesne A, Zitvogel L, Chauffert B (2007) Metronomic cyclophosphamide regimen selectively depletes CD4+CD25+ regulatory T cells and restores T and NK effector functions in end stage cancer patients. Cancer Immunol Immunother 56:641–648

Giuntoli RL II, Lu J, Kobayashi H, Kennedy R, Celis E (2002) Direct costimulation of tumor-reactive CTL by helper T cells potentiate their proliferation, survival, and effector function. Clin Cancer Res 8:922–931

Gong MC, Latouche JB, Krause A, Heston WD, Bander NH, Sadelain M (1999) Cancer patient T cells genetically targeted to prostate specific membrane antigen specifically lyse prostate cancer cells and release cytokines in response to prostate-specific membrane antigen. Neoplasia 1:123–127

Greenberg PD (1991) Adoptive T cell therapy of tumors: mechanisms operative in the recognition and elimination of tumor cells. Adv Immunol 49:281–355

Greenberg PD, Cheever MA, Fefer A (1981) Eradication of disseminated murine leukemia by chemoimmunotherapy with cyclophosphamide and adoptively transferred immune syngeneic Lyt-1 + 2- lymphocytes. J Exp Med 154:952–963

Greenberg PD, Kern DE, Cheever MA (1985) Therapy of disseminated murine leukemia with cyclophosphamide and immune Lyt-1+,2- T cells. Tumor eradication does not require participation of cytotoxic T cells. J Exp Med 161:1122–1134

Griffith KD, Read EJ, Carrasquillo JA, Carter CS, Yang JC, Fisher B, Aebersold P, Packard BS, Yu MY, Rosenberg SA (1989) In vivo distribution of adoptively transferred indium-111-labeled tumor infiltrating lymphocytes and peripheral blood lymphocytes in patients with metastatic melanoma. J Natl Cancer Inst 81:1709–1717

Groh V, Li YQ, Cioca D, Hunder NN, Wang W, Riddell SR, Yee C, Spies T (2005) Efficient cross-priming of tumor antigen-specific T cells by dendritic cells sensitized with diverse anti-MICA opsonized tumor cells. Proc Natl Acad Sci U S A 102:6461–6466

Hirooka Y, Itoh A, Kawashima H, Hara K, Nonogaki K, Kasugai T, Ohno E, Ishikawa T, Matsubara H, Ishigami M, Katano Y, Ohmiya N, Niwa Y, Yamamoto K, Kaneko T, Nieda M, Yokokawa

K, Goto H (2009) A combination therapy of gemcitabine with immunotherapy for patients with inoperable locally advanced pancreatic cancer. Pancreas 38:e69–e74

Hodi FS, Butler M, Oble DA, Seiden MV, Haluska FG, Kruse A, Macrae S, Nelson M, Canning C, Lowy I, Korman A, Lautz D, Russell S, Jaklitsch MT, Ramaiya N, Chen TC, Neuberg D, Allison JP, Mihm MC, Dranoff G (2008) Immunologic and clinical effects of antibody blockade of cytotoxic T lymphocyte-associated antigen 4 in previously vaccinated cancer patients. Proc Natl Acad Sci U S A 105:3005–3010

Holler PD, Holman PO, Shusta EV, O'Herrin S, Wittrup KD, Kranz DM (2000) In vitro evolution of a T cell receptor with high affinity for peptide/MHC. Proc Natl Acad Sci U S A 97:5387–5392

Hunder NN, Wallen H, Cao J, Hendricks DW, Reilly JZ, Rodmyre R, Jungbluth A, Gnjatic S, Thompson JA, Yee C (2008) Treatment of metastatic melanoma with autologous CD4+ T cells against NY-ESO-1. N Engl J Med 358:2698–2703

Hung K, Hayashi R, Lafond-Walker A, Lowenstein C, Pardoll D, Levitsky H (1998) The central role of CD4(+) T cells in the antitumor immune response. J Exp Med 188:2357–2368

Kalams SA, Walker BD (1998) The critical need for CD4 help in maintaining effective cytotoxic T lymphocyte responses. J Exp Med 188:2199–2204

Kershaw MH, Westwood JA, Parker LL, Wang G, Eshhar Z, Mavroukakis SA, White DE, Wunderlich JR, Canevari S, Rogers-Freezer L, Chen CC, Yang JC, Rosenberg SA, Hwu P (2006) A phase I study on adoptive immunotherapy using gene-modified T cells for ovarian cancer. Clin Cancer Res 12:6106–6115

Kessels HW, de Visser KE, Kruisbeek AM, Schumacher TN (2001) Circumventing T-cell tolerance to tumour antigens. Biologicals 29:277–283

Khammari A, Nguyen JM, Pandolfino MC, Quereux G, Brocard A, Bercegeay S, Cassidanius A, Lemarre P, Volteau C, Labarriere N, Jotereau F, Dreno B (2007) Long-term follow-up of patients treated by adoptive transfer of melanoma tumor-infiltrating lymphocytes as adjuvant therapy for stage III melanoma. Cancer Immunol Immunother 56:1853–1860

Khammari A, Labarriere N, Vignard V, Nguyen JM, Pandolfino MC, Knol AC, Quereux G, Saiagh S, Brocard A, Jotereau F, Dreno B (2009) Treatment of metastatic melanoma with autologous Melan-A/MART-1-specific cytotoxic T lymphocyte clones. J Invest Dermatol 129:2835–2842

Khanolkar A, Fuller MJ, Zajac AJ (2004) CD4 T cell-dependent CD8 T cell maturation. J Immunol 172:2834–2844

Klebanoff CA, Gattinoni L, Torabi-Parizi P, Kerstann K, Cardones AR, Finkelstein SE, Palmer DC, Antony PA, Hwang ST, Rosenberg SA, Waldmann TA, Restifo NP (2005) Central memory self/tumor-reactive CD8+ T cells confer superior antitumor immunity compared with effector memory T cells. Proc Natl Acad Sci U S A 102:9571–9576

Klebanoff CA, Gattinoni L, Restifo NP (2006) CD8+ T-cell memory in tumor immunology and immunotherapy. Immunol Rev 211:214–224

Kobari M, Egawa S, Shibuya K, Sunamura M, Saitoh K, Matsuno S (2000) Effect of intraportal adoptive immunotherapy on liver metastases after resection of pancreatic cancer. Br J Surg 87:43–48

Lafreniere R, Rosenberg SA (1985) Successful immunotherapy of murine experimental hepatic metastases with lymphokine-activated killer cells and recombinant interleukin 2. Cancer Res 45:3735–3741

Lamers CH, Sleijfer S, Vulto AG, Kruit WH, Kliffen M, Debets R, Gratama JW, Stoter G, Oosterwijk E (2006) Treatment of metastatic renal cell carcinoma with autologous T-lymphocytes genetically retargeted against carbonic anhydrase IX: first clinical experience. J Clin Oncol 24:e20–e22

Li Y, Yee C (2008) IL-21 mediated Foxp3 suppression leads to enhanced generation of antigen-specific CD8+ cytotoxic T lymphocytes. Blood 111:229–235

Li Y, Bleakley M, Yee C (2005) IL-21 influences the frequency, phenotype, and affinity of the antigen-specific CD8 T cell response. J Immunol 175:2261–2269

Liao X, Li Y, Bonini C, Nair S, Gilboa E, Greenberg PD, Yee C (2004) Transfection of RNA encoding tumor antigens following maturation of dendritic cells leads to prolonged presentation of antigen and the generation of high-affinity tumor-reactive cytotoxic T lymphocytes. Mol Ther 9:757–764

Lotze MT, Grimm EA, Mazumder A, Strausser JL, Rosenberg SA (1981) Lysis of fresh and cultured autologous tumor by human lymphocytes cultured in T-cell growth factor. Cancer Res 41:4420–4425

Lugade AA, Moran JP, Gerber SA, Rose RC, Frelinger JG, Lord EM (2005) Local radiation therapy of B16 melanoma tumors increases the generation of tumor antigen-specific effector cells that traffic to the tumor. J Immunol 174:7516–7523

Lugade AA, Sorensen EW, Gerber SA, Moran JP, Frelinger JG, Lord EM (2008) Radiation-induced IFN-gamma production within the tumor microenvironment influences antitumor immunity. J Immunol 180:3132–3139

Lutsiak ME, Semnani RT, De Pascalis R, Kashmiri SV, Schlom J, Sabzevari H (2005) Inhibition of CD4(+)25+ T regulatory cell function implicated in enhanced immune response by low-dose cyclophosphamide. Blood 105:2862–2868

Machiels JP, Reilly RT, Emens LA, Ercolini AM, Lei RY, Weintraub D, Okoye FI, Jaffee EM (2001) Cyclophosphamide, doxorubicin, and paclitaxel enhance the antitumor immune response of granulocyte/macrophage-colony stimulating factor-secreting whole-cell vaccines in HER-2/neu tolerized mice. Cancer Res 61:3689–3697

Mackensen A, Meidenbauer N, Vogl S, Laumer M, Berger J, Andreesen R (2006) Phase I study of adoptive T-cell therapy using antigen-specific CD8+ T cells for the treatment of patients with metastatic melanoma. J Clin Oncol 24:5060–5069

Maguire HC Jr, Ettore VL (1967) Enhancement of dinitrochlorobenzene (DNCB) contact sensitization by cyclophosphamide in the guinea pig. J Invest Dermatol 48:39–43

Mahnke K, Schonfeld K, Fondel S, Ring S, Karakhanova S, Wiedemeyer K, Bedke T, Johnson TS, Storn V, Schallenberg S, Enk AH (2007) Depletion of CD4+CD25+ human regulatory T cells in vivo: kinetics of Treg depletion and alterations in immune functions in vivo and in vitro. Int J Cancer 120:2723–2733

Malone CC, Schiltz PM, Mackintosh AD, Beutel LD, Heinemann FS, Dillman RO (2001) Characterization of human tumor-infiltrating lymphocytes expanded in hollow-fiber bioreactors for immunotherapy of cancer. Cancer Biother Radiopharm 16:381–390

Mandic M, Castelli F, Janjic B, Almunia C, Andrade P, Gillet D, Brusic V, Kirkwood JM, Maillere B, Zarour HM (2005) One NY-ESO-1-derived epitope that promiscuously binds to multiple HLA-DR and HLA-DP4 molecules and stimulates autologous CD4+ T cells from patients with NY-ESO-1-expressing melanoma. J Immunol 174:1751–1759

Marzo AL, Kinnear BF, Lake RA, Frelinger JJ, Collins EJ, Robinson BW, Scott B (2000) Tumor specific CD4+ T cells have a major "post-licensing" role in CTL mediated anti-tumor immunity. J Immunol 165:6047–6055

Meidenbauer N, Marienhagen J, Laumer M, Vogl S, Heymann J, Andreesen R, Mackensen A (2003) Survival and tumor localization of adoptively transferred Melan-A-specific T cells in melanoma patients. J Immunol 170:2161–2169

Mills CD, North RJ, Dye ES (1981) Mechanisms of anti-tumor action of *Corynebacterium parvum*. II. Potentiated cytolytic T cell response and its tumor-induced suppression. J Exp Med 154:621–630

Mitchell MS, Darrah D, Yeung D, Halpern S, Wallace A, Voland J, Jones V, Kan-Mitchell J (2002) Phase I trial of adoptive immunotherapy with cytolytic T lymphocytes immunized against a tyrosinase epitope. J Clin Oncol 20:1075–1086

Morgan RA, Dudley ME, Yu YY, Zheng Z, Robbins PF, Theoret MR, Wunderlich JR, Hughes MS, Restifo NP, Rosenberg SA (2003) High efficiency TCR gene transfer into primary human lymphocytes affords avid recognition of melanoma tumor antigen glycoprotein 100 and does not alter the recognition of autologous melanoma antigens. J Immunol 171:3287–3295

Mule JJ, Shu S, Schwarz SL, Rosenberg SA (1984) Adoptive immunotherapy of established pulmonary metastases with LAK cells and recombinant interleukin-2. Science 225:1487–1489

Mule JJ, Shu S, Rosenberg SA (1985) The anti-tumor efficacy of lymphokine-activated killer cells and recombinant interleukin 2 in vivo. J Immunol 135:646–652

Munn DH, Mellor AL (2007) Indoleamine 2,3-dioxygenase and tumor-induced tolerance. J Clin Invest 117:1147–1154

Murali-Krishna K, Lau LL, Sambhara S, Lemonnier F, Altman J, Ahmed R (1999) Persistence of memory CD8 T cells in MHC class I-deficient mice. Science 286:1377–1381

Muranski P, Boni A, Wrzesinski C, Citrin DE, Rosenberg SA, Childs R, Restifo NP (2006) Increased intensity lymphodepletion and adoptive immunotherapy – how far can we go? Nat Clin Pract Oncol 3:668–681

Muranski P, Boni A, Antony PA, Cassard L, Irvine KR, Kaiser A, Paulos CM, Palmer DC, Touloukian CE, Ptak K, Gattinoni L, Wrzesinski C, Hinrichs CS, Kerstann KW, Feigenbaum L, Chan CC, Restifo NP (2008) Tumor-specific Th17-polarized cells eradicate large established melanoma. Blood 112:362–373

Muul LM, Spiess PJ, Director EP, Rosenberg SA (1987) Identification of specific cytolytic immune responses against autologous tumor in humans bearing malignant melanoma. J Immunol 138:989–995

North RJ (1982) Cyclophosphamide-facilitated adoptive immunotherapy of an established tumor depends on elimination of tumor-induced suppressor T cells. J Exp Med 155:1063–1074

Overwijk WW, Theoret MR, Finkelstein SE, Surman DR, de Jong LA, Vyth-Dreese FA, Dellemijn TA, Antony PA, Spiess PJ, Palmer DC, Heimann DM, Klebanoff CA, Yu Z, Hwang LN, Feigenbaum L, Kruisbeek AM, Rosenberg SA, Restifo NP (2003) Tumor regression and autoimmunity after reversal of a functionally tolerant state of self-reactive CD8+ T cells. J Exp Med 198:569–580

Pardoll DM, Topalian SL (1998) The role of CD4+ T cell responses in antitumor immunity. Curr Opin Immunol 10:588–594

Park JR, Digiusto DL, Slovak M, Wright C, Naranjo A, Wagner J, Meechoovet HB, Bautista C, Chang WC, Ostberg JR, Jensen MC (2007) Adoptive transfer of chimeric antigen receptor redirected cytolytic T lymphocyte clones in patients with neuroblastoma. Mol Ther 15:825–833

Peggs KS, Quezada SA, Korman AJ, Allison JP (2006) Principles and use of anti-CTLA4 antibody in human cancer immunotherapy. Curr Opin Immunol 18:206–213

Perez-Diez A, Joncker NT, Choi K, Chan WF, Anderson CC, Lantz O, Matzinger P (2007) CD4 cells can be more efficient at tumor rejection than CD8 cells. Blood 109:5346–5354

Plautz GE, Mukai S, Cohen PA, Shu S (2000) Cross-presentation of tumor antigens to effector T cells is sufficient to mediate effective immunotherapy of established intracranial tumors. J Immunol 165:3656–3662

Proietti E, Greco G, Garrone B, Baccarini S, Mauri C, Venditti M, Carlei D, Belardelli F (1998) Importance of cyclophosphamide-induced bystander effect on T cells for a successful tumor eradication in response to adoptive immunotherapy in mice. J Clin Invest 101:429–441

Qian F, Villella J, Wallace PK, Mhawech-Fauceglia P, Tario JD Jr, Andrews C, Matsuzaki J, Valmori D, Ayyoub M, Frederick PJ, Beck A, Liao J, Cheney R, Moysich K, Lele S, Shrikant P, Old LJ, Odunsi K (2009) Efficacy of levo-1-methyl tryptophan and dextro-1-methyl tryptophan in reversing indoleamine-2,3-dioxygenase-mediated arrest of T-cell proliferation in human epithelial ovarian cancer. Cancer Res 69:5498–5504

Reker S, Meier A, Holten-Andersen L, Svane IM, Becker JC, thor Straten P, Andersen MH (2004) Identification of novel survivin-derived CTL epitopes. Cancer Biol Ther 3:173–179

Rosenberg SA (1984) Immunotherapy of cancer by systemic administration of lymphoid cells plus interleukin-2. J Biol Response Mod 3:501–511

Rosenberg SA, Lotze MT, Muul LM, Leitman S, Chang AE, Ettinghausen SE, Matory YL, Skibber JM, Shiloni E, Vetto JT et al (1985) Observations on the systemic administration of autologous lymphokine-activated killer cells and recombinant interleukin-2 to patients with metastatic cancer. N Engl J Med 313:1485–1492

Rosenberg SA, Spiess P, Lafreniere R (1986) A new approach to the adoptive immunotherapy of cancer with tumor-infiltrating lymphocytes. Science 233:1318–1321

Rosenberg SA, Lotze MT, Muul LM, Chang AE, Avis FP, Leitman S, Linehan WM, Robertson CN, Lee RE, Rubin JT et al (1987) A progress report on the treatment of 157 patients with advanced cancer using lymphokine-activated killer cells and interleukin-2 or high-dose interleukin-2 alone. N Engl J Med 316:889–897

Rosenberg SA, Packard BS, Aebersold PM, Solomon D, Topalian SL, Toy ST, Simon P, Lotze MT, Yang JC, Seipp CA et al (1988) Use of tumor-infiltrating lymphocytes and interleukin-2 in the immunotherapy of patients with metastatic melanoma. A preliminary report. N Engl J Med 319:1676–1680

Rosenberg SA, Lotze MT, Yang JC, Aebersold PM, Linehan WM, Seipp CA, White DE (1989) Experience with the use of high-dose interleukin-2 in the treatment of 652 cancer patients. Ann Surg 210:474–484; discussion 484–475

Rosenberg SA, Lotze MT, Yang JC, Topalian SL, Chang AE, Schwartzentruber DJ, Aebersold P, Leitman S, Linehan WM, Seipp CA et al (1993) Prospective randomized trial of high-dose interleukin-2 alone or in conjunction with lymphokine-activated killer cells for the treatment of patients with advanced cancer. J Natl Cancer Inst 85:622–632

Rosenberg SA, Yannelli JR, Yang JC, Topalian SL, Schwartzentruber DJ, Weber JS, Parkinson DR, Seipp CA, Einhorn JH, White DE (1994) Treatment of patients with metastatic melanoma with autologous tumor-infiltrating lymphocytes and interleukin 2. J Natl Cancer Inst 86:1159–1166

Sadelain M, Riviere I, Brentjens R (2003) Targeting tumours with genetically enhanced T lymphocytes. Nat Rev Cancer 3:35–45

Sakaguchi S, Sakaguchi N, Asano M, Itoh M, Toda M (1995) Immunologic self-tolerance maintained by activated T cells expressing IL-2 receptor alpha-chains (CD25). Breakdown of a single mechanism of self-tolerance causes various autoimmune diseases. J Immunol 155:1151–1164

Schiavoni G, Mattei F, Di Pucchio T, Santini SM, Bracci L, Belardelli F, Proietti E (2000) Cyclophosphamide induces type I interferon and augments the number of CD44(hi) T lymphocytes in mice: implications for strategies of chemoimmunotherapy of cancer. Blood 95:2024–2030

Schleypen JS, Baur N, Kammerer R, Nelson PJ, Rohrmann K, Grone EF, Hohenfellner M, Haferkamp A, Pohla H, Schendel DJ, Falk CS, Noessner E (2006) Cytotoxic markers and frequency predict functional capacity of natural killer cells infiltrating renal cell carcinoma. Clin Cancer Res 12:718–725

Schneck JP, Slansky JE, O'Herrin SM, Greten TF (2001) Monitoring antigen-specific T cells using MHC-Ig dimers. Curr Protoc Immunol Chapter 17:Unit 17.2

Schwartzentruber DJ, Hom SS, Dadmarz R, White DE, Yannelli JR, Steinberg SM, Rosenberg SA, Topalian SL (1994) In vitro predictors of therapeutic response in melanoma patients receiving tumor-infiltrating lymphocytes and interleukin-2. J Clin Oncol 12:1475–1483

Simpson AJ, Caballero OL, Jungbluth A, Chen YT, Old LJ (2005) Cancer/testis antigens, gametogenesis and cancer. Nat Rev Cancer 5:615–625

Specht JM, Wang G, Do MT, Lam JS, Royal RE, Reeves ME, Rosenberg SA, Hwu P (1997) Dendritic cells retrovirally transduced with a model antigen gene are therapeutically effective against established pulmonary metastases. J Exp Med 186:1213–1221

Spiess PJ, Yang JC, Rosenberg SA (1987) In vivo antitumor activity of tumor-infiltrating lymphocytes expanded in recombinant interleukin-2. J Natl Cancer Inst 79:1067–1075

Stanislawski T, Voss RH, Lotz C, Sadovnikova E, Willemsen RA, Kuball J, Ruppert T, Bolhuis RL, Melief CJ, Huber C, Stauss HJ, Theobald M (2001) Circumventing tolerance to a human MDM2-derived tumor antigen by TCR gene transfer. Nat Immunol 2:962–970

Terabe M, Ambrosino E, Takaku S, O'Konek JJ, Venzon D, Lonning S, McPherson JM, Berzofsky JA (2009) Synergistic enhancement of CD8+ T cell-mediated tumor vaccine efficacy by an anti-transforming growth factor-beta monoclonal antibody. Clin Cancer Res 15:6560–6569

Till BG, Jensen MC, Wang J, Chen EY, Wood BL, Greisman HA, Qian X, James SE, Raubitschek A, Forman SJ, Gopal AK, Pagel JM, Lindgren CG, Greenberg PD, Riddell SR, Press OW (2008) Adoptive immunotherapy for indolent non-Hodgkin lymphoma and mantle cell lymphoma using genetically modified autologous CD20-specific T cells. Blood 112:2261–2271

Topalian SL, Muul LM, Solomon D, Rosenberg SA (1987) Expansion of human tumor infiltrating lymphocytes for use in immunotherapy trials. J Immunol Methods 102:127–141

Topalian SL, Gonzales MI, Parkhurst M, Li YF, Southwood S, Sette A, Rosenberg SA, Robbins PF (1996) Melanoma-specific CD4+ T cells recognize nonmutated HLA-DR-restricted tyrosinase epitopes. J Exp Med 183:1965–1971

Topp MS, Riddell SR, Akatsuka Y, Jensen MC, Blattman JN, Greenberg PD (2003) Restoration of CD28 expression in CD28- CD8+ memory effector T cells reconstitutes antigen-induced IL-2 production. J Exp Med 198:947–955

Uyttenhove C, Maryanski J, Boon T (1983) Escape of mouse mastocytoma P815 after nearly complete rejection is due to antigen-loss variants rather than immunosuppression. J Exp Med 157:1040–1052

Van den Eynde BJ, van der Bruggen P (1997) T cell defined tumor antigens. Curr Opin Immunol 9:684–693

Van den Eynde B, Lethe B, Van Pel A, De Plaen E, Boon T (1991) The gene coding for a major tumor rejection antigen of tumor P815 is identical to the normal gene of syngeneic DBA/2 mice. J Exp Med 173:1373–1384

van der Bruggen P, Traversari C, Chomez P, Lurquin C, De Plaen E, Van den Eynde B, Knuth A, Boon T (1991) A gene encoding an antigen recognized by cytolytic T lymphocytes on a human melanoma. Science 254:1643–1647

Vierboom MPM, Nijman HW, Offringa R, Vandervoort EIH, Vanhall T, Vandenbroek L, Fleuren GJ, Kenemans P, Kast WM, Melief CJM (1997) Tumor eradication by wild-type P53-specific cytotoxic T lymphocytes. J Exp Med 186:695–704

Vierboom MP, Bos GM, Ooms M, Offringa R, Melief CJ (2000) Cyclophosphamide enhances anti-tumor effect of wild-type p53-specific CTL. Int J Cancer 87:253–260

Vonderheide RH, Hahn WC, Schultze JL, Nadler LM (1999) The telomerase catalytic subunit is a widely expressed tumor-associated antigen recognized by cytotoxic T lymphocytes. Immunity 10:673–679

Wallen H, Thompson JA, Reilly JZ, Rodmyre RM, Cao J, Yee C (2009) Fludarabine modulates immune response and extends in vivo survival of adoptively transferred CD8 T cells in patients with metastatic melanoma. PLoS One 4:e4749

Wang JC, Livingstone AM (2003) Cutting edge: CD4+ T cell help can be essential for primary CD8+ T cell responses in vivo. J Immunol 171:6339–6343

Wang J, Jensen M, Lin Y, Sui X, Chen E, Lindgren CG, Till B, Raubitschek A, Forman SJ, Qian X, James S, Greenberg P, Riddell S, Press OW (2007) Optimizing adoptive polyclonal T cell immunotherapy of lymphomas, using a chimeric T cell receptor possessing CD28 and CD137 costimulatory domains. Hum Gene Ther 18:712–725

Wang W, Lau R, Yu D, Zhu W, Korman A, Weber J (2009) PD1 blockade reverses the suppression of melanoma antigen-specific CTL by CD4+ CD25(Hi) regulatory T cells. Int Immunol 21:1065–1077

Weber KS, Donermeyer DL, Allen PM, Kranz DM (2005) Class II-restricted T cell receptor engineered in vitro for higher affinity retains peptide specificity and function. Proc Natl Acad Sci U S A 102:19033–19038

Weng DS, Zhou J, Zhou QM, Zhao M, Wang QJ, Huang LX, Li YQ, Chen SP, Wu PH, Xia JC (2008) Minimally invasive treatment combined with cytokine-induced killer cells therapy lower the short-term recurrence rates of hepatocellular carcinomas. J Immunother 31:63–71

Wherry EJ, Ahmed R (2004) Memory CD8 T-cell differentiation during viral infection. J Virol 78:5535–5545

Wrzesinski C, Paulos CM, Gattinoni L, Palmer DC, Kaiser A, Yu Z, Rosenberg SA, Restifo NP (2007a) Hematopoietic stem cells promote the expansion and function of adoptively transferred antitumor CD8 T cells. J Clin Invest 117:492–501

Wrzesinski SH, Wan YY, Flavell RA (2007b) Transforming growth factor-beta and the immune response: implications for anticancer therapy. Clin Cancer Res 13:5262–5270

Yee C, Savage PA, Lee PP, Davis MM, Greenberg PD (1999) Isolation of high avidity melanoma-reactive CTL from heterogeneous populations using peptide-MHC tetramers. J Immunol 162:2227–2234

Yee C, Thompson JA, Byrd D, Riddell SR, Roche P, Celis E, Greenberg PD (2002) Adoptive T cell therapy using antigen-specific CD8+ T cell clones for the treatment of patients with metastatic melanoma: in vivo persistence, migration, and antitumor effect of transferred T cells. Proc Natl Acad Sci U S A 99:16168–16173

Yron I, Wood TA Jr, Spiess PJ, Rosenberg SA (1980) In vitro growth of murine T cells. V. The isolation and growth of lymphoid cells infiltrating syngeneic solid tumors. J Immunol 125:238–245

Yuan J, Gnjatic S, Li H, Powel S, Gallardo HF, Ritter E, Ku GY, Jungbluth AA, Segal NH, Rasalan TS, Manukian G, Xu Y, Roman RA, Terzulli SL, Heywood M, Pogoriler E, Ritter G, Old LJ, Allison JP, Wolchok JD (2008) CTLA-4 blockade enhances polyfunctional NY-ESO-1 specific T cell responses in metastatic melanoma patients with clinical benefit. Proc Natl Acad Sci U S A 105:20410–20415

Yuen MF, Norris S (2001) Expression of inhibitory receptors in natural killer (CD3(−)CD56(+)) cells and CD3(+)CD56(+) cells in the peripheral blood lymphocytes and tumor infiltrating lymphocytes in patients with primary hepatocellular carcinoma. Clin Immunol 101:264–269

Zeng G, Wang X, Robbins PF, Rosenberg SA, Wang RF (2001) CD4(+) T cell recognition of MHC class II-restricted epitopes from NY-ESO-1 presented by a prevalent HLA DP4 allele: association with NY-ESO-1 antibody production. Proc Natl Acad Sci U S A 98:3964–3969

Zhang Y, Sun Z, Nicolay H, Meyer RG, Renkvist N, Stroobant V, Corthals J, Carrasco J, Eggermont AM, Marchand M, Thielemans K, Wolfel T, Boon T, van der Bruggen P (2005) Monitoring of anti-vaccine CD4 T cell frequencies in melanoma patients vaccinated with a MAGE-3 protein. J Immunol 174:2404–2411

Zhang L, Gajewski TF, Kline J (2009) PD-1/PD-L1 interactions inhibit antitumor immune responses in a murine acute myeloid leukemia model. Blood 114:1545–1552

Zhou J, Dudley ME, Rosenberg SA, Robbins PF (2005) Persistence of multiple tumor-specific T-cell clones is associated with complete tumor regression in a melanoma patient receiving adoptive cell transfer therapy. J Immunother 28:53–62

Index

A

A20-binding inhibitor of NF-κB activation (ABIN), 283
αβT cell depleted (αβTCD) grafts, 29
Acute lymphocytic leukemia (ALL), 396
Adaptively induced CD4$^+$ Treg cells, 196–197
Adaptive Tregs, 148
Adoptive cellular therapy, 439, 456–457
Adoptive T cell therapy
    CTLs, 415
    EBV-negative lymphomas, 426–427
    EBV-related lymphomas, 416, 417, 423, 426
    Hodgkin's lymphoma, 423–425
    HSCT, 415
    metastatic melanoma, 399
    MHC, 400
    PTLD
        CD20-specific monoclonal antibody rituximab, 418
        GVHD, 418
        HSCT/SOT, 416
        post-HSCT, 418–420
        post-SOT, 418, 421, 422
    target antigens identification, 445–446
    T-cell efficacy and safety, 431–432
    TCR, 400
    telomerase/costimulatory receptors, 400
    transgenic receptor expression
        artificial chimeric antigen receptors, 428–431
        transgenic T-cell receptors, 427
    tumor immune evasion, 432
α-galactosylceramide (α-GalCer), 8–10, 13–14
Allogeneic antigens, 342–343
Anaphylatoxin, 235–236
Antigen-induced Tr1 cells, 197
Antigen presenting cells (APCs), 121, 179, 181, 252, 291
Antigen-specific CD4$^+$ cells, 448–449
Antigen-specific CD8$^+$ cells, 446–448
Antigen-specific vaccines, 401
AOM. *See* Azoxymethane
AOM-DSS-induced colon cancer model, 79
APCs. *See* Antigen presenting cells
Artificial chimeric antigen receptors, 428–431
Azoxymethane (AOM), 73, 79

B

Bacilli Calmette–Guérin (BCG), 393, 398
4–1BB receptor
    agonistic antibodies, 258
    anti–4–1BB monoclonal antibodies, 257, 258
    B7-H1/PD–1 Immunotherapies, 262
    B16 melanoma, 259
    CD4$^+$ cells, 257, 258
    CD8$^+$ T cells, 253
    cyclophosphamide, 259
    hematopoetic and nonhematopoetic cells, 258
    lymphopenia, 259
    NF-κB and AP–1 activation, 255
    NK cell, 258
    proliferation, 253
    Treg depletion, 257
    Type I transmembrane protein, 255
B cells, 292
BCG. *See* Bacilli Calmette–Guérin
Bevacizumab, 395

B7-H1/PD–1 pathways
  4–1BB immunotherapies, 262
  blocking antibody, 261
  ITIM, 260
  LCMV, 260–261
  mRNA transcripts, 260
Blocking antibodies, 320
Bone marrow transplantation, 395–396
Bovine diarrhoea virus, 273
Bronchioloalveolar carcinoma (BAC), 353

C
Cancer immunosurveillance, 1
Cancer-testis (CT) antigens, 372
  antigen-specific cancer immunotherapy, 347
  cancer vaccine trials
    $CD8^+$ and $CD4^+$ immune response, 362
    clonal anti-NY-ESO–1 $CD4^+$ T cells, 364
    His-tagged recombinant protein, 363
    ISCOMATRIX, 363
    melanocyte antigens, 362
  functions, 359–360
  genomic organization
    CT-X antigen, 352
    self-renewing spermatogonia, 350
    X-chromosome, 350–351
  identification
    anti-CT10 antibody, 349
    CTL, 348
    MAGE-A1, 348
    MPSS, 349
    RT-PCR analysis, 350
  immunogenicity, 361–362
  MAGEA3 and NY-ESO–1, 342
  mRNA expression, 352–354
  nonviral tumor antigens, 427
  normal tissue, 352
  protein expression
    COX6B2, 355–356
    heterogeneous staining pattern, 358
    Hodgkin lymphoma, 355, 357
    polyclonal and monoclonal antibody, 355
  regulation, 358–359
  SOX6, 342
CARs. See Chimeric antigen receptors
Caspase recruitment and activation domain (CARD), 51–52, 56
β-Catenin, 339
CCL17/ CCL22 signals, 153
CCL20 chemokine, 177
CCL22 expression, 177
CCR4 integrin, 177
CCR6 integrin, 177
CCRs. See Chimeric cytokine receptors
CD137/4–1BB, 255–257
$CD8^+CD11b^-$ cDC, 100
$CD15^+CD66b^+$ granulocytes, 220
$CD4^+CD25^+FOXP3^+CD127^+$ T cells, 149
$CD4^+CD25^+FOXP3^+CD127^-$ T cells, 149
$CD4^+CD25^+FOXP3^+$ T cells, 148, 149
$CD4^+CD25^+Foxp3^+$ Treg cells, 225
$CD4^+CD25^{hi}$ T cells, 147, 150
$CD4^+CD25^-$ T cells, 152
$CD4^+$ $CD25^+$ Treg cells, 12, 205, 207
CD11c-negative, lymphoid-related cells, 122
$CD8^+$ cytotoxic T lymphocytes, 335
$CD34^+$ haematopoietic progenitors, 99
$CD14^+HLA-DR^{-/low}$ cells, 220
$CD19^+$ plasmacytoid DCs, 308
$CD8^+$ T-cell, 3
$CD4^+$ Th and Treg cells
  DNA sequencing analysis, 378
  GTE system, 378
  MHC class II-restricted melanoma antigens, 379–380
  mutated fibronectin, 379
  Th1, 379–381
  TILs, 379
$CD4^+$ Treg cells, 3
$CD8^+$ Treg cells, 197
CD3ζ chain, 222
C/EBPβ gene, 221
Cell surface co-signaling molecules
  agonistic antibodies, 254
  APCs, 252
  B7-CD28 family
    B7-DC, 252, 259
    B7-H1/PD–1 pathways, 260–262
    costimulatory and coinhibitory receptor-ligand pairs, 259
    IgV and IgC domain, 259
    PD-L1, 252–253
  CTLA4, 262
  CTL response, 253
  DCs and macrophages, 252
  lymphodepletion, 254
  monoclonal antibodies, 253, 254
  pathogenic agents detection, 251
  TGN1412, 262
  TNF superfamily
    4–1BB receptor (see 4–1BB receptor)
    CD137/4–1BB, 255–257
    homotrimers and heteromultimers, 255
    TRAF molecules, 255
  tumor antigen-based vaccines, 254
  tumor immunity, 263
Chemo-immunotherapy, 309

Index 469

Chemokines receptors, 449
Chimeric antigen receptors (CARs), 428–431, 452
Chimeric cytokine receptors (CCRs), 452–453
Chronic inflammation, 2
Chronic myelocytic leukemia (CML), 396
Classical swine fever virus (CSFV), 273
Clec9A gene, 106
Colon adenocarcinoma model (MC-38), 443
Conventional dendritic cells (cDCs)
    CD11c$^+$ myeloid-derived hematopoietic cells, 122
    GM-CSF and IL-4, 122
    immune tolerance, 123–124
    intratumoral activation, TLR ligands, 135
    major histocompatibility complex, 122
    MDSCs
        suppress antitumor immune responses, 127–128
        tolerogenic cDCs, 125–127
    neo-epitopes, 125
    protective immunity, pathogens, 124–125
    tumor-specific altered peptides, 125
Copper metabolism (Murr1) domain containing 1 (COMMD1), 282
COX-2. *See* Cyclooxygenase–2
CtBP1-binding motif, 203
CTLA4. *See* Cytotoxic T lymphocyte antigen 4
CTLs. *See* Cytotoxic T lymphocytes
C-type lectin-like domains (CTLD), 102, 106
C-type lectin-like molecules
    carbohydrate recognition, 106
    CD205 endocytic receptor, 106
    Clec12A, 107
    Clec9A gene, 106
    CTLD, 102, 106
    DC-SIGN and Dectin–1, 106
CXCR4/CXCL12 interaction, 153
Cyclooxygenase–2 (COX–2)
    inhibitors, 158, 328
    PGE2, 235, 241
    Tregs antitumor activity, 182
Cyclophosphamide, 454–455
Cylindromatosis (CYLD), 280, 281
Cytokine-based tumor vaccines, 402–404
Cytotoxic T lymphocyte antigen 4 (CTLA4), 239, 397
Cytotoxic T lymphocytes (CTLs), 348, 415

D

Damage-associated molecular patterns (DAMPs), 2
Daudi lymphoma cells, 28
DC-SIGN, 106
Dectin–1, 106
Dendritic cells (DCs)
    anti-angiogenic and prodeath molecules, 110
    blood DC, 99
    cytokine requirement, 92
    human DC, 99–100 (*see also* human dendritic cells)
    IDO, 307
    immune regulation (*see* Immune regulation, dendritic cells)
    inflammatory DC, 96, 98
    lymphoid tissues
        CD8$^-$ cDC prime Th2, 96
        CD8^{hi} Sirpα (CD172a)^{lo}, 94, 95
        CD8^{lo} Sirpα^{hi} cDC, 94
        cytokine, 96
        spleen, LN and thymus, 93–94
        tissue-associated antigens, 96
        Treg cells, 94
    naive T cells, 92
    non-lymphoid tissues, 93
    pattern recognition receptor, 100
    pDC, 98–99
    precursors
        BM HSC, 90, 91
        CD45RA$^-$CD11c^{int}CD11b$^+$ population, 91
        Flt3$^+$ myeloid progenitors, 90
        MHC class II$^{-/lo}$ CD11c^{int}CD 45RA^{lo}CD43^{int}Sirpα^{int}Flt3$^+$, 92
        monocytes, 92
        myeloid and lymphoid pathways, 90, 91
        steady-state mouse, 90
    pro-survival molecules, 110
    subset-specific functions, 93
    TGF-β, 291
    vaccines, 401–402
    VEGF secretion, 110
Denileukin diftitox, 399
5-aza-2-Deoxycytidine (5DC) inhibitor, 358
Deubiquitinating enzyme A (DUBA), 276
Dextran sulfate sodium (DSS), 73, 79
Dicerrelated helicase (DRH–1), 57
DLI. *See* Donor leukocyte infusion; Donor lymphocyte infusions
Donor innate lymphocyte infusion (DILI) therapy, 27, 30
Donor leukocyte infusion (DLI), 396
Donor lymphocyte infusions (DLI), 30, 439
Double-stranded RNAs (dsRNAs), 274
DSS. *See* Dextran sulfate sodium

E

EBV. *See* Epstein–Barr virus
Effector cells
  endogenous and antigen-specific
    adoptive T cell therapy, 445–446
    CD4⁺ cells, 448–449
    CD8⁺ cells, 446–448
    endogenous T cells, 444
    T cell differentiation, 449–450
  endogenous and nonspecific
    adoptive therapy, 440–441
    LAK cells, 441–443
    TILs, 443–444
  genetically modified
    autocrine growth factor, 452
    CARs, 452
    CCRs, 452–453
    T cell genetic modification, 450
    TCR, 450–452
Encephalomyocarditis virus (EMCV), 54
Epidermal growth factor (EGF), 395
Epstein–Barr encoded RNAs (EBERs), 416
Epstein–Barr virus (EBV), 415

F

Fibronectin (FN), 379
Flaviviridae, 54
Flavivirus, 272
Fludarabine, 454–455
Foxp3 protein, 147–148
  multiples factors, 198, 201, 202
  naïve T cells, 295
  posttranslational modification and the
    transcriptional complex, 202–203
  retroviral transduction, 198
  target genes, 203–204
  transcriptional and posttranslational levels,
    198, 200
  transcription factors and transcriptional
    coregulators, 198, 199
FOXP3⁺ T cells, 155, 165
Fragment c receptors (FcRs), 395
Francisella tularensis infection, 72

G

α-Galcer, 398
G-CSF-mobilized CD34⁺ stem cells, 133
γδ T cells
  development and implementation
    obstacles, 31–32
  development, migration, and recognition
    strategies, 24–25
  primary effectors
    adoptive cellular therapy, 27
    allogeneic cellular therapy, HSCT, 29–30
    autologous cellular therapy, 28–29
    DILI therapy, 27, 30
    in vivo activation and expansion, 27–28
    manufacturing strategies, 30–31
    regulatory γδ T cells, 27
    Vδ1+ T cells, 25–26
    Vδ2+ T cells, 26–27
Genetic polymorphisms, 304
Genetic targeting expression (GTE) system, 378
Genomic organization, cancer-testis antigens
  CT-X antigen, 352
  self-renewing spermatogonia, 350
  X-chromosome, 350–351
GM-CSF. *See* Granulocyte macrophage
    colony-stimulating factor;
    Granulocyte-monocyte colony-
    stimulating factor
Grade 2 hypophysitis, 312
Graft-*versus* host disease (GVHD), 28–30, 418
Graft *versus* leukemia (GVL), 396
Granulocyte macrophage colony-stimulating
    factor (GM-CSF), 243
Granulocyte-monocyte colony-stimulating
    factor (GM-CSF), 122
Gr-1⁺CD11b⁺ cells, 244
GVHD. *See* Graft-*versus* host disease

H

Haematopoietic stem cells (HSC), 90
Helicobacter pylori, 2, 182, 393
Hematopoietic stem cell transplantation
    (HSCT), 29–30
Hepatitis B virus (HBV) vaccine, 391, 393
Hepatitis C virus (HCV), 272
Herceptin, 158
His-tag MAGE-A3 protein, 362
Histone deacetylase (HDAC) inhibitor, 158, 358
HLA tetramer analysis, 338
Hodgkin's lymphoma, 423–425
HPV. *See* Human papilloma virus
HSCT. *See* Hematopoietic stem cell
    transplantation
Human dendritic cells
  APCs, 121
  cancer vaccines
    antigen-specific T cells, 133
    blood monocyte precursors, 133
    G-CSF-mobilized CD34⁺ stem cells, 133
    peptide-pulsing, 134
    unconjugated antigen, 135

Index 471

viral vector transductions, 134
whole protein-pulsing, 134
cDCs (*see* Conventional dendritic cells)
immune suppression, 136
pathogen-specific adaptive immunity, 122
pDCs (*see* Plasmacytoid dendritic cells)
self-reactive effector cells, 122
T-cell-mediated immune response, 133
Human papilloma virus (HPV), 273, 393
Human tumor antigens, T cells
  CD8+ CTL, 335
  CD4+ helper T (Th) cell, 335
  identification methods, 336
  immunotherapy development
    allogeneic antigens, 342–343
    clinical implications, 339–340
    CT antigens, 342
    HLA tetramer analysis, 338
    TCR, 338
    tissue-specific antigens, 341–342
    tumor-specific antigens, 339, 341
  mechanisms
    immunoproteasomes, 338
    T cell epitope generation, 336–337
    T cell recognition, 337
Hypoxia-inducible factor (HIF), 328

I

IDO. *See* Indoleamine 2,3-dioxygenase
IFI16, 66
IFN-α receptor, 123
IFN-β promoter stimulator–1 (IPS–1), 57
IFNγ+ effector T cells, 185
IFN receptors (IFNAR), 275
IFN-stimulated gene factor 3 (ISGF–3) complex, 270
IκB. *See* Inhibitors of NF-κB
IκB kinase (IKK), 277
IL–2 (NFAT), 198, 201, 203
IL–2 diphtheria toxin fusion protein, 244
IL–6 signals, 202
Imatinib mesylate, 158
Imiquimod, 398
Immune adjuvants and cytokines, 393–394
Immune-modulating antibodies
  antitumor cytotoxicity, 396
  negative regulatory receptor, 397
  TNF family costimulatory receptor, 397–398
Immune regulation, dendritic cells
  B cells, 102
  DC targeting
    immune outcomes, 109–110

    immunity induction, antigen delivery, 108, 109
    in vivo antigen, 108
    tolerance induction, antigen delivery, 109
    vaccination, 107
  functional related molecules
    cell surface molecules, 102
    C-type lectin-like molecules, 102, 106
    mouse splenic DC subsets, 102–105
    Sirp molecules, 107
  IFN-I, 102
  IL–6, 102
  IL–12, 102
  T-cell activation, 101
Immunogenic murine mastocytoma, 445
Immunoglobulin idiotype antigen, 427
Immunoreceptor-based tyrosine activation motif (ITAM), 130
Immunoreceptor tyrosine-based inhibition motif (ITIM), 260
Indium-labeled T cells, 447
Indoleamine 2,3-dioxygenase (IDO)
  cancer immunotherapy, 304
  characteristics, 304
  counter-regulatory mechanism, 310
  D–1MT, 312
  drugs and vaccines, 310
  endogenous mechanism, immune tolerance
    human cells, 306–307
    mechanism of action, 305–306
    mouse model, 305
    Tregs, 306
  human leukemia cells, 152
  1MT, D and L isomers, 311
  Treg re-programming control, 312
  tumor, 307–308
Induced Treg (iTreg) cells, 148, 198
Inducible nitric oxide synthase (iNOS), 236–237
Inflammatory bowel disease (IBD), 183
Influenza infections, 96
Inhibitor of apoptosis proteins (IAPs), 67
Inhibitors of NF-κB (IκB), 277, 279
iNOS. *See* Inducible nitric oxide synthase
Interferon-α (IFN-α), 394
Interferon γ (IFNγ), 10, 239
Interleukin–2 (IL–2), 444
Interleukin–4 (IL–4), 122
Invariant natural killer T cells (iNKT cells), 292
Ipilimumab, 364, 397
IRAK-M regulator, 153

J

JAK1 tyrosine kinases, 270

K
Kynurenine production, 306

L
Laboratory of genetics and physiology 2 (LGP2), 51
LAK cells. *See* Lymphokine-activated killer cells
L-Arginine (L-Arg), 222, 236, 322–323
Latency associated protein (LAP), 289
Latent membrane protein (LMP) antigen, 416
L-Citrulline, 222
LCMV. *See* Lymphocytic choriomeningitis virus
Leishmania infection, 96
Lenalidomide, 158
Leucine-rich repeat (LRR), 39
Lipopolysaccharide (LPS), 239, 276
3LL murine lung carcinoma model, 328
Lymphocytic choriomeningitis virus (LCMV), 260–261
Lymphokine-activated killer (LAK) cells, 441–443
Lymphoma immunotherapy, 431–432
Lymphoma-specific T-cells, 426–427

M
Macrophages, 290–291
MAGE, 1
MAGE-A3 antigen, 401
MAGE-A3 peptide vaccine, 157
MageA2 protein, 359
Major histocompatibility complex (MHC), 400
Mammalian target of rapamycin (mTOR), 201, 202
MART–1/MelanA-specific T cells, 447
Massively parallel signature sequencing (MPSS), 349
MDSCs. *See* Myeloid-derived suppressor cells
Melanocyte antigens, 362
Melanoma
  adoptive cellular therapy, 439, 456–457
  cancer, 1
  CT antigens, 440
  DLI, 439
  effector cells (*see* Effector cells)
  lymphodepletion conditioning
    cyclophosphamide and fludarabine, 454–455
    cyclophosphamide resistant lymphopma, 453
    radiation, 455–456
  melanocytes, 440

Melanoma antigen A1 (MAGE-A1), 348
Melanoma differentiation associated gene 5 (MDA5)
  CARD, 51, 56
  downstream molecules, 57
  DRH–1, 57
  dsRNA, 54, 55, 58
  EMCV, 54
Metastatic cancer, 442
1-Methyl-tryptophan (1MT), 309
Metronomic temozolamide, 158
MHC class II-restricted melanoma antigens, 379–380
MHC class I-restricted tumour antigens
  $CD4^+$ and $CD8^+$ T cells, 372–374
  peptide splicing, 375–376
  proteolytic processing, 376
  T-cell epitopes, 372, 375
  transcriptional/splicing control, 372
  translational control, 372, 374–375
MicroRNA (miRNA), 274
Mitogen-activated protein kinases (MAPKs), 290
Molecularly defined tumor antigens, 376–377
Monoclonal antibodies, 394–395
MSLQRQFLR peptide, 374
mTOR. *See* Mammalian target of rapamycin
Mucosal-associated lymphoid tissue (MALT) lymphomas, 393
MyD88 adaptor-like (Mal), 40
MyD88 deficiency, 79
Myeloid-derived suppressor cells (MDSCs)
  accumulation, chronic inflammation, and cancer, 233
  angiogenesis, 240
  antigen-specific immune response, 319
  ARG1, 222
  Arg1 and iNOS, 236, 238
  arginase expression, tumor, 325–326
  carcinogenesis, 319
  $CD4^+$ and $CD8^+$ T-cells, 3
  COX2, 225
  crosstalk with macrophages, 239
  expansion and activation, 220–221, 232, 233
  granulocytic MDSCs, 219
  $Gr-1^+/CD11b^+$ cells, 219
  human MDSCs, 220
  human tumor, 326–327
  identification, 231
  immune response alteration, 320–321
  immune suppression mechanisms, 236, 237
  immunotherapy outcome, 240–241
  immunotherapy target
    effectors, metabolite, 241–242

Index 473

T-cell tolerance, 242–243
Tregs, 244
L-Arg starvation, T cells, 323–325
monocytic MDSCs, 219–220
NKT cells, 12–13
NOS2
   gamma-glutamyl-transpeptidase enzyme, 224
   L-arginine, 222
   L-citrulline, 222
   NO-mediated cytotoxicity/cytostasis, 224
   T-cell apoptosis, 222, 223
   Th1-and inflammatory cytokines, 224
NOX2, 224–225
origin and characterization, 218–219
peroxynitrite, 238
regulation and activation
   active pulmonary tuberculosis, 329
   arginase I production, 329
   cytokines, 327
   3LL murine lung carcinoma model, 328
   4T1 breast carcinoma cell, 328
ROS, 238
suppress antitumor immune responses, 127–128
surface makers and subsets, 231–232
TACE, 240
T cell anergy mechanism
   CD3ζ, 321
   fas-fasl-induced T cell apoptosis, 321
   L-Arginine and immune response, 322–323
   tolerogenic cDCs, 125–127
Treg cells, 225–226
Treg induction, 239–240
tumor environment factors
   C5a, 235–236
   COX–2-dependent PGE2, 235
   IL-1β, 234
   S100A8 and S100A9 proteins, 235
   SCF, 234
   VEGF, 234
Myeloid differentiation factor 88 (MyD88), 39–41, 46

N
National Cancer Act, 1
Natural killer (NK) cells, 123, 291
Natural killer T (NKT) cells
   CD4$^+$CD25$^+$ T regulatory cells, 12
   clinical trials/therapeutics, 13–14
   cytokines, 7
   definition, 7
   MDSC, 12–13
   Type I cells
      CD4$^+$ and CD4$^-$CD8$^-$ double negative populations, 8
      CD1d-tetramers, 8
      IFN-γ, 10
      nonglycosidic lipid antigens, 9
      sulfatide, 12
      TCR signaling, 9
      Th1 and Th2 cells, 12
      Vα24-negative cells, 10
   Type II cells, 11, 12
Naturally occurring CD4$^+$ CD25$^+$ Treg cells, 196
Natural Treg (nTreg) cells, 148, 198
Negative regulators
   cytoplasmic receptors, 62
   DAMPs, 61
   intracellular RLRs (*see* RIG-I-like receptors)
   NF-κB (*see* Nuclear factor-kappaB)
   NLRs (*see* NOD-like receptors)
   PAMPs, 61
   positive regulators, 72, 73
   PRRs, 61, 62, 267
   signaling adaptors and regulators, 79
   TLRs (*see* Toll-like receptors)
   type I IFN (*see* Type I interferons)
Negative regulatory receptors, 397
Neuronal apoptosis inhibitor proteins (NAIPs), 67
Newcastle disease virus (NDV), 272, 276
NG-monomethyl-arginine (L-NMMA), 242
N-hydroxynor-l-Arg (nor-NOHA), 242
NKG2D ligands, 32
NKT cells. *See* Natural killer T cells
NKT regulatory T cells, 197
NOD-like receptors (NLRs)
   diverse biological functions and signaling pathways
      inflammasome activation, 70–72
      NF-κB and MAPK signaling activation, 69–70
   ligand recognition
      BIR domain, 66–67
      CARD domain, 66–67
      domain organization, 66, 68
      IAPs, 67
      LRR domains, 66, 68
      NAIPs, 67
      NALP3, 69
      NLRP4, 69
      NLRX1 and NLRP1, 68–69
      PYD domain, 66–67
      subfamilies, 68
   protein receptors/regulators, 62

Non-structural protein 1 (NS1), 272, 273
Nonviral tumor antigens, 427
Nuclear factor-kappaB (NF-κB)
   ABIN–1, 2 and 3, 283
   A20 zinc finger protein, 280–281
   CYLD protein, 281
   homodimers/heterodimers, 277
   IκB family, 277, 279
   IκB proteins, 279
   inhibitors, 277, 278
   micro-RNA 146, 283
   PDLIM2-termination, 282
   PIAS, 282–283
   pro-inflammatory cytokines, 277
   p65 subunit, 282
   SOCS1 and COMMD1, 282
   TNF receptors, 277
   ubiquitination, 280
Nucleotide-binding oligomerization domain (NOD), 62
NY-ESO–1
   antigen, 1, 401
   vaccination, 363

O

ONTAK protein, 244
Orthomyxoviridae, 54
Ovarian tumour (OTU), 276
OY-TES–1 (ACRBP) protein, 360

P

Pamolidomide, 158
Paramyxoviridae, 54
Pathogen-associated molecular patterns (PAMPs), 3, 39, 267
Pattern recognition receptors (PRRs), 2, 96, 267
PBMCs. *See* Peripheral blood mononuclear cells
PD–1-blocking monoclonal antibody, 397
PD–1 inhibitory receptor, 397
PD–1 ligand one (PD-L1), 252–253
PDLIM. *See* Protein domain LIM
Peripheral blood mononuclear cells (PBMCs), 274, 326, 372
Peroxisome proliferator-activated receptor gamma (PPARγ), 201
Peroxynitrites, 224, 238
PGE2. *See* Prostaglandin E2
Phosphodiesterase 5 (PDE5) inhibitors, 242
PIAS. *See* Protein inhibitor of activated STAT1
Picornaviridae, 54

Plasmacytoid dendritic cells (pDCs), 98–99
   cancer
      bone marrow, 132
      breast cancer, 131
      ovarian cancer, 131
      primary skin melanoma, 132
      SDF–1, 131
      squamous head and neck cancer, 132
      T cells, 131
      T regulatory cell-mediated immunosuppressive microenvironment, 133
   CD11c-negative, lymphoid-related cells, 122
   immune tolerance, 130–131
   intratumoral activation, TLR ligands, 135–136
   protective immunity, pathogens
      BDCA2 and ILT–7, 130
      hematopoietic cell type, 128
      ITAM, 130
      TLRs, 129, 130
      type I IFNs, 128–129
P815 mastocytoma model, 262
Poly-G oligonucleotides, 207
Posttransplant lymphoproliferative disease (PTLD)
   CD20-specific monoclonal antibody rituximab, 418
   GVHD, 418
   HSCT/SOT, 416
   immunoprophylaxis
      post-HSCT, 418, 420
      post-SOT, 418, 422
   immunotherapy
      post-HSCT, 418–419
      post-SOT, 418, 421
Poxviridae, 54
PRAT4A. *See* Protein associated with Toll-like receptor 4
Programmed cell death 1 (PD–1), 181
Proinflammatory cytokines, 3
Prolyl isomerase (Pin1), 275–276
Prophylactic immune therapy and tumor vaccine, 391–393
Prostaglandin E2 (PGE2), 181, 235, 241, 320
Protamines, 360
Protein associated with Toll-like receptor 4 (PRAT4A), 43–44
Protein domain LIM (PDLIM), 280, 282
Protein inhibitor of activated STAT1 (PIAS), 282–283
PRRs. *See* Pattern recognition receptors
PTLD. *See* Posttransplant lymphoproliferative disease

Index

PVIWRRAPA peptide, 378
PYHIN protein, 66

R

RA. *See* Retinoic acids
Rabies virus (RV), 272
Rapamycin, 158
RCC. *See* Renal cell carcinoma
Reactive oxygen species (ROS), 238
Receptor-interacting protein 1 (RIP1), 277, 280
Reed–Sternberg (RS) cells, 423
Regulatory γδ T cells, 27
Regulatory T (Treg) cells, 4
  antagonizing Treg cells, 399
  anticancer therapies
    cyclooxygenase-2 inhibitors, 158
    cyclophosphamide, 158
    cytokine treatments, 157
    retinoids, 158
    vaccines, 156–157
  antigen specificity, 205–206
  antigen-specific targeting, 160–161
  autoimmunity control, 151
  B7-H1 co-signaling molecules, 164
  blocking differentiation, 162
  B16 melanoma, 164
  cancer prevention, 155–156
  $CD4^+CD25^{hi}$ T cells, 147, 150
  $CD4^+FOXP3^+$ Tregs, 164
  $CD8^+$ T cells, 164
  $CD4^+$ Th
    DNA sequencing analysis, 378
    GTE system, 378
    MHC class II-restricted melanoma antigens, 379–380
    mutated fibronectin, 379
    Th1, 379–381
    TILs, 379
  content and prognosis, 154
  cytotoxic agents, 163
  cytotoxic T lymphocyte epitope, 165
  DC subsets, 94, 101
  denileukin diftitox, 163, 164
  differentiation and plasticity, 204
  effector cell suppression threshold, 161
  endogenous antitumor immunity, 159
  enhanced de novo differentiation, 152
  enhanced local proliferation, 153
  enhanced recruitment, 152–153
  Foxp3, 147–148, 295
    multiples factors, 198, 201, 202
    posttranslational modification and the transcriptional complex, 202–203
    retroviral transduction, 198
    target genes, 203–204
    transcriptional and posttranslational levels, 198, 200
    transcription factors and transcriptional coregulators, 198, 199
  IDO, 306
  IL–6 and IL–10, 156
  immune and nonimmune cells, 156
  inflammation control, 151–152
  iTreg, 148
  lymphoid tissues, 94
  management strategy, 165
  miscellaneous host factors, 153
  naïve and tumor-bearing hosts, 164
  nonspecific depletion, 159–160
  nTreg, 148
  phenotypic markers and subsets, 196–197
  potential malignancy, 165
  reduced local Treg death, 153
  subverting differentiation, 163
  suppressive function
    anti-OX40, 206
    depletion with anti-CD25, 206
    Poly-G oligonucleotides, 207
    ssRNA40, 207
    TLR8 signaling, 207–208
  suppressive functions, 162
  suppressive mechanisms, 205
  TGF-β, 294–295
  Th17 cells (*see* Th17 and Treg cells)
  therapy response, 154
  trafficking, 161
  tumor-associated Tregs
    bona fide functional tumor Tregs, 150
    $CD4^+CD25^-CD69^+$ Tregs, 149
    CD127 expression, 149
    $Nrp-1^+$ cells, 149
    tumor immunopathology, 151
    tumor tolerance, 149
  tumor prognostic indicators, 155
Renal cell carcinoma (RCC), 326
Retinoic acid-inducible gene-I (RIG-I). *See* RIG-I-like receptors (RLRs)
Retinoic acid nuclear receptor (ROR), 203
Retinoic acids (RA), 198, 201, 202
Rhabdoviridae, 54
RIG-I-like receptors (RLRs)
  activation, 56
  biological activity, 57
  future perspectives, 58
  knockout mice, 54
  ligands, 54–55, 63–64
  signaling pathways and regulation, 57, 66, 67

RIG-I-like receptors (RLRs) (cont.)
　structure
　　CARD, 51–52
　　C-terminal region, 52, 53
　　dsRNA-binding domain, 53
　　innate antiviral reactions, 51
　　molecules, signaling regulation, 52, 53
　　RNA-binding surface, 54
　　RNA helicase domain, 52
　type I IFN, 268
　　IRF3/IRF7 regulators, 78
　　MAVS regulators, 76–77
　　RIG-I and MDA5 regulators, 76
　　STING regulators, 77
　　TBK1/IKKi regulators, 77–78
　　TRAF3 regulators, 77
RIP1. *See* Receptor-interacting protein 1
RLRs. *See* RIG-I-like receptors
RNA interference (RNAi), 274
RNA silencing suppressor (RSS), 274

S
S100A8 proteins, 235
S100A9 proteins, 235
SEMG1 protein, 360
Serological analysis of recombinant cDNA expression (SEREX), 348
Short hairpin RNA (shRNA), 276
Signal transducer and activator of transcription (STAT), 221, 282
Single modality immune therapy, 403
Single nucleotide polymorphism (SNP), 336
Sipuleucel-T vaccine, 402
Sirpα molecules, 102
Sirpβ1 molecules, 102
Sirp molecules, 107
Smad proteins, 289–290
Small interfering RNAs (siRNAs), 274
SOCS–1. *See* Suppressor of cytokine signalling–1
Solid organ transplant (SOT), 416
SOX6 antigen, 342
S1P1-Akt-mTOR signaling pathway, 201
Stem cell factor (SCF), 234, 326
Stromal-derived factor (SDF)–1, 131
Suppressor of cytokine signalling–1 (SOCS–1), 45, 74, 275, 282
Systemic lupus erythematosus (SLE), 274

T
TAMs. *See* Tumor-associated macrophages
T and B lymphocytes, 123

T cell receptors (TCRs)
　CD8$^+$ cells, 326
　Foxp3 expression, 198, 201, 202
　human tumor antigens, 338
　MHC, 400
TCR-γδ$^+$ Treg cells, 197
TDFs. *See* Tumor-derived factors
TDLN. *See* Tumor-draining lymph nodes
TDO. *See* Tryptophan oxygenase
TGF-β. *See* Transforming growth factor-β
Thalidomide congeners, 158
Th17 and Treg cells, 4, 378
　actions mechanism, 185–186
　crosstalk, 179
　cytokine milieu, 178–180
　definition, 175–176
　distribution, 176, 177
　functional relevance
　　anti-inflammatory activity, 185
　　B16 melanomas, 184
　　IBD, 183
　　IL–17 cytokine, 183–184
　　IL–23 cytokine, 183
　　inflammatory milieu, 182
　　pro-inflammatory cytokines, 184
　　TGF-β, 182, 184
　　tissue damage and regeneration, 182
　　tumor vascularization, 184
　migration, 177–178
　TAMs, 180–181
TILs. *See* Tumor-infiltrating lymphocytes
TipDC. *See* TNF-α and iNOS producing DC
TIR. *See* Toll/interleukin–1 receptor
TIR-domain-containing adaptor inducing interferon-β (TRIF), 40–41
TIR domain-containing adaptor proteins (TIRAP), 39, 40
Tissue-specific antigens, 341–342
TLR9 agonists, 398
TLRs. *See* Toll-like receptors
TNF-α and iNOS producing DC (TipDC), 96, 98
TNF-α converting enzyme (TACE), 240
TNF family costimulatory receptors, 397–398
TNF-receptor-associated death domain (TRADD), 277
Toll/interleukin–1 receptor (TIR), 39, 40, 277
Toll-like receptors (TLRs)
　chaperone, 43
　ER resident molecule, 43–44
　Gp96 heat shock protein, 43
　inflammation and cancer, 78–79

Index

IRAK sequence polymorphism, 2
ligand recognition, 62–63
LRR motifs, 61
negative regulatory molecules, 45–46
NF-κB signaling
   A20, 74
   CYLD, 74–75
   IRAKM, 74
   NLRC5, 75–76
   NLRX1, 75
   SIGIRR, 72–73
   SOCS1, 74
   TRIAD3A, 73
nucleotide-sensing TLRs, 41–42
PRAT4A, 43–44
signaling molecules
   LRR, 39
   membrane-spanning receptor, 39
   MyD88, 39–40
   TIRAP, 39, 40
   TRAM, 40–41
   type I interferon, 41
signaling pathways and regulation
   IKK complex, 65
   MyD88, 64–65
   TRAF6 complex, 65
   type-I interferon, 65, 66
TLR4 activation mechanism, 41
trafficking, 43–44
type I IFN, 268
UNC93B1, endolysosomes, 44–45
TRADD. *See* TNF-receptor-associated death domain
TRAF-family member-associated NF-κB activator-binding kinase 1 (TBK1), 272–273
Transforming growth factor-β (TGF-β)
   aberrant immune response
     autoimmunity, 296–297
     cancer, 297
     immune cell regulation, 295–296
   Foxp3, 198, 201, 202
   immune system, effects
     B cells, 292
     dendritic cells, 291
     macrophages, 290–291
     NK cells, 291
   intracellular signaling, 289
   LAP, 289
   Smad proteins, 289–290
   T cells
     development, 292–293
     function, 293–294
   Th17 and Treg cells
     cytokine milieu, 178–179
     functional relevance, 182, 184
     Th17 cell expansion, 298
     Treg cell differentiation and plasticity, 204
     Tregs, 294–295
Transgenic T-cell receptors, 427
Traztuzumab, 158
Treg cells. *See* Regulatory T cells
Tremelimumab, 397
TRIF-related adaptor molecule (TRAM), 40–41
Tryptophan oxygenase (TDO), 304
Tumor antigens and immune regulation
   cancer therapy, 371
   $CD4^+$ T cell subsets, 377–378
   $CD4^+$ Th, Treg cells
     DNA sequencing analysis, 378
     GTE system, 378
     MHC class II-restricted melanoma antigens, 379–380
     mutated fibronectin, 379
     Th1, 379–381
     TILs, 379
   clinical study, 376–377
   host immune system, 371
   immune suppression blocking, 381–382
   MHC class I-restricted antigen
     $CD4^+$ and $CD8^+$ T cells, 372–374
     peptide splicing, 375–376
     proteolytic processing, 376
     T-cell epitopes, 372, 375
     transcriptional/splicing control, 372
     translational control, 372, 374–375
   myeloid-derived suppressor cell, 382
Tumor antigens and therapeutic cancer vaccines
   antigen-specific vaccine, 401
   cytokine-based vaccine, 402–404
   DC vaccine, 401–402
Tumor-associated macrophages (TAMs), 180–181, 242
Tumor-derived factors (TDFs), 220–221
Tumor-draining lymph nodes (TDLN), 176, 306
Tumor-infiltrating lymphocytes (TILs)
   endogenous and nonspecific effector cells, 443–444
   melanoma-reactive T cells, 339
   tumor-/antigen-specific $CD4^+$ Treg cell, 379
Tumor necrosis factor (TNF), 252
Tumor necrosis factor receptor-associated factor (TRAF), 57, 255
Tumor-specific antigens, 339, 341

Type I interferons
    host mechanisms
        DUBA, 276
        micro RNA–146a, 274–275
        peptidyl Pin1, IRF–3-mediated antiviral response, 275–276
        SOCS–1, 275
        STAT3, 275
    IRF–7, 270
    IRF–3 phosphorylation, 270
    JAK1 and Tyk2 tyrosine, 270
    pDCs, 123, 128–130
    RLRs, 268
    signalling pathways, 268, 269
    TLRs, 268
    viral counter attack
        dsRNA, ssRNA targeting, 272
        IRF3, 273
        IRF9 and IRF1 and Tyk2, 273–274
        recognition machinery, 272
        RSS activity, 274
        TBK–1, 272–273
        viral proteins, 270, 271
Tyrosine kinases (Tyk2), 270

U
Ubiquitination, 46

V
Vα24-negative cells, 10
Vδ1+ T cells, 25–26
Vδ2+ T cells, 26–27
VEGF. *See* Vascular endothelial growth factor
Vesicular stomatitis virus (VSV), 276
Vγ9Vδ2 $\gamma\delta$ T cells, 28, 30
Viral double-stranded RNA (Viral dsRNA). *See* RIG-I-like receptors

W
WRRAPAPGA peptide, 378

Z
Zoledronate (ZOL), 28